Biological Psychiatry

Third Edition

Biological Psychiatry

Third Edition

Biological Psychiatry

Michael R. Trimble, MD, FRCP, FRCPsych
Professor of Behavioural Neurology, Institute of Neurology,
Queen Square, London UK

Mark S. George, MD
Distinguished Professor of Psychiatry, Radiology and Neurosciences,
Medical University of South Carolina
Director, Brain Stimulation Laboratory
Director, Center for Advanced Imaging Research (CAIR)
MUSC Director, SC Brain Imaging Center of Excellence
Ralph H. Johnson VA Medical Center, Charleston, SC, USA

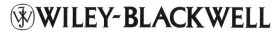

A John Wiley & Sons, Ltd., Publication

Library of Congress Cataloguing-in-Publication Data

Trimble, Michael R.
  Biological psychiatry / Michael R. Trimble, Mark S. George. – 3rd ed.
      p. ; cm.
  Includes bibliographical references and index.
  ISBN 978-0-470-68894-6
  1. Biological psychiatry. I. George, Mark M. II. Title.
  [DNLM: 1. Biological Psychiatry – methods. 2. Brain – physiology. 3. Mental Disorders – physiopathology.
WM 102 T831b 2010]
  RC341.T73 2010
  616.89 – dc22

                                                                                          2009053116

ISBN: 978-0-470-68894-6

A catalogue record for this book is available from the British Library.

Typeset in 10/12 and Palatino-Roman by Laserwords Private Limited, Chennai, India
Printed in Singapore by Markono Print Media Pte Ltd

First Impression   2010

Cover design by Jim Wilkie. Portrait of Hippocrates inspired by his words, 'Men ought to know that from the brain, and from the brain only, arise our pleasures ... as well as our sorrows ... and tears' as quoted in 'The Soul in the Brain' by Michael Trimble, 2007.

We dedicate this book to our late friend, mentor and scholar Paul MacLean.

Contents

Acknowledgements

The editors wish to acknowledge the following people for their helpful comments on various sections of the manuscript:

Andrea Cavanna, Tim Crow, Ray Dolan, Mark Edwards, Paul Johns, Eileen Joyce, Marco Mula, Karl Friston, Nick Wood.

Professor Trimble acknowledges his late friend and mentor Dr Lennart Heimer who has given him many of the images used in this text. He is also grateful for the contributions of Dr Scott Zahm and Gary van Hoesen. He thanks his wife Dame Jenifer for her continuing support to his writing activities.

Dr George acknowledges his wife, Eloise, and children, Laura and Daniel, who have allowed him to merge his hobby (brain and behavior) with his work (clinical neuroscience) and tolerated the time away, Dr Edmund Higgins, for his help with several of the illustrations and figures in this edition, Dr James Ballenger, for creating the combined residency program in neurology and psychiatry, and encouraging him to pursue research and further training, and Professors Michael Trimble and Robert Post, his research fellowship advisors who opened up so many doors and have proved such good colleagues and mentors through the years.

Both editors are grateful for the hours of work that Jackie Ashmenall has put into preparation of the final manuscript and helping with the editorial process.

Quotations

Mental disorders are neither more nor less than nervous diseases in which mental symptoms predominate, and their entire separation from other nervous diseases has been a sad hindrance to progress.

Henry Maudsley (1870, p.41)

Le Gros Clark has also drawn attention to the difficulty of judging what constitutes normality in some of these old rhinencephalic regions. It is not inconceivable that a pathological change in one or the other region has been overlooked in schizophrenic brains. In the text books of neurology and psychiatry of my student days chorea, parkinsonism and related motor disorders were treated as neuroses. When the first discoveries of their organic nature were made, there was surprise bordering on disbelief that circumscribed lesions, for instance in the substantia nigra and periaqueductal grey matter, should give rise to massive neurological and psychopathological syndromes. Such experiences should make us cautious before we give a final verdict that there is no pathological change in schizophrenic brains.

Professor A. Meyer, writing in the early 1950s

Preface to the First Edition

In the last thirty years there has been a remarkable explosion of knowledge in medicine, and psychiatry is no exception. Much of the progress is related to the exploration of the biological foundations of the discipline, and this may be referred to as biological psychiatry. It is often said, quite mistakenly, that psychiatrists are unscientific and that psychiatry has made little progress over the years, and in any case lacks an adequate foundation of knowledge. In reality, psychiatry as a discipline is one of the more critical of all in medicine, continually questioning not only its data base, but also its fundamental methodological principles. Further, it has a long and distinguished history of progress, a point of departure for this book.

Thus, Chapter 1 outlines the development of psychiatry from its early origins, noting that it is one of the oldest medical specialties. The emphasis of most practitioners has been to elucidate any underlying pathology that is related to psychopathology, an endeavour that has been highly successful. Although much of this may be more appropriately referred to as neuropsychiatry, it should be recognized that, for example, in the last century, psychopathologists were in the main neuropathologists and vice versa. The reduction in morbidity and mortality of psychiatric patients that followed discovery of the cause and treatment of general paralysis of the insane (GPI) was substantial, and the progress that was made in the first half of this century in relation to treatments such as electroconvulsive therapy had a dramatic impact on the lives of thousands of patients otherwise condemned to long-term institutionalization.

Such progress is often ignored when discussing psychiatry, and emphasis is often given to an alternative stream of thought, one of psychological theorizing, which arose on the neo-romantic tide of the turn of the century. This culminated in the psychoanalytic movement, which for a considerable time became synonymous with psychiatry. The point is made, however, that this era has provided psychiatry with a legacy that it does not deserve, the main trend of the tradition for over 2000 years being medical and neuropathologically based.

The position today is that these psychological theories of pathogenesis have been overtaken by a wealth of neurochemical and neuropathological hypotheses and findings, especially with regards to the major psychoses. Further, in addition to using knowledge accumulated in cooperation with other disciplines, biological psychiatry now seeks an understanding of psychopathology using theories and findings often based on clinical observations of patients and their effective treatment with biological remedies. Hence, the importance of the neurochemical era, ushered in by the psychopharmacological discoveries of the 1950s. These have given us not only a completely new image of the brain to work with, but also have allowed a more complete understanding of underlying functional and structural changes of the brain that accompany psychiatric illness. Functional, a misused word in the clinical neurosciences, once again may be used in its original sense, to designate a physiological disturbance, rather than as an epithet for 'psychological'.

Indeed, with our present knowledge the distinction between 'organic' and 'functional' melts away, stripped of its Cartesian dualism.

In spite of such progress, the very concept of biological psychiatry still meets with scepticism in the eyes of many. As we approach the turn of the next century, there may well be a revival of a *fin de siécle* phenomenon, in which the recent gains will become submerged and lost in a quagmire of new, old or revived psychological theorizing. The reasons for this are not difficult to understand. Thus, biological psychiatry is a complicated subject, requiring in particular an intimate knowledge of the central nervous system. Many find such knowledge hard to grasp, and the very pace of discoveries is often bewildering. The principles rely to some extent on diagnosis and measurement of biological variables, yet in the clinical area these are often ignored, thought unnecessary or counterproductive. This is in spite of them being fundamental to medicine, and psychiatry being a most important branch of medicine. The latter fact is often trivialized, many, especially of the lay public, but also sadly some practitioners, preferring to deny the medical roots of psychiatry, but in doing so confusing it with psychology.

Biological treatments, in spite of their obvious and proven efficiency, are criticized. However, the psychopharmacological revolution has given psychiatrists, not for the first time, powerful remedies. The days when multitudes of patients suffered intensely because of lack of adequate treatment are forgotten, and false arguments that compare and contrast psychotherapy to biological treatments are constructed. It is assumed that the use of such treatments implies a lack of interest in patients, and that somehow the doctor is less than adequate for prescribing them. However, in medicine it is obvious that often several approaches to patient care are appropriate and can be applied simultaneously if required. The neurologist or the chest physician know the value of physiotherapy and when it is applicable, and likewise the psychiatrist may recognize the value of other treatments for his patients, in addition to the biological ones. However, the neurologist would not hesitate to prescribe medication to his patient with Parkinson's disease, or the chest physician antituberculous remedies to a consumptive. Indeed, with tuberculosis, the remedies of 50 years ago, which relied mainly on changes in environment and the passage of time, have been superseded by more effective modern treatment regime, as is the case with many psychiatric illnesses.

One challenge for biological psychiatry is to unite information we now have regarding functional changes in the brain in psychopathology with that which we know about brain–behaviour relationships and brain structure. The latter was of great interest to the neuropsychiatrists of the last century, and has recently been an area of much research, but often referred to as behavioural neurology. This discipline has developed rapidly in the United States of America, and may come to be seen as a neurological discipline if its relevance for psychiatry is not acknowledged, and the essential value of examining patients with known structural disease for helping to understand the course and development of psychopathology is not appreciated.

In this text I have reviewed a number of key areas of importance for biological psychiatry. A strong emphasis has been placed on the work of Jaspers, and the fundamental distinction between illness, which is related to a process, and development. The whole area of personality disorders is one of continuing disagreement, although as emphasized in Chapter 7 neurochemical and neuropathological substrates of at least some personality traits are being uncovered. However, it is arguable to what extent psychiatrists are an appropriate professional group to deal with personality disorders generally, and their ready acceptance of this task in the past has led to a great deal of criticism, not the least being the failure to influence behaviour patterns in ways which the then-accepted theories, predominantly psychoanalytic, predicted they should change with treatment. An alternative argument would be that psychiatrists should deal with illness, not personality problems, for which latter group other agencies in society are readily available as a source of help.

The main diagnostic system used in this book is that of the American Psychiatric Association's DSM III. However, as noted in Chapter 2, classification is in a constant process of change, and is not immutable. However, the DSM III is likely to dominate psychiatric research for many years to come – hence the emphasis. The reader will quickly note the profusion of different terms used in the book for similar states, many of which do not even conform to the alternative ICD system. This is because in quoting papers, the original patient designation used by the authors is selected. Many of the investigations were carried out prior to the introduction of the DSM III, but reclassification of patients would be an inappropriate exercise. It is hoped that the introduction of such systems as the DSM III, and soon the DSM IIIR and DSM IV, will lead to more uniformity of patients included in research populations, making a reviewer's task easier and increasing the validity of any findings.

It is hoped that the two chapters on neurochemistry and neuroanatomy will be of interest, and give an up-to-date account of the state of knowledge. These fields are moving so rapidly that information has a danger of soon being out of date. Nonetheless, it is hoped that areas of importance for biological psychiatry are adequately outlined, and that their inclusion, essential for the text, will increase the reader's interest in exploring some of these areas further.

The main clinical chapters cover the major psychopathologies, notably affective disorders (Chapter 9) and schizophrenia (Chapter 8). Structural disorders of the limbic system are discussed separately (Chapter 6), and individual chapters are devoted to dementia (11) and epilepsy (10). This follows some other psychiatric texts, including in the contents mainly information on the major psychoses, although the neuroses are discussed where relevant (Chapters 7 and 9). These areas of psychopathology have been chosen to reflect subjects of relevance to biological psychiatry, but also relate to the author's interests. Dementia and epilepsy are of growing importance. Patients with dementia, from those with dementia praecox to those with the disorders identified by Alzheimer and Pick, are often assessed and managed by psychiatrists. The recent neurochemical findings, especially in Alzheimer's disease and the possibility of replacement therapy to hold the condition for a few years at least have encouraged renewed interest in this area. Epilepsy is included, in part reflecting the author's own area of special interest, but mainly because of the very close relationship between epilepsy and psychiatry that has existed for many years. Epilepsy has a great deal to teach us about the CNS, about psychopathology and about patient management.

There are many topics missing from this book, which no doubt will lead to comment. For example, not discussed are conditions such as alcoholism and the addictions, and eating disorders, the biological bases for which are becoming clarified, and relevant neurochemical and neuropathological findings have been reported. Inevitably, the final size of the volume, as well as the author's personal interests, are responsible for the exclusions. In addition, this volume is a companion to my earlier book *Neuropsychiatry* (Trimble, 1981a). Although there is some overlap, here the data on dementia, epilepsy and biological treatments have been rewritten and updated, and some subjects that may interest the reader, but not included here, may be found there.

Biological psychiatry is such a rapidly advancing field, and the number of papers of relevance so vast, that much selectivity has gone into the choice quoted in this book. Undoubtedly there will be those disappointed that their paper is not quoted, and others who will point to a missing reference of some negative finding not substantiating a claim made in the text. To a large extent I have quoted work that has either been independently replicated or seems to be of interest to the theme of the topic at hand. In several areas, for example the neuropathology of schizophrenia, all the findings consistently show some changes, but there is not exact replication as to the precise changes in all studies. Nevertheless, the combined findings add up to an extremely important conclusion with regards to schizophrenia, namely the obvious, but until recently ignored, relationship of the condition to structural brain lesions.

It is hoped that the text will provide an informative data base for those psychiatrists interested in exploring the biological foundations of their discipline further. It may help to stimulate the interests of students wanting to explore one of the most exciting areas of current research in psychiatry, and may provide those active in the field with ideas for future investigations that will increase our knowledge even further.

Michael R. Trimble
London, 1987

Preface to the Second Edition

It is nearly a decade since I started to write the first edition of this book, and the progress in biological psychiatry since that time has been truly remarkable. Of course many of the pieces for this progress were in place at that time, but the speed of progress, and the studies that have been completed have been, in some areas, awesome. I refer in particular to advances in neuroanatomy and neurochemistry, to progress in genetics, and to the development of high resolution neuroimaging techniques. The elegance of some of the methods, their complexity, and yet their ability to answer for us questions of principal relevance for the discipline would have left our forefathers breathless.

Attempting to harness such progress, and to interpret the findings from an ever expanding database has not been a simple task. Students over the past few years have asked me if, and when, I would be writing a second edition of this book, and I had carefully avoided any decisions or deadlines. However, it was rapidly becoming clear around 1993 that revision was essential, especially for those faithful readers who were still buying copies of the first text. The new classifications of psychiatric illness (ICD 10: DSM IV) perhaps became the final goad to action, although the wish to provide a helpful guide to the technological advances was also important.

As with the first edition, one major problem has been what to leave out. I can only apologise, once again if some researcher is aggrieved because I have not quoted him or her, and if another is upset because I have selectively quoted, and not cited all references available on a particular topic. However, for a single authored book, to achieve its aim, some selectivity is essential, and without it, the text would become quite unwieldy.

However, equally difficult has been the problem of what to remove from my first edition. Marrying new text, with something written several years ago is difficult enough, sacrificing text with scissors can be positively painful. Particularly since much of what went into the first edition still forms part of the corpus of the subject, and has become the foundation of later investigations and data.

I hope that, these faults notwithstanding, the final product is readable and informative. It will succeed for me if it stimulates even one student to find the richness and excitement of neurobiological research which has so stimulated me over the years. For others, it may provide a spur to further research in a particular area, to enhance or refute a conclusion of mine or some investigator I have quoted. Once again I am grateful to colleagues and patients alike who have helped me understand some of the complexities of human behaviour, and the relevance of biological psychiatry for contemporary medicine.

M.R.T.
London, 1995

Introduction and Preface
to the Third Edition

'Biological psychiatry' may have a modern ring to it, but the idea of seeking naturalistic origins for psychiatric disorders is part of a long-standing intellectual tradition. Hippocrates, in his writings on 'The Sacred Disease', the name given by the Greeks to epilepsy, pointed out that it was no more sacred than any other disease, and 'has a natural cause from which it originates like other affections' (Adams, 1939, p. 355). He continues with one of the more quoted historical remarks that 'men ought to know that from nothing else but thence [from the brain] comes joys, delights, laughter and sports, and sorrows, griefs, despondency and lamentations... And by the same organ we become mad and delirious, and fears and terrors assail us...' (p. 366).

It is generally accepted that with a few notable exceptions such as Galen, and the contributions of the Arab world, for the next 1300 years medicine abandoned any semblance of a scientific approach, and retreated under the combined influences of theology and demonology.

The 17th century saw a revival of the idea that the brain was the seat of many mental diseases, and the rudiments of present-day localization theories can be found in the writings of several authors, such as Thomas Willis (1671–1675), the founder of neurology and one of the first physicians of the new enlightenment to clearly equate mental disorders with brain diseases.

René Descartes (1596–1650), the 17th-century philosopher, skillfully, with deductive reasoning, was able to philosophically separate the unextended mind from the extended body. While this allowed examination and speculation about the brain and its relationship to sensation and movement to progress relatively unfettered from the religious domination over anything that had to do with the human mind, and hence the soul, it set the trend for three centuries in which psychological theories of mental illness vied with the biological.

The 19th century saw a rapid expansion of knowledge in medicine, and a continued growth of the anatomico-clinical method. Such an approach was seen especially with the attempts to localize mental functions in the brain. However, localization theories such as we are familiar with today did not emerge until the rise of the phrenological movement, the greatest exponents of which were Franz Joseph Gall (1758–1828) and his collaborator Johann Caspar Spurzheim (1776–1832). The brain was conceived of as being composed of many different organs, which could be palpated through the scalp. This last contention was the downfall of phrenology, since it quickly became taken up by all sorts of charlatans and fell into disrepute. Nonetheless, Gall was the originator of modern localization theories and, for example, suggested the presence of a speech centre, a concept revived later by Paul Broca (1824–1880). The unfortunate overdue attention to the importance of the cerebral cortex for mentation, with neglect of subcortical structures, represents a state of affairs that persisted until recently (see below). The studies of Broca also initiated a literature which emphasized lateralization. Broca in fact was unable to explain the coincidence of aphasia and right-sided hemiplegia, although, after consideration of the facts, the English neurologist John Hughlings Jackson (1835–1911) referred to the left side of the brain as the 'leading hemisphere' for speech, and concluded that there were important differences in the functions of the two brain hemispheres. Laterality differences in relationship to psychopathology, an area of study now actively pursued, underwent a revival in the 1960s with the work of Pierre Flor-Henry on psychotic patients with epilepsy.

Hughlings Jackson thoughtfully put forward four key ideas of brain function, which were the evolution of nervous functions, the hierarchy of functions, the negative and positive symptoms of dissolution and the distinction between local and uniform dissolution. For him, the nervous system was seen as developing both in space and time, and was not the static organ of the pathologist's specimen. Further, it was hierarchically organized, not merely a collection of reflexes. With any lesion there are two effects, one due to the destruction of tissue, resulting in the negative symptoms, and the other due to release of subjacent activity of healthy areas of the brain, causing positive symptoms. He discussed mental disorders and noted that in all cases of insanity the principle of dissolution, the level of evolution that remains and the positive and negative elements need to be considered. In a paper called 'The Factors of the Insanities' he stated, 'In every insanity there is morbid affection of more or less the highest cerebral centres ... [they] are out of function, temporally or permanently from some pathological process' (Taylor, 1958, vol. 2, p. 411), a statement relevant for biological psychiatry. His use of the terms 'positive' and 'negative' symptoms, as a reflection of a mechanism of nervous-system function equally applicable to a whole range of neuropsychiatric conditions, stands in contrast to the more recent reintroduction of these expressions into psychiatry, with a more-or-less descriptive use, and largely restricted to schizophrenia. The reintroduction of Hughlings Jackson's terminology into psychiatry, and the continued awareness that strict localization hypotheses have not uncovered the essential links between the brain and behaviour, has seen a renewed interest in Jacksonian ideas.

On the continent, Wilhelm Griesinger's (1817–1868) book, *Mental Pathology and Therapeutics*, was published in Berlin in 1845, and translated into English in 1867. Griesinger's thesis was that mental illness (insanity) is only a symptom of a disordered brain, and the brain is the organ that must be diseased in mental illness. He stated: '... we therefore primarily, and in every case of mental disease, recognize a morbid action of that organ' (Griesinger, 1867, p. 1). An important tenet, reflecting the essential nature of biological psychiatry, is: 'Insanity being a disease, and that disease being an affection of the brain, it can only be studied in a proper manner from the medical point of view' (p. 9).

Other substantial contributions of German psychiatry in this era come from Theodore Meynert (1833–1892), Carl Wernicke (1848–1905), Karl Kahlbaum (1828–1899) and Emil Kraepelin (1856–1926). Meynert's work stimulated a whole generation of successors, including Sigmund Freud (1856–1939). Meynert contrasted the functions of the cortex with those of the brainstem, postulating a neurophysiological foundation of the ego based on the principles of associationist psychology and the presence of different cortical 'centres'. Wernicke is well known for his aphasiology, and his contributions to the study of chronic alcoholism are recognized in the eponym Wernicke–Korsakoff syndrome. Kahlbaum insisted on the clinical method, and his attempts to clarify disease classification led to the delineation of catatonia. Later, Kraepelin developed his nosological scheme, which has had such a profound influence on modern psychiatry.

Although German psychiatry, especially the contributions to biological psychiatry (in that era, more properly referred to as 'neuropsychiatry'), was especially dominant in the second half of the 19th century, developments in France were somewhat earlier. Phillipe Pinel's (1745–1826) influence was profound, and like many others he had misgivings about philosophy and metaphysics.

Another very important figure in French psychiatry was A.L.J. Bayle (1799–1858). The late effects of syphilis, dementia paralytica, were frequent causes of mental illness in patients admitted to psychiatric hospitals. Bayle, in his doctoral thesis of 1822, related chronic arachnoiditis to dementia paralytica. This ascription of a defined pathology for general paralysis of the insane (GPI) had profound consequences for psychiatry. It reinforced somatic theories of mental illness. Further, in later writings, Bayle emphasized the stages of the disease, with a specific form and pattern of development, culminating in dementia. It was not until 1905 that Fritz Schaudinn (1871–1906) identified the spirochaete in genital lesions. In 1906, August von Wassermann (1866–1925) developed his diagnostic blood test, and in 1913 Hideyo Noguchi (1876–1928) identified the spirochaetes in the brains of patients with general paralysis of the insane. Julius von Wagner-Jauregg (1857–1940) introduced the first treatment by inducing pyrexia in patients with GPI using malaria. Although no panacea, some were helped by this, their disease process apparently arresting. For this discovery Wagner-Jauregg was awarded a Nobel Prize in 1927. He was the only psychiatrist to be so honoured until 2000, when Eric Kandel, Arvid Carlsson and Paul Greengard were also awarded the prize.

Much of the endeavour of the 19th-century neuropsychiatrists related to uncovering the causes of the more severe psychiatric disorders, especially the psychoses. However, disorders that were then referred to as 'the neuroses' also became a focus of attention, especially in France.

It was the great French neurologist Jean Martin Charcot (1825–1892) who explored the neuroses in detail, and he was particularly interested in hysteria. It is interesting that at this time, the latter half of the 19th century, neuroses were considered the province of the neurologist. This in part reflected the fact that most severe pathology was seen in hospitals, and the neuroses presumably, as today, were largely found in out-patients, and tended to be seen by a different group of physicians, usually privately. An example of this was the development in the USA of the concept of neuraesthenia by George Miller Beard (1839–1883), and the interest of Silas Wier Mitchell (1829–1914), one of the earliest and most influential of the American neurologists, in conditions of nervous debility. His 'rest cure' became widely known and used as a treatment for these disorders. Neuraesthenia evolved from ideas such as those of Marshall Hall (1790–1857), who in 1850 defined the reflex actions of the spinal cord, applying his definition to various disease states. The concept of spinal weakness found a counterpart in brain weakness, and hence cerebral neuraesthenia.

Charcot was appointed Médecin de l'Hospice de la Salpêtrière at the age of 37. It was his belief that the neuroses should be examined and investigated as any other disorders. Charcot experimented with hypnosis, which he felt induced a specific pathological state, and his influence on Freud and the development of psychoanalysis is well known. Zilboorg summed up this era, stating:

The fundamental contribution of the School of the Salpêtrière and its essential historical value lie in the fact that it was the first to capture for psychiatry the very last part of demonological territory, which up to the middle of the 18th century had belonged to the clerical and judicial marshals of theology and from the middle of the 18th century to the last quarter of the 19th had remained for the most part a no man's land (Zilboorg, 1941, p. 365).

Sadly, the first half of the 20th century saw an apparent eclipse of progress in biological psychiatry, and psychological theorizing dominated psychiatry. This had the disastrous effect of accelerating the divisions between neurology and psychiatry, and held up the development of effective treatments, especially for the more severe psychiatric disorders. It was not until the second half of the 20th century that biological approaches to psychiatry flowered again. This has provided a new generation of psychiatrists with a wide range of fascinating and important findings, which place psychiatry once again securely as a medical discipline. This has resulted in part from a vastly increased knowledge of the anatomy and chemistry of the central nervous system, the development of brain imaging and a renewed interest in genetics.

The role that encephalitis played in the development of biological psychiatry has yet to be fully appreciated. The most significant contribution initially came from Constantin von Economo (1876–1931). He studied with Wagner-Jauregg in Vienna, and towards the end of 1916 he reported on a number of patients who presented with an unusual variety of symptoms which followed an influenza-like prodrome. Some had marked lethargy and disturbance of their eye movements, and on post-mortem examination they invariably had inflammation almost exclusively confined to the grey matter of the midbrain. Von Economo defined this as a new entity, and referred to it as encephalitis lethargica. It was attributed to influenza pandemics which occurred in the first years of the 20th century. A wide range of psychopathology was noted in the survivors, especially obsessive–compulsive and psychotic disorders. The importance of this was emphasized by von Economo:

> The dialectic combinations and psychological constructions of many ideologists will collapse like a house of cards if they do not in future take into account these new basic facts ... Every psychologist who in the future attempts to deal with psychological phenomena such as will, temperament, and fundamentals of character, such as self-consciousness, the ego, etc., and is not well acquainted with the appropriate observations on encephalitic patients, and does not read the descriptions of the psychological causes in the many original papers recording the severe mental symptoms, will build on sand (von Economo, 1931, p. 167).

The last sentence of his book is 'Encephalitis lethargica can scarcely again be forgotten' (p. 167), but this prophesy was quickly to be proved wrong. This elegant work was ignored by at least two generations of psychiatric theorists, although the viral hypothesis of psychiatric illness has recently been revived (see Chapter 7).

Epilepsy has always had close links with psychiatry (see Chapter 10). Hughlings Jackson established significant clinical associations and Kraepelin, in his *Lectures on Clinical Psychiatry* (Kraepelin, 1904), included epileptic insanity as a variety of mental illness. The Hungarian Ladislas von Meduna (1896–1964), impressed by his own pathological studies, which suggested different pathological changes in the brains of patients dying with epilepsy versus schizophrenia, reasoned that there was an antagonism between the two disorders. He postulated that the artificial induction of a seizure may have a beneficial effect on the psychosis. He initially used camphor injections, but later Ugo Cerletti (1877–1963) and Lucio Bini (1908–1964) introduced electric stimulation, and the efficacy of this form of treatment in a variety of conditions was soon reported (see Chapter 12).

Another bridge between epilepsy and psychiatry was the introduction into clinical practice of the electroencephalogram (EEG). The psychiatrist Hans Berger (1873–1941), in a series of publications from 1928 to 1935, made regular observations of the electrical patterns he recorded from human brains. The identification of different forms of epilepsy followed; the significance of this disorder for biological psychiatry cannot be overemphasized. The identification that patients with temporal-lobe epilepsy were more likely to have psychiatric disorders than those with other seizure disorders, and the realization that psychic symptoms typified the onset of temporal-lobe seizures, coincided with the rediscovery of the limbic lobe of the brain by Paul MacLean (1913–2007). He recognized the importance of the temporal–limbic anatomy as a neurological framework for emotional feelings, and while he initially referred to this as the 'visceral brain', he later, in 1952, introduced the term 'limbic system'.

Before MacLean there were others who had discussed how it is that we experience emotions. The hypothesis independently developed by William James (1842–1910) and Carl Lange (1834–1900) had implied that emotions were derived from sensory inputs to the brain, but without an obvious cerebral localization. Walter Cannon (1871–1945) had noted subcortical areas which on stimulation led to emotional release, and James Wenceslas Papez (1883–1858) had outlined a harmonious mechanism which he considered elaborated emotion. MacLean's work took the important step of revealing how exterosensory inputs obtained access to limbic structures to allow for the elaboration of their emotional content. However, with his concept of the triune brain,

MacLean set the developed structures of the mammalian brain into a firm evolutionary mould, in a modified Jacksonian framework.

Since MacLean's conceptualizations, the connectionist views of brain function have overtaken an outmoded modularity, and our knowledge of cortical–subcortical circuits, networks and the developed understanding of limbic connectivity have altered our perspective on the limbic-system concept entirely (see Chapter 2). Perhaps fundamental has been the *re*-realization that the limbic areas of the brain are not, as often diagrammatically portrayed in the human brain, small and hidden, but are large and very prominent. Limbic connectivity, via the basal ganglia and frontal cortex, drives the organism forward in time and space. Importantly, emotion and limbic tone pervade many actions, and in the case of *Homo sapiens*, tinge most thinking.

One very important consequence of a biological approach to psychiatric disorders was the progress of biological treatments (see Chapter 12). In the first part of the 20th century pellagra was found to be caused by a deficiency of nicotinic acid, phenylalanine deficiencies were identified in certain mentally handicapped children and endocrine replacement therapies, for example thyroxine, became possible. Neurosurgical approaches to treating psychiatric disorders were initiated by the Portuguese neurologist Antonio Egas Moniz (1874–1955). In 1952, Jean Delay (1907–1987) and Paul Deniker (1917–1998) successfully gave chlorpromazine to psychotic patients. Soon after, antidepressant medications were developed and in 1949 John Cade (1912–1980) introduced lithium, the first prophylactic treatment in psychiatry. 'Librium', the first of the benzodiazepines, was marketed in 1960. With these new and largely effective treatments, based on medical models of normal and pathological behaviour, the future of biological psychiatry was secure, and the societies followed. The Society for Biological Psychiatry and its journal were founded in 1954 and the first World Congress of Societies of Biological Psychiatry was held in 1974. The World Federation of Societies of Biological Psychiatry today has 50 affiliated nationalities and nearly 5000 members.

Looking back on this history of fits and starts and forgotten lessons, one can even wonder if the field of biological psychiatry can continue and evolve. In point of fact, it has, and quite exuberantly. In the 13 years since the last edition of this book, the field of neuroscience has exploded. The Society for Neuroscience annual meeting has gone from 400 attendees in 2000 to over 20 000 now, with each attendee presenting new data. It is thus almost impossible for a clinical, biologically-oriented psychiatrist to even keep up with all this new information. In this edition, we have done our best to integrate new information with the older wisdom, thoroughly revamping and changing broad aspects of the text where needed. Many of the chapters have been completely restructured, and we have included a new chapter on disorders of motivation and addiction (Chapter 9). There are few authored books (not edited) that attempt to cover the full range of biological psychiatry with a single comprehensive voice. We apologize to anyone whose specific work is not directly cited, but we have tried to overview the important contemporary themes in this field. Understanding how the brain organizes thoughts and consciousness is the most important scientific issue facing humanity, and many believe that biological psychiatry is the most dynamic and interesting area in all of medicine and psychology, with profound philosophical implications. We hope the reader will enjoy and be informed by this new edition.

M.R.T.
M.S.G.
2402 Happy Acres Rd.
Cedar Mountain, NC, USA

1
Principles of Brain Function and Structure: 1 Genetics, Physiology and Chemistry

INTRODUCTION

It has become fashionable periodically to ascribe much psychopathology to the evils of modern society, and the resurgence of this notion from time to time reflects the popularity of the simple. Often imbued with political overtones, and rarely aspiring to scientific insights, such a view of the pathogenesis of psychiatric illness ignores the long tradition of both the recognition of patterns of psychopathology and successful treatment by somatic therapies. Further, it does not take into account the obvious fact that humanity's biological heritage extends back many millions of years.

In this and the next chapter, consideration is given to those aspects of the neuroanatomy and neurochemistry of the brain that are important to those studying biological psychiatry. Most emphasis is given to the limbic system and closely connected structures, since the understanding of these regions of the brain has been of fundamental importance in the development of biological psychiatry. Not only has a neurological underpinning for 'emotional disorders' been established, but much research at the present time relates to the exploration of limbic system function and dysfunction in psychopathology.

GENETICS

Every cell in the human body contains the nuclear material needed to make any other cell. However, cells differentiate into a specific cell by expressing only partially the full genetic information for that individual. While it is beyond the scope of this book to fully explain all of modern genetics, it is important to grasp several basic aspects that are involved in building and maintaining the nervous system, and which may impact on psychiatric diseases.

Modern genetic theories are based on knowledge of the deoxyribonucleic acid (DNA) molecule, its spontaneous and random mutations and the recombination of its segments. DNA is composed of two intertwined strands (the double helix) of sugar-phosphate chains held together by covalent bonds linked to each other by hydrogen bonds between pairs of bases. There is always complementary pairing between the bases, such that the guanine (G) pairs with cytosine (C), and the adenine (A) with thymine (T). This pairing is the basis of replication, and each strand of the DNA molecule thus forms the template for the generation of another. Mammalian DNA is

Biological Psychiatry 3e   Michael R. Trimble and Mark S. George
© 2010 John Wiley & Sons, Ltd

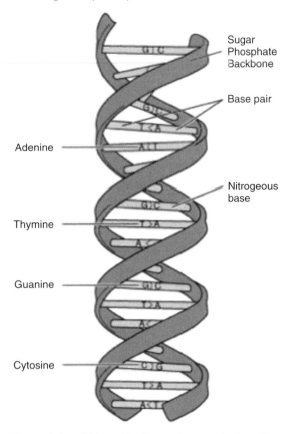

Sugar
Phosphate
Backbone

Base pair

Adenine

Nitrogeous
base

Thymine

Guanine

Cytosine

Figure 1.1 DNA replication and transcription. During transcription, the DNA strands separate, and one is transcribed. The primary mRNA transcript is a copy of the DNA strand, except that a U has been substituted for every T (reproduced with permission from Professor Nick Wood)

supercoiled around proteins called histones (Figure 1.1). Recently it has been discovered that histones can be modified by life experiences. The actual protein folding of the genetic materials changes as a function of histones or methylation on the DNA. Early life experiences can actually cause large strands of the DNA to become silent and not expressed (McGowan *et al.*, 2008 ; Parent and Meaney, 2008).

On the DNA strand are many specific base sequences that encode for protein construction. Thus, proteins are chains of amino acids, and one amino acid is coded by a triplet sequence of bases (the codon). For example, the codon TTC codes for phenylalanine.

DNA separates its double helix in a reaction catalysed by DNA polymerase. In the synthesis of protein, ribonucleic acid (RNA) is an intermediary. RNA is almost identical to DNA, except that uracil (U) replaces thymine, the sugar is ribose, and it is single-stranded. Thus, an RNA molecule is created with a complementary base sequence to the DNA, referred to as messenger RNA (mRNA). This enters the cytoplasm, attaches to ribosomes, and serves as a template for protein synthesis. Transfer RNA (tRNA) attaches the amino acids to mRNA, lining up the amino acids one at a time to form the protein. The tRNA achieves this by having an anticodon at one end attach to the mRNA and the amino acid at the other (see Figure 1.2). Coding occurs between the start and stop codons.

Much is now known regarding the various sequences of bases that form the genetic code. In total, chromosomal DNA in the human genome has approximately 3 billion base pairs. There are 20 amino acids that are universal constituents of proteins, and there are 64 ways of ordering the bases into codons (Wolpert, 1984). Most amino acids are represented by more than one triplet, and there are special techniques for starting and stopping the code. Although it was thought that the only direction of information flow was from DNA to RNA to protein, investigations of tumour cells have revealed retroviruses: RNA viruses that can be incorporated into host DNA.

The genetic programme is determined by DNA, and at various times in development, and in daily life, various genes will be turned on or off depending on the requirements of the organism. There is a constant interplay between the genetic apparatus and chemical constituents of the cell cytoplasm.

In the human cell there is one DNA molecule for each chromosome, and there are some 100 000 genes on 46 chromosomes. This constitutes only a small portion of the total genomic DNA, and more than 90% of the genome seems non-coding. About 50% of human DNA consists of short repetitive sequences that either encode small high-abundance proteins such as histones, or are not transcribed. A lot of these are repetitive sequences dispersed throughout the genome, or arranged as regions of tandem repeats, referred to as satellite DNA.

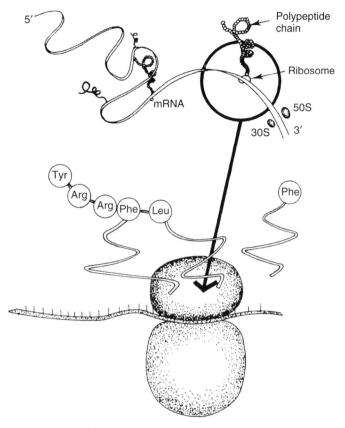

Figure 1.2   RNA translation. The mRNA (top) acts as a template that specifies the sequential attachment of tRNAs: amino acid complexes to make a protein shown in the bottom of the figure. Coding occurs between the start codon (3′) and ends at the stop codon (5′) (reproduced with permission from Lowenstein *et al.*, 1994; *Biol Psych*, 2 Ed, p. 44)

Such repeats are highly variable between individuals, but are inherited in a Mendelian fashion. These variations produce informative markers, and when they occur close to genes of interest are used in linkage analysis. Complimentary cDNA probes are produced using mRNA as a template along with the enzyme reverse transcriptase. The latter is present in RNA viruses; HIV is a well-known example. Reverse transcriptase permits these viruses to synthesize DNA from an RNA template. It is estimated that 30–50% of the human genome is expressed mainly in the brain.

Retroviruses enter host cells through interaction at the host cell surface, there being a specific receptor on the surface. Synthesis of viral DNA then occurs within the cytoplasm, the RNA being transcribed into DNA by reverse

transcriptase, and the viral DNA becoming incorporated into the host's genome.

Oncogenes are DNA sequences homologous to oncogenic nucleic acid sequences of mammalian retroviruses.

In the human cell the chromosomes are divided into 22 pairs of autosomes, plus the sex chromosomes: XX for females and XY for males. Individual genes have their own positions on chromosomes, and due to genetic variation different forms of a gene (alleles) may exist at a given locus. The genotype reflects the genetic endowment; the phenotype is the appearance and characteristics of the organism at any particular stage of development. If an individual has two identical genes at the same locus, one from each parent, this is referred to as being a homozygote; if they differ, a heterozygote. If a heterozygote develops traits as a homozygote then the trait is called dominant. There are many diseases that are dominantly inherited. If the traits are recessive then they will only be expressed if the gene is inherited from both parents. Dominant traits with complete penetrance do not skip a generation, appearing in all offspring with the genotype.

If two heterozygotes for the same recessive gene combine, approximately one in four of any children will be affected; two will be carriers, and one unaffected. When there is a defective gene on the X chromosome, males are most severely affected, male-to-male transmission never occurs, but all female offspring of the affected male inherit the abnormal gene.

Many conditions seem to have a genetic component to their expression, but do not have these classic (Mendelian) modes of inheritance. In such cases polygenetic inheritance is suggested.

Mitochondrial chromosomes have been identified. They are densely packed with no introns and they represent around 1% of total cellular DNA. They are exclusively maternally transmitted. Unlike nuclear chromosomes, present normally in two copies per cell at the most, there are thousands of copies of the mitochondrial chromosomes per cell.

In the gene there are coding sequences, called exons, and intervening non-coding segments referred to as introns. Some sequences occur around a gene, regulating its function. It is not unusual for the genes of even small proteins to be encoded in many small exons (under 200 bases) spread over the chromosome. Most genes have at least 1200 base pairs, but are longer because of introns. Further, important sequences precede the initiation site (or 59), and the end of the gene (39). A model of a generic gene is shown in Figure 1.3. The promotor region is at the 59 end, containing promotor elements and perhaps hormone binding sites. These activate or inhibit gene transcription. The coding region consists of sequences that will either appear in the mature mRNA (exons) or be deleted (introns).

During meiosis, the strands from the two chromosomes become reattached to each other, but each chromosome carries a different allele. There is then a new combination of alleles in the next generation, this exchange being referred to as recombination. The frequency of a recombination between two loci is a function of the distance between them: the closer they are, the less is the likelihood that a recombination will occur between them (Figure 1.4).

Linkage analysis places the location of a particular gene on a chromosome; physical mapping defines the linear order among a series of loci. Genetic distance is measured in centimorgans, reflecting the amount of recombination of traits determined by genes at the two loci in successive generations.

In mutations, unstable mRNA is produced and cannot be translated into a functional polypeptide. Mutations may be referred to as point mutations (substitution of single

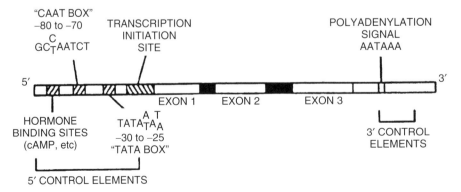

Figure 1.3 A 'generic gene'. Three exons (white) and two introns (black) are shown (reproduced with permission from Ciaranello *et al.*, 1990; *Biol Psych*, 2 Ed, p. 46)

Crossing–over and Recombination During Meiosis

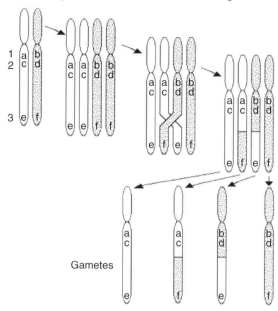

Figure 1.4   The principle of crossover. If there are two genes A and C, the closer together they are, the more likely they are to remain together during meiosis (reproduced with permission from Professor Nick Wood)

incorrect nucleotide), deletions, insertions, rearrangements or duplications.

Molecular cloning techniques allow for the study of gene structure and function. Restriction endonucleases cut the DNA molecule at specific sites, allowing the fragments to be replicated on a large scale by transfecting other organisms, which produces multiple copies of an inserted DNA section. Foreign fragments of DNA are inserted into a plasmid, a cosmid or a bacteriophage vector capable of autonomous replication in a host cell: the process of cloning. Recombinant DNA molecules are amplified by growth in the host (e.g. bacteria) and then subsequently isolated and purified. Once isolated, complementary DNA (cDNA) can be chemically sequenced, introduced into a host cell to produce encoded protein, or hybridized to genomic DNA to examine the structure of the genes encoding for the target protein.

Complementary DNAs are made from mRNAs, prepared from the tissue of interest, and then propagated *in vitro* to form cDNA libraries. A gene probe is a fragment of DNA that detects its complementary sequence. Often such cDNA probes are produced from animal protein, and for most diseases they are not specifically related to a disease gene, but may be linked to it genetically.

The 'lod' score refers to the 'log of the odds' and expresses the relative probability that two loci are linked as opposed to not linked. Thus, given a disease gene and a known DNA marker, if they co-segregate together more than by chance, they may be linked; the tighter the linkage, the greater the probability. The log value of the relative probability of linkage is the lod score, and a positive score of >3 is usually taken as proof of linkage. This means that the odds are 1000 to 1 that the correlation is the result of gene linkage, rather than chance. A lod score of −2 excludes linkage.

Lod scores from independent family observations are added together, overcoming the problem of the small size of the human families that are usually available for observation. Lod scores are calculated with available computer algorithms, and thus quantify probable linkage, but are most effective for conditions with Mendelian inheritance.

In modern genetics, restriction enzymes are used to split the DNA segments, which can then be recognized by gene probes. Restriction-fragment-length polymorphisms (RFLP) are DNA fragments that differ in length between individuals. Tandem repeated sequences vary between individuals, and smaller sequences of repeats are referred to as mini-satellites. Micro-satellites are very short sequences of repeated dinucleotides, usually GT, that are useful for mapping (Figure 1.5).

These satellite sequences and mutations are detected as RFLPs. The technique involves taking tissue – the origin is immaterial – and splitting the DNA into fragments. These are then displayed by a hybridization blot method (Southern blot), which depends on the ability of DNA to bind to nitrocellulose paper. The fixed DNA fragments are then hybridized with a radioactive DNA probe and detected by the subsequent band pattern dependent on

Step 1: Digestion. Amplicons (PCR-amplified DNA segments) are cut (▲) with a restriction enzyme wherever a specific DNA sequence occurs.

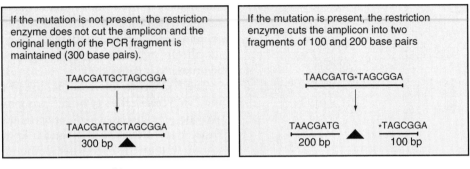

Three outcomes are possible:

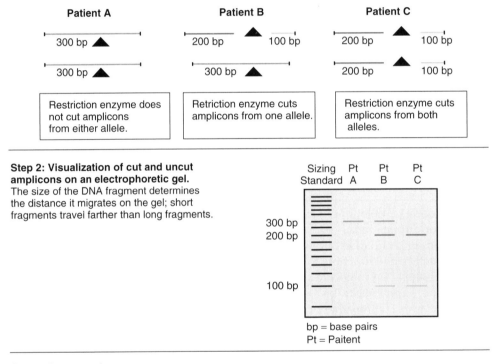

Figure 1.5   Restriction fragment-length polymorphism method to test for genetic variants (reproduced with permission from www.genetests.org and the University of Washington, Seattle)

the speed of migration with electrophoresis. Libraries of DNA probes are available from across the spectrum of the human genome.

Recently, the discovery of the polymerase chain reaction has revolutionized the analysis of RFLPs. In this technique, sufficient high-quality DNA is produced by biological amplification using DNA polymerase, increasing the speed and power of analysis.

The RFLPs are used as genetic markers for inherited diseases if they can be shown to be linked to a gene that is thought to be abnormal and responsible for the condition. Families in which there are several affected members are investigated and RFLPs are probed to detect only those that are present in affected individuals. When found, the chromosome on which the abnormal gene resides can be identified, and the linked marker, which may be the gene itself, is used to detect genotypes likely to become phenotypes. There have been three generations of marker loci used for genetic linkage mapping. The first was the RFLPs described above, followed by the micro-satellites. More recently the single-nucleotide polymorphisms (SNPs, pronounced 'snips') have been used for the same purpose of tracking genetic variants in pedigrees. A SNP is a silent genetic variation in which one nucleotide (AGTC) is replaced by another, often not affecting the expression of the gene. These minor changes are useful in tracking genetic changes over time and in different populations.

Linkage studies are complicated by incomplete penetrance, age of onset of disease, variable expression of that disease and genetic heterogeneity (more than one gene leading to the phenotype).

The identity of a gene marker linked to Huntington's chorea in 1983 provided the first example of the locating of an autosomal dominant gene in neuropsychiatry. This is known to be on chromosome 4, and encodes a structurally unique protein of 348 kd (huntingtin). There is a specific trinucleotide repeat (CAG), which varies from 9 to 37 copies in normals, but can be massively expanded (>100 copies) in Huntington's chorea. It is also possible to pinpoint genes for specific enzymes and receptors; for example, the D_2 receptor at 11q22, and tyrosine hydrolase at 11p15.5.

Despite now having mapped the entire human genome, as well as the genome of many other plants and animals, there has been considerable difficulty in locating specific genes for psychiatric illnesses. The initial breakthroughs (see chapters on individual diseases) have not been replicated in many cases. This relates partly to difficulties of clinical diagnosis and partly to problems of genetic modelling. Thus, the same data set is used to generate the lod score that is used to construct the model for inheritance in the first place.

Building on the world of genomics (study of genes), scientists are now investigating the world of proteomics (the study of the proteins an individual expresses, which change over time). This is immensely richer than even genetics, as the proteins that the RNA transcribes at any given moment are even more variable than the 'largely' static genetic information. In the example above, in Huntington's disease the abnormal protein made by the gene variation is huntingtin; the build-up of toxic proteins then goes on to impair intracellular dynamics and receptor and neuronal function, resulting in disease. A surprising finding of the Human Genome Project is that there are far fewer protein encoding genes than there are proteins in the human body. How can this be? Obviously there must be other factors – where the environment interacts with how genes make proteins – that explain this paradox. The whole study of how the micro-environment within the cell can impact back on which genes are expressed and when is called 'epigenetics'. Some of the more interesting new theories about stress and trauma involve the lifelong effect of the social environment (childhood stress) on gene expression (see Chapters 6 and 8).

It is important to remember that genes code for some facet of a disorder, and not a DSM category. Recently the concept of endophenotypes has emerged. This refers to a biomarker which is intermediate between the genotype (pure gene) and the phenotype (the individual with a disease). The endophenotype is closer to the genetic variation, and represents a risk factor or propensity for a behaviour that then leads to the development of a syndrome (Chapter 4). For example, someone might inherit a gene that codes for a particular cognitive profile (abnormal sensory gating or startle or problems with executive function) which predisposes someone to develop psychosis.

The genes that code for proteins make up about 1.5% of the human genome, and at least some of the rest regulates gene expression. The transcription factors turn on DNA sequences called enhancers, which determine that genes are expressed only where they are wanted and at the time that they are wanted. The enhancers are often hundreds of base pairs in length, and may not be sited near the gene itself. They allow the same gene to be used over and over in different contexts, and from an evolutionary point of view may allow individual traits to be modified without changing the genes themselves. In understanding genetics, the study of the role of enhancers is in its infancy (Carroll *et al.*, 2008).

BRAIN CHEMISTRY AND METABOLISM

In order to function adequately, the brain requires energy which is derived from the catabolism of the food we eat. The major nutrient for the brain is glucose, which, in the process of oxidization to carbon dioxide (CO_2) and water gives up energy. This process results in the formation of adenosine triphosphate (ATP) from adenosine diphosphate (ADP). In the course of energy use through cellular transport and biosynthesis the ATP is degraded to ADP (see Figure 1.6).

Glucose enters cells via transporters, and glucose utilization is higher in astrocytes than neurones. Glycogen in the brain is stored mainly in astrocytes, and the latter release energy to neurones via pyruvate and lactate. Glycogen turnover is rapid and coincides with synaptic activity. Several neurotransmitters (such as the monoamines) are glycogenolytic, releasing energy from the astrocytes. Another important

function of astrocytes is to remove glutamate from the synaptic space, which is recycled via glutamine back to neurones to replenish the glutamate pool. The metabolism of glucose in the brain is highly temporospatially specific and linked to neuronal-glial (the neutropil) activity, a property which has been used in the theories of glucose PET imaging (see Chapter 4) and is also important for understanding functional MRI.

The oxidation of one molecule of glucose generally gives 36–38 moles of ATP (Siesjo, 1978). It is obvious that ATP has a central role in cellular metabolism, being the product of oxidation and the substrate for further chemical reactions requiring energy. It is composed of a nitrogenous base (adenine), a five-carbon sugar and attached phosphate groups; it is one of several triphosphonucleotides in the cell that yield energy.

As noted, the main energy requirements are those of cellular transport mechanisms and biosynthesis. The former includes the movement of both charged and uncharged particles across cell membranes and the transport of molecules intracellularly. Biosynthesis involves the formation of simple and complex molecules required for cellular function, in addition to such energy storage molecules as glycogen.

A related molecule is adenosine 3,5-monophosphate (cyclic AMP), which has one phosphate molecule and forms a ring structure with links between the sugar and phosphate molecules. It is formed from ATP in a reaction

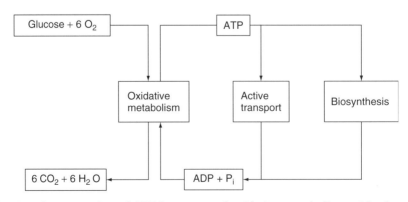

Figure 1.6 Showing the generation of ATP by means of oxidative metabolism with glucose as substrate. Oxidation of 1 mole of glucose yields 36–38 moles of ATP (reproduced with permission from Siesjo, 1978; *Biol Psych*, 2 Ed, p. 50)

that utilizes adenyl cyclase as a catalyst. It is activated by adrenaline and is known to be involved, via the intermediary phosphorylase, in the activation of glycogen. Further, cyclic AMP appears to act as an intermediary in many other cellular reactions, including those stimulated by hormonal or neurotransmitter stimuli (see below).

Chemical reactions in the body are facilitated by enzymes, some of which themselves are activated by coenzymes which transfer atoms or groups of atoms from one molecule to another. Since the quantity of active enzyme present is the essential ingredient that determines the rate of a biochemical reaction in the presence of appropriate substrates, activation and inhibition of enzymes regulates the metabolic activity of cells. One method of inhibition of a particular metabolic reaction is by feedback from a resulting metabolite (feedback inhibition).

THE METABOLISM OF GLUCOSE

Glucose and glycogen catabolism result in the production of ATP via the well-known tricarboxylic acid (Krebs) cycle (see Figure 1.7). Glucose is first phosphorylated by hexokinase

to yield glucose-6-phosphate. This is converted, via the several intermediary steps of glycolysis, to lactic acid. This yields two molecules of ATP thus:

$$\text{Glucose} + 2\,\text{ADP} + 2\,\text{phosphate}$$
$$\rightarrow 2\,\text{lactic acid} + 2\,\text{ATP} + 2\,\text{water}$$

Lactic acid is converted to acetyl-coenzyme A via pyruvic acid, and the former is oxidized by the tricarboxylic acid cycle to citrate and ultimately oxaloacetate, which itself is incorporated with acetyl-coenzyme A to yield citrate. Hydrogen atoms that are generated react with oxygen to form water, and further molecules of ATP are generated. Since other products of digestion undergoing catabolism also utilize the tricarboxylic acid cycle, it represents a final common path, and almost two-thirds of all energy released in the breakdown of food occurs during the reactions of this cycle.

PROTEINS AND FATTY ACIDS

While glucose is the most important food involved in metabolism, proteins and fatty acids are also involved. Protein is broken down

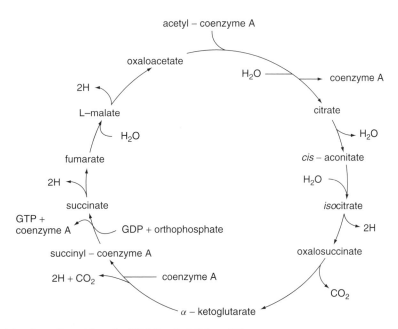

Figure 1.7 The tricarboxylic acid cycle (*Biol Psych*, 2 Ed, p. 52)

Table 1.1   Some essential amino acids

Histidine
Arginine
Ornithine
Valine
Methionine
Lysine
Phenylalanine
Tyrosine
Tryptophan
Homocysteine
Cysteine
Glycine
Amino butyric acid

to amino acids, which can be oxidized through the tricarboxylic acid cycle. Degradation reactions common for several amino acids include deamination, in which an amonia group is removed, transamination, in which there is exchange between amino and ketonic acids of amino and keto groups, and decarboxylation, in which a carbon dioxide radical is given up. Only some amino acids are broken down for energy, others being involved in the synthesis of neurotransmitters, and most in the building of proteins.

There are only a limited number of amino acids in living cells, some of the most important being shown in Table 1.1.

Fats are hydrolysed to free fatty acids and glycerol. The fatty acids are chains of carbon atoms terminated with a carboxylic acid (—COOH) group. Glycerides are esters (compounds formed by the interaction of an acid and an alcohol) of fatty acids and glycerol, and phospholipids are esters of fatty acids and alcohol, the latter containing a phosphate group. Sphingolipids have the base sphingosine instead of glycerol, and sphingomyelines contain choline. The cerebrosides and gangliosides are sphingolipids with a hexose, and in the case of gangliosides, a polyhydroxy amino acid. All of these are found in abundance in nerve tissue.

CELL MEMBRANES

Neurones, in common with other cells, are bounded by a membrane. It is now known that

this is a continuous double structure with two electron-dense layers separated by an interzone. The thickness is approximately 100 Å, and similar membranes are seen in the cell, forming, for example, the endoplasmic reticulum or the mitochondria.

They are mainly formed from lipids (whose central components are fatty acids) and proteins. One end is hydrophilic and the other hydrophobic, and these align to form a structure suggested to look like that shown in Figure 1.8. The inside is hydrophobic, and proteins seem embedded in the structure, carrying out such functions as aiding active transport, forming the structure of receptors and enzyme activity. Channels in the membrane are thought to be protein aggregates, and they help regulate permeability. These are either active (which can be open or closed) or passive (which remain open all the time). Active channels may be influenced by various stimuli including electrical or chemical ones such as the neurotransmitters.

The primary structures of sodium, potassium and calcium channels have been revealed following cloning, and they are all similar, with four homologous transmembrane domains surrounding a central ion pore, which sits in the centre of the square array.

In the technique of patch clamping, a small micropipette with a polished end is pushed into the cell and then sucked. The membrane forms a tight seal on the pipette, and if it is then pulled the small patch of membrane remains intact

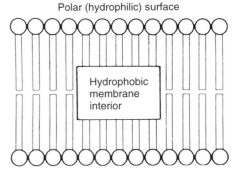

Figure 1.8   A schematic representation of a cell membrane (reproduced from Shaw *et al.*, 1982, by permission of Butterworth & Co; *Biol Psych*, 2 Ed, p. 54)

and is used to study receptor function in detail, including ion flow through channels.

In order that the cell is excitable, a potential difference across it must exist (polarization). This membrane potential is positive on the outside and negative on the inside. It is due to electrolyte differences on the two sides of the membrane, and in most neurones is in the region of 50–60 mV. This is referred to as the resting potential; to generate the action potential the membrane must be depolarized by alteration of the ion distribution on the two sides of the membrane.

There are four main ions in the cells: sodium (Na^+), potassium (K^+), chloride (Cl^2) and organic anion (A^2). Sodium and chloride are at lower concentrations on the inside of the cell; the other two have higher concentrations. At rest, the potential is maintained by the action of the sodium pump, which, at the expense of energy, forces the sodium out and draws the potassium in. The resting potential acts as the energy store of the cell, and neuronal action is dependent on it. The electrical signals of the nerve cells result from a change in the resting potential with alteration of the distribution of ions on either side of the membrane.

The action potential is generated by depolarization, during which sodium flows into the cell and, with slight delay, the potassium moves out. This process is initiated by the opening of the sodium channel, allowing sodium to flow in: a process that opens more sodium channels. Then, as sodium channels begin to close, the potassium voltage-regulated gated channels begin to open and repolarization occurs. The resulting phases of the action potential are shown in Figure 1.9.

These action potentials are generated by such stimuli as synaptic transmission, and propagation of the current along the membrane proceeds as adjacent portions of the membrane become depolarized by electronic conduction. Generally, the larger the diameter of the axon of the cell, the more rapid the current flow; however, in myelinated axons (see below), where the resistance at the nodes of Ranvier is low compared with that at the internodes, current travels along intracellular fluid from node to node, a process referred to as saltatory conduction. Following the action potential there is a brief refractory period during which the sodium channels return to their closed state. The entire neuron firing and refractory period take 5–6 milliseconds, allowing neurone to potentially

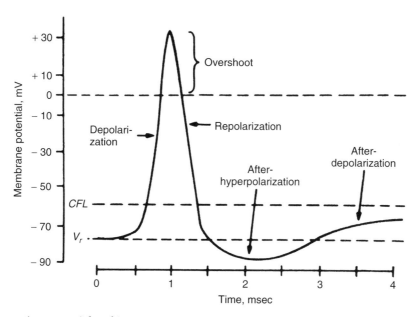

Figure 1.9 The action potential and its components. Vr, resting membrane potential; CFL, critical firing level (*Biol Psych*, 2 Ed, p. 55)

refire or oscillate at very high frequencies (several hundred events per second). This is in contrast to the megahertz frequencies sometimes used in modern electronics or computers. However, neurone also have the ability to amplify their signal; that is, once the axon is triggered, it can spread to the full tree of the axon, and potentially interact with thousands of other neurone. Axonal information can travel at $0.5–50\,\mathrm{m\,s^{-1}}$.

Although the most important ions for the generation of the action potential are sodium and potassium, others exert influences, such as calcium and magnesium.

SYNAPSES

The main link between one neurone and the next is the synapse, and in the human central

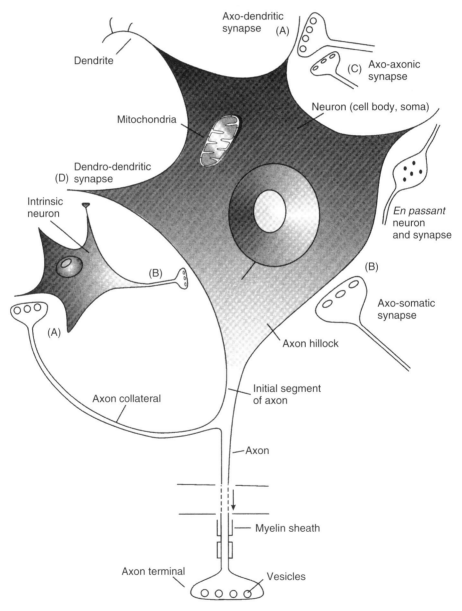

Figure 1.10   Schematic representation of a neuron (Webster, 2002)

nervous system (CNS) transmission is mainly chemical. However, it is recognized that electrical synapses occur (bridged junctions) with only small gaps (around 20 Å) separating the presynaptic and postsynaptic membranes. In contrast, chemical synapses (unbridged junctions) have a larger gap (200 Å), the synaptic cleft, and specialized vesicles are identifiable in the presynaptic terminals. Information flow across the electrical synapse is more rapid than across chemical junctions, although the latter are more flexible.

Postsynaptic potentials are either inhibitory (IPSP) or excitatory (EPSP). The former prevent the initial area of the axon from reaching the threshold required to generate an action potential (hyperpolarization) by increasing the influx of potassium and chloride. These IPSPs can summate either temporally or spatially, and interact with EPSPs to determine the ultimate excitability of the postsynaptic cell. EPSPs result from an influx of sodium via chemically gated channels, and the spike discharge is generated not at the postsynaptic membrane, but at the axon hillock, which has a low electrical threshold (see Figure 1.10).

In addition to these postsynaptic events, presynaptic factors which control transmitter release also affect postsynaptic activity. These include presynaptic inhibition or facilitation via activity in synapses on the presynaptic boutons (axo-axonic synapses) and ionic influences such as calcium (Ca^2) influx. The presynaptic terminals come from interneurones, and they provoke an EPSP or IPSP in the terminal of the afferent nerve fibre. In the case of inhibition, this partial depolarization reduces the amplitude of the oncoming afferent action potential. Since the transmitter release is proportional to the amplitude of the action potential, less transmitter is released and a smaller EPSP results in the postsynaptic cell. Although first discovered in relation to spinal cord afferents, this form of inhibition has been shown to exist in many CNS areas. Varieties of presynaptic connections are shown in Figure 1.11. Where the neurone has receptors to its own transmitter on these terminals they are called autoreceptors.

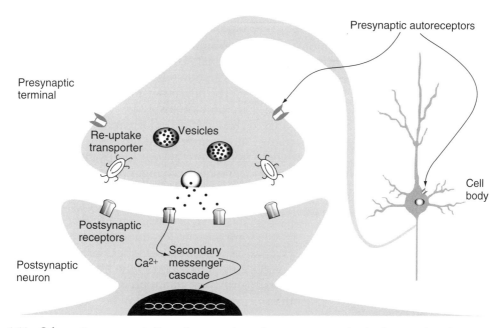

Figure 1.11 Schematic representation of a generic excitatory synapse in the brain. This shows glutamate released by fusion of transmitter vesicles at the nerve terminal and diffusing across the synaptic cleft to activate AMPA and NMDA receptors. Glutamate also binds to metabotropic G-protein-coupled glutamate receptors, initiating secondary messenger intracellular signalling through the G-protein complex (Webster, 2002)

Calcium has been shown to be essential for transmitter release. During depolarization of the presynaptic terminal the calcium channels open and calcium moves into the cell. This allows the presynaptic vesicles that contain neurotransmitters to bind to releasing sites on the postsynaptic membrane. Control of calcium currents by presynaptic receptors is thought to be an important mechanism of their action.

The amount of transmitter released is related to the calcium levels and the presynaptic input. The response is thus plastic, and further varied by the postsynaptic variation in ion channels. Single vesicles can release up to 5000 molecules of a neurotransmitter.

A further consideration is the retrograde control of presynaptic activity by diffusible messengers from the postsynaptic cell. Nitrous oxide (NO) is a gaseous messenger involved in long-term potentiation (LTP). NO is synthesized in the postsynaptic cell following calcium influx at the N-methy-aspartate (NMDA) receptor, and diffuses back to the presynaptic terminals, altering transmitter release. Other candidates are arachidonic acid and carbon monoxide. A possible target for these messengers is the presynaptic calcium influx.

There are two types of communication between cells: classical, with fast transmission, in which highly specialized regions of the presynaptic cell make contact with discrete areas of the postsynaptic cell; and more diffuse, with transmitter released over a broader area. The latter is less readily removed, and transmission is slower. Transmitters such as amines and opiates use this latter, slower method and set the level of a response.

RECEPTORS

In recent years much attention has been paid to the structure and function of receptors. These are proteins to which transmitters bind, and are located on the outer surface of the cell membranes. Two types are defined, the transmitter-gated ion channel (called ionotropic) and the G-protein-coupled receptor (called metabotropic). The former act very

quickly, while the latter initiate a series of postsynaptic intracellular events which alter either intracellular proteins or the DNA of the nucleus, altering gene expression. The latter will lead to alteration of the configuration of the cell, for example by activating growth factors or receptor activity (see Figure 1.12).

The genes for many receptors have been cloned and their polypeptide structures identified. Many have a similar conformation, perhaps suggesting a common evolutionary precursor. Since the sequence of the amino acids is known for the Dopamine D_1 receptor, it is possible to look at which parts of the sequence will interact with the lipid-rich membrane, and at the hydrophobic and hydrophilic parts identified. The general model is of five subunits, a channel, a gate and a receptor bound in a pocket. Some receptors have many subunits, and these are selected in different combinations to give different responses, the length of time the channel is open and the number of ions that flow through it (Sibley and Monsma, 1992).

G-protein-coupled receptors share a generic pattern of protein folding, with seven hydrophobic transmembrane helices joined by alternating intracellular and extracellular loops, an extracellular amino terminal and a cytoplasmic carboxyl terminal. The protein folding of several receptors is shown in Figure 1.13.

The neurotransmitter binds with the receptor to form a transmitter–receptor complex, which changes the conformation of the latter. With the transmitter-gated ion channels, opening up the ionophore allows ion exchange to occur with consequent changes of the membrane potential. An influx of negative ions such as Cl^- leads to IPSPs, while an influx of positive ions such as Na^+ will encourage EPSPs. Some ionophores are specific for chloride or sodium, others are less selective. With the G-protein-coupled receptors, interaction of the transmitter and receptor provokes alteration of intracellular metabolism by the stimulation of second messengers.

In addition to neurotransmitter receptors, there are receptors for other chemicals, some of which help with the early development of neuronal systems, such as for nerve growth factors (NGF) and steroid receptors. The latter

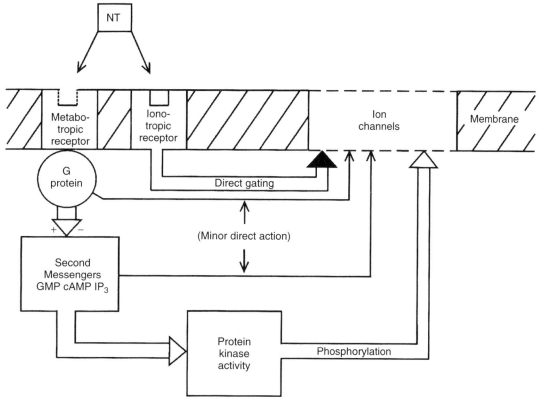

Figure 1.12 The difference between ionotropic and metabotropic mechanisms. With the former, the neurotransmitter combines with the receptor, leading to opening of the ion channel. With the latter, G-protein is activated, leading to a secondary messenger cascade. The image also shows how the intracellular activations can feed back, affecting ion channels (Webster, 2002)

are intracellular molecules which carry the steroid to the nucleus.

Ligands (transmitters or synthesized chemicals that act on receptors), which are agonists, antagonists, partial agonists (exhibiting less than a maximal response) and inverse agonists (leading to the opposite response to a full agonist) have been identified, depending on the receptor type.

There are several second messenger systems. Following contact between the receptor and a neurotransmitter, a G-protein is activated (a GTP-binding protein), which in turn activates further proteins, leading to the conversion of ATP to cAMP.

One secondary messenger system is via adenylate cyclase to cyclic AMP. There is an intermediary G-protein which binds with the receptor–transmitter complex and alters its configuration; it then links with adenylate cyclase and activates it, leading to cyclic AMP formation. An important feature of this system is amplification, whereby each activated receptor protein stimulates many molecules of G-protein, which in turn activate many molecules of adenylate cyclase, each further generating many cyclic AMP molecules. Protein kinases are enzymes which phosphorylate (add phosphorous to) proteins and help physiologically activate them (Figure 1.12).

Another second messenger system is via the hydrolysis of a membrane phospholipid (phosphatidylinositol biphosphate), which leads to the production of diacylglycerol and, via phospholipase C, inositol triphosphate (IP_3). Diacylglycerol activates protein kinase C and

(a) (b) (c)

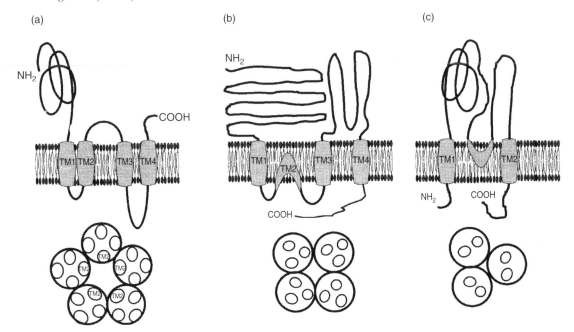

Figure 1.13 How transmembrane subunits are conceived. The subunits are embedded in the cell membrane. The example in (a) reflects the structure, for example, of a GABA$_a$ receptor. Below is shown pentameric stoichiometry of the domain receptors lining the central ion channel. (b) shows the structure of ionotropic glutamate receptors. (c) shows a subunit of an ATP receptor (Webster, 2002)

IP$_3$ causes release of calcium from the endoplasmic reticulum, which activates a protein kinase called calmodulin-dependent protein kinase. G-proteins can also elevate intracellular calcium, thus indirectly activating kinases. Calcium is intimately related to these secondary messenger systems, and a calcium-binding protein, calmodulin, mediates these events and release of neurotransmitters from synaptic vesicles.

Thus, phosphorylation modifies the action of intracellular enzymes and cell regulatory proteins; signals mediated through second messengers influence protein kinases and protein phosphatases, which in turn modify the action of genes via transcription factors in the cytoplasm that bind to DNA. Genes encoding transcription factors have been referred to as third messengers. Genes such as *c-fos* are actively switched on quickly, having binding sites for the transcription factor CREB. The receptors for steroid hormones are also transcription factors, acting in the cell cytoplasm.

Calcium Channels

Calcium channels are essential because they allow the influx of calcium into the synapse, calcium being involved in the attachments of vesicles to the synaptic membrane, which is essential for neurotransmitter release. Thus, calcium channels, and their proper functioning, can affect many different neurotransmitter systems. Several different types of calcium channel have been identified, some of which, such as the T-type, or the subcomponent alpha-2-delta, have been implicated in the action of some anticonvulsant medications. There is evidence that calcium-channel blockers may be effective in stabilizing mood in bipolar patients, particularly those who are treatment-resistant or are rapid-cycling.

Third Messengers and Other Proteins

Recent research has unravelled many other intracellular proteins involved in either

Table 1.2 Types of dopamine receptors

	DA_1	DA_2	DA_3	DA_4	DA_5
Coupled	adenylate cyclase	<	phospholipase C	>	adenylate cyclase
Chromosome	5	11	3	11	4
Highest CNS	<neostriatum>		paleostriatum		hypothalamus
Density	nucleus accumbens olfactory tubercle		archicerebellum hypothalamus	frontal cortex	hippocampus
Adenylate cyclase	activate	inhibits	?	inhibits	activates
Pituitary	no	yes	no	yes	no
Affinity for DA	micromol	micromol	nanomol	submicromolar	submicromolar

the biology of psychiatric disorders or the action of psychotropic drugs, for example DARPP (dopamine- and cyclic-AMP-regulated phosphoprotein) and CREB (cAMP-response-element binding) proteins. These form part of a complex intracellular machinery, leading to longer-term genetic and synaptic changes in cells. It is now known that receptors under the influence of these factors can actually move in and out of synapses. Genes encoding transcription factors have been referred to as third messengers. The receptors for steroid hormones are also transcription factors, acting in the cell cytoplasm. New research is focusing on whether these systems are abnormal in psychiatric disorders, and if so, whether they might be targets for novel therapies.

A single receptor in a homogenous cell population may couple differently to different effector systems, allowing for a range of activity from near antagonism to full agonism.

At the present time many different receptors have been classified and subclassified, although there is not universal agreement. It should be noted that, when receptor binding studies are presented, usually either receptor agonist affinity (Kd) or receptor number (BMax) is referred to. Receptor reactivity, a third but crucial variable, is poorly investigated owing to the limitations of *in vivo* techniques. Some of the more relevant receptors for psychiatry are now presented.

Dopamine

It is now accepted that there are five types of dopamine receptor (DA_{1-5}). They are all linked with a binding protein, and all have been cloned.

There are two subfamilies: DA_1 and DA_5, and DA_2, DA_3 and DA_4 (see Table 1.2). The first subfamily of receptors couples with adenylate cyclase, and the other subfamily couples with phospholipase C, which then inhibits adenylate cyclase.

The distribution of the D_1 and the D_2 receptors is wide compared with the others, but this does not relate to functional significance. D_3 has a limited distribution in the limbic striatum, especially in the olfactory tubercle and nucleus accumbens, while D_4 is found in the prefrontal cortex.

D_2, D_3 and D_4 are also autoreceptors. They may inhibit DA cell firing, DA release or synthesis.

Individual cells have been shown to contain both D_1 and D_2 receptors. D_2 receptors have high affinity for traditional antipsychotic drugs, D_1 less so. Interestingly, there are less abundant dopamine transporters in the frontal cortex, which suggests that dopamine may act differently there than in the basal ganglia.

Receptors for Excitatory Amino Acids (EAA)

Glutamate and aspartate are the main EAAs. The glutamate receptors are of two main types, AMPA and NMDA. The former have fast kinetics and are coupled to a sodium channel; the latter are slower, having high calcium permeability, which activates intracellular processes. Others include the kainate receptor and the trans-ACPD receptor. Excessive NMDA receptor activity can lead to excess calcium influx and neuronal death.

Table 1.3   Agonists and antagonists of adrenoceptors

	α-1	α-2	β-1	β-2
Agonists	Adrenaline	Adrenaline	Adrenaline	Adrenaline
	Noradrenaline	Clonidine	Isoprenaline	Isoprenaline
	Methoxamine		Noradrenaline	Salbutamol
	Phenylephrine			Terbutaline
Antagonists	Phenoxybenzamine	Yohimbine	Practolol	Propranolol
	Phentolamine		Atenolol	
	Prazosin		Metoprolol	
			Propranolol	

The molecular structure of these receptors is known, and subtypes have been defined. It is thought that NMDA receptors are involved in synaptic plasticity, and probably with LTP and memory storage.

The NMDA receptor has within it a glycine binding site, and occupancy of this is necessary to allow opening of the channel by glutamate. Phencyclidine, some anaesthetics and MK-801 have high-affinity binding for sites in the ionic channel. The channel is normally blocked by magnesium, which is removed on depolarization.

Many glutamate synapses have two receptor sites – NMDA and non-NMDA – with an interaction between them. If the non-NMDA receptor fires once, because of the presence of the magnesium, the NMDA receptor ion channel remains closed. The latter is opened only by the cell firing in bursts, with sufficient voltage change in the post-synaptic neurone to remove the magnesium ion and allow an influx of sodium and calcium.

Glutamate receptors are widely distributed in the cortex, and are linked to activity in the CA_1 cells in the hippocampus.

Adrenoceptors

In the same way that dopamine receptors can be subdivided, so can those for several other neurotransmitters. The adrenergic receptors are divided into three main subtypes: α_1, α_2 and β. Each of these has three subtypes: $\alpha_{1a}, \alpha_{1b}, \alpha_{1d}, \alpha_{2a}$, etc. α_1 receptors are postsynaptic and excitatory, and α_2 are both post- and presynaptic and inhibitory. At the presynaptic location they are involved in noradrenaline release, and their postsynaptic role is undetermined. Relatively selective agonists and antagonists have been defined for all subtypes (see Table 1.3). The α_1 receptor is believed to play a role in smooth muscle contraction and has been implicated in effecting blood pressure, nasal congestion and prostate function. Although widely expressed in the CNS, the central role of the α_1 receptor remains to be determined. Locomotor activation and arousal have been suggested by some studies. Stimulation of the α_1 receptor may synergistically increase the activity of the 5-HT neurone in the raphe nucleus, although stimulation of the α_2 receptor may have the opposite effect. α_1 receptors stimulate the IP_3 system; α_2 inhibit adenylate cyclase.

The α_2 receptor subtypes in the CNS inhibit the firing of the noradrenaline neurone through autoreceptors. This mechanism of action is believed to mediate the sedative and hypotensive effects of the α_2 receptors agonist clonidine. Additionally, stimulation of the α_2 receptors decreases sympathetic activity, which may explain the therapeutic utility of clonidine for suppressing the heightened sympathetic state of patients in opiate withdrawal.

The β receptor subtypes are more famous for their part in slowing cardiac rhythm and lowering blood pressure. The functions of the β receptors in the CNS, although widely distributed, are not well understood. It is not uncommon to use a β blocker, such as propranolol, to treat performance anxiety or antipsychotic-induced akathisia. Whether these benefits come from a central or peripheral blockage (or both) of the β receptor is not known. All β subtypes interact with adenylate cyclase.

Histamine Receptors

There are now four histamine receptors, although H_4 is predominately in the periphery and was only recently discovered. The H_1 receptor is the target for the classic antihistamines, which highlights its role in sedation and, conversely, arousal. Of great interest to psychiatrists is the role of H_1 in weight gain. Recent analysis has shown that the potential to gain weight with antipsychotic agents correlates with their antagonism for the H_1 receptor; examples include clozapine and olanzapine (Han *et al.*, 2008; Nasrallah, 2008).

The H_2 receptor is more traditionally associated with the gut. Blockade of the H_2 receptor has been a widely used treatment for peptic ulcer disease. The H_3 receptor functions as an inhibitory receptor on the histamine neurone as well as on other non-histamine nerve terminals. The role of this receptor is not clearly understood, but may be involved in appetite, arousal and cognition.

5-HT Receptors

The original discovery of the 5-HT receptor led to two subtypes: 5-HT_1 and 5-HT_2. Further discoveries, especially the application of molecular cloning techniques, have resulted in multiple subdivisions of these two receptors and the addition of several new ones, for a total of 14. While the prospect of activating or blocking the various receptors for further refinement of psychopharmacological treatment is enticing, the clinical results, with a few exceptions, have been limited (see Table 1.4).

The 5-HT_1 receptors make up the largest subtype, with 5-HT_{1A}, 5-HT_{1B}, 5-HT_{1D}, 5-HT_{1E} and 5-HT_{1F}. 5-HT_{1A} has received the most interest and seems to play a prominent role in depression and anxiety. It is an autoreceptor on the cell body. Stimulation of this receptor reduces cell firing and curtails the release of 5-HT. How this would improve mood is unclear, but blocking this receptor has decreased the effectiveness of tricyclic antidepressants in rat models of depression. The anxiolytic buspirone is a partial 5-HT_{1A} agonist, which suggests that 5-HT_{1A} has some role in anxiety. The development and distribution of buspirone is an example of specific 5-HT-receptor targeting, which has had only a marginal effect on clinical practice.

The 5-HT_{1D} receptor is also an autoreceptor but is located on the nerve terminal at the synapse. There it appears to function to sense the 5-HT in the synaptic cleft and turn off release of more 5-HT when stimulated. The 5-HT_{1D}

Table 1.4   5-HT receptor subtypes

Main type	Sub-main site type	Second messenger	Agonist (AG)[*] antagonist (ANT)
5-HT_1	a raphe; hippocampus	ac	buspirone (a) propranolol (ant)
	b substantia nigra: globus pallidus	ac	propranol (ant)
	d basal ganglia	ac	metergoline (ant) sumatriptan (ag)
5-HT_2	a cerebral cortex; caudate; limbic system	IP_3	ritanserin (ant) ketanserin (ant) spiperone (ant) cyproheptadine (ant) mianserin (ant) methysergide (ant) metergoline (ant)
	c choroid plexus	IP_3	m-CPP (ag)
5-HT_3	entorhinal cortex	ion channel	quizapine (ant) ondansetron
5-HT_4	limbic system; basal ganglia; frontal cortex	ac	

[*]Only limited ones given. Note that drugs like quizapine (ag), L-tryptophan (ag), fenfluramine (ag), p-chloroamphetamine (ag), methysergide (ant) and metergoline (ant) act at multiple 5-HT receptors. Ac is adenylate cyclase, IP3 is phosphatidyl inositol.

receptor is stimulated by the antimigraine drug sumatriptan, although the importance of this effect in the overall efficacy of the medication is unclear. Some researchers are exploring the effectiveness of a $5\text{-}HT_{1D}$ receptor antagonist for the treatment of depression. The goal is to block the negative feedback mediated through the $5\text{-}HT_{1D}$ receptor so that more 5-HT is released into the synapse.

Other important 5-HT receptors for the psychiatrist are $5\text{-}HT_{2A}$ and $5\text{-}HT_{2C}$. The $5\text{-}HT_{2A}$ receptor has been identified as playing an important role in the 'atypical-ness' of the second-generation antipsychotic agents (clozapine, risperidone, olanzapine, etc). These newer agents have a greater capacity to block $5\text{-}HT_{2A}$ than the traditional agents like haloperidol and it is speculated that this results in the observed decrease in extrapyramidal side effects (EPS) and greater cognitive improvements.

5-HT receptors are involved in the regulation of dopamine and acetylcholine release. $5\text{-}HT_{1A}$ is an autoreceptor on the cell body and reduces 5-HT release; $5\text{-}HT_3$ activation stimulates striatal and mesolimbic dopamine release, and it is in mesolimbic areas that many of the $5\text{-}HT_3$ binding sites are to be found. In contrast, this receptor decreases the release of acetylcholine. $5\text{-}HT_{1D}$ is also an autoreceptor, but at the nerve terminal, and also inhibits 5-HT release. There has been much interest in the $5\text{-}HT_{2A}$ receptor, because it is involved in the action of the atypical antipsychotics (Chapter 12).

GABA and Benzodiazepine Receptors

Multiple types of the GABA receptor exist. This receptor is composed of three subunits, alpha, beta and gamma, each with its own isoforms. There are at least six for the alpha, four for the beta, and two for the gamma. There seem to be around 48 possible structures of the receptor, although it has to be noted that these have been identified with the techniques of molecular biology, not pharmacology. These subunit types differ with respect to their sensitivity for GABA and recognition sites for other molecules such as the benzodiazepines. For the latter, binding occurs at the alpha subunit, although it requires the presence of the gamma subunit

for stabilization. Two types of benzodiazepine receptors are described, BZ_1 and BZ_2, depending on the alpha subunits from which they are composed (Doble and Martin, 1992). Other important modulators of the GABA receptor include neurosteroids and alcohol.

$GABA_a$ receptors are ligand-gated ion channels composed of five subunits, the recognition site for GABA being present on the beta unit. Picrotoxin and bicuculline are antagonists, and they contain a benzodiazepine and a barbiturate binding site. They are linked to chloride channels.

$GABA_b$ receptors are coupled to G-protein and activated by baclofen; they may decrease the flow of calcium and are not linked to the benzodiazepine recognition site. The distribution of the subunits in the brain reveals GABA receptors to be widespread; indeed, GABA is one of the most common neurotransmitters, occurring in over 30% of all synapses (Leonard, 1992). Ethanol enhances the function of the GABA receptor. Long-term use of ethanol decreases the expression of the GABA receptor, which may explain the tolerance that develops with alcoholism. Whether the receptor alterations contribute to the propensity for seizures when the alcohol is withdrawn remains unclear. The steroid hormones can also modulate GABA receptors (sometimes called neurosteroids when they have effects on neurone). The distribution of GABA receptors with different subunits varies widely in brain; alpha subunits localize especially with 5-HT and catecholamine neurone.

More recently, extra-synaptic GABA receptors have been identified, which are thought to act by using the overspill of GABA from the synapse, and provide tonic background inhibition. This tonic conduction is activated by low ambient levels of GABA. Research is underway to find selective agents that act extra-synaptically. These compounds (e.g. gaboxadol) would increase inhibition and perhaps be useful as a hypnotic or anticonvulsant.

Acetylcholine

Acetylcholine has four protein subunits (alpha, beta, gamma and delta). Muscarinic and nicotinic subtypes are recognized, and five molecularly distinct muscarinic proteins (M_1–M_5) have been cloned. They transduce their intracellular signals by coupling with G-proteins.

It was with the cholinergic receptor that scientists first realized that one neurotransmitter (ACh) could have different receptors. The initial subtypes were identified and named after the drug that distinguished their effects. For example, nicotine will stimulate cholinergic receptors in skeletal muscle but not the heart. Conversely, muscarine will stimulate the heart but has no effect on skeletal muscle. Thus the two receptors can be identified by the actions of different drugs and the receptors were named after those drugs: nicotinic and muscarinic. Unfortunately, it has been hard to find a drug with unique action on each receptor subtype, so we have designations such as 1A, 2B and so on.

Many more subtypes of the nicotinic and muscarinic receptors have been identified since the early days of receptor delineation, but the significance of these various subtypes remains obscure. Clearly, ACh is important in cognition and memory, as shown by the benefits of inhibiting acetylcholinesterase as a treatment for Alzheimer's disease (Chapter 12). Likewise the blockage of the muscarinic receptor by tricyclic antidepressants and antipsychotic medications results in troublesome dry mouth, constipation and urinary hesitancy (which are generically referred to as the anticholinergic side effects). However, the importance of one receptor subtype over another has not been shown.

Other Receptors

Many other receptors and their subtypes have been identified in the CNS, although often their functional significance is unknown.

Peptide and opiate receptors have been identified. There are at least three classes of opiate receptor (Reisine and Bell, 1993): delta, kappa and mu. The delta and kappa bind enkephalins and endorphin, and the kappa receptors bind dynorphins. Mu receptors are selectively sensitive to morphine. All three types couple to adenylate cyclase, inhibiting cAMP.

Receptors for substance P, enkephalins, prolactin, steroids, adenosine (A_1–A_3) and even some drugs such as imipramine, have also been described. In the latter instance, it is the case that the imipramine, or another drug such as paroxetine, binds to the 5-HT transporter site. Sigma receptors, once considered to be opiate receptors, are well represented in limbic structures, and have a high affinity for some neuroleptics.

The body and brain produce endogenous endocannabinoid substances. The cannabinoid receptors are of two types: CB_1 is found in the brain and the heart, CB_2 in immune and hematopoetic cells. They work through G-protein receptor mechanisms.

Transporters

Neurotransmitter transporters collect released transmitters from the synaptic space, bringing them back to the presynaptic terminals. Transport is sodium-dependent, and their regional distributions are consistent with those of their released neurotransmitters. Many drugs, for example antidepressants, cocaine and amphetamine, act at such sites. The DNA structures of many transporter sites have now been identified, and while most seem to be situated on neurones, glial localization has also been shown for some transmitters. Reversal of flow through the transporter from the cell back to the synaptic space is known to occur.

The genes coding for the 5-HT transporter (5-HTT), which removes 5-HT from the synaptic cleft, have been identified. A polymorphism 5-HTTLPR in the promoter region has 22 base pair repeats, consisting of a short (s) and a long (l) version, which influences the function of the transporter, the s variant leading to less 5-HTT mRNA and thus higher concentrations of 5-HT in the synaptic cleft.

NEURONES

The main types of cell in the CNS are the neurones and the glial cells. The neurone has dendrites, an axon, the soma or cell body, and sites for synapses (see Figures 1.10 and 1.14). Essential metabolic molecules are synthesized in the soma and transported to other regions of the neurone. The difficult process of moving products down the long axon is accomplished

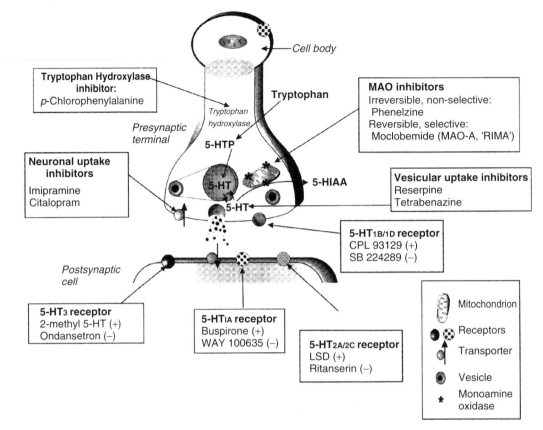

Figure 1.14 Example of the manufacture and distribution of 5-HT and various 5-HT receptors and sites of drug action (Webster, 2002)

by a microtubular system composed of a protein called tubulin. The larger axons are surrounded by a myelin sheath, which aids the speed of electrical conduction.

The glial cells vastly outnumber the neurones, and while they play a structural supportive role, they are also involved in metabolic processes and the manufacture of myelin. Five types are identified: astrocytes, oligodendrocytes, microglia, Schwann cells and ependyma cells, the latter of which line the inner surface of the brain.

The role of glial cells in cerebral activity is still largely unknown, but astrocytes, which are closely enmeshed with synapses, also have receptors for some neurotransmitters, especially glutamate and GABA. Astrocytes have several functions within the CNS in addition to transmitter uptake and release. These include metabolic support for the neurone, modulation

of synaptic transmission, phagocytosis (microglia) and gap-junction syncitiation for Ca^{++} wave propagation for astrocytic glutamate release. By regulating glutamate metabolism the astrocytes are central for glutamate homeostasis.

The synaptic region of the neurone is highly specialized for the storage and release of neurotransmitters. The latter are contained in storage vesicles along with ATP and proteins, and are there protected from breakdown by intracytoplasmic degradation enzymes. Release of the transmitter into the synaptic cleft is by exocytosis, and quanta of transmitter are shed into the synaptic cleft. This process requires calcium, which interacts with presynaptic release areas, facilitating fusion between the vesicle and cell membranes. Calcium enters the cell terminals through voltage-dependent calcium channels. The interaction of transmitter with receptors then takes place, and IPSPs or EPSPs are generated. The synaptic contacts can be to an opposing soma (axo-somatic), dendrite (axo-dendritic) or axon (axo-axonic), and the position of contact has relevance for the postsynaptic effect: the nearer to the axon hillock, the greater the effect.

In contrast to the rather rigid anatomical structure shown in cartoons of the neurone, the neurone – especially the dendrites and the synapses – must be seen as part of a dynamic system (Smythies, 2002). The electronic structure of the dendrites is forever shifting: signals spread from dendrites to soma and vice versa, and the electronic properties of the latter alter with the resting membrane potential. Synaptic responses are often nonlinear, and related to prior activity.

The synapses themselves should be viewed as quite plastic; they are continually pruned and replaced. Their receptors are modulated in number and location, endocytosis- and exocytosis-redistributing membrane components, and the highly regulated intracellular processes directing cell growth, including synaptic modification (Smythies, 2002).

Neurodevelopment and Neurogenesis

It used to be believed that an individual was born with a fixed number of neurone and lost them as they aged. New research has established that the brain is not such a fixed structure: although the rate of change and development is especially prominent early in life, alteration of the structure of the brain in response to environmental factors remains a feature across the entire life span.

A single fertilized egg develops into 100 billion neurone with 100 trillion connections in a short amount of time. *In utero*, this process is largely activity-independent and genetically driven. After birth, interactions with the environment begin to modify development and play a greater role. Unequivocally newly created neurone have been identified in the hippocampus of elderly subjects whose brains were examined shortly after death.

Undifferentiated neural stem cells remain in the CNS and continue to divide throughout life. They divide into more neural stem cells as well as neural precursors that grow into neurone or glial cells. But they must migrate away from the influence of the stem cell before they can differentiate and only about half the cells successfully move and transform.

Neurotrophic factors are chemicals that are essential for neuron survival and differentiation. Nerve growth factor (NGF) is a prototypical neurotrophin, and NGF receptors are found on cells which when activated lead to rapid intracellular phosphorylation events. Programmed cell death seems to be a process that occurs across vertebrates and invertebrates alike, and the two main mechanisms are necrosis and apoptosis.

Clear evidence for adult neurogenesis has been limited to the granule cells of the dentate gyrus and olfactory bulb. Newly formed cells are identified by tagging them with a molecule such as bromodeoxyuridine (BrdU), a thymidine analogue that can be incorporated into newly synthesized DNA. A florescent antibody specific for BrdU is then used to detect the incorporated molecule and thus indicate DNA replication.

The rate of neurogenesis is modulated by various factors. It is known that enriched environments and exercise will increase neurogenesis. Additional research suggests that gonadal steroid hormones may also enhance new cell production. There is more research showing the positive effects of oestrogen on mammal brains, but testosterone will stimulate nerve-cell production in songbirds (Duman, 2005). Stress, on the other hand, has an inhibitory effect on neurogenesis. Extended maternal separation is a well-characterized model of early-life stress for a rodent. As adults, such rodents will show protracted elevations of CRF, ACTH and corticosterone (cortisol in a rat), as well as behavioural inhibition in response to stress. Rats exposed to prolonged maternal separation will have a long-lasting blunting of neurogenesis (Fabricius *et al.*, 2008).

Stem Cells

One potential way of rebuilding neurone is to implant human embryonic stem cells that have been isolated from a very immature embryo, placenta or bone marrow (only 100–200 cells). So far it has been difficult to get these immature cells to differentiate into functioning neurones outside of the olfactory bulb and hippocampus. The problem may be the absence of biochemical signals that normally prompt the developing stem cell to migrate and differentiate.

As noted above, it used to be considered that the synapse was fixed and static. Indeed, many cartoons of synaptic function falsely reinforced this view. In fact, however, the synapse is a constantly changing and dynamic concept and structure. Synaptogenesis describes the extensive growth of axons and dendrites to make synaptic connections – a process that primarily occurs early in life but continues even in adults. During development, the tips of axons and dendrites have growth cones that appear to reach out with finger-like structures, filopodia, and literally pull the growth cone to its destination. The axon is guided in a specific direction by chemical signals that attract and repel the growth cone; that is, chemoattractants and chemorepellents.

Another important phase of neuronal cell development is pruning or synaptic elimination, which entails retraction and elimination of excessive connections. Some refer to this constant struggle of neurones to connect as 'neural Darwinism'. The evolution of cortical connectivity reflects an adaptation to sensory inputs in a constantly competitive fashion, with winners and losers depending on the environmental surroundings of importance to the organism and input to the brain (Edeleman, 1989). Disordered pruning may be the pathological basis for such conditions as autism and schizophrenia.

Apoptosis is referred to as programmed cell death, which reflects the fact that the cells actually carry genetic instructions to self-destruct, leaving no scars or damaged tissue.

Neurotrophic Factors

Neurotrophic or nerve-growth factors (NGFs) are best defined as any molecule that affects the nervous system by influencing the growth or differentiation of neurones or glia. Neurotrophic factors are the stimulus behind neurogenesis and synaptogenesis (see Figure 1.15). NGFs

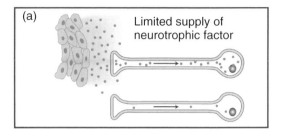

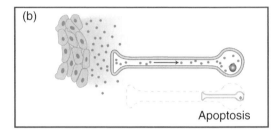

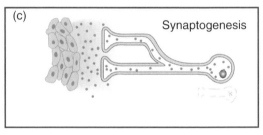

Figure 1.15 Neurotrophic factors mediate cell proliferation and elimination by promoting cell growth, stimulating synaptogenesis and preventing apoptosis (reproduced with permission from Higgins and George, 2007, Figures 7–8, p. 82)

mediate cell survival, and cells that do not receive enough NGFs die. Target organs produce NGFs and specific NGF receptors are present on nerve terminals which attract afferant input.

Several other growth factors have been discovered and are being studied, including neurotrophin-3 (NT-3), glial cell-line-derived neurotrophin factor (GDNF) and insulin-like growth factor (IGF) to name a few, but the one of most interest is brain-derived neurotrophic factor (BDNF).

NEUROTRANSMITTERS

A neurotransmitter is a substance that is manufactured by a cell, released into the synaptic cleft in response to stimulation and has a specific effect on another cell. In the CNS this cell is a neurone, but peripherally it may be a secretory cell. Further, to qualify, the substance should, when applied experimentally, mimic the effect of the natural release, and some mechanism should be available to remove it from the synaptic cleft (Schwartz, 1981).

Although it was at first thought that a single neurone used only one transmitter, it is now known that two or more transmitters can be identified in many neurones, especially with the coexistence of a peptide and an amine (see below). In fact, different neurotransmitters sometimes share the same vesicle. Further, while the criteria given for neurotransmitter status have been identified, the situation is not so clearly defined. Thus it is possible to see all levels of chemical communication between cells, from direct neurone–neurone contact, through to neurosecretory cells that release neurohormones either into the hypophyseal portal system, which influences pituitary cell output, or directly into the circulation via the posterior pituitary gland (neurohypophysis). Receptors for some neurohormones have been identified in the brain, and the possibility of feedback from release into the peripheral circulation exists. Finally, as in the autonomic system, neurones make contact with adrenal medulla cells, directly influencing hormonal output.

The situation is further complicated by the concept of neuromodulators. Thus, the action of neurotransmitters is considered to be brief and to operate over a short distance. However, some neurotransmitter candidates, especially the peptides, lead to longer alterations of synaptic tone, modulating the environment of other ongoing neurotransmitter events.

Of the many potential transmitters, the synthesis of a few key ones is described.

Acetylcholine

This is synthesized from choline and acetyl coenzyme A, the reaction being catalysed by choline acetyltransferase. Following release into the synaptic cleft, it is broken down by acetylcholinesterase. It is the main transmitter used by motor neurones in the spinal cord and is the transmitter for all preganglionic autonomic neurones and for postganglionic parasympathetic neurones. In the CNS it is found in high concentration in the caudate nucleus and hippocampus, and an ascending cholinergic system has been defined innervating the thalamus, the striatum, the cerebellum, the limbic system and the cerebral cortex. The basal nucleus of Meynert is an important CNS location of acetylycholine.

GABA

GABA is synthesized from L-glutamate, utilizing the enzyme glutamate decarboxylase (GAD). It is metabolized by GABA transaminase to glutamic acid and succinic semialdehyde, which, following oxidation, enters the citric acid cycle. It is involved in the activity of some 30–50% of CNS neurones, especially of interneurones. The highest concentrations of GABA are in the substantia nigra, globus pallidus, hippocampus, hypothalamus and cortex. In the spinal column it is in the spinal grey matter. It is an inhibitory transmitter, and antagonists such as bicuculline provoke convulsions. It is one of a group of amino acid transmitters that have a ubiquitous distribution, some of which serve as substrates in metabolic cycles. These include glycine, beta-alanine, glutamate and aspartate.

Glycine

Glycine is another inhibitory transmitter, especially in the spinal cord and brainstem. It inhibits neuronal firing by gating chloride channels. It can modulate the action of glutamate at the NMDA receptor.

Serotonin (5-HT)

This is one of the amine neurotransmitters; others include dopamine and noradrenaline. It is synthesized from tryptophan under the influence of the enzyme tryptophan hydroxylase, which converts it to 5-hydroxy-tryptophan. This is decarboxylated to 5-HT. It is metabolized to

5-hydroxyindole acetic acid (5-HIAA) by the enzyme monoamine oxidase.

The main nuclei containing 5-HT are the raphe nuclei of the brainstem, from which fibres ascend and descend to influence many areas of the brain, especially the neocortex, limbic system, thalamus and hypothalamus. In the pineal gland, 5-HT is converted to melatonin.

Catecholamines

These are metabolized from tyrosine. Conversion to DOPA occurs under the influence of tyrosine hydrolase. DOPA is then decarboxylated to dopamine. In the presence of dopamine-beta hydrolase this is converted to noradrenaline. In a few areas, *N*-methylation of the latter results in adrenaline.

Breakdown involves two main enzyme systems: monoamine oxidase and catechol-*O*-methyl transferase. The former acts mainly intraneuronally, the latter in the synaptic cleft. The main metabolites of dopamine are homovanillic acid (HVA) and DOPAC, while noradrenaline (NA) breaks down to vanillomandelic add (VMA) and methoxyhydroxy-phenylglycol (MHPG).

Noradrenaline is the transmitter at post-ganglionic sympathetic neurones, but in the brain the main synthesizing neurones are in the brainstem, the locus coeruleus and related nuclei. The ascending neurones terminate widely to influence the cerebral cortex, limbic system and hypothalamus. Catechol *O*-methyl transferase, responsible for breaking down the catecholamines, is regulated by the COMT gene, which has polymorphisms, and of importance is the Met (methionine)–Val (valine) substitution at codon 158 of chromosome 22q. The Met allele is associated with low enzyme activity, and the Val with high activity.

Dopamine derives from nuclei in the brainstem (notably the substantia nigra and the ventral tegmental area), but its output is more restricted than noradrenaline or 5-HT. In particular, it involves the striatum and the limbic system. It is of interest that cortical dopamine projections in primates suggest a functional specialization. The major influences are motor rather than sensory: sensory association areas have more dopamine than primary sensory regions, and auditory association cortex has more than visual association areas (Lewis *et al.*,1986). A further location of dopamine is in the tuberoinfundibular system of the hypothalamus, which is involved in the regulation of prolactin release, with stimulation leading to inhibition.

Peptides

Many peptides that may have a central role, either as neurotransmitters or as neuromodulators, have been recognized. In contrast to classic neurotransmitters, they are large molecules and are composed of chains of aminoacids. A list of these is given in Table 1.5. At present the evidence that many are actually transmitters awaits confirmation. Moreover, attempts at developing treatments based on peptides have been disappointing to date. Most peptides are formed by

Table 1.5   Potential peptide neurotransmitters

ACTH
Angiotensin
Bombesin
Bradykinin
Calcitonin
Carnosine
CCK (cholecystokinin)
CRF (corticotrophin releasing factor)
Dynorphin
Beta-endorphin
Met-enkephalin
Leu-enkephalin
Gastrin
Glucagon
Growth hormone
Lipotropin
LHRH
Alpha-MSH
Motilin
Neuropeptide Y
Neurotensin
Oxytocin
Prolactin
Secretin
Somatostatin
Substance P
TRH
Vasopressin
VIP

cleavage of larger precursors and understanding of the functional significance of the fragments is quite incomplete.

An interesting feature of the peptides is their wide distribution throughout the body, identical ones being found, for example, in the gut and the brain. These include cholecystokinin, vasoactive intestinal peptide (VIP) and gastrin. It can be seen that several are hormones.

Peptide receptors are coupled mainly with secondary messenger systems.

Enkephalins

These were the first morphine-like (endorphin) substances to be discovered in the brain, being penta peptides. They were shown to possess opiate-like activity, along with other peptides such as beta-endorphin and dynorphin. Enkephalin neurones and opiate receptors have been identified in the limbic system and striatum, and receptors in such areas as the hippocampus, nucleus accumbens, thalamus and amygdala. They occur in several areas of the spinal cord, including the substantia gelatinosa. Beta-endorpin distribution is more restricted, the highest concentration being in the pituitary, which structure is almost devoid of enkephalins. Mu receptors are more related to sensory events, being found in the cerebral cortex, whereas the limbic system has an abundance of delta receptors.

Neurotensin

This is found in high concentrations in the hypothalamus, basal ganglia and amygdala. It inhibits neuronal firing in the locus coeruleus, where neurotensin is abundant. Receptor sites in the brain are widespread.

Substance P

This occurs in dorsal root ganglia, with terminals in the substantia gelatinosa, a region of the spinal cord thought to be involved in the pain pathways. It is found in high concentrations in the striatal–nigral system, the habenula, the amygdala and the bed nucleus of the stria terminalis.

Cholecystokinin

This is found in high concentrations in the cortex, it and VIP being brain peptides well represented within cells in the cortex. It is found in the hypothalamus, and terminals are in the amygdala. It also is seen in the periaqueductal grey region and, like substance P, in the dorsal root ganglia cells.

Vasoactive Intestinal Peptide

Highest levels are found in the cerebral cortex, and terminals containing it are identified in the amygdala and the hypothalamus. In the body it has several functions, including vasodilation and enhancing lipolysis and pancreatic secretion.

Angiotensin

This has for some time been known to be involved in vasoconstriction and sodium regulation by the kidney. It is found centrally in several regions, including the hypothalamus, and many angiotensin receptor sites have been identified. Complementing its peripheral action, it is involved in the central regulation of drinking.

Releasing Factors

These are found in the median eminence of the hypothalamus, and pass through the portal capillaries to influence hormonal release from the anterior pituitary. They include thyrotropin-releasing hormone (TRH), a tripeptide, the majority of which is found outside the hypothalamus. Somatostatin inhibits growth hormone release and is found in the amygdala, hippocampus and cortex, with terminals in these sites and in the striatum. Luteinizing hormone-releasing factor (LHRH) stimulates LH and FSH release, and is found primarily in

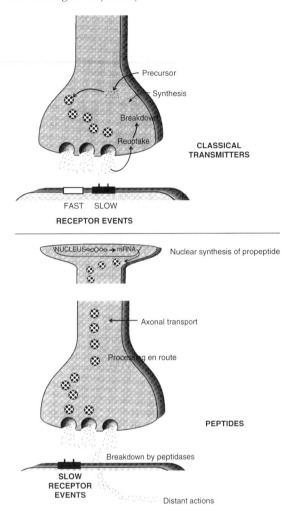

Figure 1.16 Comparison of the manufacture and release of classical neurotransmitters and peptides (Webster, 2002)

the hypothalamus. Corticotropin-releasing factor (CRF) releases ACTH. Various medications modifying CRF were once considered promising candidates as anxiolytics or antidepressants but were disappointing in clinical trials.

Other Central Peptides

The posterior pituitary hormones oxytocin and vasopressin seem to have a central role, with pathways projecting to some brainstem and limbic-system structures. These two peptides appear to act selectively in some animals in terms of promoting or inhibiting interpersonal bonding (Stein and Ythilingum, 2009; Young *et al.*, 2008). Active investigation involves administering synthetic oxytocin and observing changes in interpersonal behaviour, and in disorders of bonding such as autism. Adrenocorticotrophic hormone (ACTH) is found throughout the brain, especially in the hypothalamus, thalamus, periaqueductal grey and reticular formation.

Some of the differences between the peptide transmitters and the more classical ones are summarized by Hokfelt *et al.* (1980) and are shown in Figure 1.16. In particular, peptides are produced in the cell soma and not synthesized at synaptosomes, unlike other transmitters, and there are no re-uptake mechanisms from the synaptic cleft. This may be compensated for by their effective action at much lower

Table 1.6 The coexistence of classical and peptide transmitters

Transmitter	Peptide	Location
Dopamine	Enkephalin	Carotid body
Dopamine	CCK	Ventral tegmental area
Noradrenaline	Somatostatin	Adrenal medulla
Noradrenaline	Enkephalin	Adrenal medulla
Noradrenaline	Neurotensin	Adrenal medulla
5-HT	Substance P	Medulla oblongata
5-HT	TRH	Medulla oblongata
Adrenaline	Enkephalin	Adrenal medulla
Acetylcholine	VIP	Autonomic ganglia, sweat glands

concentrations, their more prolonged action and their intermittent rather than tonic release.

INTERRELATIONSHIPS AMONG TRANSMITTERS

Dale's principle, namely that one neurone synthesizes and releases only one neurotransmitter, has had to be modified in the light of recent data. Although it has been known for some time that certain neurones probably released both acetylcholine and noradrenaline, the coexistence of peptides and other neurotransmitters has been reported for several neurone groups. A list is shown in Table 1.6. However, not all neurones possessing one classical transmitter contain the same peptide, and vice versa. The functional significance of such arrangements has been a matter of speculation. For example, in one group of neurones from sympathetic ganglia involved in sweat gland secretion, both acetylcholine and VIP are present (Hokfelt *et al.*, 1980). It is suggested that the VIP may be the mediator of vasodilation aiding the acetylcholine-primed secretion. A further example is the coexistence of CCK in a subpopulation of dopamine neurons. These are mainly in the substantia nigra and related ventral tegmental area (VTA), and project to the limbic forebrain (Hokfelt *et al.*, 1980).

Other examples of interaction include the influence of monoamine release by peptides, such as the association between substance P and dopamine, the former acting as an excitatory transmitter for some dopamine neurones (Iversen and Iversen, 1981), or peptides interacting with peptides as in the case of opiate receptors located on substance P terminals.

TRANSMITTER DISPERSAL

Following interaction with the postsynaptic cell, transmitters are either broken down by enzyme systems in the synaptic cleft or taken back up by the neurone for degradation for re-use. Some are lost by simple diffusion away from the cell. The intracellular enzymes, monoamine oxidase and catechol-*O*-methyl transferase, are of importance to the amine transmitters, and the major extracellular mechanism for the degradation of acetylcholine is acetylcholinesterase. Peptides are degraded by peptidases.

CNS INFLAMMATION

Cytokines are produced by activated macrophages, and are either proinflammatory (interferon, INF, and tumour necrosis factor, TNF) or anti-inflammatory (interleukin 4 or 10, IL4/ IL10). A cascade of events leads to T-helper lymphocyte activation, and these release cytokines. There are receptors for these cytokines in the brain, and they have been shown to activate the CRF system. The ratio between proinflammatory and anti-inflammatory cytokines can be measured, and has been shown to relate to psychopathology.

2
Principles of Brain Function and Structure: 2 Anatomy

INTRODUCTION

This chapter concentrates on those areas of the brain of most importance to biological psychiatry. After a brief introduction to neuroanatomy, the limbic system, the basal ganglia, the thalamus and some important cortical areas are discussed. In the past it was common to refer to different areas of the brain using modular models. However, theories using strict localization of function to adequately explain behaviour, especially with regard to psychiatry, failed. It then became popular to consider systems, such as the limbic system, but renewing localization theories with respect to 'systems' would also likely fail.

The most recent concepts of brain behaviour relationships have to some extent developed from the era of artificial intelligence. Although some have been led to adopt an unusual view, namely that cognition is similar in process to a computer algorithm and therefore there is no necessity to understand the hardware (i.e. the brain itself) in order to understand how the brain works and how consciousness develops, this is clearly illogical. There are indeed many differences between brains and current modern computers. While the latter are good at arithmetical computations, logical thinking and exhaustive memory searching, brains are better at pattern recognition and the use of context to interpret the whole (as in language,

for example). Processing is in parallel, not in sequence, hence the development of models referred to as parallel distributed processing (PDP). As information is added to a computer, it gets slower; the exact opposite occurs with the brain.

In PDP, information is no longer thought of as being represented by a sequence of numbers, but by a pattern of activation. Information is stored in connections among processing units, each with a graded activity value, a probability of firing. There is a weighted connection with other units, and it is the pattern of the activation that is relevant (Figure 2.1). Learning is thus a change in connection weights over time. Crucial to the development of these models has been the concept of back propagation, which allows for computations in multilayer networks continually adjusting connection weights depending on output patterns. The system can literally learn on its own, in keeping with the concept of neural Darwinism (Edelman, 1989). As discussed in Chapter 1, during development many neurones die, and competition leads to unique wiring repertoires as the strengths of certain synapses amplify, allowing organisms to respond to experience. These circuits (maps) have interconnections with others, leading to higher-order maps that map maps, with parallel re-entrant signalling between them. This allows different properties of an input, for example visual and

Biological Psychiatry 3e   Michael R. Trimble and Mark S. George
© 2010 John Wiley & Sons, Ltd

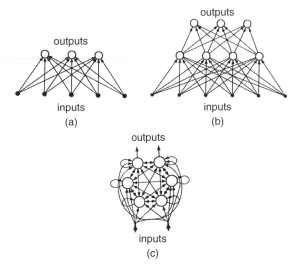

Figure 2.1   Three types of network. (a) Feedforward, with one layer of weights connecting the input to the output units. (b) Feedforward, with two layers of weights and one hidden layer of units between the input and output units. (c) Recurrent, with reciprocal connections (reproduced with permission from Churchland and Sejnowski, 1992; *Biol Psych*, 2 Ed, p. 77)

tactile, to be connected in the response of higher-order networks, explaining such cognitive phenomena as categorization and generalization.

THE NEUROANATOMY OF EMOTION

Although great strides were made in neuroanatomy and neurophysiology in the 19th century, little progress was made in understanding how emotions were represented neurologically. William James suggested that the emotions are derived from sensory inputs to the brain, which activate motor outputs, which the brain perceives as the emotion. We do not run away from something because we are frightened; we experience fear because we are running away. However, there was no obvious cerebral location for the generation of emotion, although the sensory experiences were known to be received cortically, namely in the parietal regions of the brain.

The James-Lange hypothesis was soon tested and shown to be wrong from two avenues.

First, it was shown in animals that removal of the cortex of the brain on both sides did not abolish the expression of emotion. Second, it was revealed that direct electrical stimulation of various structures buried deep within the brain could lead to the release of emotion.

The Brain

The CNS axis is composed of several identifiable components: the cerebrum, the cerebellum (the smaller lobe at the posterior base of the cerebrum), the brainstem and the spinal cord. Information flows up the spinal cord from peripheral sensory receptors, which send signals to the brain concerning the external and the internal environments of the organism; many such afferent nerve tracts have been identified within the spinal cord. Information travels to the muscles from the brain down the spinal cord, again in identified pathways referred to as 'efferent'. In the brainstem reside many of the nerves which control autonomic functions such as breathing, heart rate and so on, and several of the cranial nerves begin or terminate there.

Divisions of the Brain

The brain itself has been divided, purely on visual anatomical grounds, into four main lobes: the frontal, the parietal, the occipital and the temporal. Some also refer to the insula component as a lobe. The neocortex, so called because in phylogenetic terms it is the most recent, is that which is generally seen on surface inspection of the brain. The gyrae and sulcae form the irregular, undulating patterns of the cortical mantle, the former being composed of grey and white matter, the latter forming the spaces in between. The grey matter is formed by the neurones, and the white matter is composed of the fibre bundles of myelinated axons, which stretch from one neurone population to another, interconnecting circuits of information.

Most sensory data initially terminate in a collection of nuclei situated subcortically in the thalamus. This is one of several identifiable subcortical collections of nuclei which are important to an understanding of the cerebral representatives of emotion. Others include the basal ganglia (striatal structures), the accumbens and the limbic system, referred to by some as the limbic lobe.

From the thalamus, information is passed on to the neocortex, arriving in a primary sensory area, such as one selective for vision or for touch. These are mainly in the occipital and parietal areas of the brain. There then occurs a cascade of information flow, from these primary receptive areas to the secondary, tertiary and then association cortices of the brain, during which transfer the representations are fused, amalgamated and combined, such that while artificial stimulation of say the first visual receptive area will lead to the experience of flashes of light, stimulation in the temporal lobe association areas can sometimes lead to complex visual (and other) hallucinations. Information then flows to the limbic related cortex (Figure 2.2). An exception to the above generalization is the olfactory system; this first enters the brain at one of the limbic nuclei, as will be discussed below.

Information flow out of the brain descends from the motor areas of the neocortex, down the pyramidal tracts to the spinal cord (the pyramidal system), where neurones emerge to influence movements by connecting with muscle cells. Other key structures which influence movement and permit the smooth pursuit of action are the cerebellum and the basal ganglia, the motor paths of the latter being referred to as the extrapyramidal motor system.

There is also much cross-talk within the brain, with some white matter commissures connecting areas within one hemisphere, and others connecting points across the hemispheres. The largest of the latter is called the corpus callosum.

The four main domains of the cerebral hemisphere of mammals are then the neocortex, the limbic lobe, the thalamus and the basal ganglia. The neocortex (also referred to as isocortex) is six-layered, with extensive subcortical connections, and provides the mantle for the structures of the other three divisions. Within the limbic lobe, the most relevant structures are the amygdala and the hippocampus, and their afferent

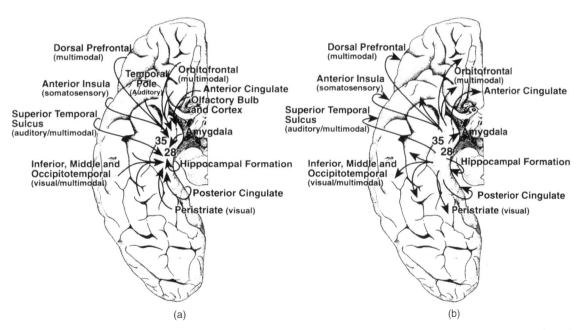

(a) (b)

Figure 2.2 Input (a) and output (b) connections of the human entorhinalcortex (area 28). Area 35 is referred to as the perirhinal area. The input is multimodal and known to be associated with episodic memories. The output connections are associated with memory consolidation in association cortices (courtesy of Dr van Hoesen)

and efferent connections. These and related structures are referred to as allocortex (essentially 'older cortex'). The very oldest cortex is referred to as archicortex. The medial forebrain bundle is a continuum of interconnected neurones and pathways extending caudally to the midbrain and hind brain (Figure 2.3).

The term 'agranular cortex' refers to isocortex that lacks a clear layer 4 (internal granular layer). The layers and columns of the isocortex have allowed neuroscientists to parcel out the cortex into various regions. The number has varied from as low as four (Bayley and Bonin) to over 150 (Vogt). The most popular scheme in use is that of Constantin Brodmann (see Figure 2.33), but it must be noted that this method does not take into account intersubject variability, and only considers one third of the cortex, missing all the tissue buried within the sulci. The Talairach Atlas is a widely used three-dimensional atlas, taking its starting point for defining coordinates from the anterior commissure (0, 00). However, this too does not take sulci into account, and cannot identify borders between histologically defined areas (as per Brodmann). In imaging studies, it has become fashionable to refer from the Talairach coordinates to a putative Brodmann area, transforming the latter into a three-dimensional space. This extrapolation from individual results into a morphed three-dimensional atlas and then on into a two-dimensional projection (Brodmann) should be viewed with caution. It is really little more than an educated guess (see Chapter 4). Recently, attempts have been made to define borders within the brain more precisely using chemical markers. Radioactive ligands are used for high-resolution quantitative *in vitro* receptor autoradiography, which outlines receptor architechtonics, allowing a neurochemical 'fingerprint' of brain areas to be developed.

The basal ganglia are a collection of structures (the corpus striatum: the putamen and the globus pallidus, connected with the substantia nigra and the subthalamic nucleus) whose efferents remain largely within the forebrain, forming so-called parallel distributed circuits, whereby the termination of a loop in the cortex is near to or at the site of the cortical origin of the loop (see below) (Figure 2.4).

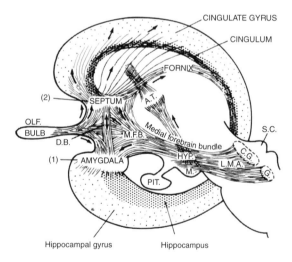

Figure 2.3 The main limbic structures as envisioned by MacLean. MacLean added the amygdala to the limbic concept of Papez. MFB = Medial Forebrain Bundle. AT, Anterior Thalamus; 1 and 2, ascending pathways to the limbic lobe; CG, Central Grey of midbrain; G, dorsal tegmental nucleus of Godden; DB, Diagonal Band of Broca; Hyp, hypothalamus; LMA, Limbic Midbrain Area; M, Mamillary body; Pit, Pituiatry gland; SC, Superior Colliculus

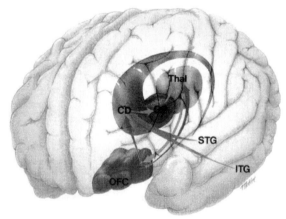

Figure 2.4 The circuits linking the frontal cortex with the basal ganglia, the basal ganglia with the thalamus, and the thalamus with a re-entrant circuit back to frontal cortex. Note: the temporal-limbic inputs to the circuitry

The Limbic System

As already noted, James had no idea how emotions could be represented in the brain other than by suggesting the sensory neocortex as a site of integration of bodily sensations representing an emotional state. The concept that certain brain structures could form the foundation of an emotional brain system was a stunning departure for neurology, and the launch pad of the disciplines of biological psychiatry and behavioural neurology (that branch of neurology which tries to understand how neurological disorders relate to behavioural changes).

Papez delineated his proposed cerebral mechanism of emotion in 1937. The key components of his now-famous circuit were the hippocampus, the cingulate gyri, the mammillary bodies and the anterior thalamus. For him, the cingulate cortex was a receptive area for experiencing emotion, in the same way that the visual areas of the brain are receptive for visual information. While the hypothalamus was essential for the expression of emotion, the experience required the cortex, 'the stream of feeling' depending on strong interconnections between the cortex and the hypothalamus. He summed this up with the famous quote that 'the hypothalamus, the anterior thalamic nuclei, the gyrus cinguli, the hippocampus and their interconnections constitute a harmonious mechanism which may elaborate the functions of central emotion, as well as participate in emotional expression' (Figure 2.5).

The key structures of the limbic system, as originally outlined by MacLean but elaborated on by others, are the amygdala and the hippocampus, both neuronal aggregates of considerable complexity, and their immediate connecting structures, such as the orbital part of the frontal cortex and the so-called ventral striatum: that part of the brain's extrapyramidal system that relates to emotional motor expression. In humans, on account of the migration of the temporal lobes posteriorly, inferiorly and then anteriorly, and the large increase in size of the corpus callosum in development, much of the archicortex (evolutionary older cortex) lies folded and buried in the medial temporal lobe in the hippocampus.

The cingulate gyrus surrounds the corpus callosum, forming a C-shaped band, linking posteriorly with the parahippocampal gyrus and connecting extensively with neocortical structures. The frontal lobes of the brain have many demarcated subregions, but the orbital, medial and dorsolateral are the most frequently referred to. The orbitofrontal cortex lies over the floor of the anterior cranial fossa and has intimate connections with the anterior insula, the amygdala, the ventral striatum and the sensory projection pathways. The ventromedial frontal cortex is a part of the cingulate region. The insula is a large limbic structure, which in contrast to most limbic components is not visible from the medial surface of the brain, and lies laterally, but buried beneath folds of neocortex (Figure 2.6). Many have found cause to cavil with the term 'limbic system'. Some neuroanatomists now prefer to use the term 'limbic lobe' after the original designation of Broca, an aid to breaking down the concept of an isolated system (Heimer *et al.*, 2007). It was the development of new techniques in neuroanatomy, such as the use of horseradish peroxidase (HRP), histofluoresecence, autoradiography and improved silver-staining methods that led to a Renaissance in interest in and understanding of the structure, connectivity and functions of the limbic lobe, especially its cortical–subcortical interactions, and the

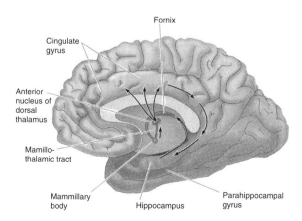

Figure 2.5 Circuit of Papez. A coloured version of this figure can be found on the colour plate

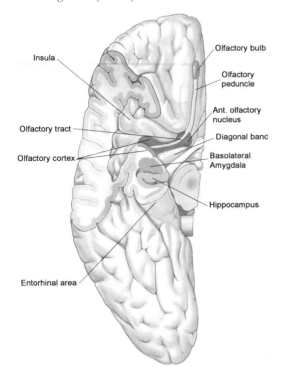

Figure 2.6   The insula, buried beneath the cortex following removal of the frontal and temporal polar opercula. The position of the amygdala, hippocampus and entorhinal cortex are shown (courtesy of Dr Gary van Hoesen). A coloured version of this figure can be found on the colour plate

relevance of these to an understanding of the neuroanatomy of emotion and behaviour.

Although Broca's term was topographical, the limbic lobe may be differentiated from other cortical structures by cellular-staining methods and susceptibility to certain disease processes. A recent definition of the limbic lobe is given by Heimer *et al.* (2007) as: 'composed of the olfactory allocortex, hippocampal allocortex, and transitional cortical areas that intervene between these and larger isocortices. The transitional areas are numerous, and form the bulk of the limbic lobe, and depart in terms of structure in one or more ways from the isocortex... Limbic lobe cortical areas form the cingulate and parahippocampal gyri as well as the bridging caudal orbitofrontal, medial frontal, temporopolar, anteroventral insular and retrosplenial cortices... We also favour inclusion of the laterobasal–cortical complex of the amygdala...' (Figure 2.7).

An extension of the original limbic system concept was suggested by Nauta and Domesick (1982). They included the posterior orbitofrontal cortex and the temporal pole, which project to the amygdala and hippocampus, and some subcortical structures linked by reciprocal pathways. These include the accumbens

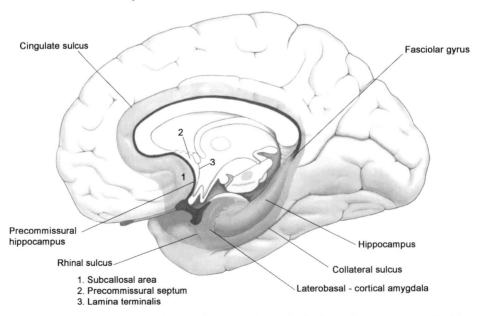

1. Subcallosal area
2. Precommissural septum
3. Lamina terminalis

Figure 2.7   Medial view of the human brain. The areas shown in darker colours represent limbic structures (courtesy of Dr L. Heimer). A coloured version of this figure can be found on the colour plate

and such midbrain structures as the ventral tegmental area (VTA) and the interpeduncular nucleus. The inclusion of the latter has led to the designation of a midbrain limbic area, the mesolimbic system.

Nieuwenhuys (1996) has introduced the term 'greater limbic system', which also includes pontine and medullary neuronal groups that relate to autonomic and somato-motor integration. He pointed out that this

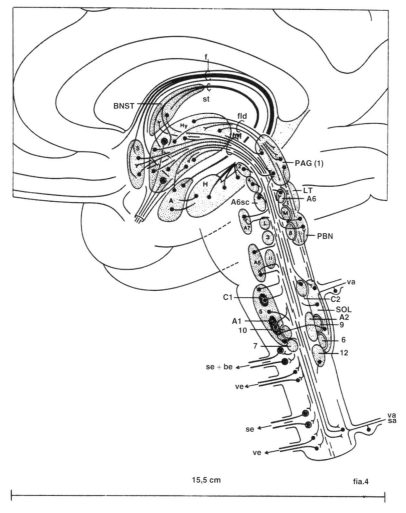

Figure 2.8 Extended limbic circuitry. Note how the limbic connections output to diencephalic, midbrain and brain-stem structures. Abbreviations: A, amygdala; A1, A2, A5, A7, noradrenergic cell groups; A6, the noradrenergic locus coeruleus; A6sc, the noradrenergic locus subcoeruleus; bc, branchial efferent fibres; BNST, bed nucleus of stria terminalis; C1, C2, adrenergic cell groups; f, fornix; fld, fasciculus longitudinalis dorsalis; fmt, fasciculus medialis telencephali; H, hippocampus; Hy, hypothalamus; L, L-region of Holstege *et al.* (1986); LT, lateral pontine tegmentum; M, M-region of Holstege *et al.* (1986); PAG, periaquaductal grey; S, septum; se, somatic efferent fibres; ve, visceral efferent fibres; 1, loci for defence reactions, vocalization and lordosis; 2, mesencephalic attack site; 3, pontine attack site; 4, mesencephalic locomotor region; 5, area reticularis superficialis ventrolateralis or 'lateral medulla', implicated in cardiovascular and respiratory regulation; 6, dorsal respiratory group; 7, ventral respiratory group; 8, Kölliker-Fuse nucleus: pneumotaxic centre; 9, dorsomedial swallowing area; 10, ventrolateral swallowing area; 11, pontine swallowing area; 12, nucleus retroambiguus, containing loci for vocalization and lordosis (reproduced with permission from R. Nieuwenhuys, and from Nieuwenhuys, 1996; *Biol Psych*, 2 Ed, p. 93)

'system' is composed of masses of thin and ultrathin nerve fibres, and has embedded into it neuronal groups related to monoamine and peptide activity, and contains loci from which integrated patterns of behaviour can be elicited (see Figure 2.8).

It is important to recognize that anatomically, the limbic lobe is non-isocortical, not six-layered, and consists of allocortex and belts of agranular or dyslaminar (layer 4 missing, poorly organized or atypical) transitional cortex. In other words, one possible definition of limbic cortex is those areas of cortex that are NOT isocortical (six-layered).

The inputs to the limbic system have been shown to be both interoceptive (visceral) and exteroceptive (conveying information about the environment). The former derive from many structures that give information about the internal state of the organism, and include modulating influences from neurotransmitter pathways, which originate in the mid and hind brain, which help drive behaviour and modulate mood, such as dopamine, 5-HT and noradrenaline. The exteroceptive afferents derive from all sensory systems, and ultimately present complex integrated sensory information to the cortex of the hippocampus and the amygdala (see Figure 2.2).

The Basal Ganglia

The demonstration that the basal ganglia extend all the way to the ventral surface of the brain, and that the inputs to the corpus striatum involve not only the whole of the cortical mantle but also limbic structures, allowed for a differentiation between the ventral and dorsal striata, respectively receiving their main inputs from the limbic lobe and the neocortex (see Figures 2.9 and 2.10). A main area of the ventral striatum is referred to as the accumbens, which is heavily afferented from the cortical amygdala and hippocampus, and the prefrontal and temporal association cortices. The main output from the ventral striatum is to the ventral globus pallidus and thence to the thalamus, which then projects back to the frontal cortex. This is but one of several cortico–striatopallidal–thalamic–cortical

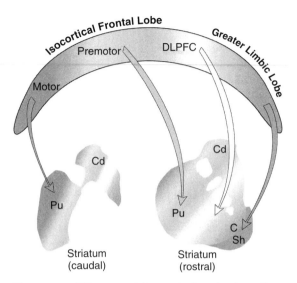

Figure 2.9 Diagram of the cortical projections (from frontal and limbic cortices), showing how the cortex projects to the basal ganglia and how this process is continuous; in essence there is no discrete break between the frontal inputs and limbic inputs. It should be noted that this figure helps to emphasize that cortico-striatal projections come from the entire cerebral cortex. Cd = caudate nucleus; Pu = putamen; C = core and Sh = shell of accumbens (courtesy of Dr L. Heimer). A coloured version of this figure can be found on the colour plate

re-entrant loops to have been defined, which have important regulatory properties governing behaviour (Figure 2.11). The loop from the motor cortex (dorsal striatum) is involved with somatomotor activity, while the ventral limbic–striatal circuits modulate reward and motivation. Figure 2.12 shows a cartoon of these loops, and inserted are the indirect and direct loops. Essentially these refer to two different projections through the basal ganglia, which through inhibition and excitation balance output from the globus pallidus internus to the thalamus and hence back to the cortex. Disturbance of this balance results in symptomatology, such as the motor manifestations of Parkinson's disease or the compulsive phenomena of obsessive-compulsive disorder. There is a close anatomical association between the globus pallidus interna and the substantia nigra pars reticulata.

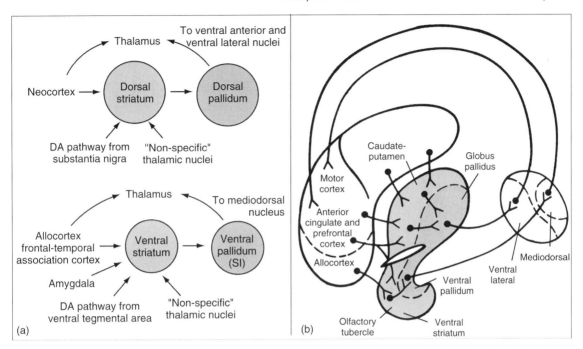

Figure 2.10 (a) Cartoons showing the classical distinction between the ventral and dorsal cortico-striato-pallido-thelamic re-entrant circuits. Image (b) emphasizes the parallel character of the re-entrant circuits (courtesy of Dr L. Heimer)

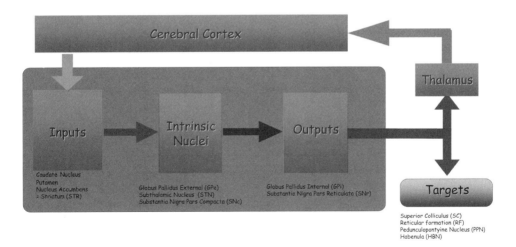

Figure 2.11 The basic anatomy of the cortico-striato-thalamic re-entrant loops

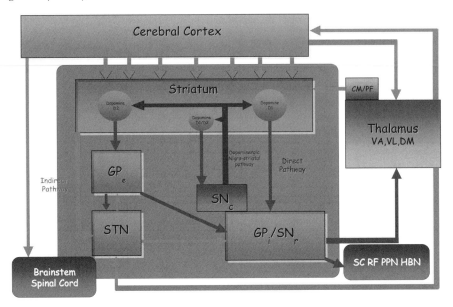

Functional Organisation of the Basal Ganglia

Figure 2.12 A similar anatomy to that in Figure 2.11, but emphasizing the external as well as the internal globus pallidus connections, and the role of the subthalamic nucleus in regulating the output from the globus pallidus internus to the thalamus and hence the cortex. GP_e = globus pallidus externus; GP_i = globus pallidus internus; STN = subthalamic nucleus and SN = substantia nigra

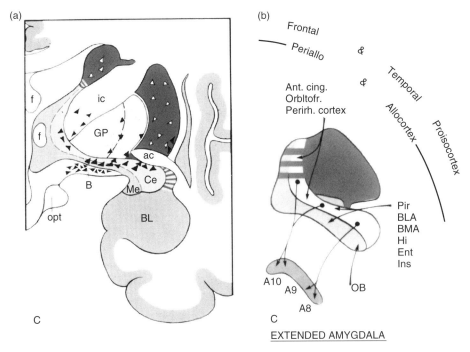

Figure 2.13 (a) The extended amygdala, connecting the central and medial nuclei of the amygdala with limbic forebrain structures notably the bed nucleus of the stria terminalis. (b) Outputs from the extended amygdala influencing autonomic and neuroendocrine function (courtesy of Dr L. Heimer)

The so-called extended amygdala refers to those components of the amygdala (central and medial nuclei), which bridge its temporal lobe components, with the limbic forebrain and the ventral striatum, and the hypothalamus, with its autonomic and endocrine influences (see Figure 2.13). However, the outputs also flow through the stria terminalis posteriorly and then loop anteriorly so as to from a ring-shaped structure that encircles the internal capsule (Figure 2.14). The most relevant point to note is that the amygdala is not an isolated temporal lobe structure, but intimately linked with the basal forebrain. The extended amygdala has been distinguished from the laterobasal and cortical amygdala nuclei, especially by its neurochemical differences and its outputs to the hypothalamus and brainstem autonomic and somatomotor structures (Heimer *et al.*, 2007).

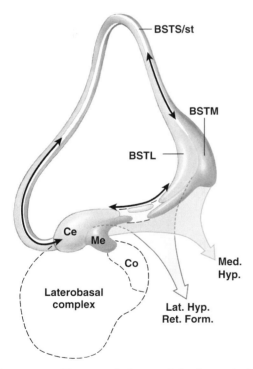

Figure 2.14 The extended amygdala shown in isolation from the rest of the brain. Ce, Central and Me, Medial amygdaloid nucli; BSTL and BSTM, lateral and medial divisions of the extended amygdale; Co, cortical amygdala nucleus; BSTS/st, supracapsula part of the bed nucleus (courtesy of Dr L. Heimer). A coloured version of this figure can be found on the colour plate

INDIVIDUAL ANATOMICAL STRUCTURES

Amygdala

The amygdala is located at the anterior part of the temporal lobes, in front of and above the temporal horn of the lateral ventricle (see Figures 2.2 and 2.3). It abuts the rostral part of the hippocampus. It is a composite of several neuronal aggregates and has two main components: a larger basolateral complex, which has extensive connections with the neocortex and from which it receives polysensory information, and a central-medial division, extending medially, establishing continuity with the bed nucleus of the stria terminalis (extended amygadala; see below). The laterobasal complex is cortical, whereas the centromedial nucleus is striato-pallidal-like. The basal nucleus has a high acetylcholine content, which it receives from the basal nucleus of Meynert (see below).

The main afferent and efferent pathways traverse the stria terminalis and the ventral amygdalofugal pathway. The latter is a longitudinal association bundle linking to the ventral striatum (see below) and the medial frontal cortex. There is also a caudal part going to the lateral hypothalamus and, via the MFB, to the brainstem.

The uncinate fasciculus projects to the frontal cortex. The connections to the brainstem come almost exclusively from the central nucleus, the fibres ending in structures that serve autonomic and visceral functions. These include the catecholamine and 5-HT brainstem nuclei, the VTA and the substantia nigra, the central grey, the dorsal nucleus of the vagus and the nucleus of the solitary tract (NTS). There are also connections to the midbrain and medullary tegmentum. The basolateral nuclei have cortical and ventral striatal links, and the medial and central groups connect to the hypothalamus. In the cortex, amygdaloid fibres are found in the orbital and medial frontal lobe, the rostral cingulate gyrus and most of the temporal lobe (Price, 1981).

It is further appreciated that the amygdala has extensive distributions to sensory cortical areas, especially visual cortex, which presumably modify early sensory inputs (Amaral *et al.*, 1992). The connections from the amygdala to the hippocampus are primarily via the entorhinal cortex (see below), which is a major source of hippocampal afferents. There are direct connections to the subiculum part of the hippocampus. Those to the hypothalamus may influence the control of pituitary hormone release, especially the projections to the ventromedial nucleus,

which itself projects to the arcuate nucleus. Some of the widespread connections of the amygdala are shown diagrammatically in Figure 2.15.

GABA is an important inhibitory transmitter in the amygdala, and other neurotransmitters identified within it include acetylcholine, histamine, dopamine (especially in the basolateral and central nuclei), noradrenaline, 5-HT,

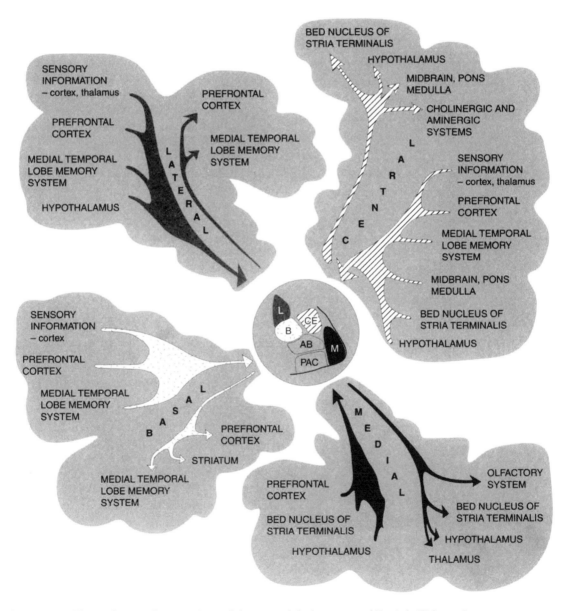

Figure 2.15   The widespread connections of the amygdala (courtesy of Dr Asla Pitkänen)

glutamate and peptides such as substance P, metenkephalin, somatostatin, VIP, CRF and neurotensin (Ben-Ari, 1981).

As noted above, the amygdala has extensive afferent and efferent connections. When the amygdala speaks, the rest of the brain listens. The amygdala provides affective valence to sensory representations and is crucial for the emotional tone of memories. The reciprocal connections with the cortical structures it receives information from, including even the primary sensory cortical areas, allow for a direct influence of emotional tone on cortical sensory impressions (Figure 2.16).

Hippocampus

The hippocampus is also situated in the temporal lobe, but is an elongated structure composed of several subdivisions, together referred to as the hippocampal formation (with the dentate gyrus). The main outflow path of the hippocampus is called the fornix, which like several other of the limbic components curves around the thalamus and then descends to the mammillary bodies of the hypothalamus, forming a crucial link in the Papez circuit. In the human brain, the right hippocampus is larger than the left, but much of this relates to the uncus, that anterior

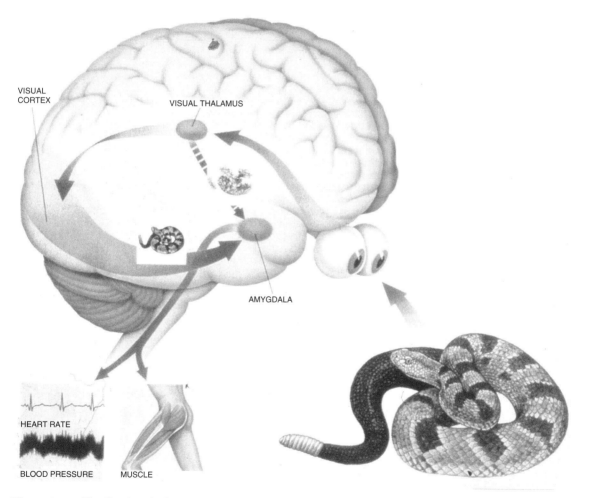

Figure 2.16   The 'fast' and 'slower' routes to the amygdala in response to a frightening stimulus. The latter uses cortex, and is less direct than the former. For further explanation see page 75 (adapted from Le Doux JE, *Scientific American*, 1994, 270, 6, 50–57)

portion closely related to piriform cortex, amygdala and extended amygdala, and interlinked with emotion. The posterior hippocampus is more uniquely human, related to the development of the temporal cortex, and the expansion of association cortices.

The hippocampal structures are closely linked to the septal nuclei, sometimes referred to as the septohippocampal system. The expansion and development of the human brain has led to separation of these two structures, but in lower animals they are closely linked. Gray (1982) likens this to a pair of joined bananas,

the joint being the septal area, with progression from anterior to posterior accompanied by the structures spreading laterally as they descend into the temporal lobes. The main fibre systems connecting the two are the fimbria and the fornix, and the two hippocampi are interconnected by the hippocampal commissures (Figure 2.17).

The structure of the hippocampus displays a constant architectural pattern, and three main divisions are recognized. These are the fascia dentata, Ammon's horn and the subiculum (Figure 2.18).

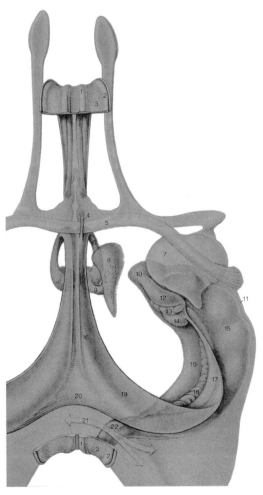

1 Stria longitudinalis medialis
2 Stria longitudinalis lateralis
3 Indusium griseum
4 Fornix precommissuralis
5 Commissura anterior
6 Columna fornicis
7 Corpus amygdaloideum
8 Nucleus anterior thalami
9 Tractus mamillothalamicus
10 Subiculum
11 Ventriculus lateralis, cornu inferius
12 Cornu ammonis (gyrus uncinatus)
13 Limbus Giacomini
14 Cornu ammonis (gyrus intralimbicus)
15 Cornu ammonis (digitationes hippocampi)
16 Corpus fornicis
17 Fimbria hippocampi
18 Gyrus dentatus
19 Crus fornicis
20 Commissura fornicis
21 Site of corpus callosum
22 Gyrus fasciolaris

Figure 2.17   The way in which the hippocampus loops round to join its opposite number in the hippocampal fornix. Relevant numbers: 5, anterior commisure; 7, amygdala; 8, anterior thalamic nucleus; 9, mamillothalamic tract; 10, subiculum; 12, 14 & 15, Ammon's horn; 16, fornix; 17, fimbria of the hippocampus; 18, dentate gyrus; 20, commisure of the fornix (reproduced with permission from Nieuwenhuys *et al.*, 1978)

(a)

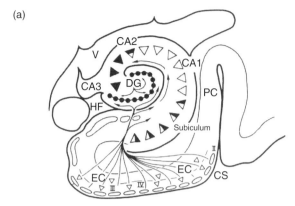

HIPPOCAMPAL CORTICAL INPUT

(b)

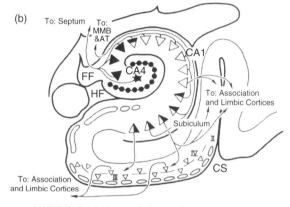

HIPPOCAMPAL CORTICAL OUTPUT

Figure 2.18 (a) Details of the hippocampal formation. The inputs from the entorhinal cortex are shown. (b) Outputs from subiculum and CA1. AT, anterior thalamus; CS, collateral sulcus; DG, dentate gyrus; EC, entorhinal cortex; FF, fimbria-fornix; HF, hippocampal fissure; MMB, mamillary bodies; PC, perirhinal cortex (reproduced from Heimer *et al.*, 2007, Figure 4.8, p. 88; courtesy of Dr van Hoesen; *Biol Psych*, 2 Ed, p. 93)

The fascia dentata consists of a compact layer of granular cells, which forms a U-shape and embraces the pyramidal cells of Ammon's horn (see Figure 2.19). The latter is sometimes subdivided into four areas, CA1–4, the CA1 area in humans being particularly prominent and susceptible to damage by anoxia (an alternative name is Sommer's sector). The subiculum is a transitional structure between CA1 and the parahippocampal gyrus. On sections it is found where the neat structure of Ammon's horn

breaks down as it merges with the six-layered neocortex, and is an exit region for many hippocampal efferents.

The laminar organization of the hippocampus is derived from its regular cell layers, notably the pyramidal cells, granular cells and interneuronal inhibitory basket cells.

Essentially the circuit of information flow from the neocortex is from the parahippocampal gyrus and entorhinal cortex via the perforant path to the dentate gyrus, then from CA3 to the CA1 areas and the subiculum. The latter feeds into the fornix, and back to the parahippocampal gyrus and neocortex. As noted, interoceptive information flows via the fornix to and from the hypothalamus, septum, accumbens, thalamus and midbrain limbic areas. The CA3 region is rich in connectivity, and it forms an excellent funnel for diverse exteroceptive and interoceptive inputs to coalesce.

The intrinsic connections of the hippocampus are largely unidirectional. The granular cells of the dentate gyrus send mossy fibres to CA3, and the pyramidal cells of CA3 give rise to collateral axons (Schaffer collaterals) to CA1. The pyramidal cells of the latter project to the subiculum.

The principal outputs are back to the entorhinal cortex and to the ventral striatum (see below).

The main neurotransmitter associated with inhibition in the hippocampus is GABA, but the structure receives dopaminergic, serotoninergic and noradrenergic afferents. Peptides such as VIP, CCK, neurotensin, somatostatin, substance P and metenkephalin have been identified in the hippocampus (Roberts *et al.*, 1984).

Parahippocampal Gyrus

The parahippocampal gyrus links posteriorly with the descending cingulate gyrus. Anteriorly it contains part of the cortical amygdala, while the entorhinal cortex forms a substantial component posterior to this. The entorhinal cortex inputs much integrated polysensory information to the hippocampus via the perforant path.

This structure is of central importance in the limbic system. It is adjacent to the hippocampus and includes, progressing caudally, the piriform, entorhinal and parahippocampal cortices. In Brodmann's system, the entorhinal cortex is represented by area 28 (see below). It has extensive projections to the hippocampal formation via the perforant pathway and, most importantly, receives afferents from many cortical sites. Thus, the association cortices project to this region, providing a direct limbic system input of visual, auditory and somatic information. Further, as noted, the amygdala projects to the entorhinal area such that the hippocampus receives, via the parahippocampal gyrus, multimodal sensory information derived from the external and internal world.

The subiculum also projects to the parahippocampal gyrus, and the latter in turn has widespread limbic and association cortical projections in frontal, parietal, temporal and occipital lobes (see Figure 2.19).

Septal Area

The septal nuclei are situated below the corpus callosum, ventrally bounded by the olfactory tubercle and the accumbens. The lateral boundary is made by the lateral ventricle, and the caudal boundary by the third ventricle and hypothalamus (see Figure 2.20). In humans, the dorsal part is elongated by the development of the corpus callosum to form the septum pellucidum, which forms a glial and fibre attachment to the corpus callosum. The septal nuclei of the human are often referred to as the precommissural septum.

The septal area is usually subdivided into medial and lateral groups, and the medial septal area is further divided into the medial septal nucleus and the nucleus of the diagonal band of Broca. Both contain acetylcholine and project to the hippocampus and entorhinal cortex via the fimbria and fornix. The lateral nuclei receive hippocampal afferents mainly from CA3 and the subiculum. Since the lateral and medial septal nuclei interconnect, a functional circuit is derived as follows: hippocampus–lateral septum–medial septum–hippocampus. The septal area receives rich monoamine projections, especially dopamine, from the VTA via the

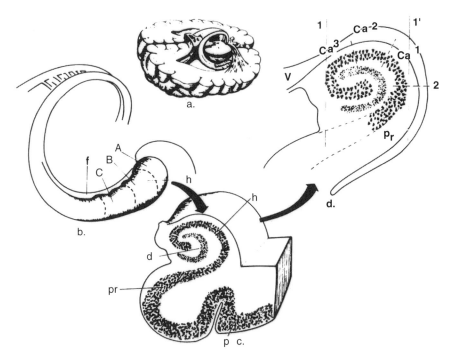

Figure 2.19   The hippocampus within the hemispheres and after dissection (reproduced from Kovelman and Scheibel, 1984; *Biol Psych*, 2 Ed, p. 85)

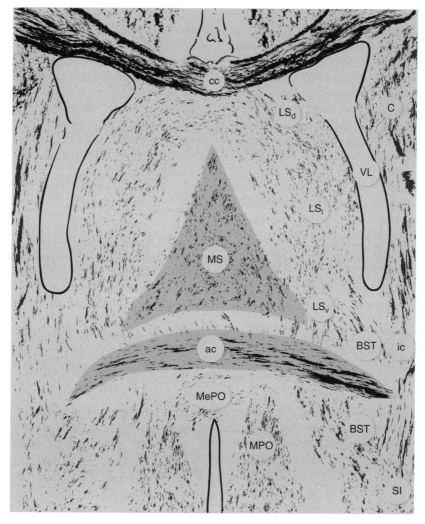

Figure 2.20   The septal area. BST, bed nucleus of stria terminalis; C, caudate nucleus; LS, lateral septal nucleii; MePO, median preoptic nucleus; MPO, medial preoptic nucleus; MS, medial septal nucleus; VL, lateral ventricle; ac, anterior commissure; SI, substantia innominata; cc, corpus callosum (*Biol Psych*, 2 Ed, p. 88)

MFB. VIP, CCK, somatostatin, metenkephalin, neurotensin and substance P are all found in the septum.

Extended Amygdala

Shown in Figure 2.20 are the bed nucleus of the stria terminalis and the substantia innominata. There has been some confusion over the innominata, the substance with no name, since neuroanatomical advances in recent years have unravelled at least some important structures within this complex. The ventral striatal territory, located beneath the temporal limb of the anterior commissure, contains the accumbens and the basal nucleus of Meynert; the region of the innominata has thus been shown to contain a collection of cholinergic and noncholinergic neurones referred to as the magnocellular basal forebrain complex, which also contains extensions of the basal ganglia and the amygdaloid complex (Heimer *et al.*, 2007).

The extended amygdala has been defined by Alheid and Heimer (1988) as a collection of cells forming a continuum from the amygdala (notably the centromedial nuclei) to the bed nucleus of the stria terminalis and the intervening sublenticular portion of the substantia innominata. The concept is of a broad sheet of interconnected neuronal structures which receives a rich monoamine input from ascending midbrain afferents, but also, by its efferents, broadly influences hypothalamic, autonomic and somatomotor functions (see Figures 2.13 and 2.14).

However, with outputs through the stria terminalis, the extended amygdala can be visualized as a ring formation encircling the internal capsule and per definition is distinct from the basolateral amygdala, is not a part of the limbic lobe, and is characterized by its projections to hypothalamic and brain-stem structures.

Cingulate Gyrus

This runs dorsal to the corpus callosum, following a C-shaped curve as it progresses posteriorly. The anterior cingulate region is the area outlined by Brodmann as areas 23, 24, 25, 31 and 33. The retrosplenial region is Brodmann's areas 26, 29 and 30, and here the cingulate gyrus becomes narrow and continuous with the lingual gyrus, a dorsal extension of the parahippocampal gyrus. The cingulate cortex is continuous with the frontal cortex anteriorly, is rich in dopamine fibres and contains CCK and opiate receptors.

The cingulum has important connections with the parietal cortex, including an area referred to as the precuneus, a part of the brain involved in visuo-spatial processing and somehow in an appreciation of our sense of self. However, the widespread cingulate connections with the entorhinal area, the amygdala, the ventral striatum, the hypothalamus and other subcortical structures allow the cingulate gyrus to have an important role in attention, motivation and emotion.

Insula

A large portion of the insular cortex is located in the depths of the Sylvian fissure, and it has a key position linking the temporal pole with the posterior orbitofrontal cortex (see Figure 2.6). It is a bridging area in the continuous ring of cortex that forms the limbic lobe. It has many functions, including integration of limbic and cortical information, and forms a part of what may be called the 'visceral cortex'. It links with the frontal cortex anteriorly and with the hippocampal structures posteriorly, and receives direct input from brainstem structures such as the tractus solitarius.

Thalamus

This, as with many other identifiable cellular groups in the brain, is a collection of nuclei with a wide variety of motor and sensory functions. The anterior thalamic nucleus was identified by Papez as a part of his circuit. However, the thalamic nuclei are part of the re-entrant pathways from strital outputs to the cortex, the parallel, segregated cortico-basal ganglia-thalamocortical circuits that have become important to understanding the functional anatomy of a range of neurological and psychiatric disorders (see below). The thalamus is usually considered to play a key role in the transmission of somatic sensory impulses on their way to the cerebral cortex. It is composed of three main nuclear groups, the medial, lateral and anterior (Figure 2.21). The ventral posterolateral nucleus conveys medial lemniscal and spinothalamic information to the primary and secondary sensory cortical areas. The basal ganglia afferents project mainly to ventrolateral, ventroanterior, mediodorsal and so-called intralaminar nuclei (located within white matter laminae that transect the thalamus); these thalamic nuclei also receive cerebellar projections. Reciprocal connections with the frontal cortex are made by the ventral anterior and mediodorsal nucleus, the anterior nucleus connecting to the cingulate gyri as part of the Papez circuit. The reticular formation – that loosely assembled, closely packed network of neurones in the brainstem – activates many thalamic neurones, and continues by relay and direct connection to influence all fields of the cortex; the midline intralaminar nuclei and

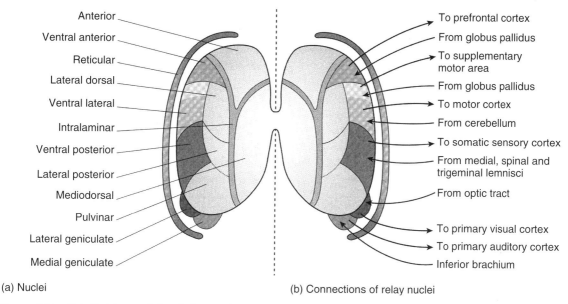

Anterior
Ventral anterior
Reticular
Lateral dorsal
Ventral lateral
Intralaminar
Ventral posterior
Lateral posterior
Mediodorsal
Pulvinar
Lateral geniculate
Medial geniculate

To prefrontal cortex
From globus pallidus
To supplementary motor area
From globus pallidus
To motor cortex
From cerebellum
To somatic sensory cortex
From medial, spinal and trigeminal lemnisci
From optic tract
To primary visual cortex
To primary auditory cortex
Inferior brachium

(a) Nuclei

(b) Connections of relay nuclei

Figure 2.21 Subdivisions of the thalamus (reproduced from Clarke *et al.*, 2009, with permission of Wiley Blackwell)

the thalamic reticular nuclei with their cortical outputs thus influence cortical arousal.

The principal afferents from the thalamus to the cortex are glutaminergic. The cytoarchitecture of the thalamus is unique, in that the GABA inhibitory neurone are not typical interneurons; rather they form a shell around the nucleus, which is called the reticular nucleus and may have an important role in gating the massive sensory and cortical information passing through the thalamus. This is probably relevant in regulating thalamocortical oscillations and rhythms (Buzsaki, 2006).

Hypothalamus

The hypothalamus, positioned dorsal to the pituitary gland, is a site of convergence for much limbic-system and extended-amygdala activity. Posterior are the mammillary bodies and anterior are the optic chiasm and the preoptic area. The descending fornix divides the hypothalamus into medial and lateral areas. The medial border of the medial hypothalamus is formed by the third ventricle, and several nuclear groups are defined (Figure 2.22). Three zones are identified: the periventricular, with essentially

neuroendocrine output (paraventricular and arcuate nuclei); the medial, connected to the limbic system and extended amygdala; and the lateral zone, which contains many fibres of passage of the monoamine brainstem and midbrain nuclei travelling with the MFB, but the fornix, stria terminalis and mammillothalamic tracts connect anteriorly, and the mammillotegmental tract posteriorly.

The suprachiasmatic nucleus is thought to be a regulator of rhythmic activity, a sort of biological clock. The axons of neurones from the supraoptic and paraventricular nuclei are neurosecretory fibres travelling mainly to the posterior pituitary gland.

Several of the hypothalamic nuclei secrete neuropeptides, some of which release hormones. These are released into the hypophysial portal blood vessels, which carry them to the anterior pituitary where they stimulate or inhibit various pituitary hormones. A list of some of these and the accompanying releasing hormones is shown in Table 2.1.

The neurohormones are typically released in a pulsatile fashion. They are found in brain areas other than the median eminence and also influence the pituitary gland via secretion into

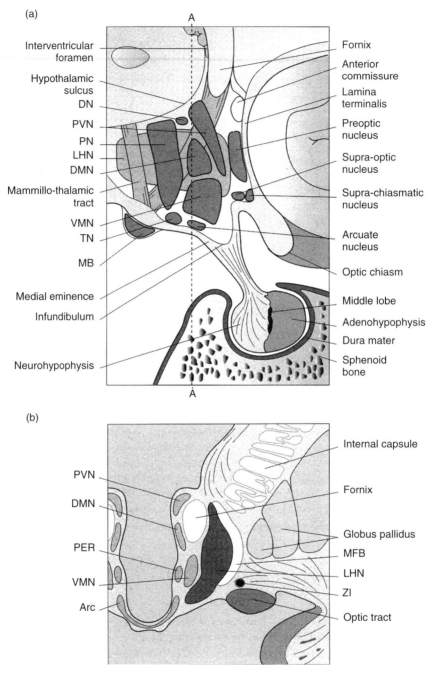

Figure 2.22 The hypothalamic nuclei: (a) sagital and (b) coronal sections. ARC = arcuate nucleus; DN = dorsal nucleus; DMN = dorsomedial nucleus; LHN = lateral hypothalamic nucleus; MB = mammillary body; MFB = medial forebrain bundle; PER = periventricular nucleus; PN = posterior nucleus; PVN = paraventricular nucleus; TN = tuberomammilary nucleus; VMN = ventromedial nucleus and ZI = zona incerta (reproduced from Clarke *et al.*, 2009, with permission of Wiley Blackwell)

Table 2.1 Hypothalamic releasing and inhibiting factors and pituitary hormones

Neurohormone	Pituitary hormone
Thyrotropin-releasing hormone	TSH, prolactin
Corticotropin-releasing hormone (CRF)	ACTH, beta-endorphin
LH/FSH-releasing hormone	LH, FSH
Growth hormone-releasing factor	Growth hormone
Melanocyte-stimulating hormone-releasing factor	MSH
Prolactin-inhibitory factor (PIF)	Prolactin
Somatostatin	Growth hormone, TSH
MSH-inhibiting factor	MSH

the CSF. The extrapituitary influence is exerted on limbic system structures, the thalamus, the periaqueductal grey region and the brainstem catecholamine nuclei.

Monoamine transmitters are also present in the hypothalamus, some of which impinge on the median eminence to influence hormone release. Indeed, catecholamines have been linked to the release of virtually all anterior pituitary hormones. Of importance is the intrahypothalamic dopamine pathway with cell bodies in the arcuate nuclei. Here the dopamine is thought to inhibit prolactin release, dopamine being a prolactin-inhibitory factor (PIF). 5-HT is thought to stimulate both growth-hormone and prolactin release.

Habenula

The habenula is located in the dorsal diencephalon, in the sides of the third ventricle, and receives afferents from the hypothalamus and the ventral pallidum – part of the cortical basal ganglia re-entrant circuits – especially those areas innervated by the accumbens shell. The main efferents descend to the midbrain nuclei, which contain the monamine and cholinergic neurones. The habenula has been shown to be involved in stress responses, reward, learning and addiction (Figure 2.23) (Geisler, 2008).

Autonomic Nervous System

The arrangement of the autonomic system, responsible for much of the body's homeostasis, is substantially different from that of the somatomotor system. There are sympathetic and parasympathetic divisions, but both have pre- and post-ganglionic components. The former are located in the CNS, in the brainstem and spinal cord; the latter are located either distant from the target organ (sympathetic) or close to it (parasympathetic). The main features of the two systems are shown in Table 2.2.

Sympathetic preganglionic neurones are located in a cell column which lies in the lateral

Table 2.2 Classical comparisons of sympathetic and parasympathetic divisions of ANS[a]

	SNS	PSNS
Location of preganglionic somata	Thoracolumbar cord	Cranial neuroaxis; sacral cord
Location of ganglia (and postganglionic somata)	Distant from target organ	Near or in target organ
Postganglionic transmitter	Noradrenaline	Acetylcholine
Length of preganglionic axon	Relatively short	Relatively long
Length of postganglionic axon	Relatively long	Relatively short
Divergence of preganglionic axonal projection	One to many	One to few
Functions	Catabolic	Anabolic
Innervates trunk and limbs in addition to viscera	Yes	No

[a]Langley (1921) stressed the contrasting and distinguishing traits of the two divisions of the ANS. Since his time, most discussions have identified several contrasting features. Most of these distinctions apply generally but not universally. Although many of these distinctions have blurred (e.g. transmitter) or may be completely unfounded (e.g. divergence), they are often discussed.

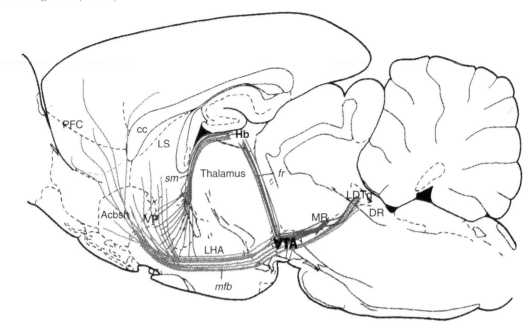

Figure 2.23   The connections of the habenula. The habenula is part of the dorsal diencephalic circuit, conveying information from several forebrain nuclei to ascending brain-stem systems. HB, habenula; MFB, medial forebrain bundle; LHA, lateral hypothalamic area; PFC, prefrontal cortex; CC, corpus callosum; Fr, Fasciculus retroflexus; Acbsh, Accumbens shell; VP, ventral pallidum; MR and DR, medial and dorsal raphe; VTA, ventral tegmental area (reproduced with permission from Stefani Geisler)

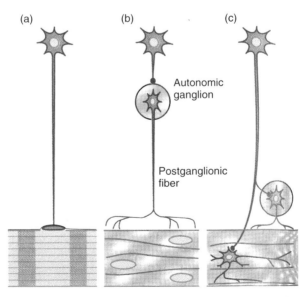

Figure 2.24   Differences between the somatic motor output and the sympathetic output to effector end points. (a) Motorneurones project directly to the muscles. (b) The sympathetic nervous system projects first to preganglionic neurones, which then project to post-ganglionic motor neurones in para- and pre-vertebral autonomic ganglia. (c) The parasympethic nervous system has preganglionic neurones in brain-stem cranial nerve nuclei (and in spinal cord) that project to post-ganglionic motor neurones in ganglia located near or inside viscera (reproduced with permission from APA Press)

Brainsteam Slices With Vagus Nerve Connections

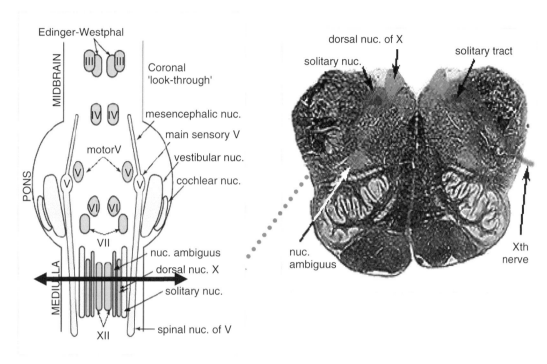

Figure 2.25 The autonomic nuclei that relate to control of autonomic function in the lower pons and medulla. Central to this arrangement are the nuclei related to the vagus nerve, the nucleus of the tractus solitaries, the nucleus ambiguous and the dorsal motor nucleus of the vagus. The section indicated on the right relates to the slice of the arrow on the left

horn of the spinal grey matter between the first thoracic (T1) and the third lumbar (L3) segments. The post-ganglionic cells are in either paravertebral (adjacent to the spinal cord) or prevertebral (situated close to where major abdominal arteries leave the aorta) ganglia. The sympathetic postganglionic fibres then supply target organs such as skin and blood vessels (Figure 2.24).

Parasympatheric output stems from two columns of cells, one in the brainstem and one in the spinal cord (S2–4). The brainstem, visceral division comprises a number of cell groups adjacent to the central aqueduct, which send efferents through cranial nerves to the head (III, VII and IX), thorax and abdomen (X – the vagus nerve), providing innervation that controls pupil size, lacrymation and salivation, for example. The vagus innervates the digestive

tract and the two main nuclei are the dorsal motor nucleus of the vagus and the ventral vagal nucleus (nucleus ambiguus) (see Figure 2.25). As shown in Table 2.2, the two divisions of the autonomic nervous system use different neurotransmitters at the post-ganglionic site, but most preganglionic neurones are cholinergic.

There are extensive visceral afferent inputs to the autonomic nervous system, many ending in the nucleus of the solitary tract.

ASCENDING AND DESCENDING LIMBIC-SYSTEM CONNECTIONS

Knowledge of the anatomy and functional unity of the limbic system has altered radically in recent years. It is now accepted that a limbic forebrain–midbrain circuit exists which unites the monoamine- and peptide-rich zones of the midbrain with rostral structures such as the hippocampus, amygdala and the accumbens, and a limbic midbrain area has been defined in the paramedian zone of the mesencephalon (Nauta and Domesick, 1982). The main connecting structure is the MFB, a poorly defined fibre system with a loose arrangement, characteristic of brainstem reticular formation. It receives contributions from such structures as the septal nuclei, accumbens, hypothalamus, olfactory tubercle, amygdala, bed nucleus of stria terminalis and the orbitofrontal cortex. Caudally it projects to the VTA, the interpeduncular nucleus, the raphe nuclei, the locus coeruleus and the midbrain reticular formation. Nieuwenhuys (1996), with his concept of the greater limbic system, emphasizes the caudal projections to and from the rostral medulla, and further connections with the spinal cord which influence autonomic function (Figure 2.8). Included are several regions from which behavioural and autonomic symptoms can be elicited by stimulation.

The final common pathway for emotional expression is through the autonomic nervous system, and some authors refer to the 'emotional motor system' (see below). The periaqueductal grey matter (PAG) is situated immediately below the superior colliculus, surrounding the aqueduct between the third and fourth ventricles. Stimulation leads to a variety of expressed emotions, especially threat and flight, and it is involved in pain perception (Bandler and Keay, 1996). It receives projections from the limbic lobe, and outputs both centrally, but also to the rostroventral medulla and spinal cord.

In the rostral medulla, and at the junction between the medulla and the pons, lies a group of neurone clusters that seem to directly control autonomic function (see Figure 2.25). These include neurones regulating cardiac and respiratory function and micturition. Some of the neurones (presympathetic cells) have direct monosynaptic inputs to the preganglionic sympathetic cells. The areas involved include the C1, A5 and the nucleus ambiguus. The nucleus ambiguus is part of the vagus nerve efferent motor system. The nucleus of the

tractus solitarius (NTS) receives afferent fibres from the vagus and glossopharyngeal nerves and is reciprocally connected to the nucleus ambiguus, which, with the dorsal nucleus of the vagus, provides efferents to the vagus nerve, supplying the GI tract with autonomic nerves. The NTS also relays information rostrally to the insula, hypothalamus and several other structures involved in monoamine regulation and limbic function. It is now appreciated that the majority of fibres in the vagus nerve are afferent, and this has been exploited in vagus nerve stimulation (see Chapter 12).

It is now known that there is an extensive system of interneurones at the spinal level which interact with the sympathetic and parasympathetic preganglionic neurones and use neurotransmitters such as glycine and GABA. The final output of the autonomic system is therefore both supraspinal and spinal and is dependent on visceral and somatic afferents as well as descending influences from the cortex, hypothalamus and mesencephalon, ultimately reflecting limbic and cortical information.

The ascending components of the limbic forebrain–midbrain circuit arise from the ventral tegmental area (VTA), the raphe nuclei and the locus coeruleus. The VTA occupies the basomedial midbrain, dorsal to the substantia nigra, and is continuous rostrally with the lateral hypothalamus. It borders on the ventral periaqueductal grey substance, the nucleus ruber (red nucleus), the dorsal raphe nuclei and other nuclei of the limbic midbrain (see Figure 2.26).

The ascending connections to the limbic forebrain include the dopamine-rich cells which innervate the accumbens, olfactory tubercle, the extended amygdala, entorhinal area, hippocampus, frontocingulate cortex and septal area. The catecholamine nuclei are found in relatively discrete areas of the brainstem, and were first identified using fluorescent histochemical techniques. On the basis of animal work they have been designated as A1, A2, ... up to A13 (Ungerstedt, 1971), and those arising from the substantia nigra and the VTA are referred to as A9 and A10 respectively. From these the majority of dopamine neurones that project to the

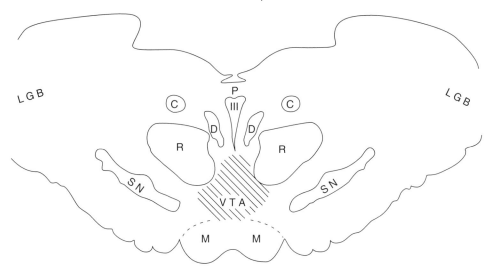

Figure 2.26 Location of the ventral tegmental area in the midbrain. C, nucleus of Cajal; D, nucleus of Darkschewitsch; LGB, lateral geniculate body; M, mammillary bodies; P, posterior commissure; R, red nucleus; SN, substantia nigra; VTA, ventral tegmental area

limbic areas, striatum and cortex arise. Using this terminology, the locus coeruleus is A5 and A6. In a similar fashion the serotoninergic neurones are confined virtually to the brainstem raphe nuclei. The A10 projection also innervates the striatum and the thalamus and has connections with the locus coeruleus and raphe nuclei, although not all paths are thought necessarily to be dopaminergic (Nauta and Domesick, 1982).

The locus coeruleus lies ventrolateral to the fourth ventricle, and has widespread connections to the neuroaxis, probably more extensive than those of any other nucleus (Vertes, 1990). It innervates the spinal cord, the thalamus and the limbic system, with a particularly dense projection to amygdala and cortex. This distribution is in marked contrast to the relatively restricted termination of fibres from A9 and A10. The ascending catecholaminergic system is thought to exert a tonic modulatory influence on cortical neurones, and locus coeruleus neurones are sensitive to sensory input, stress increasing their activity.

5-HT distribution is intermediate, being more extensive than that of dopamine and projecting to the hippocampus and amygdala, parahippocampal gyrus, habenula, thalamus and cortex.

Raphe cells are unresponsive to arousing sensory stimuli, and high-frequency firing occurs with repetitive movements and with feeding. Their descending influences increase the excitability of motor neurones and are antinociceptive (see Figure 2.27).

MACROSYSTEMS

Based on cytoarchitectural and neurochemical properties, functional basal forebrain anatomical systems can thus be identified, and have been referred to as macrosystems. These include the ventral and dorsal striato pallidal system, the extended amygdala and the septal-preoptic system.

Macrosystems are processing units that receive information from the cortex and project to somatic and autonomic motor outputs in the lateral hypothalamus or brainstem, or via re-entrant paths back to the cortex. They are hypothesized to detect the positive or negative valence of stimuli and via their outputs they compete and cooperate to influence resulting behaviour (Heimer *et al.*, 2007).

They have a common template, with largely cortical inputs, terminating predominately in inhibitory neurones (especially medium-sized

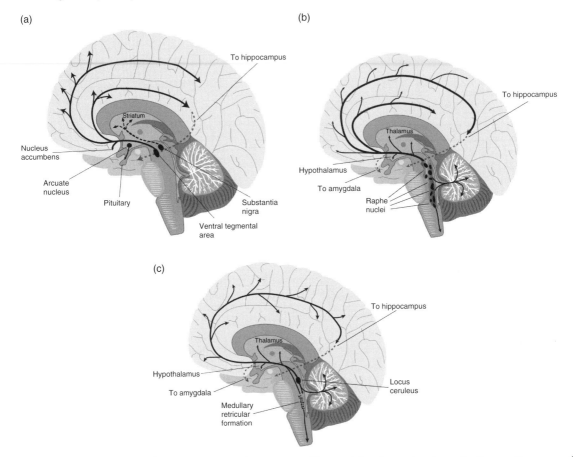

Figure 2.27   Distribution of various monoamines output fibres arising from structures in the pontine area of the brain: (a) dopamine, (B) 5-HT, (c) noradrenaline (courtesy of Dr Ned Higgins)

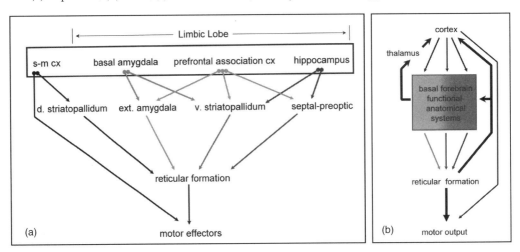

Figure 2.28   The connections underpinning the concept of basal forebrain macrosystems. (a) Outputs from greater limbic lobe structures, which converge in the reticular formation, and in addition to outputs from the cortex (CX) converge on motor effectors. (b) Re-entrant pathways returning to cortex (courtesy of Dr Scott Zahm)

spiny neurones), which project on to other GABA neurones in structures such as the pallidum, extended amygdala and preoptic area, which then send projections back to the cortex via thalamo-cortical re-entrant pathways (see Figure 2.28). They also have projections to forebrain cholinergic and monoaminergic cell groups, and influence somatomotor, autonomic and endocrine systems (Heimer *et al.*, 2007). Since the thalamus, pivotal in this scheme, has no direct motor outputs, and the striatum lacks direct projections back to the cortex, funnelling information through the thalamus, the intrinsic macrosystem circuitry modifies cortical activity. Since the macrosystems under consideration here have substantial limbic inputs, they are situated to synthesize multiple somatic and emotional information and thus regulate output behaviours.

THE BASAL GANGLIA AND THE RE-ENTRANT CIRCUITS

The term 'basal ganglia' usually refers to the caudate nucleus, putamen and globus pallidus but may also include the subthalamic nucleus and the substantia nigra. 'Striatum' refers to the caudate nucleus and putamen, divided as they are by the internal capsule. In lower animals the separation is less complete, and the structure is referred to as the caudatoputamen. The caudate

nucleus is a large curved nucleus which adheres throughout its length to the lateral ventricles, anteriorly being continuous with the putamen. The putamen and globus pallidus are referred to as the lenticular nucleus.

The substantia nigra has two components, the pars reticulata and the pars compacta. The former is a part of the pallidum, and uses GABA as its main efferent neurotransmitter; the pars compacta is the origin of the nigrostriatal dopamine pathway.

Recently, concepts of the organization of the basal ganglia have undergone profound changes. Previously discussed as if they used serial processing, they are now viewed as being parallel in nature, with structurally and functionally distinct circuits that act in parallel linking cortex, basal ganglia, thalamus and frontal cortex – the macrosystem template just referred to (Alexander *et al.*, 1986; Heimer *et al.*, 2007). Six such circuits are postulated, targeting different areas of the frontal lobe. Representative structures of three circuits especially involved in regulating emotional behaviour are shown in Figure 2.29. These involve prefrontal, orbital and medial frontal cortex. The features that are shared by all the circuits are shown in Figures 2.11, 2.12 and 2.29. The cortical output is glutaminergic, and projects to the striatum, with an enkephalin link to the globus pallidus. The latter structure is defined by at least two

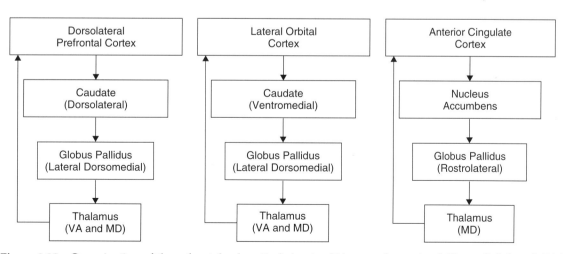

Figure 2.29 Organization of three frontal-subcortical circuits. VA, venral anterior; MD, medial dorsal (*Biol Psych*, 2 Ed, p. 98)

segments, the internal and the external. The projection to the internal segment utilizes GABA and connects with the thalamus, feeding back to frontal cortex. The globus pallidus externus loops with the subthalamic nucleus back to the internal segment. The final thalamocortical link returns to the same area of cortex where the original corticostriatal connection began.

Activation of the direct pathway through the internal pallidum excites the thalamocortical projection (via GABAergic inhibition of an inhibitory pathway), while that of the external pallidum, which activates the STN, increases inhibition of the thalamus, and the balance between the external and internal loops modulates output to the cortex (see Figures 2.11 and 2.12).

In this context, the basal ganglia facilitate movement by a process of disinhibition.

The nigrostriatal pathways are dopaminergic, exciting the GABAergic striatal neurones and inhibiting the projections to the internal and external pallidal segments. The net effect could be to enhance the output. Acetylcholine has effects antagonistic to dopamine in the striatum.

Essentially all of the cortical mantle projects to the basal ganglia structures (see Figure 2.9). Thus, the caudate/putamen receives widespread, somatotopically organized projections from the cerebral cortex and the cortical association areas, including temporal cortex projecting to caudate. The main striatal structure of the 'motor circuit' is the putamen, that of the 'limbic circuit' being the caudate and the ventral striatum (see below). 'All of cortex uses basal ganglia mechanisms' (Heimer *et al.*, 2007, p. 43).

The cytoarchitecture of the striatum has functional significance. Striosomes, zones lacking acetylcholine, exhibit enkephalin-like, opiate-like, substance P-like and somatostatin-like reactivity, and are contrasted with the matrix. The striosomes seem more related to limbic inputs, the matrix to sensorimotor processing (Graybiel, 1990). While the matrix outputs to the pallidum, the striosomes project largely to the pars compacta of the substantia nigra, perhaps modulating dopamine input to the striatum. D_1 binding is greater in the striosomes, and D_2 greater in the matrix.

It seems that in the human striatum, striosomes predominate (50%) (Saper *et al.*, 1996), suggesting a profound limbic component, which must have functional significance. The main neurones (70%) identified in the basal ganglia are called medium spiny neurones. The rest are interneurones and contain neurotransmitters such as acetylcholine, neuropeptide Y and GABA.

The name of the spiny neurones relates to the approximately 13 000 spiny dendrite protruberances, which have a head sticking out at the end of a neck. Excitatory input (glutamate) synapses to the head, while the dopamine input (mainly from the substantia nigra) is to the neck. This arrangement allows the dopamine to modulate the glutaminergic input. This microcontrol within the striatum is disturbed in many basal ganglia diseases such as Parkinson's disease.

THE VENTRAL STRIATUM AND 'LIMBIC STRIATUM'

Much attention has been focused on dopamine-rich structures lying ventral and medial to, and associated with, the head of the caudate nucleus. The ventral striatum is contrasted with the dorsal striatum in the circuitry outlined above mainly by its limbic inputs, and crucially by output to the mediodorsal nucleus of the thalamus, as opposed to the ventrolateral, ventromedial and centromedian nuclei (see Figure 2.10). The accumbens and the closely associated olfactory tubercle are the main nuclear groups of the ventral striatum. The accumbens has a caudal boundary with the bed nucleus of the stria terminalis, which is difficult to establish, emphasizing the interconnectedness with the extended amygdala. Anteriorly it extends into the ventromedial portion of the frontal lobe, and it lies lateral to the septal region (White, 1981) (see Figure 2.30).

It has recently been appreciated that there are two components of the accumbens, a core and a shell (see Figure 2.31). The core is striatal and projects to the ventral pallidum, and hence to the loops of the thalamus and back to cortex. The shell is essentially continuous with the extended

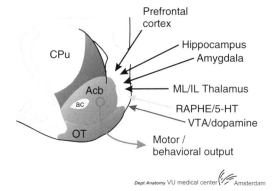

Convergence of prefrontal cortical,
limbic and dopamine inputs

Prefrontal
cortex

CPu

Hippocampus
Amygdala

Acb
ac

ML/IL Thalamus

RAPHE/5-HT
VTA/dopamine

OT

Motor /
behavioral output

Dept Anatomy VU medical center Amsterdam

Figure 2.30 The connections of the accumbens, emphasizing the central position of the accumbens, which receives cortical and limbic input and has widespread outputs that influence behaviour (courtesy of Dr Groenewegen)

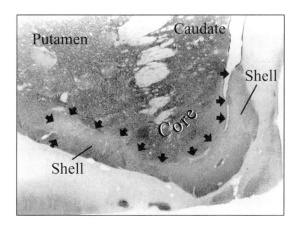

Figure 2.31 Shell and core of the accumbens (courtesy of Dr L. Heimer)

amygdala and projects both to the globus pallidus and to the hypothalamus and brainstem motor and autonomic nuclei. Further, the core and the shell project directly to the VTA and the substantia nigra reticulata. D_1 receptors are abundant in the shell.

Substance P, enkephalin and CCK are found in both ventral and dorsal striatum, while VIP, TRH and neurotensin are found mainly in the accumbens. Other peptides located in the accumbens include somatostatin

and melanocyte-stimulating hormone (MSH) (Johannsson and Hokfelt, 1981). There are also high concentrations of acetylcholine, glutamate and GABA.

Nauta repeatedly emphasized the cross-talk between the limbic system and the basal ganglia (Nauta and Domesick, 1982). This is of great importance for biological psychiatry, not least because of the close links between motor and emotional behaviour (Trimble, 1981a). Direct connections exist between the hippocampus, amygdala, cingulate cortex and ventral striatum and the habenula, a nucleus at the caudal end of the midbrain which projects to the raphe nuclei and has both limbic and pallidal afferents (Figure 2.23). Hypothalamic MFB efferents impinge on the VTA and substantia nigra. Further, indirect links by way of the substantia nigra and raphe nucleus exist, both being influenced by the descending fibres of the MFB and the fasciculus retroflexus from the habenula. In contrast, direct connections in the opposite direction, from striatum to limbic system, are very limited.

One further point of anatomical interest is that three limbic projections converge on the anterior ventral component of the striatum, namely the dopaminergic fibres from the VTA, the projection from the amygdala and fibres from the frontal cortex (Figure 2.32).

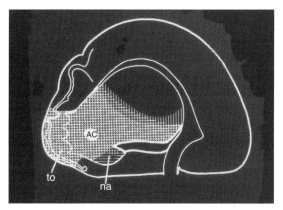

Figure 2.32 Inputs to the accumbens overlapping from the ventral tegmental area (vertical lines) prefrontal cortex (horizontal lines) and amygdala (stipple). NA, nucleus accumbens; AC, anterior commisure (courtesy of Dr L. Heimer)

THE ASCENDING CHOLINERGIC SYSTEMS

The nuclear groups including the medial septal nucleus, the basal nucleus of Meynert and the nucleus of the diagonal band are all sites of origin of cholinergic ascending systems that project to the cerebral cortex and hippocampus (septal). The area forming a rostroventral extension of the globus pallidus, the ventral pallidum, is coextensive with the basal nucleus of Meynert, and it is difficult to draw discrete boundaries between these structures (see the discussion above concerning the substantia innominata). The main inputs to this cholinergic system come from the cortex, limbic system and hippocampus, and the efferents terminate in all layers of cortex. As with the basal ganglia macrosystems the projection is back to the cortical areas from which their input derives. Acetylcholine excites cortical neurones, modulating the effect of incoming information, and increased activity desynchronizes the electroencephalogram (EEG). Deficits of cholinergic input, as associated with Alzheimer's disease for example, lead to attentional, as opposed to pure memory, deficits.

Additional cholinergic neurones arise from the mesencephalic reticular formation in the pedunculopontine and dorsolateral tegmental nuclei. These are also part of an arousal system influencing the thalamocortical system.

CORTICAL REGIONS OF INTEREST

As already noted, there are two main divisions of cortex, the six-layered isocortex (neocortex) and the non-isocortex. The isocortex, especially in humans, has developed rapidly and extensively in the latter phases of evolution and is attributed a dominant role in human higher cerebral processes. Much work of relevance for biological psychiatry and neuropsychiatry has highlighted the frontal and temporal areas of the cortex, although here further emphasis is given to parietal cortex.

The human isocortex has been divided into various areas dependent on microscopic differences, such as those described by Brodmann (see Figure 2.33). The layer of cortex closest to the pia mater contains mainly dendrites of the deeper-lying cells. The pyramidal cells, with long axons that traverse the internal capsule to form part of the pyramidal tract, are found in layer 5. It is the granular cells of layer 4 that mainly receive the thalamic sensory afferents, and this layer, in contrast to layer 5, is best developed in primary sensory cortices. The cerebral cortex is made up predominantly of pyramidal cells, which use glutamate as their neurotransmitter. Betz cells are large pyramidal cells found in the motor cortex of hominids.

The primary sensory somatocortex is located posterior to the central sulcus in the postcentral gyrus, equivalent to Brodmann's areas 1 to 3. More posterior, corresponding to areas 5 and 7, is the somatic sensory association area. The visual receptive areas are the striate and peristriate cortex (area 17, the primary visual cortex, and areas 18 and 19, the visual association areas). The auditory cortical areas are in the superior temporal gyrus (Brodmann's areas 41 and 42). Heschl's gyrus (the transverse temporal gyrus) is located on the dorsal surface of the superior temporal gyrus. It forms the anterior border of the planum temporale and is part of the temporal operculum. It is also part of the primary auditory cortex and receives auditory information from the medial geniculate of the thalamus, and has efferents to the association auditory cortex in the superior temporal gyrus.

The main motor cortex is situated in the precentral gyrus, immediately rostral to the central sulcus (area 4), its main afferents coming from area 6, adjacent to it, which itself receives prefrontal projections. Area 8, another region anterior to the precentral gyrus, is referred to as the frontal eye field, and on stimulation eye movements are provoked. The supplementary motor area is Brodmann's area 6. This is highly involved in motor planning and pre-rehearsal.

It is now known that the cerebral cortex has a columnar arrangement, which has functional significance. The cortical neurones form connections within a column, but also ramify with cells in adjacent columns. This arrangement allows for an amplifying effect on afferent impulses, in the motor cortex permitting sufficient neurones to discharge for movement

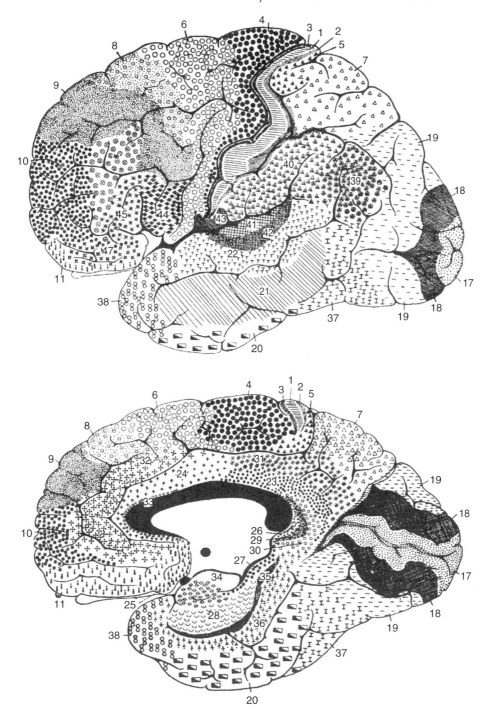

Figure 2.33 The cortical areas as defined by the Brodmann system

and in the sensory cortex distinguishing two closely related stimuli. Further, by allowing for the development of positive-feedback loops and inhibition of neighbouring columns, the columns are self-excitatory, sharpening their effect by surround inhibition. In the visual cortex, columns of orientation-selective cells have been identified, many of which are developed and present at birth.

A large proportion of intrinsic cortical neurones are GABAergic, many of which receive thalamic afferents. Cortical peptides include somatostatin, VIP, CCK and neuropeptide Y. In the cortex, cholinergic neurones have been shown to contain VIP.

The noradrenergic innervation of the neocortex is extensive and tangential to the columnar arrangement. The fibres run longitudinally through the cortical grey matter, in laminaae VI, V and I, and branch widely, thus affecting activity over wide areas of cortex. They are activated by a novel stimulus, and interact with the thalamocortical inputs impinging on pyramidal and interneuronal dendrites. VIP is also released, which enhances the activity of the pyramidal neurones and influences cerebral microcirculation. Thus VIP exerts specific local effects, possibly complementary in terms of information processing, with the influence of monoamines.

The frontal lobes are anatomically represented by those areas of cortex anterior to the central sulcus, including the main cortical representations for the control of motor behaviour. The term 'prefrontal cortex' designates the most anterior pole, an area sometimes referred to as the frontal granular cortex or the frontal association cortex (Brodmann's areas 9–15, 46 and 47; see Figure 2.33). The prefrontal cortex is amongst the last to myelinate in development. One definition of the prefrontal cortex is that region which receives projections from the mediodorsal thalamic nucleus (Fuster, 1980). These are topographically organized such that the medial part of that nucleus projects to the medial and orbital frontal cortex, and the lateral to the lateral and dorsal cortex. The medial thalamic area receives afferents

from the mesencephalic reticular formation, and from the amygdala, entorhinal and inferior temporal cortex, whereas the lateral nuclear area only has afferents from the prefrontal cortex (Fuster, 1980).

Other important prefrontal connections are made by the mesocortical dopamine projections from VTA. Unlike the subcortical dopamine projections, these neurones lack autoreceptors (Bannon *et al.*, 1982). Further links are to the hypothalamus (the orbital frontal cortex alone in the neocortex projects to the hypothalamus), the amygdala, the hippocampus, and the retrosplenial and entorhinal cortices. On the basis of primate data, Nauta (1964) suggested that the orbital frontal cortex makes connections with amygdala and related subcortical structures, whereas the dorsal cortex links more to the hippocampus and parahippocampal gyrus. Certainly there seems to be a comparable circuit to the Papez circuit, but based on the amygdala instead of the hippocampus; thus: Amygdala–thalamus (mediodorsal nucleus)–orbitofrontal cortex–inferior temporal cortex–amygdala. In the same way that sensory information from the primary sensory cortex, after passing to adjacent secondary areas, cascades to the anterior temporal areas (Jones and Powell, 1970), the prefrontal cortex is also a projection area for extensive somatic, auditory and sensory information from parietal areas.

The prefrontal cortex has efferents to, but does not receive afferents from, the striatum, notably the caudate nucleus, globus pallidus, putamen and substantia nigra.

The flow of motor information is from prefrontal to premotor to primary motor areas, with further loops to the basal ganglia and lateral thalamus via the circuits described above. Thus, with the exception of some primary sensory and motor areas, the prefrontal cortex is interconnected with every other cortical region (Fuster, 1993).

The area of the prefrontal cortex that receives the dominant dorsomedial thalamic nucleus projection overlaps with that from the dopaminergic VTA. The internal connectivity of the prefrontal cortical structures is complicated. In summary, the medial cortex shows few connections with orbital cortex and vice versa. The orbital networks mainly communicate with each other, and such internal connectivity is the case with medial frontal areas. The orbital networks receive somatosensory and visceral inputs, including taste, and have been shown to possess cells which respond to taste and the sight of food (Buckley *et al.*, 2001; Rolls, 2001). Output is to the basolateral amygdala and accumbens. In contrast, the medial networks have few olfactory inputs, and important outputs to the hypothalamus and periaqueductal grey region (which has very limited output from the orbital region), a descending visceral control.

The OFC with information from the accumbens, amygdala and hippocampus may attribute salience to the environment. The lateral PFC reciprocally interacts with parietal cortex, supporting working memory and planning action sequences, and since the OFC through intrinsic connections influences the dorsolateral prefrontal cortex (DLPFC), these structures along with the ventral striatal re-entrant circuits provide a cerebral substructure for coordinated motivated action plans.

THE CEREBELLUM

This structure lies posteriorly over the brainstem, and its cortex is divided into the central vermis and the cerebellar hemispheres. It receives afferents from both peripheral sense receptors and sensory and motor cortices, and projects to the thalamus, spinal cord and the same areas of cortex. Direct influences of the cerebellum on limbic system structures have been reported, notably at the hypothalamus, limbic midbrain and amygdala. These may be mediated via the fastigial nucleus of the vermis (Heath *et al.*, 1978). Although traditionally considered purely motor in function, recent work has suggested that it plays an important role in cognition and possibly also in emotional behaviour (Schmahmann, 1991). Attention has also recently focused on important projections from the cerebellum to the frontal cortex.

3
Important Brain–Behaviour Relationships

INTRODUCTION

Three clinical neuroscience discoveries in the middle of the 20th century have revolutionized our view of brain–behaviour relationships, with profound therapeutic, conceptual and philosophical implications. The first was the development of the limbic system concept, the second was the discovery of so-called 'pleasure pathways' in the brain and the third was the tranquilizing antipsychotic effect of chlorpromazine. The first two are discussed in more detail in this chapter.

The Limbic System and Beyond

Paul MacLean's (1913–2007) original concept of the limbic system involved what he referred to as the 'triune brain'. This was a three-layered structure, in which each layer had differing behavioural repertoires, but all were interconnected (see Figure 3.1). There was the protoreptilian complex, in humans referred to as the striatal complex (basal ganglia), the paleomammalian formation (the limbic system), and the neomammalian formation (the neocortex and its connections to the thalamic apparatus). This triune brain represented the achievements of millions of years of evolution of the neural axis, but also of behaviour.

The striatal elements of the brain are involved in mastering daily behavioural routines and subroutines. These are repetitive and perseverative motor programmes but also include rituals and communicative displays, best observed in reptiles, but obviously applicable to much human behaviour.

The limbic system in MacLean's scheme was involved in three key mammalian behaviours, namely nursing and maternal care, audio-vocal communications – vital for maintaining maternal–offspring contact – and play. These neuronal structures, rudimentary in reptiles, but developed extensively in mammals, lead to MacLean's important dictum that 'the history of the evolution of the limbic system is the history of the evolution of the mammals, while the history of the evolution of the mammals is the history of the evolution of the family' (MacLean, 1990).

A well-developed limbic system is thus a common denominator in the brains of all mammals, and the evolutionary development of the limbic system was an essential prerequisite for the development of characteristic mammalian behaviours. The key feature of being a mammal is of course the presence and need of a mother, and all that goes with having a mother. A reptile hatching from an egg must not cry out for its mother or else it will be readily detected

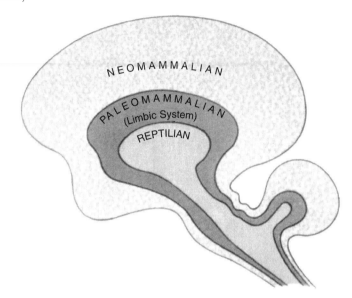

Figure 3.1   The triune brain. This diagram from Paul MacLean (1968) illustrates the evolution of the human forebrain and how it expands along the lines of three basic formations that anatomically reflect an ancestral relationship to reptiles, early mammals and late mammals (reproduced from Maclean, 1990). A coloured version of this figure can be found on the colour plate

by predators and eaten either by them or by its mother. In contrast, a mammalian infant depends on the separation cry for security and succour. Further, the development of family-, sibling- and later peer-relevant behaviours, including interpersonal bonding, relates to the phylogenetic and ontological development of these limbic structures.

MacLean outlined three main subdivisions of the limbic lobe, which he referred to as an amygdalar division, a septal division and a thalamocingulate division (see Figure 2.3). These divisions had to do with feeling and expressive states relating to self-preservation, to procreation and to maternal care and play, respectively. MacLean's contributions to unravelling the neural basis of emotional and social behaviour were central to a revolution in the neurosciences that took neurology not only towards mental illness, but also in the direction of understanding normal as well as abnormal social behaviours. It was pointed out in Chapter 2 how in the past half-century, the underlying concepts of the limbic system have altered considerably, not least due to the anatomical explorations of neuroanatomists

such as Walle Nauta (1916–1994) and Lennart Heimer (1930–2007).

A problem with the earlier conceptions of the limbic system was the then-accepted anatomical belief that the hypothalamus was to be regarded as the principal subcortical projection of the limbic system. Indeed, for some people, a relationship to the hypothalamus became a defining factor of a limbic structure (Heimer *et al.*, 2007, p. 20). Now we know that the major outputs from the limbic system are to the basal ganglia. The former view led to an interesting but rather damaging conclusion, which had implications not only for understanding brain–behaviour relationships, but also for the developing specializations of behavioural neurology and neuropsychiatry. Thus, those neurologists who, a half-century ago, might reluctantly have conceded that there was an underlying neurology of emotional behaviour, could acknowledge that the limbic system–hypothalamic axis was explanatory enough for a neurology of the emotions (and hence psychiatry), but this was very different from the neuroanatomy of neurological disorders. The latter involved essentially the neocortex and its main outputs, especially the basal ganglia and the pyramidal motor system. A fundamental flaw in this scheme however was that it did not correspond to many clinical observations. Included were the obvious behavioural problems and psychiatric illnesses that accompanied movement disorders (such as Parkinson's disease or Huntingtons's chorea), and the obvious abnormal movements that were a part of the clinical picture of psychiatric disorders across the spectrum from anxiety (tremor) to schizophrenia (tics, dystonias, dyskinesias and catatonias). Further, it failed to connect with common English and everyday observations, namely that emotion is six-sevenths motion (e-motion), and that we express our states of distress and emotion with motion, including of course speech.

Nauta (1986) challenged the belief that cortical and subcortical systems were so distinctly separated, and noted how anatomical studies had revealed not only that nearly all of the neocortex is connected to the basal ganglia by extensive efferent connections, but that there was serial linkage between the limbic structures, the basal ganglia and the neocortex (as discussed in Chapter 2). Further, it became appreciated that the rostral parts of the basal ganglia, far from being exclusively motor in function, were actually innervated by the limbic system. There was in fact a much stronger connectivity between limbic structures and the basal ganglia than with the hypothalamus, overthrowing entirely the idea that the limbic system was a discrete system devoted to the hypothalamus and unable to influence the basal ganglia (motor systems) or the cortical mantle.

As has been discussed, Nauta and others also extended the influence of the limbic system caudally, through the medial forebrain bundle (a limbic traffic artery) and other structures to the midbrain (limbic midbrain) and hind brain, including the cell structures we now know to be the origin of the ascending monoamine systems. These innervate not only the ventral striatum itself but the frontal cortex and indeed, for some neurotransmitters like 5-HT, probably the whole of the neocortex.

Nauta also noted how limbic efferents influenced autonomic neurones and the cranial nerves that innervate the muscles of facial expression. Further, since the frontal lobes (especially the orbital and cingulate divisions) were also by this time revealed as being limbic-related, Nauta speculated that the fronto–limbic connections enabled the frontal cortex to monitor and modulate the activities of the limbic system.

The ventral striatum, which is a striatal structure, is now seen as essentially limbic. What this means, conceptually, is that the regions of the brain that modulate emotion and motivation have direct access to its motor systems, down as far as the brainstem and beyond even to the neurones that control somatic and autonomic muscular activity.

Pleasure Pathways

The second important neuroscience discovery of the 20th century was that of James Olds (1922–1976) and Peter Milner in the early 1950s (Olds and Milner, 1954). For centuries, the brain had been viewed as a passive recipient of sensory impressions, which led in a Pavlov-type sequence to motor action, with, in some philosophies (the behaviouralists) the assumption of little else of relevance in between stimulus and response. And yet a growing undercurrent of knowledge was emphasizing the prepared brain, the brain not as a receptacle and *tabula rasa*, but as an active organ, a synthesizing and creating brain. Proceeding from the psychology of Freud and his successors, the very drivenness of human activity, by unconscious and in some theories unknowable forces, became common currency, but these hollow frames lacked a neurological basis, a neurobiology of the emotions and movement.

What Olds and Milner did was uncover cerebral circuits for pleasure and reward, endowing hedonic tone to percepts and behaviour. This research was being conducted at the same time that Papez and MacLean were unravelling the additional neuroanatomical structures already discussed. The identification of such a neuroanatomy of the emotions opened the possibility of altering emotional expression, and hence of providing amelioration of neurobehavioral disturbances by influencing such circuitry. The discovery of dopamine and other neuromodulators ushered in the era of psychopharmacology and heralded brain stimulation: the ability to influence crucial neuroanatomical circuitry, whether indirectly across the scalp or directly by application of electrodes to the brain itself.

IMPORTANT ANATOMICAL STRUCTURES FOR UNDERSTANDING BEHAVIOUR

Hypothalamus and Peptides

The role of the hypothalamus in regulating eating and drinking has been well investigated. Destruction of the ventromedial nuclei results in hyperphagia, and destruction of the lateral hypothalamus, to aphagia. Stimulation leads to the opposite. In part the effects are due to alteration of activity in fibres of passage passing through the region, and it is now known that dopamine projections from substantia nigra are involved. An interesting observation is that CCK, injected in small amounts intraperitoneally or intraventricularly, leads to satiety in hungry animals. Another example of the central and peripheral action of a peptide neurohormone is in the regulation of drinking: the hypothalamus contains cells sensitive to osmotic signals and sodium levels, however angiotensin 2, the active form of angiotensin, peripherally causes vasoconstriction and renal sodium retention, and centrally stimulates drinking. Findings such as these emphasize that the brain is a target organ for hormones released peripherally and centrally, and may explain the presence of central receptors that bind hormones, especially in limbic and hypothalamic structures.

The increasing relevance of peptides becomes clearer as peptide circuitry is worked out. This is similar to the catecholamine systems, where the cell bodies of the neurone originate from a few discrete sites but influence wide areas of the brain. In the CNS, peptides can be divided into two groups depending on the origin of their cell bodies (Roberts et al., 1984): one group from the hypothalamus, the other has extrahypothalamic as well as hypothalamic neurones. The hypothalamic ones project to a variety of mainly limbic structures, including the limbic forebrain, the amygdala, the thalamus and the VTA. In contrast, the extrahypothalamic ones are less diverse, with local projections and longer fibre bundles suggesting more specific functions.

Some other specific roles for peptides can be defined. Thus substance P is thought to be involved with sensory transmission, being present in the dorsal roots of the spinal cord. Afferent fibres are seen in the substantia gelatinosa, an area known to be linked to pain perception, and in other areas related to pain such as the pain fibre-receptive region of the trigeminal nuclear complex (Iversen and Iversen, 1981). Release of substance P leads to intense pain. Enkephalin has been shown to exist in proximity to substance P neurones, and opiates inhibit the release of substance P. This suggests functional links between this peptide, opiates and pain appreciation.

There is an extensive network of CRF fibres running from the central amygdala to the hypothalamus, the parabrachial nuclei and on to the brainstem, notably the dorsomotor nucleus of the vagus. This transmitter and vasopressin seem linked with stress responses. CCK is also found in similar situations, and CCK antagonists have anxiolytic properties. CCK is now thought to be involved in the neurobiology of panic attacks and anxiety (Harro et al., 1993). Oxytocin receptors are plentiful in the forebrain, and this peptide, along with vasopressin, has aroused much interest recently. Oxytocin stimulates maternal behaviour in animals, while vasopressin has been shown to relate to pair bonding, revealed in differences in behaviour between two types of vole. The prairie vole forms longstanding pair bonds with a partner, while the montane vole does not, being more independent and promiscuous. Vasopressin infused into the cerebral ventricles of the male montane voles increases their bonding behaviour, an effect replicated by increasing (by DNA vector manipulation) their central vasopressin receptors. In contrast, female vole partner preference seems related to oxytocin (Lim et al., 2004).

Orexin A and B (hypocretin 1 and 2) are found in the lateral hypothalamus and regulate sleep and appetite. The latter is partly related to the efferent projections of orexin neurones, which include the cholinergic and monoaminergic cell clusters. Orexin deficiency is found in CSF in narcolepsy, especially when accompanied by cataplexy.

Neuron clusters in the lateral hypothalamus, such as the tuberomammillary nucleus and a cluster in the perifornical area, project widely to thalamus, basal forebrain and cortex and are involved with the sleep–wake architecture. The perifornical cells synthesize orexin, an excitatory neuropeptide which is involved in maintaining wakefulness. Neurones from the ventrolateral preoptic hypothalamic nucleus are reciprocally connected with the tuberomammillary nucleus, and also influence sleep–wake cycles via projections to hindbrain ascending monoamine, histaminergic and cholinergic arousal systems.

Insula

The insula occupies such a key position in the limbic lobe, anteriorly connected to the orbitofrontal cortex, and posteriorly to the parietal and temporal lobes, that it should not be surprising that it seems to play a part in many neuropsychiatric disorders. This has become especially apparent with brain-imaging studies. Polysensory inputs make the insula a site of multimodal convergence, interrelating events of the external world with relevant internally generated motivational states, but also providing affective tone and hedonic valence to perceptual experiences. In insula epilepsy, a variety of sensory symptoms may occur, including gustatory and olfactory ones, but also epigastric gurgling, rising epigastric sensations, nausea and even vomiting – truly visceral. The insula is also involved in the processing of pain and in addictive behaviours, being activated by salient visual cues (Shelley and Trimble, 2004). Deficits of emotional expression have been noted in patients with insula lesions. The insula has been regarded as the receptive cortex for visceral inputs, from vagus influences for example. One of the important insula efferents is to the central nucleus of the amygdala, with outputs to the bed nucleus of the stria terminalis and thence to the hypothalamus (the extended amygdala). These descending influences to the brainstem allow for reciprocal interplay on the afferent autonomic tone. Further, since the insula receives information from sensory cortex and the sphlanchnic vagal input reaches sensory cortex via the thalamus, there is scope for much integration of autonomic and sensory information within the brain.

Cingulate Gyrus

The cingulate gyrus is an extensive structure in the human brain, but from a neuropsychiatric point of view most attention has been paid to the anterior cingulate. It embraces cortical areas 23, 24 and 25 of Brodmann. The anterior cingulate-related disorders have much to do with motivation and movement, with the extensive dorsal and ventral striatal connections.

In the past the cytoarchitectural differences between the anterior granular cortex (area 32) and the posterior agranular cortex (area 24) were emphasized, but other distinctions are also realized. At least four functional divisions are suggested: a viscero-motor region (including area 32), a cognitive-effector region, a motor region (area 24) and a sensory processing region, as found progressing from anterior to posterior cingulate, respectively (Figure 3.2).

In animal models, the cingulate cortex is one limbic area which has been shown to be associated with vocalizations and primate calls on stimulation. Release of autonomic activity, including changes of breathing and heart rate, sexual arousal and automated oral behaviours, can also be observed. Cingulate epilepsy is characterized by brief episodes of alteration of consciousness, but signs may include vocalization, rapid onset of motor activity (axial flexion and limb extension) and gestural automatisms (Devinsky and Luciano, 1993).

In humans, the cingulate has been shown to be nociceptive, probably related to its thalamic afferents, and a wide variety of affective responses, including fear, euphoria, depression

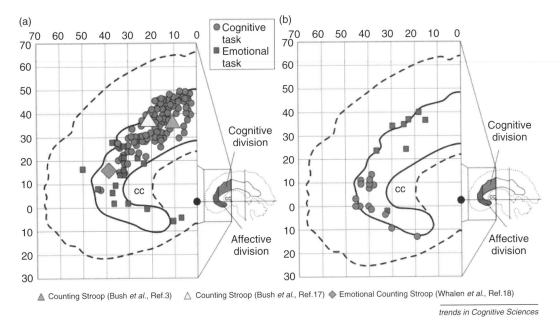

Figure 3.2   Meta-analysis of the different imaging studies carried out, highlighting the differences between the cognitive and affective divisions of the anterior cingulate. Note that the studies employing cognitive tasks, (a) commonly employing multitasking, cause activations in the upper cingulate (in circles), while studies manipulating emotion, (b) cause activation in the lower affective division (in rectangles) (reproduced from Bush *et al.*, 2000). A coloured version of this figure can be found on the colour plate

and aggression, have been elicited by stimulation in individual patients, as have behaviours characterized by disinhibition, hypersexuality, tic-like movements and obsessive and/or compulsive activity. Lesions of the anterior cingulate, which will lead to a pattern of behaviour characterized by emotional blunting and decreased motivation, are considered as one of the frontal lobe syndromes (see Figure 3.3).

Area 25, the subgenual cingulate area, has become a focus of considerable interest following observations that increased activity in this area is strongly associated with depression (Wu *et al.*, 1992), and it has become a target for surgical ablation for intractable depression and more recently for deep brain stimulation (see Chapter 12 and Figure 3.3). This area has reciprocal connections with other frontal areas, with the hypothalamus, the ventral striatum, the amygdala and the autonomic outputs of the brainstem (Johansen-Berg *et al.*, 2008).

New target for depression provided by functional imaging

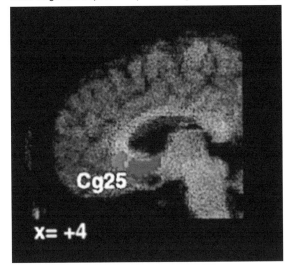

Figure 3.3   The position of the subgenial cingulate area, which has become a target for deep brain stimulation (courtesy of Dr Wayne Drevets)

The posterior regions of the cingulate gyrus have been less studied. They are less involved with motor functions and have more to do with visuospatial function and learning and memory, the latter being linked to the cingulate projections to the subiculum. Posteriorly, the cingulate gyrus blends with an area of parietal area cortex now thought to be involved with self-consciousness, the precuneus (see below).

Hippocampus

The hippocampus only has major cortical connections with the entorhinal cortex, but has extensive subcortical afferents and efferents, and thus is a conduit for multi-informational cortical influences on behaviour and is altered in structure or function in many neuropsychiatric disorders. It has been estimated that there is a 5% chance of a CA3 neurone synapsing with another hippocampal neurone, emphasizing the rich connectivity of the area and its role in memory. Many of the structures surrounding the hippocampus, such as the entorhinal, parasubicular and retrosplenial parts of the limbic lobe, are continuous with the hippocampus, rendering the hippocampus larger that it appears from surface anatomy. The hippocampus is involved in many neuropsychiatric disorders. One paradigm is temporal lobe epilepsy, but changes of structure or function have been noted in schizophrenia, the dementias and affective and anxiety disorders.

Thus it seems established that apoptosis (cell death) occurs in the postnatal hippocampus, and that in animal models psychotropic drugs such as antidepressants and electrical cortical stimulation (ECS) can stimulate neurogenesis. The plasticity within the structure is therefore substantial, perhaps interlinked with its central role in the modulation of so many behaviours, especially memory. A memory circuit, which includes the hippocampus, the fornix and the hypothalamic mammillary bodies, has long been identified, and bilateral removal of the hippocampi leads to a severe amnestic syndrome, with complete failure to lay down new episodic memories (anterograde memories).

A similar picture is seen after bilateral fornix damage.

Another hippocampal function relates to its function as a comparator of novel and familiar stimuli, matching to expectation or prediction, and in the initiation or inhibition of behavioural strategies as appropriate to the situation. It becomes linked therefore to emotions such as anxiety, and to motor responses as evoked by its ventral striatal outputs (Gray, 1982).

Parahippocampal Gyrus and Entorhinal Cortex

It was a puzzle for a long time how sensory inputs gained access to the limbic structures; this was part of the problem of the concept of the 'isolated' limbic system. In the 1960s cortico–cortical connections were unravelled, which revealed the projections from primary sensory areas to frontal association cortices, to multimodal cortical areas (parieto–temporo–occipital) and to temporal cortex. A cascade of increasingly complex sensory information thus reaches the limbic lobe from these primary, secondary and tertiary sensory inputs. These convey further integrated data about the environment to the limbic lobe. The input targets include the amygdala and the hippocampus, and the parahippocampal gyrus, overlaying these structures, provides a relay. Extensive processing of information occurs, in which real-time information about the environment integrates with past-time stored data of memory.

The entorhinal cortex (Brodmann's area 28), the anterior part of the parahippocampal gyrus, which can be identified with the naked eye in some brains by the surface warty protuberances called the verrucae hippocampi (which overlie an island of multipolar neurones), may be viewed as the great gate through which neocortical information reaches the hippocampus and thence other limbic system structures. The main conduit of this is the perforant pathway (see Figures 2.2 and 3.4).

There is clear evidence that this region has access to specific sensory and multimodal sensory representations. The links with the

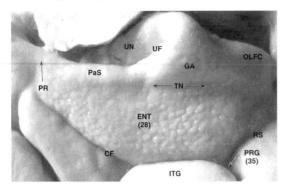

Figure 3.4   The ventromedial temporal lobe in the left hemisphere. The anterior parahippocampal gyrus is shown with small wart-like elevations. CF, colletral fissure; ENT, enterhinal cortex; GA, gyrus ambiens; ITG, inferior temporal gyrus; OLFC, primary olfactory cortex; PaS, parasubiculum; PR, perirhinal cortex; PRG, perirhinal gyrus; RS, rhinal sulcus; TN, tentorial notch; UF, uncle fissure; UN, uncus (courtesy of Dr van Hoesen)

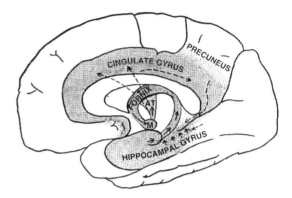

Figure 3.5   The parahippocampal gyrus and the precuneus. Note how the former has direct inputs to the latter. M, mammillary body; AT, anterior thalamic nucleus (reproduced from MacLean, 1949)

amygdala, and hence the hypothalamus and forebrain limbic structures, imply that the entorhinal cortex is another meeting point for integrating information regarding the affective and internal state of the organism with current and past sensory information. The traffic is two-way, however, both from sensory cortex to the limbic system and vice versa, allowing for limbic influences on sensory experiences.

Precuneus

The precuneus, occupying part of the medial parietal cortex, is continuous with the cortex of the posterior cingulate gyrus, and connected with the inferior parietal lobule (Figure 3.5). The precuneus links the limbic structures with the parietal neural apparatus involved with the body image and with exterior space. The posterior cingulate, the retrosplenial cortex and the precuneus area of the medial parietal lobe have been suggested to be linked to a neural network which correlates with autobiographical memories and self-consciousness. The precuneus is one of the sites where increased metabolic activity occurs while the brain is idling, when

the individual is self-reflecting, and activity decreases when attention is engaged in other tasks. Further, activity decreases in states of diminished self-awareness, such as anaestheaia, dementia or sleep (Cavanna and Trimble, 2006). This so-called default cerebral circuitry links the precuneus with medial frontal areas.

Amygdala, Extended Amygdala and Ventral Striatum

Two main divisions of the amygdala group of nuclei have been noted: the projections of the basolateral amygdala and the continuous bridge of cells from the central and medial nuclei through to the bed nucleus of the stria terminalis: the extended amygdala. The former have extensive outputs to the ventral striatum, a ventral extension of the basal ganglia, with connectivity to frontal cortical structures, with a central position in the cortico–striato–thalamocortical re-entrant circuits and with strong downstream connections to midbrain and hindbrain structures. Here limbic and frontal projections (serving cognitive executive functions) overlap, and this 'limbic loop' of the re-entrant circuits seems well suited for selecting appropriate adaptive behaviours for action (Heimer *et al.*, 2007).

The extended amygdala, which receives input from the laterobasal amygdala, projects to hypothalamus and other autonomic output structures. It is thought to coordinate the activities of multiple limbic regions in determining autonomic behavioural output.

A further area of anatomical interest has been the identification of two components of the accumbens, namely a core and a shell with distinguishing neurochemistry and connectivity (see Figure 2.31). The shell has basal ganglia connections, is closely linked to the extended amydala and has outputs to the hypothalamus and brainstem motor and autonomic structures. The shell has an abundance of D1 and mu-opioid receptors, which may be relevant to a role of the shell in addiction (see Chapter 9).

Nauta emphasized the integration between the limbic system and the basal ganglia (Nauta and Domesick, 1982), a project developed much further by Heimer and colleagues (2007). Thus, the structures of the limbic system, especially the amygdala, so vital for emotional interpretation of sensory stimuli, have direct pathways influencing motor output, which are additional to the somatic motor loops described above. The extended amygdala projects directly to autonomic and endocrine outflow areas, but can also modulate the circuitry of the motor loops and hence pyramidal outflow by influences on the gate setting of the VTA and substantia nigra. A further direct pathway is from the amygdala to prefrontal cortex, and hence to the motor area M3 and pyramidal tracts.

The ventrostriatopallidal system is thus seen not only as a radical alteration of our traditional views of the basal ganglia but also as an expansion of cortical output. The entire cortex projects to the basal ganglia, and all cortex uses basal ganglia mechanisms (Heimer *et al.*, 2007).

A reliable finding from *f*MRI studies is that emotional stimuli enhance amygdala activity, especially such stimuli as fearful faces, and evidence is accumulating that the amygdala is also associated with decision-making and thus through its output channels is central to guiding or even driving human behaviour. The latter may include the social appraisal of the emotional state of others, and value judgments in complex social situations.

Autonomic Nervous System

The autonomic nervous system has long been known to regulate such bodily activities as sweating, heart rate and respiratory rate, and to be involved in fear responses and the so-called 'flight and fight response'. In the course of phylogeny, the vagus nerve of mammals has developed two efferents: a myelinated one, originating in the nucleus ambiguus, and an unmyelinated one, originating in the dorsal motor nucleus of the vagus (see Figure 2.25). The myelinated fibres provide the primary vagus regulation of the heart and bronchi, while the unmyelinated fibres provide the primary vagus regulation to subdiaphragmatic organs.

Unique to mammals is the neuroanatomical and neurophysiological link in the brainstem between the source nuclei of the nerves controlling the striated muscles of the face and head, including the muscles of the middle ear, and the source nuclei of the myelinated vagus. Thus, in mammals there is a close connection between the regulation of the facial muscles and the visceral state. This provides a neurophysiological explanation for the covariation between facial emotional expression and changes of bodily state and feelings. The sensory pathways from the trigeminal and the facial nerve provide potent input to the nucleus ambiguus.

With development, the infant has more and more myelinated vagus fibres, as social communication and facial expressions and responses develop. There are facial-recognition areas in the fusiform and superior temporal gyri, which appear to detect intentionality of movement and may modulate the amygdala, leading to flow of neural activity to the appropriate output channels (macrosystems) for the required response to the facial expressions encountered. This explains the amygdala and fusiform responses to fearful faces shown with brain imaging.

The insula is central to this behaviour, with its vagus visceral afferents and outputs to amygdala, the bed nucleus of the stria terminalis (extended amygdala) and thence down to pontine and brainstem nuclei, influencing some of the very same nuclei that provided the autonomic input, including the nucleus ambiguus (Porges, 2007).

Subthalamic Nucleus

This area of the basal ganglia circuitry has excited much interest recently as it has become a target for DBS, especially in movement disorders. It lies close to the substantia nigra and is reciprocally connected to the globus pallidus externa and interna. However, it is suggested that as with other basal ganglia structures it is divided in its afferents and efferents, having a definable limbic component, which is connected to forebrain limbic structures and frontal cortical areas including the subgenual cingulate. This may explain why occasional patients suddenly develop emotional displays during subthalamic DBS (Bejjani et al., 1999).

SOME SPECIFIC BEHAVIOURS

Aggression

The relationship of the amygdala to aggression seems well established, although a reciprocal link with the hypothalamus and frontal cortex seems important. In one of the earliest studies of brain–behaviour relationships, Klüver and Bucy (1939) and then Schreiner and Kling (1956) tamed various aggressive feline species with bilateral amygdala lesions, an effect abolished by additional lesions in the ventrolateral hypothalamus. The Klüver–Bucy syndrome was one of the first limbic syndromes to be recognized. The main features were an alteration of personality with loss of aggressivity and taming, a tendency to repetitively explore the environment orally (hypermetamorphosis), hypersexuality and visual agnosia.

Aggression can be provoked by stimulation of the amygdala, the hypothalamus and the area around the fornix in the diencephalon, and hypothalamic elicited aggression can be inhibited by stimulation of the ipsilateral frontal cortex (Siegel et al., 1975). Delgado (1966), using implanted intracerebral multilead electrodes to stimulate various regions of the brain in monkeys, also recorded aggressive responses from the ventral posterolateral nucleus of the thalamus and the central grey area. Rosvold et al. (1954) demonstrated how amygdala lesions lead to loss of dominance in a social hierarchy.

Adamec, based on studies with kindling, introduced the concept of 'limbic permeability'. Thus kindling is an experimental procedure in which small, brief, high-frequency currents are passed across electrodes in an area of brain. At first no effects are seen, but after several trials, usually given on a daily basis, an after-discharge develops, and behaviour changes are seen. As the process continues, eventually the animal, in spite of still receiving subthreshold doses, will have a generalized seizure. The associated changes in brain physiology, as yet not well identified but thought to be related to LTP, are long-lasting, and the animal remains susceptible to a seizure on passing the current for the rest of its life. Kindling occurs best in limbic-system structures, especially from the amygdala and hipocampus.

Adamec and Stark-Adamec (1983) used cats to kindle lasting behavioural changes, notably aggressiveness or defensiveness. Limbic permeability, the degree and facility of seizure propagation from limbic to hypothalamic areas, could be related to these behaviour changes.

The frontal cortex is also part of the circuitry that modulates aggressive responses. Stimulation of frontal cortex at the same time as the hypothalamus increases the time to an aggressive episode in cats (Siegel et al., 1975), and in patients with epilepsy, very aggressive behaviour interictally has been shown with MRI imaging to be associated with thinning of the left lateral frontal cortex (Tebartz van Elst et al., 2003).

The literature on the role of various transmitters in aggressive behaviour is confusing and highly species-dependent. It is further complicated by the differing models of aggression involved. Generally, decreasing the turnover of 5-HT, and increasing cholinergic or catecholaminergic drive, facilitates aggressive behaviour. Tricyclic antidepressants and monoamine oxidase inhibitors (MAOI) are likewise facilitatory (Eichelmann, 1979), as are hormonal influences, for example the increase in aggression associated with testosterone.

In summary, while the spontaneous display of aggression is obviously dependent on environmental stimuli from many sources, the central roles of the amygdala and the hypothalamus in its neural organization seem established from animal studies. Since the frontal cortex has intimate connections with the hypothalamus and the amygdala, these findings hint at a behavioural circuit, although the details, especially in humans, remain to be elucidated.

Anxiety and the Septohippocampal Link

The existence of a behavioural inhibition system which modulates anxiety responses has been proposed (Gray, 1982). The neural counterpart of this is the septohippocampal circuit, and anxiolytic drugs are thought to act by inhibiting this system. Briefly, lesions of the septal area or the hippocampus lead to a pattern of behaviours similar to that seen after giving anxiolytic drugs, and stimulation of the septal area creates the opposite effect. The septohippocampal system forms an extensive interconnected neural network, and acts, with the associated Papez circuit, as a comparator, generating predictions about anticipated events and matching them to actual events. Mismatch allows the behavioural inhibition system to dominate, interrupting behaviour and generating a search for alternatives by increased arousal and attention. The ascending monoaminergic systems, especially noradrenaline and 5-HT, modulate information flow into the hippocampus.

A shortcoming of this model is the lack of reference to the amygdala. However, amygdala lesions dramatically influence anxiety responses (as in the Klüver–Bucy syndrome), and benzodiazepine receptors are plentiful in the amygdala. Microinjections of benzodiazapines into the amygdala, but not the hippocampus, reduce fear (LeDoux, 1992).

Neural circuits for the conditioning of autonomic and fear responses have been worked out in animal models using auditory stimuli (LeDoux *et al.*, 1988). There are essentially two pathways involved. The first is from auditory cortex to inferior colliculus to medial geniculate to amygdala, extended amygdala and the autonomic and somatomotor outputs. This direct subcortical pathway does not involve cortical associations and is essentially rapid but crude. The second circuit involves the neocortical auditory system, feeding to the amygdala via association cortices, giving a more delayed route, with refinement of the message. LeDoux tries to resolve the issue of the relative contributions of the amygdala and hippocampus by drawing a distinction between fear and anxiety. The former relates more to interactions between sensory processing areas and the amygdala, and affective implications are assessed. Hippocampal inputs to the amygdala contribute cognitive information, leading to anxiety for specific situations (see Figure 2.16).

Memory

Other functions assigned to the hippocampus, in light of electrophysiological stimulation and lesion experiments, mainly relate to memory. Although severe memory problems after hippocampal destruction were first defined in humans, animal studies produced conflicting data. Several competing theories now exist, although all ascribe to the hippocampus a role in higher cognitive function. One suggestion is that it is involved in the construction of spatial maps (O'Keefe and Nadel, 1978); an alternative is that it subserves spatial memory. Its precise role in human memory is unclear, but relates either to the consolidation of short-term memory or to the retrieval of information once remembered.

Squire *et al.* (1989) have suggested that the CA1 and CA3 fields of the hippocampus are especially involved in receiving and transmitting highly integrated information to and from the neocortex, sites of permanent memory being cortical.

The role of neuronal plasticity is crucial. The NMDA receptor is related to the development of LTP (increased postsynaptic excitability after a volley of impulses) in the CA1 region. Depolarization of the non-NMDA glutamate receptor is required to open the NMDA channel, but only with synergistic firing of adjacent synapses or burst firing. This leads to synapse modification with strengthening of synaptic connections and the potential for the laying down of memory traces. Acetylcholine is another neurotransmitter involved in the laying down of episodic memories.

The amygdala also plays a crucial role in memory, notably for emotionally influenced memories. Fear learning is inhibited by injection of protein synthesis inhibitors into the amygdala. In laying down memory traces, the hippocampus and amygdala are thought to synchronize in the encoding of information, the hippocampus encoding through time and space while the amygdala provides emotional valence and contributes to reinforcement. Other crucial areas are the entorhinal and perirhinal cortices, the fornix and the mammillary bodies.

However, memory consolidation involves a progression of trace migration from these allocortial structures to the neocortex, and frontal, cingulate and parietal areas are especially involved. The neural correlates of memories decrease their dependence on the hippocampus, and become widely distributed in cortex. With time, due to the continued plasticity of the brain and the recharging of memories through recall (each time different from the time before), remodelling occurs. Memory is actually only one way of forgetting.

Sexual Behaviour

The changes in sexual activity seen with the Klüver–Bucy syndrome were confirmed in other species. The amygdala seems to be important in its regulation, and hypersexuality induced by amygdala destruction can be reversed by septal lesions (Kling *et al.*, 1960), supporting the role of the latter in pleasurable sexual experiences. Penile erection in monkeys can be seen after stimulation of the septum (MacLean and Ploog, 1962), and electrical activity is recorded here in female rabbits and humans with orgasm (Heath, 1972; Sawyer, 1957). The hypothalamus is clearly involved in sexual behaviour, and lesions in the anterior hypothalamus prevent the hormonal activation of sexual activity (Heimer and Larsson, 1966).

There are many steroid-binding sites in hypothalamic regions that interact with systemic hormones to modulate behaviour, further interrelated with the influence of monoamine and peptide systems (Herbert, 1984).

Arousal, Sleep and the Reticular Formation

Arousal and consciousness are related to the tonic control of the ascending reticular formation, extending from the medulla upwards to the thalamus. On stimulation of this area there is desynchronization of the EEG and behavioural arousal. Lesions in this area lead to permanent sleep, although regions within it, such as the median raphe, when destroyed lead to a state of permanent insomnia. Thus, the homogeneous mass of reticular neurones referred to originally as the reticular activating system has now been shown to contain within it many different neuronal groups, including the origins of the long-ascending monoamine and peptide pathways, and nuclei sensitive to sensory information from the cardiovascular and respiratory system. Some of its efferents descend to the spinal cord, influencing motor neurones and sensory afferents. Thus, the reticular formation receives input fibres from adjacent ascending and descending tracts and nuclei, the hypothalamus, the limbic system and cortex, and moderates arousal, conscious activity and sleep–wake cycles. Cholinergic transmission, especially via relays in the thalamus, is important in arousal and in generating REM sleep (the period of sleep associated with dreaming and cortical desynchronization on the EEG).

Motion, Emotion and Motivation

Even today, exploration of the neurobiology of one of the most fundamental attributes of behaviour, namely what makes you tic(k), is in its infancy. The most significant advances in this field have derived from the discoveries of Olds and Milner (1954), and those of Nauta (1964, 1986; Nauta and Domesick, 1982), Heimer and others, who unravelled the essential links between the limbic system and the basal ganglia, revealing the role of the latter in motivation. Thus, traditionally the basal ganglia were viewed as being solely related to motor behaviour. However, emotional display involves motor patterns (hence e-motion), motor abnormalities are seen in patients with psychiatric illness as a part of their symptomatology (Trimble, 1981a) and motor disorders are frequently associated with psychopathology (Trimble, 1981a). Movement and emotion are linked in common speech (hence 'a moving experience').

The extended amygdala and the accumbens (limbic basal ganglia) are central to these concepts. The limbic efferents to cerebral cortex relate both to the development of memories and, especially from the amygdala, to the emotional valence of ongoing sensory stimuli. The hippocampal and amygdala outputs to the ventral striatum serve to gate information in cortico–striatal–pallidal–thalamic circuits, and hence the outflow to both the motor pathways and also association and frontal cortices. Further, autonomic activity is coordinated with this by the extensive network of rostrocaudal connections from the extended amygdala through hypothalamus, periaqueductal grey, ventrolateral medulla and on to the efferent nuclei of the vagus nerve and sympathetic nervous system. These CNS sites seem to cooperate and coordinate visceral and motor functions, allowing for a comprehensive emotional motor output, and the term 'emotional motor system' has been used to describe the autonomic components of this (Holstege, 1996).

In this scheme, the dorsal striatum is seen as being involved with neocortically derived motor behaviours, and the ventral striatum is related to emotional arousal and expression. These striatal structures are filters of limbic and cortical information, permitting appropriate signals to gain access to motor pathways (Mogenson *et al.*, 1980). The role of dopamine is crucial here. The mesolimbic–prefrontal dopamine system lacks autoreceptors, has a higher cell-firing rate than the other dopamine neurones and is the only one to show an increased turnover in response to stress.

The limbic output to the basal ganglia structures is massive, and until this became realized (with the new anatomical investigations of the past 40 years) there was a failure to understand the neurology of behaviour in any complexity. 'A greater portion of behaviour is nondeterministic, an outcome governed by genetic predispositions, societal norms, learning, reward and motivation. It is this aspect of behaviour with which the limbic lobe and basal forebrain are largely concerned ... neural output derivative of higher order, cortically derived cognitive representations, is channelled from the greater limbic lobe through several macrosystems, each of which may read messages differently and redistribute them back in altered form to the brainstem and, via re-entrant circuits, back to the cognitive apparatus...' (Heimer *et al.*, 2007, pp. 100, 104).

It is interesting in this context that disorders of motivation are barely considered in classifications of psychopathology. Yet essential to behaviour is action, giving direction and change to the status quo. Included would be impulse, desire and striving towards goals, individual motivations being variously consciously available or not. Patients with primary amotivational states are frequently encountered in clinical practice, and secondary disorders of motivation are noted in a wide variety of psychopathologies (see Chapter 9). The unravelling of the neuroanatomy of the limbic forebrain allows for an understanding of these behaviours, which correlate closely with that prime biological and notably human force, the will, once seen as an independent psychological faculty, now viewed as tightly bound with identifiable neuroanatomical and neurochemical substrates.

LIMBIC LOBE DISORDERS IN A CLINICAL CONTEXT

In clinical neurology it is customary to ascribe certain signature syndromes to various cortical lobes. Thus there are well-recognized parietal-lobe syndromes, such as the apraxias or the alexias, and there are the frontal-lobe syndromes (see below). However, few texts describe specific limbic-lobe disorders. An exception is temporal-lobe epilepsy, which is discussed in detail in Chapter 10.

Limbic encephalitis is a rare disorder, secondary to certain viral infections, notably rabies (rarely), and more commonly herpes simplex. Following a prodromal phase of nonspecific symptoms, behavioural changes occur with herpes simplex which include bizarre out-of-character behaviour, sometimes hallucinations, and also epileptic seizures. The EEG may reveal unilateral or bilateral changes in temporal leads. The HSV-1 virus leads to marked pathology in frontal and temporal areas, and the chronic state is characterized by dense amnesia, irritability and aggression, distractibility, emotional blunting and features of the Klüver–Bucy syndrome. It is possible to look for autoimmune antibodies to human brain intracellular or membrane antigens to establish diagnosis.

A variant is seen in some patients with carcinoma. This also presents with disturbances of affect, depression, anxiety, and sometimes hallucinations and/or seizures. It is seen most commonly with bronchial oat-cell carcinomas, and pathology is noted in the amygdala, hippocampus, fornix and mammillary bodies. It is thought to be secondary to an immunological process, but the observations that such relatively selective pathologies target the limbic lobe suggests that their anatomical location and underlying neuronal constitution have some specific defining biological markers.

In the Urbach–Wiethe syndrome there is selective bilateral degeneration of the amygdala, and relatively selective temporal pole – medial temporal limbic damage can be seen after head injuries.

RE-ENTRANT CIRCUITS IN A CLINICAL CONTEXT

The theory of the parallel cortical–subcortical re-entrant circuits (see Figures 2.11 and 2.12) has had an important impact on the understanding of several neuropsychiatric disorders. As should now be clear, they are central not only to motor systems, but also to a broad understanding

of the behavioural ramifications of limbic function and dysfunction. Altered activity in the descending cortical–striatal–thalamic loops influences motor output via the cascade of inhibitory and excitatory neurotransmitters which regulate activity in these circuits. In general, the parallel distributed nature of the circuits suggests that interventions or lesions at one of the nodal points (e.g. the pallidum) will lead to a similar clinical picture to a lesion at another point within the same circuit. Secondly, the implication is that a lesion in one circuit will be somewhat self-contained, and that the resulting behavioural effects will be different to those noted with changes in an adjacent circuit. Quite how segregated such 'basal ganglia loops' are in reality is however unclear, and there is good evidence of cross-talk between them. Nonetheless, they have formed a paradigm which has been used effectively to explain many clinical observations. This is illustrated for example with the descriptions of three different prefrontal syndromes, noted following lesions of one of the three prefrontal described circuits, namely the dorso–lateral, the orbital and the medial frontal–cingulate circuit (Figure 2.29).

Thus, central to the above three syndromes is alteration of motor, emotional and motivational behaviours and involvement of the ventral striatum. In contrast, the syndromes related to the dorsal circuitry, such as Parkinson's disease – in which the dopamine input to the dorsolateral caudate-putamen degenerates – present initially with motor symptoms, some tremor and muscle stiffening. However, because these disorders, as they progress or are influenced by treatment, involve ventral striatal structures, behaviour problems then also emerge as a significant part of the clinical picture. In Parkinson's disease, 40% of patients will develop depressive syndromes, and as the disease progresses, psychoses may appear. It is estimated that 30% of patients will have hallucinations, and about 10–20% develop frank psychoses, often exacerbated by dopamine agonists.

In a psychiatric context, these circuits have been used to help understand the underlying neuroanatomy of several disorders. A paradigm is obsessive–compulsive disorder (OCD), often linked to neurological disorders involving these structures and with alteration in fronto-basal ganglia activity revealed using brain-imaging techniques (see Chapter 6). Neurosurgical operations and direct brain stimulation for OCD and a number of other neurological and psychiatric disorders involve interfering with these circuits (see Chapter 12).

THE FRONTAL LOBES IN A CLINICAL CONTEXT

Recognition of the strategic importance of the frontal lobes in understanding human behaviour is often attributed to the observations of John Martyn Harlow, who described the case of the now famous Phineas Gage. The unfortunate man had a tamping iron driven at high velocity through the frontal part of his skull; he survived the injury but was left with severe personality changes. The site of the injury has recently been reconstructed, and shown to involve the ventromedial region of both frontal lobes, a part of the frontal cortex connected with subcortical structures such as the amygdala and hypothalamus; however, since the injury left the rest of the frontal lobes intact, Gage developed no speech or general intellectual impairments. It was his social judgement that was affected, leaving him 'no longer Gage' (Damasio *et al.*, 1994).

It is now customary to refer to three rather distinct frontal-lobe syndromes, based on the underlying neuroanatomy of any lesions or functional disturbances. In reality, many patients with frontal pathology show a combination of symptoms, partly based on the clinical fact that injuries such as head injuries or tumours fail to obey natural lines of dissection, but also on a relative fragility of the links between anatomy and behaviour in general, and the nature of the cortical–subcortical circuitry. In other words, the manifestations of a frontal syndrome may differ with the extent of subcortical tissue involvement. Further, so-called executive functions, while perhaps driven by activation in the frontal areas, involve the brain in a much broader context. Motor knowledge,

the ability to perform and contain on-line a continuous sequence of desired movements and their operation, implicates also executive attention and memory: so-called working memory. In considering activity in frontal networks, it is important to consider their extensive input from posterior cortical areas, notably linking sensory association areas with motor equivalents, which are reciprocated in what Fuster refers to as a perception–action cycle (Bodner *et al.*, 2005; Fuster, 2004). Thus, the so-called corollary action of frontal activity, the anticipatory monitoring of ongoing sensory and motor action in response to an action, with feedback and feed-forward loops having corrective and modulating attributions, is related to frontal efferent discharge to the association cortices of the parietal and temporal cortices via the longitudinal and arcuate fasciculi. The additional reciprocal limbic–frontal connectivity allows memory and motivational components of the cognitive hierarchy to be incorporated into an action sequence.

The three main syndromes of neuropsychiatric interest are the orbital, the dorsolateral and the medial syndromes. The dorsolateral syndrome, involving isocortex, with anatomical conectivities to the thalamus, hypothalamus, amygdala and hippocampus, and prominent outflows to the caudate nucleus, is often complex and can be variable in presentation. It may involve problems with motor facility and temporal integration, leading to perseverations and motor persistence, such that performing sequenced hand positions (such as the Luria three-hand-position test) is impaired, or patients may have difficulty copying from design templates with alternating patterns, such as multiple loops. The mental inflexibility is revealed with such tests as the Wisconsin card-sorting test, in which sorting of cards into different groups is achieved only by the examinee detecting an undisclosed rule; the rule is then changed by the examiner, and the new one must be followed. The failure to shift the mental set with perseveration is then revealed in someone with a lesion involving this dorsolateral circuit.

Representations of the world must be held on-line, prior to action (working memory), and when disturbed this leads to problems with tasks of short-term and intermediate memory. There is poor spontaneous recall and a 'forgetting to remember'; however, recognition memory and memory for implicit tasks (motor acts) remains intact. Language tasks such as word-list generation are impaired more following dominant hemisphere lesions, while design-fluency tasks (generating as many different designs in a one-minute time interval) are impaired with nondominant lesions.

With the dorsolateral syndrome, planning is impaired, and shows up in tasks such as the Tower of London test and variants, in which patients are asked to rearrange objects in as few moves as possible to achieve a specified pattern. Sometimes the inability to inhibit a response is shown; the Stroop test is one such task, in which the patient has to state the colour of a word where the colour in which it is printed (say blue) is different from the word itself (say green). The natural tendency is to read 'green', which has to suppressed. They may be unable to inhibit a motor response; for example, when asked to tap once in response to the examiner tapping twice, and tap twice when the examiner taps once, they will tend to tap as the examiner. Estimating answers to unusual questions may be awry ('How tall is the Empire State Building?'), as may proverb interpretation, which becomes concrete.

Stimulus binding and environmental dependence are key features of the dorsolateral syndrome, shown by poor attention with easy distractibility, poor planning abilities and concretization of thought. Attentional problems lead to a reduced digit span and failure on continuous performance tasks. Further, a number of patients will show either utilization behaviour or imitation behaviour, where attention is captivated and dominated by environmental stimuli. In utilization behaviour, patients use objects placed in front of them even if they do not need to. The classic example is giving a patient a pair of glasses to wear when they already have a pair on; they will put on the second pair without removing the first. In imitation behaviour, the patient copies even complex movements of the examiner (such as picking up a patella hammer

that the examiner has used and tapping the examiner with it).

The dorsolateral syndrome is summed up by the expression 'executive function'. The term 'dysexecutive syndrome' has become popular to short-hand this clinical picture. Unfortunately this term suggests some overarching supervisory system, which fails to emphasize the flexible and dynamic nature of the neuronal systems involved, and the important roles of the basal ganglia and parietal cortex in integrating behaviour.

The medial frontal syndrome is related to lesions involving the anterior cingulate cortex, with extensive connections to limbic and subcortical structures, and is associated with apathy and loss of drive for many or most of an individual's daily activities. Affect is flattened, there is an emotional emptiness, social contacts are diminished, and lack of interest in others and the self are seen. Self-neglect, reduced spontaneous behaviour and speech, increased dependence and sometimes abulia (complete loss of will) may be seen, with patients sitting doing nothing for long periods of time, not getting bored at all. In bilateral cingulate lesions, akinetic mutism appears, with virtual lack of spontaneous interaction with the world, in spite of being awake and following events visually. The medial syndrome is summed up by the expression 'apathy'.

In the orbital frontal syndrome, patients like Gage display a lack of social concern and judgement. They are disinhibited, tactless and aggressive in social interactions, and lack insight into their coarseness. Their capacity for empathy is diminished and they display poor risk assessment. This clinical picture is sometimes referred to as 'pseudopsychopathic'. The key anatomical connectivities are again limbic and subcortical, especially the amygdala, hippocampus, thalamus and hypothalamus. The orbital syndrome is summed up by the expression 'disinhibition'.

Disturbed affect is common in people with frontal lesions. This may be a lability, which to the uninitiated may seem at times like a bipolar disorder. Depressive-like behaviour seems common, but testing may reveal the associated cognitive stamps of a frontal lesion. However, there are clear associations between disorders of affect and frontal activity, as revealed particularly with neuroimaging studies and discussed in Chapter 6.

LATERALITY

It is now well accepted that in the human brain there is lateralization of functions within the cerebral cortex. Potentialities to lateralization, which are suggested in some other species, have actualized in our evolution with huge consequences. Many aspects of speech are linked, in right-handed people, to the left hemisphere, while spatial and emotional processing is more a function of the right hemisphere. This skewing of the brain's functional allocation must have had evolutionary advantages, placing representations that did not need to be bilateral, as for example those regulating vision or the motor functions of the two hands obviously do, in one or other hemisphere. This would minimize brain size and energy consumption, and allow for continued safety of the process of birth in mammals. Neurones with the same type of computational activity are placed together, aiding the developing brain and minimizing the need for long-distance connecting axons. It seems that functional asymmetry in humans begins early in life, blood flow showing a right-hemisphere predominance until about age three, when a shift to the left occurs. What is less clear is whether or not the primitive cortical, limbic and subcortical structures of the brain also have lateralized functions, and if they do, how this may influence, or have influenced in the course of evolution, the overlying cortical development. The animal experimental literature suggests that lateralization of even limbic and subcortical structures is indeed the case (Vallortigara, 2006a, 2006b).

Thus some suggestion of lateralization of function can be found in species all the way along the phylogeny from fish to nonhuman primates, which relates not only to basic behaviours but also to everyday social repertoires, and the overall conclusion seems to be that lateralization of function in the brain is found across many vertebrate species. With regards to limbic structures, there is good evidence from primates, from human brain stimulation studies and from patients with epilepsy of lateralization. It has been shown for example that in rhesus monkeys and marmosets there is a population bias for the right hemisphere to control emotional expressions. In humans, the right amygdala is associated with fear and panic. Tachycardia recorded during seizures is associated with right-temporal-lobe epilepsy, and human micturition seems regulated by a group of cortical and subcortical structures predominantly right-sided. There is evidence for lateralization of function in the human insula, especially with regards to the control of autonomic activity.

Several of the major neurotransmitter systems in the brain, which drive and regulate behaviour, seem asymmetrically distributed in animal and human brains, including dopamine, acetylcholine and GABA (all with a left-hemisphere predominance), and 5-HT and noradrenaline (which have right-sided predominance). Separate processing abilities of the two hemispheres may relate to these observations, since such neurotransmitters, involved with the expression of motor behaviour and attention, may link with the differing hemisphere capabilities, and the right hemisphere's capacity in *Homo sapiens* for maintaining holistic, global representations, which are closely related to arousal and attentional mechanisms.

4

Classifications and Clinical Investigations

INTRODUCTION

Although it is readily apparent in case conferences, it is often poorly appreciated that our concepts of disease are not immutable, and various models may be proposed. It is customary to assume that a disease has some independent existence of its own, visiting our healthy bodies and altering them in some way. Physicians note these changes, establish the pattern that they assume, ascribe a diagnosis and prescribe a remedy that will influence the disease process. Earlier theories using this model attributed disease to the intrusion of spirits and evil forces, often as a punishment for wrongdoing. Later theories were given the most powerful boost by the discovery of microorganisms, and their cure by antibiotics. However this led, in many instances, especially of infections, to disease being seen as having a single cause, and, ideally, a single treatment.

Hippocrates (c. 460–c. 380 BC) introduced the historical dimension to disease, and the first case histories in medicine were from this era. A disease has signs and symptoms, a beginning, a course, a duration and an outcome. Recognition of diseases as independent entities did not come until the 17th century, however, and the works of Baglivi and Sydenham, who felt that diseases in their natural states were subject to the same laws of observation and description as other natural phenomena. The final step was made by Virchov, who combined his cellular pathology with the new knowledge of anatomicoclinical medicine, completing the notion of disease as a local affection. The research for classification systems as well as aetiology became predominant.

Entwined with the development of the concept of a disease as an independent local entity has been the principle of reaction: Sydenham (1740), in spite of his attempts to study the natural history of diseases, recognized this important element: '. . . a disease is nothing else but Nature's endeavour to thrust forth with all her might the morbifick matter for the health of the patient. . .' (p. 1). Thus intrinsic, as opposed to extrinsic, factors assume importance in the pathogenesis of symptoms. The reactions of the organism were seen as healing.

This 'biographic' conception of disease stands in obvious contrast to the 'ontological' one, in the sense that it admits only diseased individuals, and not diseases *per se*. It has had a marked influence in psychiatry. The testimony of individuals, as opposed to clinical observation, assumes with this model an ever-increasing significance. The introspective techniques of the psychoanalytic method took this to its extreme, devaluing diagnosis, elevating the subjective and, in most cases, allowing its practitioners the excuse not even to physically examine their patients! The phrase 'reaction types' became an accepted nomenclature, especially in the United States, under the influence of both psychoanalytic thinking and the contributions of Adolf Meyer. Extreme conclusions of this stance have been taken by some

Biological Psychiatry 3e   Michael R. Trimble and Mark S. George
© 2010 John Wiley & Sons, Ltd

authors, such as Szasz, who would deny the very existence of psychiatric illness.

Finally, the technology of the 20th century saw statistics used in attempts to define disease. It was Galton who, in the 19th century, successfully applied mathematical and statistical methods to the measure of biological phenomena, and demonstrated how this could also be done for psychological data. The use of statistical models for the definition of normality was adopted by psychiatry, especially for personality disorders, and the development of a large range of rating scales of psychopathology derived from these techniques.

SIGNS, SYMPTOMS, SYNDROMES AND DISEASE

In clinical medicine we recognize two fundamental kinds of data. *Symptoms* are those complaints of the patient that are spontaneously reported or are elicited by the clinical history. *Signs* are observed by the physician, the patient, or a friend or relative of the patient, and indicate the presence of some abnormal functioning of one or more body systems. A *syndrome* is a constellation of signs and symptoms which seem to coalesce to provide a recognizable entity with defining characteristics. Syndromes may be classified, and are the clinical representatives of illness. The latter implies some biological change or variation of the organism, and the task of medical science has been to explore this. A clear distinction has to be drawn between illness and disease: illness is that with which the patient presents, which only in part represents the expression of disease. Biological psychiatry attempts to understand psychiatric illness through defining syndromes and ultimately diseases, based on a knowledge of the associated changes of the structure and function of the central nervous system and their provoking factors.

At the present time, classification of disease in medicine generally represents a potpourri of notions, some being defined by symptoms (such as epilepsy, migraine or schizophrenia), others by aetiology (such as syphilis) and still others by pathology (such as Alzheimer's disease).

Indeed, with regard to the CNS, no attempt has been made to provide a comprehensive classification since that of Romberg in 1853. In general, in medicine progress has led from syndrome delineation and the classification based upon it to an understanding of pathology and a new classification. General Paresis of the Insane (GPI) is now classified as a syndrome of syphilis. Unfortunately, for many psychiatric syndromes, the underlying aetiologies and pathogeneses are unclear, and reliance on syndrome classification has led to a multitude of different classification systems. An important question is why psychiatry largely remains at the level of syndrome classification, when much of medicine, and even neurology, has moved beyond syndromes to disease classification. This is likely due to the until-recent inability to examine the main organ of interest (namely the brain) while patients are alive, the lack of readily identifiable neuropathological changes at autopsy, mistaken notions about the mind and brain, and the sheer complexity of the brain and its links to behaviours. Advances in brain-imaging techniques, combined with the search for endophenotypes and more refined genetics, hold the promise that biological psychiatry may rapidly regain lost ground. As Hughlings Jackson noted (Taylor, 1958), there are two ways to classify flowers: as a gardener or as a botanist. At present we still use the techniques of the gardener, but are progressing towards the position of the botanist.

CLASSIFICATION IN PSYCHIATRY

The two main diagnostic systems in use at present are the International Classification of Diseases (ICD), which derives from the World Health Organization, and the American Psychiatric Association's Diagnostic and Statistical Manual of Mental Disorders, 4th edition TR (text revised). It is important to emphasize that, although diagnostic fashion changes frequently, some of the categories that we use today were recognized by many earlier generations, and have a degree of constancy over time. Further, the classifications discussed will themselves soon be modified in the light of clinical experience and the accumulation of knowledge, particularly as more biological correlates of clinical syndromes become manifest.

Kraepelin's textbook of psychiatry went through nine editions, and his views evolved with time and experience. Prognosis was an essential feature of his system, and this was related to diagnosis. Dementia praecox and manic–depressive psychosis were his two main groupings, involutional melancholia and paranoia being considered as separate entities. Three forms of dementia praecox were described, namely the hebephrenic, the catatonic and the paranoid. These fundamental categories of psychopathology form the framework of the system in use today. The ideas of the Kraepelinian system were opposed to the unitary psychosis model, and reaffirmed the disease concept firmly for psychiatry.

One more term should briefly be discussed, namely 'endogenous'. The meaning of this is unclear though unfortunately it is still in popular use. Aubrey Lewis (1971) pointed out that the term 'endogenous' is often merely a cloak for ignorance. Its introduction was strongly linked to the 19th century European degeneration theory, and Lewis felt its use 'should be openly linked to presumptive evidence of a powerful hereditary factor in causation' (p. 196).

Karl Jaspers (1883–1969)

Although Jaspers' *Allgemeine Psychopathologie* was first written in 1913 and went through nine editions, the English translation did not become available until 1963. Nonetheless, the influence of his thinking has been widespread, especially in Europe. His approach was strongly empirical, despite being rooted in the philosophical school of phenomenology. Jaspers developed a method for examining the mental state of another person, which, in its purest form, attempts to delineate psychic events as sharply as possible. Central to his theme is the distinction between the psychological development of the individual (psychogenic development) and an organic disease process. He also makes a clear distinction between understanding a psychological process (*Verstehen*) (e.g. why someone is sad following

a loss) and providing a causal neurobiological explanation (*Erklären*) (e.g. a tumour in the frontal cortex causally explains the features of a frontal lobe syndrome).

Some quotations from his book (Jaspers, 1963) emphasize these issues:

> *Phenomenology . . . gives a concrete description of the psychic states which patients actually experience and presents them for observation (p. 55).*
>
> *Form must be kept distinct from content . . . from the phenomenological point of view it is only the form that interests us. . . (p. 58).*

Jaspers was clearly opposed to those who confused form and content, and he emphasized how the theories of Freud provided psychological understanding but were not biologically causal. Freud was concerned only with the content of the mental state and not the underlying causal neurobiology or endophenotypes. Jasper's approach differed from that of Kraepelin in emphasizing a descriptive psychopathology rather than actual diseases. It was continued by Kurt Schneider (1887–1967), who further developed criteria to distinguish development from process and introduced what are now referred to as the first-rank symptoms of Schneider. From these developments diagnostic tools such as the earlier 'present-state examination' (PSE) of Wing and colleagues (1974) and the currently-used Structured Clinical Interview for DSM IV (SCID) emerged.

Current Classifications

The classification schemes currently in use in psychiatry are based almost entirely on symptoms. Various operational definitions have been introduced and are widely employed, the basis of which is the completion of a checklist of symptoms, signs and historical facts which must be satisfied before a diagnosis is made. ICD 10 came into use in 1992, DSM IV in 1994. In the section that follows, emphasis is given both to DSM IV and ICD 10. A 'text revision' of the DSM IV, known as the DSM IV-TR, was published in 2000. The diagnostic categories and the vast majority of the specific criteria for diagnosis were unchanged, but the text sections giving extra information on each diagnosis were updated, as were some of the diagnostic codes, in order to maintain consistency with the ICD. DSM V has had initial comments in 2010. DSM IV-TR adopts a multi-axial classification, but this is not overemphasized. However, it is in keeping with the distinction drawn by Jaspers between personality disorder and psychiatric illness. Axis 1 refers to clinical syndromes, axis 2 covers developmental and personality disorders, and axes 3, 4 and 5 refer to physical disorders, psychosocial stressors and global assessment of functioning respectively. It is not intended that a comprehensive classification be given here, and attention is given to the disorders that relate to subsequent chapters.

The newer versions of these ICD and DSM systems, although perhaps slightly improved, still fundamentally represent committee-derived consensus about classifications of symptoms, and continue to fail to make the needed leap, at some point, into disease definitions based on firm understanding of pathophysiology. The rest of medicine has progressed to disease classifications based on endophenotypes defined by genetics, or biomarkers such as imaging data, but ICD and DSM systems are fundamentally symptom-based systems. The updated versions of these systems, while perhaps necessary for some issues, are fundamentally incomplete in not moving into a pathophysiological, endopheno-type approach, as is used in the rest of modern medicine and neurology (see Chapter 13 for an attempt at a new classification scheme).

An example of this evolution has occurred in the area of multiple sclerosis (MS). Twenty years ago MS was a disorder diagnosed on purely clinical grounds, with lesions separated in time and space. There were a few helpful confirmatory tests, but nothing definitive. The ability to give individual prognosis was limited, and treatments were largely ineffective. Now the disease is almost 100% identifiable with brain imaging, and other ancillary tests can exclude rare forms. This newfound ability to diagnose based on endophenotype

(imaging) (rather than mere constellation of signs and symptoms), coupled with more complete knowledge of the pathophysiology, has allowed for much-improved individual diagnosis, prognosis and treatment monitoring for those suffering from MS. It is hoped that this biological approach will gain favour in the psychiatric classification schemes of the near future. Currently, the larger symptom-based approaches are being progressively modified based on new science information. For example, in DSM IV-TR there is a new section under 'Dementia' entitled 'Dementia with Lewy Bodies'. This incremental change is helpful, and may represent a gradual transformation of symptom-based into more endophenotype- and pathophysiologically-based systems.

Organic Mental Disorders

The muddles with regards to this category in earlier editions of the ICD and DSM have to some extent been resolved, although much more work needs to be done to clarify this important area of psychiatric nosology.

The term 'organic mental disorders' of DSM IIIR has been replaced, and, as noted, some of these disorders are classified in the diagnostic section with which they share phenomenology (for example, anxiety disorder due to a general medical condition). In this scheme, the underlying condition can be specified in axis 3. Delirium, dementia and amnestic and other cognitive disorders are allocated a separate category. Sub-categories of dementia and amnestic disorders are then given.

There is a further overall category of mental disorders due to a general condition that have not been specified elsewhere. This includes catatonia, personality change and mental disorder not otherwise specified, which embraces post-concussional disorder.

ICD 10 has a category labelled 'organic', including symptomatic mental disorders. This includes the dementias, delirium and other mental and personality disorders due to brain damage and dysfunction and to physical disease. In the latter category are found the disorders secondary to a general medical condition in the

DSM IV. The retention of the term 'organic' in ICD 10 seems unfortunate, as it leads to a semantic muddle over the biological basis of other mental disorders, and the decision of DSM IV to drop this seems logical.

More concerning, perhaps, is the DSM approach of requiring a separate designation of an axis 1 (psychiatric condition), a comment on axis 2, and then a separate listing of medical conditions (axis 3). This Cartesian splitting of the psychiatric from the somatic forces an artificial separation of what is the reality. Brain and body are interconnected, as are brain and mind. Having a classification system that separates these realms runs the risk of perpetuating an underinformed, incomplete and impoverished view of diseases that affect the brain.

CLINICAL INVESTIGATION

It is not intended in this chapter to outline the basic or essential features of the neuropsychiatric examination, nor to discuss the various methods that are available for the quantification and documentation of the mental state. Accounts of these are given elsewhere (Cummings and Trimble, 2002; Roberts, 1984; Trimble, 1981a). Here some of the more important clinical investigation techniques are presented, including biochemical markers, EEG and brain-imaging techniques.

The importance of careful history-taking in the evaluation of patients cannot be overemphasized in psychiatry, as in other branches of medicine. This should, where possible, extend to third-party accounts of the patient's behaviour, and in particular must concentrate on change of behaviour. An understanding of the more regular patterns of the patient's activities is derived from information about their past, including any previous change in behaviour that led to psychiatric referral. Genetic diatheses must be sought by careful questioning. The essence, however, is the delineation of change; the identification of the point in time at which a process intervened. Personality – its style and development – has to be dissociated from process. The manifestations of the latter are then analysed for their form, noting the problems that occur if form and content

are confused. Diagnosis proceeds through documentation of psychopathology, the combination of signs and symptoms, and the application of some recognized nomenclature. As in medicine generally, the essential point of the initial patient evaluation in psychiatry is to draw up a differential diagnosis so that a plan of investigation and treatment can be initiated.

In the clinical setting, the initial diagnostic process should be accompanied by a search for aetiology and if possible an understanding of pathogenesis. As noted, many of the conditions that once formed a significant part of psychiatric practice now have a clarified disease base, often associated with structural brain change. However, the fact that the signs and symptoms of psychiatric illness are reflections only of disturbed brain function, and alteration of function arises either from intrinsic alteration of function (functional disorder) or as a consequence of structural change (structural disorder), requires us to examine the CNS in our patients.

Since psychiatry is a branch of medicine, it is reasonable to offer to psychiatric patients the same facilities for medical investigation as they would expect from other specialists. In particular, their clinical evaluation should always be accompanied by appropriate laboratory tests, many of which are routine. Thus all patients should have assessment of their basic haematology profile, an ESR measurement and certain biochemical tests. The latter include urea and electrolytes, liver function tests, calcium, phosphate and thyroid function tests (T3, T4, TSH). The liver function tests are important since alcohol intake is usually underestimated and under-revealed and may be significant in the patient's pathology. If alcoholism is suspected, estimation of red-cell transketolase activity may be of value, as well as gamma glutamyl transpeptidase (GGT) or carbohydrate-deficient transferrin (CDT). In many situations it may still be wise to test the patient's syphilis serology. This is usually tested with a Treponemal enzyme immunoabsorbant assay (EIA) combined with a Treponema pallidum haemaggultination assay (TPHA). The flourescent Treponemal antibody absorption (FTA-ABS) may be used as a confirmatory test. Depending on the clinical question, and local policy, testing for human immunodeficiency virus (HIV) is often carried out. If the initial antibody test or tests are positive, one should also assess for the viral load and CD4 count.

Routine skull and chest X-rays are not now recommended unless there is a suspicion that they may be revealing (for example, when there are concerns about tuberculosis or occult tumours). Measurement of vitamin B_{12} and folic acid status, thyroid function studies and blood glucose are often indicated, and in cases of 'funny turns' an extended glucose tolerance test is often done. On occasion, rarer investigations will be indicated, such as measurement of plasma and urine osmolality, tests for LE cells and antinuclear factors, C-reactive protein, further endocrine evaluation, and tests for infectious mononucleosis or other disorders such as brucellosis. In a patient with chronic fatigue syndrome, Lyme disease serology should be examined. In patients with movement disorders and psychopathology, copper and caeruloplasmin and acanthocyte screening will help rule out Wilson's disease and neuroacanthocytosis. In patients with suspected autoimmune or vasculitis problems, one should order a test for an anti-nuclear antigen (ANA) or anti-neutrophil cytoplasmic antigen (ANCA) (both for vasculitis), or anti-voltage gated potassium channel antibodies or anti-neuronal antibodies (both associated with limbic encephalitis as part of a primary autoimmune or paraneoplastic syndrome).

Urine investigations include screening for drugs if any state of intoxication is suspected, ruling out infections (especially in the confused elderly) and rarely testing for urinary catecholamines in suspected phaeochromocytoma or searching for metachromatic material in suspected cases of metachromatic leucodystrophy. Testing for porphyrins when porphyria is suspected still occasionally yields rewarding results.

Serum-level monitoring of certain drugs has now become routine, especially for lithium and anticonvulsants. Antidepressant monitoring can be of value, especially if a patient is responding poorly to good oral doses of the drug. Low levels may indicate a rapid metabolism or poor compliance. In addition, measurement when there is a complaint of toxic side effects on small doses may allow the physician to determine if this is related to unexpectedly high levels, especially helpful in the elderly, who often show reduced clearance of drugs. Serum alcohol or barbiturate levels are helpful in cases of suspected dependence.

One neuropeptide that is useful to assess is prolactin. This is elevated by drugs that block dopamine receptors and thus may be helpful in detecting compliance in patients on some neuroleptic drugs. Although there is tolerance to the initial higher levels of prolactin over four weeks of treatment, a period of stability is reached which lasts for months thereafter (Brown and Laughren, 1981). Prolactin levels tend to be elevated in patients on intramuscular therapy (Chalmers and Bennie, 1978), and while not correlating with the serum levels of the neuroleptics, may be a predictor of the dopamine blockade at the hypothalamopituitary axis. Patients who develop extrapyramidal side effects to these drugs tend to have higher prolactin levels (Kolakowska *et al.*, 1979), and hyperprolactinaemia is often associated with sexual disorders, especially in men (Schwartz *et al.*, 1982). Serum prolactin estimations will often help differentiate epileptic from non-epileptic seizures and thus may be useful in the investigation of intermittent behavioural disorders. Although there are some exceptions (frontal lobe seizures, simple partial seizures), a significantly raised prolaction 15–20 minutes after the episode, in the presence of normal baseline prolactin, may be confirmatory of an epileptic event (Dana-Haeri and Trimble, 1984).

The dexamethasone suppression test (DST) has a rather specific application to psychiatry. The details of this and some other neuroendocrine tests are reviewed in Chapter 8.

Finally, lumbar puncture is of value in psychiatric practice. Thus, in cases of suspected cerebral syphilis, serological investigation is required, and in some cases of undiagnosed dementia the presence of, for example, an oligoclonal immunoglobulin pattern may lead to a diagnosis of multiple sclerosis. More recently, CSF measures of amyloid-beta protein and tau protein can be helpful in early diagnosis of Alzheimer's disease.

Biochemical Investigations

In recent years the ability to measure substances of biological importance in body fluids – plasma, saliva, CSF and urine – has increased considerably. Further, the detection of small quantities with reliable, quick and relatively inexpensive techniques has been important in expanding the use of biological tests in psychiatry. Gas chromatography and high-performance liquid chromatography (HPLC) use the separation of compounds on columns and their analysis by sensitive detectors. In the former, the substance to be measured is carried in a gaseous phase into a column in which the separation takes place. Detectors at the end of the column measure and quantify the compounds. A particularly powerful detection method is mass spectroscopy. In this technique the substance to be measured is ionized electrically or chemically, and the application of magnetic and electrical forces separates the fragments in relation to their mass and electrical charge. In HPLC the contents of the separation column are forced in under high pressure, and their subsequent density allows excellent separation of compounds when the sample is injected rapidly through them. Unlike gas chromatography, there is no need to create gaseous derivatives. When combined with mass spectroscopy, HPLC is capable of quantifying picomolar concentrations.

Radioimmunoassay (RIA) has also been important. Here a biologically radiolabelled compound is combined with a very specific immunoglobulin molecule – the complex – which is then quantified by competitive binding to antibody. After an incubation period, when the binding of the labelled and unlabelled substances have equilibrated, the bound and the unbound portions are separated. As the concentration of the unlabelled portion increases, the amount of bound radioactivity decreases

and the appropriate quantitative calculations can be made from standardized curves.

EMIT assay, fluorescent polarization immunoassay and OPUS immunoassay are more newly developed highly specific immunoassays, which can be quickly performed on a small amount ($< 50 \, \text{m} \, \text{l}^{-1}$) of plasma or serum.

Many RIAs are available in kit form and are widely used in the assessment of neurohormones. There are many difficulties, however, with RIA, not the least being the specificity of the antibodies, and often there are discrepancies between the results obtained with biological assays (bioassay: the direct measurement of changes in isolated tissue responsive to the substance, for example a hormone) and the results of RIA.

Another technique is the radioreceptor assay, in which binding to a specially prepared suspension of receptors is calculated. Again, the biologically active compound competes with known radioactively labelled ligands for the receptor, and the bound portion is assessed and compared to a standard. This technique has been especially helpful in the measurement of serum drug levels.

The newest category of biochemical testing involves measuring specific genes. This can be done either to test for a specific disease under question (e.g. Huntingtin Gene, HTT, in Huntington's disease), as a risk factor, or to determine pharmacological response (called genomic pharmacology). In the field of oncology, for example, patients are routinely assayed for the BRAC1 gene, the results of which determine each patient's prognosis and dictate the invasiveness of the treatment course. For diseases where the genetics are well known, and with appropriate counselling and physician overview, this testing can help refine diagnosis and treatment. A particularly concerning area however involves direct-to-consumer (DTC) genetic testing that patients can order over the Internet. This area is ripe with fraud, with very little government oversight or regulation. Even when the tests are legitimate, without proper interpretation by a physician they often increase patient anxiety, and actually interfere with medical care.

EEG

The EEG signal

The signal finally reflected on the EEG trace represents only an average of the electrical events generated by the dendrites of neurones in the superficial cortical layers. It thus represents the graded sum of the excitatory and inhibitory potentials from many thousands of neurones lying under the recording electrode. Theoretically, if the cells are firing at random, the potentials should average out. The fact that there is a recordable rhythm implies that synchronization has occurred, suggesting the existence of some pacemaker. The thalamus is one structure from which EEG generators derive, although the genesis of the synchrony required for the spike of an epileptic focus is likely to be different from that leading to the generation of the normal alpha rhythm. The existence of multiple origins for synchrony may be postulated, and similar waveforms may not necessarily be derived by the same mechanism.

EEG Traces

In the laboratory the patient has electrodes attached to the scalp, and usually 8 or 16 channels are recorded. These are referred to by a standardized notation known as the International 10–20 system. It should be noted that an average electrode spacing is some 5–6 cm, and, since much cortex is buried in the sulci of the brain or is too medial to influence the surface EEG, in a typical examination only some 20% of the cortex is sampled, usually for only a small period of time. Better recordings from such structures as the medial temporal lobes can be obtained by using special electrode placement such as nasopharyngeal or sphenoidal leads. The former requires electrodes to be placed through the nares to rest in the nasopharynx under the base of the skull. With sphenoidal electrodes, the tip is placed in the region of the foramen ovale. Activation procedures for enhancing normal and abnormal features of the EEG are usually employed and include hyperventilation, photic stimulation, sleep inducement or sleep

deprivation, and the administration of epileptogenic agents such as pentylenetetrazol.

Interpretation of the recordings involves recognition not only of the type of waveform but also of its voltage, frequency and polarity. The EEG is, in general, composed of relatively high-voltage slow waves of up to 20 hertz (Hz, or cycles per second), and traditionally several different rhythms are recognized. The alpha rhythm has an 8–13 Hz frequency, and tends to appear in the relaxed-but-awake state. It is most prominent occipitally, and is attenuated or blocked by eye opening. Theta rhythm is 4–7 Hz, and delta is below 4 Hz. Rhythms faster than 13 Hz are beta, and are more prominent frontally. Many psychotropic agents such as barbiturates or benzodiazepines increase beta. The mu rhythm is a central rhythm of the same frequency as alpha which does not block with eye opening but does with movement.

Age is an important determinant of the normal EEG, especially in early years. At birth theta and delta rhythms dominate, increasing in frequency with maturation, alpha becoming established around the age of 13. The full adult pattern is not reached until the mid-twenties. Paroxysmal activity, including focal spikes or sharp waves, may be seen in nearly 3% of normal children, increasing to nearly 10% if provocative techniques or sleep studies are done (Eeg-Olofsson *et al.*, 1971). Frontal and in particular posterior temporal theta activity is not infrequently recorded in younger people, and its presence is thought to reflect brain immaturity. Its detection should not be interpreted as evidence of epilepsy in patients having 'funny turns'.

An individual's EEG is characteristic, and studies of twins reveal important genetic determinants (Hill, 1950). The correlation with intelligence is poor. Level of awareness is crucial to the EEG wave pattern, and marked changes occur with the onset of sleep. Thus, in the drowsy state, alpha waves tend to come and go, and as sleep supervenes, the rhythms slow. Deeper sleep is characterized by delta activity, while in paradoxical sleep (REM) there is fast desynchronized activity. During the orthodox, slow-wave stage, a number of other

EEG events may be observed. Sleep spindles are bursts of low-voltage 13–15 Hz activity, and K-complexes – delta waves associated with spindles – may be seen. During a night's sleep, REM activity occurs in four to six periods of up to 30 minutes approximately 90 minutes apart. Typically, the first REM period starts after about 90 minutes, and the total REM time for the average adult is 20–25% of total sleep time.

Evoked Potentials

The electrical events generated by the brain following a simple stimulus are small, and in the sea of background activity will not be detected. By the technique of averaging the results of many similar stimuli, the signal-to-noise ratio is enhanced and the so-called evoked potential recorded. Thus, visual, auditory or somato-sensory stimuli are repetitively presented, and after each event the electrical activity of the brain is recorded. The averaged evoked potential is derived from computer analysis of the data and is a series of waveforms of negative and positive voltage. The actual form of the event-related potential varies with the sensory stimulus, its modality and the cognitive processes involved in its perception. The first waves represent the arrival of the signals by the specific sensory pathways, the later waveforms reflecting activation over slower, polysynaptic paths. The former seem independent of the psychological state of the individual, while the latter vary with the state of the subject and the meaning and relevance of the stimulus. The latency and amplitude of the early response seem related to the strength of the stimulus, such that amplitudes increase and latencies decrease with increasing stimulus intensity. This, however, is not invariable, and in some subjects increased intensity leads to smaller responses (Shagass, 1972). The presentation of a stimulus and the evocation of a response alter a subsequent evoked response for a short period of time. It has been suggested that alteration in the recovery of this change may relate to psychopathology (Shagass, 1972). Changes in the waveforms of evoked potentials are widely used in the diagnosis of various diseases, an obvious example being multiple sclerosis. Other, more specific tests have largely superseded the routine use of evoked potentials in clinical, as opposed to research, biological psychiatry.

In addition to the shorter 'exogenous' latency responses, a number of the 'endogenous' event-related slow potentials have been described. These include the P300 wave, the contingent negative variation (CNV) and motor potentials such as the Bereitschaftspotential. The P300 wave refers to a positive response component seen some 300–500 ms after the stimulus, said to relate to a process of cognitive appraisal of the stimulus. It has a centroparietal distribution for all sensory modalities, and its latency increases with diminishing discrimination of presented stimuli. It has been suggested that it may be related to the laying down of memory traces (Karis *et al.*, 1984).

The CNV is derived by giving a subject a stimulus, followed some brief time later by another which requires some response. The first serves as a warning stimulus in expectancy of the second ('expectancy wave' is an alternative name). The wave consists of a slow negative shift in potential, especially in the vertex and frontal regions. Originally described by Walter and colleagues in 1964, it relates to such psychological processes as motivation, attention and heightened attention (see Figure 4.1). It is increased by such factors as certainty that the stimulus will occur and interest in the stimulus. It is diminished by distraction and boredom, and its character may be altered in psychopathology. The CNV should not be confused with the 'readiness potential' or Bereitschaftspotential, which is a similar slow negative potential that arises about one second before voluntary movement. It is maximal in the precentral parietal region, and may be broken down into a number of separate components (Shibasaki *et al.*, 1980).

Some Other Techniques

In recent years other sophisticated variations of EEG recording have come into use, including prolonged monitoring and computerized analysis leading to continuous mapping of brain electrical activity.

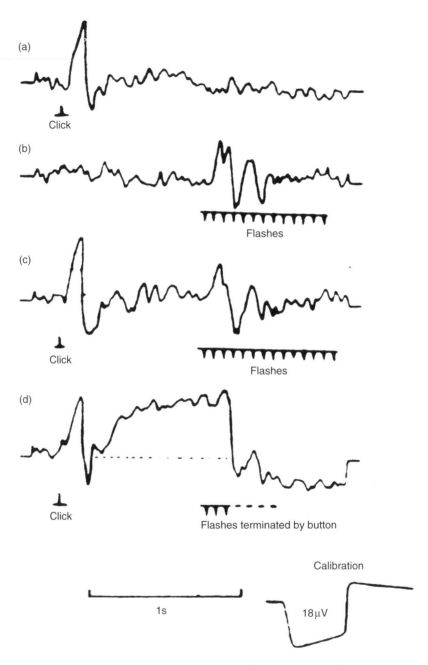

Figure 4.1 Contingent negative variation (CNV). Averages of responses to twelve presentations: (a) response in frontovertical region to clicks; (b) flicker; (c) clicks followed by flicker; (d) clicks followed by flicker terminated by the subject pressing a button as instructed. The CNV appears following the conditional response and submerges the negative component of the imperative response (reproduced with permission from Walter *et al.*, 1964)

There are two main forms of prolonged monitoring, namely videotelemetry and ambulatory monitoring. In the former the patient is filmed by a video camera, usually in a specially designed laboratory or ward, and the EEG is recorded simultaneously. Both the picture and the EEG trace are sent to an adjoining room where they are displayed on a split screen to be viewed together. The EEG and the patient's behaviour can thus be correlated.

With ambulatory monitoring, the EEG is recorded for a prolonged period of time using a portable cassette recorder strapped to the patient's body. The technique requires the use of special head-mounted amplifiers that diminish muscle and other artefacts. Although with this method there is no accompanying visual image of the patient, the apparatus can be worn at home or in the school without interference to daily activities.

A disadvantage of both these investigations is the limited number of channels that can be recorded and the interference that still occurs on the record at crucial times, such as during a seizure.

The use of computerized EEG methods allows profiles of the average amount of activity in various wavebands over time to be derived. The EEG record can be broken down into frequency components which are quantified using electronic filters and integrators, and electrical power determined according to selected frequency bands by using the mathematical technique of Fourier analysis. This has been particularly useful in psychopharmacology, noting for example the influence of different classes of drugs on these measurements.

Brain electrical activity mapping (BEAM) is a topographic mapping technique that condenses information from the EEG or evoked potential and presents it as a coloured map. Data are broken down into a matrix of some 4000 elements and a map is coded depending on the amount of electrical activity at each point. The resulting image can be an average of a series of images from a group of patients, and these data can be compared with those collected from another group. Areas of statistical differences between groups can be displayed as coloured maps, a technique known as statistical probability mapping (SPM).

One of the limitations of EEG is that it is unclear which brain regions are contributing to the recordings on the scalp. LORETA (low-resolution electromagnetic tomography) is one of several recent attempts to solve the inverse problem (i.e. where within the brain are the dipoles that drive the surface EEG?) and 'map' the surface EEG changes onto deeper brain structures.

There is an exciting new application of quantitative EEG over the prefrontal cortex as a potential early biomarker of antidepressant response. This method examines hemispheric differences in prefrontal coherence and activity (Bares *et al.*, 2007; Cook *et al.*, 2005; Hunter *et al.*, 2006; Kopecek *et al.*, 2007). One commercial company (Aspect Medical) has applied for FDA approval to market this clinically.

Magnetoencephalography (MEG), which measures extra-cranial magnetic fields derived from the brain's electrical potentials, has been introduced. The magnetic fields are not influenced by the scalp as EEG potentials are, and are more localized. It is thus possible using MEG to provide information from deeper cortical structures, which is at present impossible with the EEG without using depth electrodes. MEG has high spatial resolution and, since it detects tangential dipoles, can 'look' into a sulcus. This, combined with coregistration of MRI images, may provide a powerful technique for determination of structure–function brain relationships. MEG has not fully penetrated into routine neurological or psychiatric practice as it requires an expensive magnetically shielded room, while EEG can be performed in a routine setting. As with EEG, it is hard to determine exactly which regions in the brain under an electrode causes the signal on the surface of the brain. Some researchers are therefore combining MEG, with its high temporal resolution, with MRI or PET to determine the brain source of the MEG surface signal.

Brain-imaging Techniques

Computerized Axial Tomography (CAT or CT) Scans

Both angiography and pneumoencephalography, widely used prior to the introduction of the CT scan, provided only indirect information and did not show brain tissue directly. In contrast, the CT scan provides a computerized reconstruction of the brain image and around 1985 began transforming our ability to noninvasively visualize the brain prior to autopsy.

A typical CT scanner is composed of an X-ray source, a detector, a computer for image construction and an image display system. A fine beam of X-rays is generated and projected through the patient's head. The apparatus then rotates through one or more degrees and another projection is made. The process is repeated until all points in a plane, around 180°, have been probed from many directions. During the passages of the X-ray photons through the tissues of the head they will interact with intrinsic electrons and be either scattered or captured. In either case they will not reach the detector on the opposite side of the head. The more important event is scattering, which is dependent on tissue density. The final image represents a matrix display, a kind of grid map composed of many adjacent squares. Each square represents the average density of the tissue in the area of the square and a volume of tissue lying underneath it. The small square as seen is called a pixel, and the volume of tissue it represents is the voxel.

It is obvious that if the voxel is composed of all the same tissue then the density reflected in the pixel will faithfully reflect the quality of the represented area. However, if within the voxel there are, in addition to the soft tissue elements, bone, fluid or air, the average reading will be altered, which may lead to a misinterpretation of the presence of pathology in that tissue. This is known as the partial volume effect, and is an important source of error in CT data. The depth of the voxel varies with different machines from 2 to 13 mm. The usual matrix is made up of a 160×160 or 320×320 matrix. Although the original scanners used single beams, later models use multiple collimated beams and detectors and allow reconstruction of the X-ray data to produce sagittal and coronal, as well as axial, views. Even more common now are 'rapid' CT scanners with spiral techniques that make image acquisition more efficient, reducing both the time of the scan and the total radiation needed.

The units of density on one of the scales used are referred to as Hounsfield units, named after a pioneer of the CT technique. On this scale zero is the representative of water, air being $+2500$ and brain tissue in the region of $+15$ to $+18$. An alternative is the EMI unit, which is half the value of the Hounsfield unit. Some machines allow for direct assessment of densities in the selected region of interest (ROI).

The scan can be contrasted by using an iodinated contrast medium, which, on account of its efficient electron capture, deletes X-rays and increases tissue radiodensity.

A grey scale, ranging from white to black, allows the ultimate visual display, and the scale is set to allow maximum visualization of tissues of interest. This procedure relates to window width and level. The latter refers to setting the scale so that it is centred on the attenuation (X-ray absorption) value of most relevance, and the width refers to the range of other tissue attenuations to be included in the grey scale. Thus, if the window width is set at 20 and it is equally weighted to either side of the level then 10 units above and the same below will be included in the grey scale. Values outside of this range will appear either as all white or as all black.

The advent of CT scans in 1985 dramatically altered neurological practice and had a major indirect impact on psychiatry. However, because CT involves radiation, and is less sensitive than MRI for many clinical questions, it is now largely restricted to trauma units and trauma evaluations. CT scans are useful in imaging the two 'B's – bone and blood – where they are not supposed to be. Thus emergency room physicians use CT scans after road traffic accidents or other trauma to investigate skull fractures, subdural hematomas or haemorhagic strokes. Some newer units combine CT scans with PET cameras; these are increasingly used in cancer diagnosis and monitoring.

Magnetic Resonance Imaging (MRI) Scans

The elegant demonstration of the brain's structure by the CT scan has been superseded by MRI. While more expensive, MRI is a more powerful and diverse technology and has largely replaced conventional CT technology except in some clinical situations following trauma.

Although the technique, also referred to as nuclear magnetic resonance (NMR), has been used in spectroscopy for some time, the formation of images derives from the work of Lauterbur (1973), who used the term 'zeugmatography'. The principle involves the examination of the physicochemical environment of proton nuclei in tissue based on the inherent electromagnetic forces that exist in such electrically charged particles.

Briefly, any object that has charge and velocity produces a magnetic field perpendicular to it. A charged nuclear particle spinning in the body's tissues thus produces a magnetic field, although in this case the field is referred to as the angular magnetic moment, with a vector perpendicular to the axis of rotation. A charged nuclear particle, spinning about its axis, acts like a tiny bar magnet; before the application of an external magnetic field, the sum total magnetization of many of these spinning in human tissues is zero, since their direction of movement is random. On application of an external magnetic force the tiny magnets are aligned, just as an ordinary compass needle will align in the Earth's magnetic field. The alignment is parallel (or antiparallel) to the external field. The protons in such a setting actually spin, like a spinning top, around the alignment of the applied field, a process referred to as precession. Protons, which possess their own inherent specific precession, once aligned can be excited by the momentary application of a radio signal broadcast at their own specific frequency (the Larmour frequency) from a radiofrequency transmitter. This process may be likened to a tuning fork: if we have six guitar strings tuned to different frequencies and a tuning fork for one of those frequencies is struck nearby, only that string will resonate; if we have a series of guitars, all the strings of that frequency will respond. So it is with protons in human tissue. If now the tuning fork is silenced, the guitars will continue to give off a sound, and this can be picked up by a receiver and measured (see Figure 4.2).

The procedure of imaging makes use of the fact that waves emitted from the nuclei differ in both frequency and amplitude, the former locating the position of the particular nucleus in the body and the latter reflecting the number of nuclei present at that position. Thus, within the static externally applied magnetic field, energy is imparted to the parallel protons, exciting them to a higher energy level by radiofrequency waves of exactly the right frequency, and after the signal is finished, electromagnetic energy of the same frequency will be given off, detected by a receiver coil. After the application of the radiofrequency pulse, the magnetization returns exponentially to its pre-excitement level, a process referred to as relaxation. This may be defined by two time constants, referred to as T_1 and T_2, where T_1 is always greater than T_2.

The T_1, or spin-lattice, relaxation time, representing relaxation along the longitudinal axis, is the time taken for the protons to recover their previously aligned position in the static field after excitation in this axis by a $180°$ pulse. In practice, due to the configuration of most scanners, a so-called inversion recovery image is used to give a T_1-weighted image.

The T_2 relaxation time, representing relaxation in the transverse plane (hence transverse relaxation time), is the exponential time constant which results from decay of coherence, due to the interaction of the spinning nuclei. It relates to energy exchange between protons, and is also referred to as the spin–spin relaxation time. T_2 is thus a measure of the length of time for which the tissue maintains its temporary transverse magnetization, perpendicular to the external magnetic field, following a $90°$ pulse. The spin echo is proportional to the proton density and T_2, and is frequently used for T_2 measurement.

Thus, each tissue has a specific T_1 and T_2 value, essentially reflecting the physicochemical

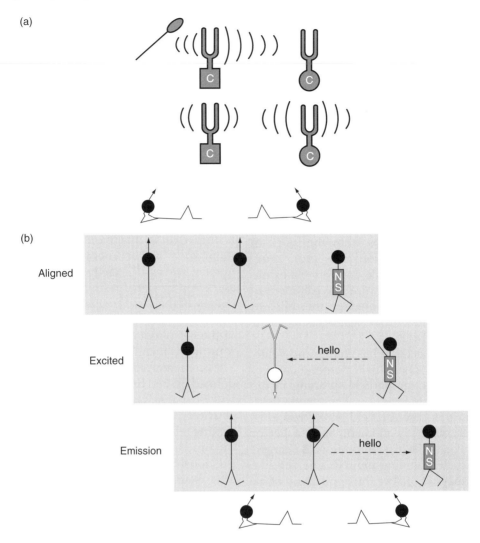

Figure 4.2 (a) The principle of resonance. If a tuning fork is struck, an adjacent one of the same tone will vibrate and emit sound (upper). This will persist after the first tuning fork is removed (lower). (b) Principles of MRI (*Biol Psych*, 2 Ed, p. 127)

environment of the proton nuclei, especially the water density of the tissue. T_1 relates to the interactions of protons with surrounding nuclei; T_2 depends on interactions of protons with each other. In the brain, the proton behaviour measured relates to the hydrogen nucleus, most commonly of CNS water. Thus the spinning atomic nucleus will behave like a spinning top only if it has an odd atomic mass or number, an atom with an even number being nonmagnetic. While NMR spectroscopy can image ^1H, ^{13}C,

^{15}N, ^{19}F, ^{23}Na and ^{31}P, most clinical and research imaging at present is largely confined to hydrogen nuclei.

In practice, the requirements for clinical brain imaging are a large superconducting bore magnet, a radiofrequency transmitter coil that may also act as a receiver, a computer and a display system. The actual imaging technique involves a series of choices for sequencing related to the direction and timing of the radiofrequency pulses delivered, the data being spatially encoded to provide information on proton density and T_1 and T_2 times. The echo time refers to the time taken to generate the echo signal after the initial $90°$ pulse, while the repetition time states the pulse signal to be repeated. Since it is an electronic process, reconstruction can be done in any direction, and is usually slice encoding. Inversion recovery and spin-echo techniques are the most widely employed. By exploiting differences between the relaxation times of different tissues, heightened contrast

between them is achieved, and hence better images. The use of contrast media such as gadolinium DTPA further aids tissue differentiation. These cross the blood–brain barrier in small quantities and alter the relaxation time of tissues, inversion recovery images being particularly sensitive (Figure 4.3).

A static magnet activates all protons, and gradient magnets activate specific cuts. The derived images have a low spatial resolution, in some machines as low as 0.8 mm square. Most

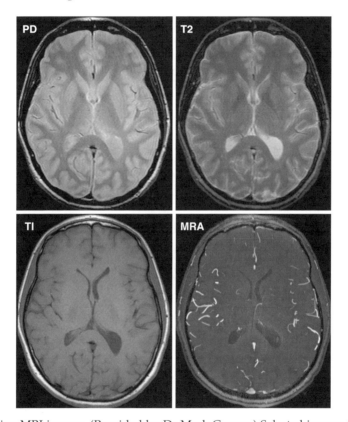

Figure 4.3 Contrasting MRI images. (Provided by Dr Mark George.) Selected images from a healthy brain MRI, all at the same level through the head. Proton density (PD, top left), T_1-weighted (T_1, bottom left), T_2-weighted (T_2, top right), and MR angiography (MRA, bottom right) scans have varying image contrast that reveals specific information about various structures in the brain. The T_1 scan is considered the 'Rembrandt' as it shows high-resolution anatomy in health, and depicts the brain as one would see it at dissection, with the skull present, grey matter as grey, white matter bright, and CSF dark. In contrast, the T_2 scan is useful to detect pathology, and things are 'non-obvious'. The skull is sometimes not even imaged, and grey matter is bright, white matter is dark, and the CSF is very bright, almost radioactive. The proton density scan is a hybrid between these two. In the MRA scan, bottom right, blood flowing in arteries or veins is very bright (reproduced with permission from Christopher P. Hess MD, PhD; Purcell, Derk D. BRAIN: CT, MRI: noninvasive imaging of the central nervous system [Internet]. Version 46. Knol. 2008 Aug 6. Available from: http://knol.google.com/k/christopher-p-hess-md-phd/brain-ct-mri/biWBkaDv/wqrGdg)

pathological conditions increase the length of T_1 and T_2, free water having even higher values. Since on T_1 images increasing the time darkens the image, and on T_2 images it lightens the image, on T_1 images, CSF and pathological areas are relatively darkened, and the opposite is true on T_2 images. Both T_1 and T_2 are shorter in white matter than in grey, but the signal from bone is very weak and is not well visualized on images. This conveys an enormous advantage for imaging in neuropsychiatry since the bony structures of the cranial vault, which on CT imaging so often obscure the structures of interest, such as the temporal lobes, are not present.

Table 4.1 Advantages and disadvantages of MRI

Advantages	*Disadvantages*
No radiation	Noise discomfort
Minimal risk[1]	Claustrophobic
Good grey/white discrimination	Limited discrimination between pathologies
Less degradation of image with movement	Length of scan time
No bone artefacts	Artefacts from ferromagnetic material (e.g. tooth filling,
Clear structural images	air sinuses)
Potential for functional imaging	
Ability to visualize several planes	

[1]Only patients with cardiac pacemakers, intracranial magnetic clips or in the first trimester of pregnancy should not be scanned.

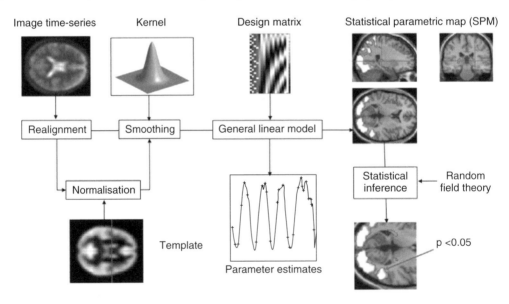

Figure 4.4 Method of statistical parametric mapping. This schematic depicts the transformations that start with an imaging data sequence and end with a statistical parametric map (SPM). An SPM can be regarded as an 'X-ray' of the significance of regional effects. On the left, voxel-based analyses require the data to be in the same anatomical space; this is effected by realigning the data. After realignment, the images are subject to nonlinear warping so that they match a spatial model or template that already conforms to a standard anatomical space. After smoothing, the statistical model is employed to estimate the parameters of a temporal model and derive the appropriate univariate test statistic at every voxel. The test statistics (usually t or F-statistics) constitute the SPM. The final stage (right) is to make statistical inferences on the basis of the SPM and Random Field Theory and characterize the responses observed using the fitted responses or parameter estimates (courtesy of Dr Mark George)

A disadvantage is that calcified lesions are not well visualized. A summary of the advantages and disadvantages of MRI is given in Table 4.1.

There is the potential to use quantitative information from the scans, especially actual T_1 and T_2 measurements for studying structural changes, and, with higher-strength magnets, to image other atoms such as ^{31}P.

It is possible to reconstruct images in three dimensions (see Figures 4.4 and 4.5). Echo-planar imaging ('fast MRI') and the use of low-flip-angle techniques which tip protons rapidly through very small angles (FLASH, or fast low-angle shots) are leading to image acquisition in short times compared with older conventional imaging.

The real expense of an MRI machine is that it requires a large superconducting magnet to create a static magnetic field big enough for a human body. A conventional electromagnet would require enormous energy, and generate a great deal of heat, to produce the magnetic field. By cooling the entire electromagnet to near zero degrees kelvin, the electricity is able to flow with less resistance (supercon-duct), requiring much less energy and not creating heat. However, the scanner must be

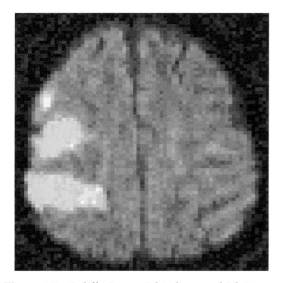

Figure 4.5 A diffusion-weighted scan, which is very sensitive to acute changes in water content, and increasingly used for detection of acute strokes (courtesy of Dr Mark George)

'refrigerated' with liquid helium or hydrogen. A breakthrough in superconducting materials would fundamentally reduce the cost of MRI scanners and expand their use. Unfortunately, there is nothing on the short-term materials horizon that might cause this change in the next decade.

MRI has so fundamentally transformed medicine in general, and neuropsychiatry in particular, that in 2003 Sir Peter Mansfield and Dr Paul Lauterbur were awarded jointly the Nobel Prize in Physiology or Medicine (not physics) for their pioneering work with MRI. There is a dizzying array of MRI methods in use in psychiatry research and clinical practice, most of which are discussed below, though it is certain that this list will continue to grow. The techniques are artificially divided into those that are used to assess structure and those that indirectly measure brain function.

Structural MRI

As noted above, conventional MRI is used to gather structural information about the size and shape of the brain. The T_1 scans are anatomically correct (sometimes called the 'Rembrandts' of scanning because they resemble the tissue they image). The T_2 and other proton-density scans are not anatomically correct but instead convey crucial information about subtle changes in water density associated with pathological states. For example, small areas of ischemia or demyelination are invisible on T_1 scans but are visible on T_2 scans. These are referred to as 'white matter hyperintensities'. There is a robust research literature on the potential relation-ship between these and new-onset, late-onset depression, sometimes referred to as 'vascular depression' (see Chapter 8). Many biological psychiatry researchers have used MRI scans to investigate the size or shape (morphology) of key brain regions like the amygdala and hip-pocampus. Early research on regional brain size or shape required trained researchers to actu-ally manually and somewhat laboriously outline and sample each region for each subject, a pro-cess resembling the work of medieval monks copying illuminated manuscripts. More com-monly now scans are manipulated by computers and boundaries are determined by sophisticated thresholding algorithms. One of the more popular recent computerized techniques is referred to as voxel-based morphometry or VBM. Briefly, in a given patient, the brightness level of a region, say the right amygdala, might be a constant X. If we were to take this subject, and several others, and morph their brains into a common atlas (a process called stereotactic normalization), then for example for those subjects with a small right amygdala, their overall brightness counts would have to be stretched into a larger common space and the overall brightness or signal intensity would be diluted. For those with a large right amygdala, their brightness level would be crowded into a smaller common space region and their relative brightness would thus increase. Researchers can thus use VBM to perform whole brain comparisons of the size of the brain in one group compared to another, or to compare a group over time to examine increases or decreases in regional brain size or shape. This VBM method is being used extensively in studies examining plasticity or changes over time with interventions and treatments. Because it is relatively easy to perform, and does calculations on the entire brain (literally thousands of comparisons), researchers struggle to make sure that results are not false positives resulting from the statistical complexity of the data. This problem of how to correct for multiple statistical comparisons plagues much of MRI imaging research (Figure 4.4).

Another new technique, called diffusion tensor imaging (DTI), yields indirect information about the structure of white-matter fibres and local water diffusion (diffusion-weighted imaging, DWI). Remember that a particle will move randomly inside a confined space (called Brownian motion): the same is true of water molecules in the brain, but the brain has hydrophobic compartments and barriers, most notably myelin. By imaging water molecules repeatedly as they migrate over time, researchers can examine their local migrations and then determine whether the movement is purely random or is constrained and thus directional. Water will tend to move more freely within a myelin sheath rather than across a sheath. Thus diffusion imaging uses

the local migration of water to infer information about local neuronal integrity. One of the first events following ischemia or trauma is a loss of cell membrane integrity, when water moves more randomly than in healthy functioning tissue. Thus DWI is now becoming the imaging modality of choice in assessing acute ischemic strokes (see Figure 4.5). The membrane integrity of a given portion of brain is called the fractional anisotropy (FA). Building on this concept of water diffusion, one can compute the average direction of water movement for a given brain voxel. Thus each voxel can be given a vector value of the direction and magnitude of water flow. This vector is called a tensor, hence diffusion tensor imaging. This indirectly correlates with the white-matter fibre tracts in that voxel. Creatively, one can then 'connect the dots'. That is, each voxel has a vector pointing to another voxel, and then to another. By mathematically tracing these vectors one can create images of 'likely' fibre tracts in the brain. There are however many different mathematical algorithms for fibre-tract tracing, and each different rule then highlights different pathways. It is important to remember that these are not real fibres being imaged, rather they are mathematical analogues. Figure 4.6 shows a diffusion tensor image, where this directional information for the entire brain is contained in the colours. Red shows water (and fibres) flowing right to left, blue shows water travelling head to toe, and green denotes vectors pointing anterior to posterior. Reassuringly, the corpus callosum is red, internal capsule blue, and arcuate fasciculus green. By planting a 'seed' one can obtain theoretical fibre tracts (shown in Figure 4.6). While these are compelling images, it is important to remember that they are simply mathematical vectors of aggregate water direction and are not the actual white-matter fibres. However, they do provide interesting indirect information about structural connectivity and directionality.

Functional MRI

Different types of MRI scanning can also be used to assess the function of the brain, not just its size, shape and structure. There are currently three main approaches: those that assess general blood flow or perfusion, those that examine

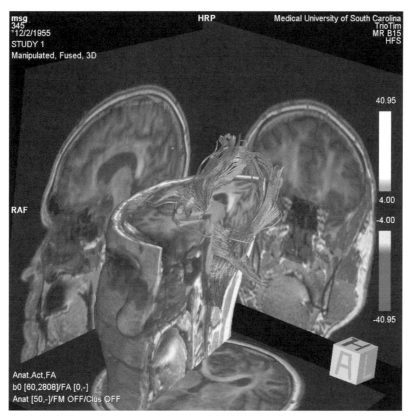

Figure 4.6 Structural MRI scan shown in 3D, with diffusion information superimposed and DTI tracts arising from brainstem. To generate the DTI tracts, 'seeds' were placed in the brainstem with a computer model (courtesy of Dr Mark George). A coloured version of this figure can be found on the colour plate

subtle changes in tissue haemoglobin use during performance of a task, and finally the classical use of MRI as MR spectroscopy, where one can directly measure chemical composition.

One MR technique for measuring large-scale blood flow is called MR angiography, where blood molecules are magnetically tagged, and then reimaged as they flow through large vessels (arteries and arterioles). In biological psychiatry MR angiography can be used to image a vasculitis, arteriovenous malformation or infection where there is a change in vessel integrity (such as herpes simplex encephalitis). For actual calculation of regional blood flow, investigators initially used bolus injections of contrast agents and measured their flow through large vessels. More recently physicists have devised methods of magnetically labelling blood and then measuring the speed and quantity of its flow into other brain regions, a technique called arterial spin-labelling or ASL. Large-vessel blood flow changes as a function of heart rate and can be modified by certain drugs, such as cocaine. ASL or perfusion is not sensitive enough to reflect subtle changes in regional brain activity associated with higher cognitive processes, however.

By far the most common MRI research technique (in terms of publications) is examining changes in tissue haemoglobin concentration before and then during various activities. Briefly, the brain uses oxygen, which is carried by haemoglobin (oxyhaemoglobin). After the oxygen leaves the haemoglobin, the deoxyhaemoglobin has a different magnetic signal. When a brain region becomes active it initially becomes anaerobic and sends chemical signals that cause a fairly rapid compensation response, and the full region is flooded with oxyhaemoglobin to replenish it. This compensation takes about 3–6 seconds (called the haemodynamic response) and is not spatially precise. As Malonek and Grinvald (1996) wrote, 'the entire garden row is flooded for want of one thirsty rose'. Serially measuring the oxy/deoxy haemoglobin ratio is referred to as blood oxygenation level-dependent functional MRI, or BOLD fMRI. This technique has allowed an explosion of research concerning what regions are 'activated' or 'deactivated' during various mental states. However, it is still not clear how local brain activity relates to the BOLD signal. That is, a brain region that is working very hard to inhibit or gate another region would have increased BOLD signal and would be an 'activation' even though its activity

is to inhibit other brain regions. Importantly, the change in BOLD signal with a task is only about 3% of the background signal, so it is not a large effect. Thus, researchers will typically have a subject perform a task, then rest, and then repeat the task and rest numerous times over a typical 10 minute scan. The images are then digitally manipulated through a series of steps in order to generate the final statistical map of the regions that have changes in activity correlating with the behaviour. These steps involve correcting for small movement that might have occurred in the scanner, lining up all the images and then morphing or spatially normalizing the scans into a common brain atlas. There are several common

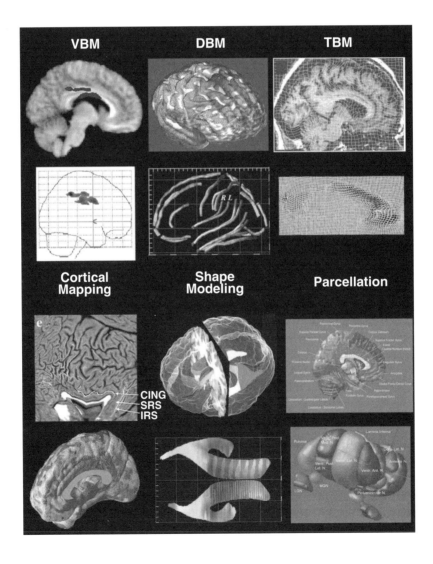

statistical software packages that researchers use: statistical parametric mapping (SPM), FMRIB Software Library (FSL) and Analysis of Functional Neuroimages (AFNI). BOLD MRI scans are then spatially smoothed and statistical tests are performed comparing brain activity during a task with the control or rest condition. Essentially the raw images undergo a series of statistical procedures which first of all stereotactically reorganize the brain image into standard stereotactic space; the resultant image has noise variance smoothed, and analysis of covariance is used to remove the contribution of underlying global activity. The SPMs are then created by statistical analysis, using **t** maps, comparing repeated measurements between groups of images on a pixel by pixel basis (see Figure 4.7) (Friston *et al.*, 1991, 1996).

Typically the areas that are statistically significantly different during the task compared to the control condition are displayed in colour and then on top of a grey-scale structural MRI. It is important to realize that the size of the activation is totally a function of where one

draws the statistical threshold, which is not at all consistent in the literature. Some other notes of caution are needed in order to make sense of this 'blobology' literature, where it is easy to be enthralled by a coloured 'blob' in the brain. Is the merged and displayed image true to all of the data, or have the investigators conveniently masked out activations in other regions? This post-hoc masking and selective presentation of results is deceptive, bordering on dishonesty. An alternative way to analyse these data is to perform a correlation analysis, seeking evidence of a distributed brain system with high covariance.

In the early days of BOLD fMRI, the signals were weak, with smaller magnets. One could only find statistically significant task activations by pooling data from multiple subjects who were all doing the same task and control condition. These were thus group statements, and one could not use them for individual diagnosis or prognosis. More recently, with higher field strengths and multiple receiver coils combined into one unit (multichannel head coils), it has

Figure 4.7 (a) The concept of inter- and intra-subject averaging, following spatial normalization. All scans are first fitted into a standard space, and subsequent comparison of pixel values is based upon standard parametric statistical techniques. Areas of significant difference between groups are illustrated as statistical maps in three formats. These are (left to right): T-maps, orthogonal projections showing areas of significant difference or surface renderings onto a standard brain template (reproduced with permission from Dr K. Friston, Wellcome Department of Cognitive Neurology, Queen Square). (b) Six major types of analysis of structural images, showing some of the main types of data used in each case. Voxel-based morphometry (VBM; top-left panels) compares anatomy voxel by voxel to find voxels (shown here in blue) where the tissue classification (grey, white matter, CSF) depends on diagnosis or other factors. Results are typically plotted in stereotaxic space (lower panel), and their significance is assessed using random field or permutation methods. Deformation-based morphometry (DBM) can be used to analyse shape differences in the cortex or brain asymmetries (coloured sulci; red colours show regions of greatest asymmetry). Tensor-based morphometry (TBM) uses 3D warping fields with millions of degrees of freedom (top) to recover and study local shape differences in anatomy across subjects or over time (red colours indicate growth rates in the corpus callosum of a young child). Other methods focus on structures such as the cerebral cortex, which can be flattened to assist the analysis (bottom left), or the lateral ventricles (shape modelling). If anatomic structures are represented as parametric surface meshes, their shapes can be compared, their variability can be visualized and they can be used to show where grey matter is lost (e.g. in Alzheimer's disease; bottom-left panel, red colours denote greatest grey-matter loss in the limbic and entorhinal areas). Fine-scale anatomical parcellation (lower right) can be used to compare structure volumes across groups, or to create hand-labelled templates that can be automatically warped onto new MRI brain datasets. This can create regions of interest in which subsequent analyses are performed (reproduced from Lawrie *et al.*, 2003, with permission of Oxford University Press). A coloured version of this figure can be found on the colour plate

become possible to make reliable and repeatable within-individual BOLD maps for some cognitive, sensory and motor tasks. This within-individual BOLD fMRI mapping is now FDA approved and used by neuroradiologists for pre-surgical planning of motor, sensory, visual and to some degree language areas. Currently BOLD scans are not able to make individual diagnoses, although they can predict, better than a polygraph and above chance, when someone is lying (Kozel *et al.*, 2005).

The third form of functional MRI involves using the MRI to image chemical spectra and is called magnetic resonance spectroscopy (MRS). Whereas MRI provides largely spatial information based on hydrogen or water content, MRS details chemical information. The principle is the same as that for structural imaging, except that the peaks for water are removed from the spectrum, and no tomographic reconstruction techniques are applied. The resolution is not as good as in conventional MRI, around 1 cm, and image acquisition is typically much longer.

^{31}P MRS reveals a number of peaks, and since phosphorus is essential for energy metabolism, several directly reflect on, for example, the activity of ATP, ADP, Pi: inorganic orthophosphate.

Proton (^{1}H) MRS gives a more complicated spectrum than ^{31}P imaging, partly because nearly all brain metabolites contain protons. Amino acids, inositol and creatine are all represented, and it is therefore possible to obtain information on excitatory and inhibitory amino acids (e.g. glutamate and GABA) and membrane precursors (choline/phosphocholine). The main localization of n-acetyl aspartate (NAA) is in neurone, and its value will fall with neuronal degeneration (Figure 4.8).

There are other spectra, including those for ^{13}carbon, ^{19}fluorine, ^{23}sodium and ^{7}lithium, and their value in CNS research is at present under investigation.

Cerebral Blood Flow (CBF) and Metabolism

Several techniques described above for brain imaging provide essentially anatomical data, and to the present have given information about structural changes in the brain. In contrast, CBF and metabolism reflect on the function of the brain. It is important to emphasize that the resulting images are based on complicated mathematical modelling, itself based on

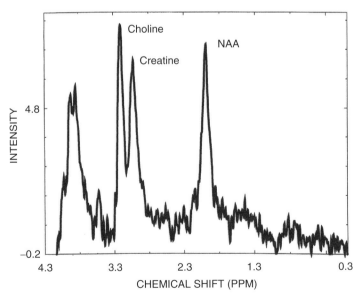

Figure 4.8 MRS from a 6 cm volume in the hippocampus. Signals measured are from NAA, creatine and choline (*Biol Psych*, 2 Ed, p. 133)

suppositions about the biochemical activity of the brain in nondiseased states, and that the resolution of current machines is far less than for MRI. Although assessment of whole-brain CBF has been available for many years, it was the development of regional analysis in the 1960s and the combination of these techniques with computed imaging to provide PET that revolutionized our knowledge in this area.

The use of radioactive isotopes to aid in diagnosis initially involved the administration of gamma ray-emitting compounds such as technetium 99 to outline blood–brain barrier defects and enhance the visualization of, for example, cerebral tumours. The first successful measurement of CBF was with the nitrous oxide technique, introduced by Kety and Schmidt (1948).

The second-generation methods, rapidly developed, relied on the rates that isotopes were cleared from the brain, traced by recording the decline in radioactivity over the scalp with scintillation counters. The isotopes were given by either inhalation or intracarotid injection, and included 85-krypton and 133-xenon. The number of detectors available has increased, and it is now possible to image regional CBF (rCBF) from many areas on both sides of the brain. In practice, a tracer is given, and the 'clearance curve' of its arrival and elimination from the region is plotted. By comparison to theoretical values obtained from a physiological model, the CBF is derived. The initial slope index (ISI) is an early flow index frequently used. Tracer is monitored for approximately 10 minutes after administration and calculations of both grey- and white-matter flow are derived. The spatial resolution of the technique is limited, and interference from the contralateral hemisphere reduces the sensitivity, especially for detecting asymmetries. Early artefacts, such as the problem of contamination of blood from extracerebral sources, have been overcome, but haemoglobin values, due to the affinity of xenon for haemoglobin, and the arterial CO_2 tension have to be taken into account in analysis. CO_2 is a potent vasodilator of cerebral vessels, and hyperventilation, for example due to anxiety, may lower the $PaCO_2$ and the CBF.

In normal healthy adults, the mean CBF is around 50 ml/100 g of brain tissue per minute, the values for grey and white matter being approximately 80 and 20 ml/100 g per minute respectively. Normally a tendency to greater values frontally is found, as is a slow decrease with advancing age (Frackowiak *et al.*, 1980).

CBF, especially xenon inhalation, has many advantages: it is a noninvasive procedure, it is quick to perform, it is possible to repeat images after a short time interval and, especially compared to PET, it is inexpensive. Its limitations are the low spatial resolution (2–4 cm), its inability to provide three-dimensional imaging and its failure to give information on deep cerebral structures. It has been largely replaced by three-dimensional SPECT and PET technology (see below).

PET

As noted above, the main source of cerebral energy is glucose, but provided that there is coupling between oxygen consumption and ATP production, energy metabolism can be deduced from measuring oxygen use. Although under normal conditions there is coupling between the CBF and the cerebral metabolic rate of oxygen use ($CMRO_2$), and thus assessment of CBF may provide information regarding metabolism, in pathological states or with hypercapnia or hyperventilation the relationship is lost. Measurement of $CMRO_2$ using the technique of Kety and Schmidt was possible, but, with the autoradiographic work of Sokoloff *et al.* (1977) and the technology of computed tomography, the development of PET has allowed for the assessment of both CBF and metabolism, *in vivo*, on a regional basis.

In PET, radioactive isotopes of biological substances are created by a cyclotron, which fires protons at a nucleus of, for example, carbon. The latter gains protons and becomes unstable, being an 'antiparticle' to a negatively charged electron. When in tissue, it combines immediately with an electron, the two particles converting their mass into radiation energy. They subsequently annihilate. The latter gives rise to the release of two coincident gamma rays of equal

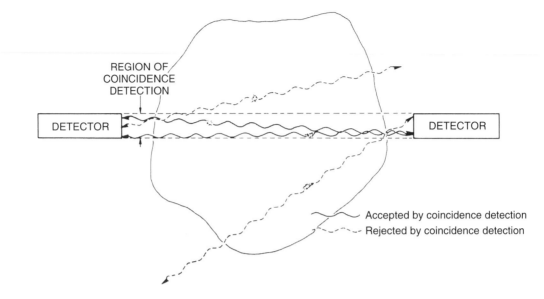

REGION OF
COINCIDENCE
DETECTION

DETECTOR

DETECTOR

Accepted by coincidence detection
Rejected by coincidence detection

Figure 4.9   Release of coincidence rays following positron annihilation, and detection of coincidence rays by the scanner (*Biol Psych*, 2 Ed, p. 135)

energy which travel at $180°$ to each other (see Figure 4.9).

The presence of these rays is picked up by the detectors of the scanner, positioned such that they only record coincident events, these being separated from other nonsimultaneously released gamma rays. Thus the decay event is known to have taken place on a line connecting the two detectors, a process called coincidence detection. Detection cameras are placed in a ring around the patient's head, the exact structure being dependent on the system used. Computerized reconstruction of the image is performed using technology similar to that of CT scanning. However, it is essential to recognize a fundamental difference between the two techniques, namely that in CT, rays from an external source are passed through the patient's brain, while in PET, rays are emitted from the brain, detected and quantified. Further, the image of PET is indeed an image, and one of tissue-tracer distributions. It is not an anatomical map as provided by MRI and CT.

The spatial resolutions of the machines vary, but typically are between 7 and 15 mm. For technical reasons related to the finite range of the decay of positrons, the maximum resolution is in the region of 2–3 mm. In order to obtain accurate readings from a structure, it should have a size twice that of the resolution of the machine.

The main biologically interesting positron emitters created include carbon-11, nitrogen-13, fluorine-18 and oxygen-15. In practice, since all but fluorine-18 have short half-lives, the patient has to be in close proximity to the cyclotron for the investigations to be carried out. With fluorine-labelled isotopes, with a half-life of 110 minutes, the substance can be transported to the patient over considerable distances.

Depending on the isotope used, PET provides information on several parameters, including cerebral blood volume, CBF, cerebral metabolism and neuroreceptor function.

At present there are two main systems for imaging metabolism, one based on oxygen and the other on glucose or deoxyglucose. In the oxygen-15 technique, the patient continuously inhales trace amounts of oxygen-15-labelled carbon dioxide (CO_2) and oxygen. The CO_2 is rapidly converted in the lungs to $H_2^{15}O$ and is distributed throughout the arterial tree, about 20% reaching the brain, where it equilibrates rapidly with tissue water. Since this is removed continuously by the venous system, at steady state the concentration of radioactivity measured will reflect both the delivery to and the decay from the tissue. Thus, at steady state, it is possible, using mathematically derived formulae with various corrections, to calculate the blood flow.

Similarly, the ^{15}O is delivered to the brain attached to haemoglobin, and is there used to fuel the Krebs cycle for the production of ATP, the radioactive oxygen appearing in water as a result of the metabolism. Again, with sophisticated mathematics and correction for sources of error (Lammertsma *et al.*, 1981), it is possible to define the oxygen-extraction fraction (OEF) – the fraction of available oxygen extracted from the blood – and from this and the CBF the $CMRO_2$ is calculated.

The fluorodeoxyglucose (FDG) method relies on the ingenious yet simple principle developed by Sokolof *et al.* (1977). Glucose, when administered, is taken up into tissue and rapidly metabolized to CO_2 and H_2O and cleared from the brain. However, deoxyglucose is taken up and phosphorylated to deoxyglucose-6-phosphate, but this is not metabolized further as there are no available enzymes for its further degradation. In addition there is no functional dephosphorylase, so it cannot re-enter the precursor pool. As a consequence it gets trapped in the tissue, and its presence is directly measured and quantified since the radioactive deoxyglucose emits positrons, which lead to the production of coincidence annihilation gamma rays detected by the scanner. In contrast to the short half-life of ^{15}O (123s), that of FDG is in the region of 110 minutes; hence its use entails a longer study and requires careful control and monitoring of the patient's state during the uptake period. The metabolic handling of this analogue of glucose has then to be equated with that of glucose if the derived measurements are to be used to reflect neuronal metabolism. The relationship has been found constant under many conditions, mathematically referred to as the lumped constant, but the latter has been derived essentially from animal models and may break down in certain pathological states, leading to erroneous calculations.

Interpretation of the data accumulated with PET is subject to a multitude of errors, which at present are probably responsible for the confusion in some of the data, especially with regard to psychiatric illness. Some of these are listed in Table 4.2.

Innovations of PET technology have been progressing rapidly. State-of-the-art cameras can collect data in seconds from many contiguous transaxial planes and have a resolution approaching 5 mm. Many measurements can be taken in one session, scanning every few minutes. Activation tasks, which will increase activity in specified areas of cerebral function, have been used to study responses to pharmacological or behavioural stimuli. The technique requires at least two data sets generated in conditions that differ for the specific function examined. Motor tasks might be simple repeating of a specific movement, while cognitive tasks might include the administration of a psychological test such as the Stroop test.

Positron-emitting radioligands are used to examine neuroreceptor and neurotransmitter function. The ligand must be selective for a receptor and have high affinity, with good blood–brain barrier penetration. Typical compounds in use include ^{11}C flumazenil for benzodiazepines, ^{11}C methyl spiperone and ^{11}C raclopride for dopamine, ^{11}C carfentanil for opiates, and ^{18}F ritanserin for 5-HT. Carbon- and fluorine-labelled L-dopa are now available to detect the precursor pool of dopamine. Newer compounds, for other systems, and receptor subtypes are in development. One of the more exciting areas is the development and testing of amyloid ligands for the diagnosis and study of Alzheimer's disease. The most widely used at present is the Pittsburgh Compound B (PIB), which is being used in several large trials for diagnosis, correlation with clinical disease burden and as a potential surrogate marker for new drug development. These amyloid ligands are not yet commercially available. A dopamine

Table 4.2 Potential artefacts in the interpretation of PET. (From De Lisi and Buchsbaum, 1986)

Compound as tracer

1. Half-life and breakdown rate of label
2. Purity of the compound
3. Differences between oxygen and glucose
4. Differences between labels, e.g. $^{18}F/^{11}C$

Experimental conditions

1. Variation in anxiety and emotional state of subject
2. Psychiatric state of patient
3. Task performed during the uptake period
4. Variation in sensory inputs, e.g. eyes open/closed
5. Prolonged uptake period with inconstant physiological changes
6. Variation in blood sampling procedures
7. Failure to control for age and sex

Instrumentation

1. Limited resolution
2. Non-uniform resolution
3. Scatter and partial volume effects
4. Inadequate number of planes sampled
5. Need to standardize adequately to phantoms
6. Variation in head size and shape
7. Head movement
8. Change in distribution of tracer compound during the scan procedure from first to last slice

Data analysis

1. Inaccuracy of models for describing biochemical kinetics
2. No appropriate model for some substances
3. Kinetic constants used derived from animals
4. Differences in the kinetics between white and grey matter
5. Difficulties in matching some slices among individuals
6. Undersampling of anatomical structures
7. Overinterpretation of assumed anatomical details
8. Computerized methods failing to account for anatomical differences among individuals
9. Accounting for cortical folding
10. Lack of serial determinations of data in the same individual over time, so normal variation unknown

D4 agonist and 5-HT$_{1a}$ antagonist, the WAY ligand, is available and is used for research.

Single-Photon-Emission Tomography (SPECT or SPET)

This technique has proved to be more useful than its early detractors predicted. Instead of positron-emitting isotopes, SPET uses single-photon emitters. The image is obtained by a rotating gamma camera. This rotates through $360°$, and a series of images are acquired representing the sum of radioactivity along a line parallel to the hole in the detecting collimator. These are reconstructed by filtered back-projection. Multidetector cameras are now in use, which give much better resolution (8 mm), as are safe, reliable tracers. The latter include ^{133}xenon, ^{123}-p-iodo-N-isopropylamphetamine, ^{99m}TcHMPAO and several neuroreceptor ligands. ^{99m}TcHMPAO has proven of particular value. Once given, it is taken up by neurones, where it remains for a few hours, giving a snapshot of cerebral activity at the time of administration (George *et al.*, 1991, 1992).

The advantages of SPECT over PET include its more ready availability and its low cost. The tracers generally have longer physical and biological half-lives, not requiring an on-site cyclotron. However, quantification of data is much more complicated, ratios between differing brain areas often being used, with one structure, such as the cerebellum, being used as a standard reference. Multiple rapid images of the type now available for PET studies are not possible, although sophisticated activation protocols can be performed.

As with PET, several SPECT ligands are useful clinically, although they are not widely used. β-CIT SPECT is used to assess dopamine function in Parkinson's disease. In general, it is more difficult to create specific ligands for SPECT than it is for PET, because of the need to couple the ligand with one of the technetium transport tracers, as opposed to simply inserting a labelled carbon or oxygen molecule.

As discussed above, it is easy to overinterpret brain-imaging results, and many patients and clinicians wish that brain imaging could do more than it can in terms of making diagnoses and guiding treatments. As will be discussed in the chapters that follow, there are several promising areas in psychiatry where brain-imaging techniques are starting to aid clinically (not just as a research tool). In classical neurological disorders such as multiple sclerosis, brain imaging has revolutionized diagnosis and treatment monitoring. One example of the likely misuse of brain imaging is in the claims that brain SPECT scans can diagnose ADHD, and predict which treatment a patient should receive (Amen and Carmichael, 1997). Unfortunately, there are no class I data showing that this is the case and many published trials show that brain imaging is not clinically useful in ADHD (Zametkin and Liotta, 1998). Biological psychiatrists should attempt whenever possible to practice evidence-based medicine, and in areas where there is no data and there is potential harm from radiation exposure, 'first do no harm'.

Near-Infrared Spectroscopy (NIR)

This approach uses a fairly small and often portable machine and a movable wand, much like an ultrasound machine. Unlike ultrasound, the fibre-optic wand transmits energy in the electromagnetic spectrum (from about 800 to 2500 nm), which interacts uniquely with tissue and is able to penetrate through bone (skull). It can thus examine changes in haemoglobin concentration in the cortical tissue just below the skull. As with fMRI and PET, brain regions that become activated have relatively rapid changes in local oxygen and haemoglobin concentrations. The advantages of NIR are that it is noninvasive, relatively inexpensive and portable. Its main disadvantage is that it can only reveal information about the cortical regions directly under the wand, and thus cannot provide a full image of brain activity. It is currently mostly a research tool.

Transcranial Magnetic Stimulation (TMS)

A common method in science to help understand causality is to eliminate something, and then see if the behaviour or disease changes. Thus, researchers 'knock out' genes and examine the effects on the animal or system they are studying. Building on the knowledge provided by PET and fMRI, many biological psychiatrists and cognitive neuroscientists are starting to use TMS as a knockout method. TMS is a technique in which a powerful small electromagnet is placed on the scalp (George and Belmaker, 2006). The brief but powerful magnetic field passes unimpeded into the outer layers of the brain and induces electrical currents in the cortex. This noninvasive approach can temporarily 'activate' brain regions, making them temporarily unavailable for normal cognitive processing (Muggleton *et al.*, 2006; Stewart *et al.*, 2001; Walsh and Cowey, 2000). Thus, TMS can be used as a research tool to 'knock out' or interrupt a brain region and observe the changes in behaviour. This is easiest to demonstrate over language areas, where brief TMS can produce a temporary speech arrest resembling a Broca's aphasia.

Cognitive Neuroscience

The introduction of the new imaging techniques has led to a revolution in understanding of brain–behaviour relationships, and the rapid development of this discipline. Using MRI techniques it has been possible to confirm and expand data about areas of cerebral cortex that respond to sensory stimulation, and relationships between multiple brain areas of activation. This in part has stimulated the approach towards circuits and parallel distributed processing (PDP) as a model of brain function. One interesting application of functional MRI has been to note signal changes during mental imagery. The brain uses much the same regions when imagining doing an action as it does actually doing it.

Despite all the advances in brain imaging and brain-stimulation knockout techniques, there is still inadequate understanding of some of the more important and basic questions. How does one form a mental image? What is the brain basis of consciousness? While these questions remain largely unanswered, many recent studies are beginning to emphasize, for example, the role of the precuneus in studies of 'self awareness of mental acts'. Thus, in addition to designing ever more clever experiments or paradigms in an attempt to understand self-awareness or consciousness, others are attempting to tackle this question using different statistical approaches and novel imaging methods. One of these approaches is called resting BOLD fMRI. In these studies, rather than the usual 'task–rest–task...' paradigms, subjects are instructed to simply 'do nothing'. Serial BOLD scans over 5–10 minutes are then analysed for brain regions that either positively or negatively

change with each other over time. This is an attempt to examine functional connectivity. Some have speculated that these functioning circuits become dysregulated in disease states or with different levels of 'consciousness' or self-awareness. The main regions of interest are the medial frontal cortex and the precuneus.

It is beyond the scope of this work to review all of brain imaging. But suffice it to say that over the past 20 years PET and fMRI data have allowed numerous cognitive operations to be mapped, for example the brain regions associated with memory, language and even emotional recognition of faces (Figure 4.10)

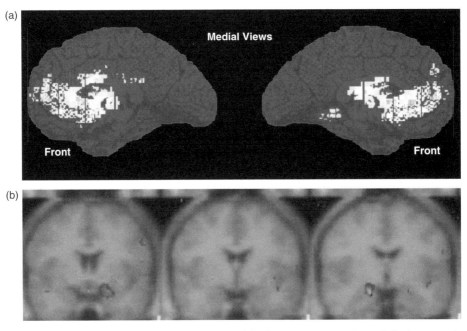

Figure 4.10   (a) Statistical parametric maps (O15 PET) of the brain regions activated during transient sadness induced by remembering sad events and viewing sad faces. The control task consisted of remembering neutral events and viewing neutral faces. Note that anterior limbic structures (septum, anterior cingulate) and left prefrontal cortex are activated. All points in dark tone represent significant increases in activity ($p < 0.01$) (courtesy of Dr Mark George). (b) Three consecutive coronal slices through the brain of the group brain activation that occurs when healthy subjects are unconsciously exposed to ultra-brief (subliminal) pictures of human faces which look fearful. The subjects were unaware after the imaging study that they had even been exposed to anything unusual. Note that the 'early warning system for danger', the amygdala, bilaterally show activation during the time the subjects are exposed to the fearful faces, compared to when they are not. This was one of the first demonstrations of the rapid fear response system of the amygdala (reproduced from Whalen *et al.*, 1998). A coloured version of this figure can be found on the colour plate

(George *et al.*, 1993). While confirming much that was previously known, these studies have enriched our knowledge of potential neuronal networks, and have emphasized the holistic nature of cerebral activity associated with cognitive tasks. Interestingly, although referred to as cognitive, many of the areas investigated might better be referred to as emotional, but such studies are now exploring the fundamentals of human thinking from decision making to rationality and consciousness.

5
Personality Disorders

GENERAL INTRODUCTION

Here, and in the following chapters on the affective disorders and the psychoses, the biological underpinnings of psychopathology will be reviewed. Following an introduction to each topic, genetics, metabolic and biochemical findings, neurochemical and neuropathological information, and the literature on neuro-logical illness – including the abnormalities from special investigations – will be referred to. Each chapter ends with a discussion of outstanding issues.

INTRODUCTION TO THE CONCEPT OF PERSONALITY

We see the personality in the particular way an individual expresses himself, in the way he moves, how he experiences and reacts to situations, how he loves, grows jealous, how he conducts his life in general, what needs he has, what are his longings and aims, what are his ideals and how he shapes them, what values guide him and what he does, what he creates and how he acts (Jaspers, 1963, p. 428).

It is thus by the personality traits that we know someone; they are enduring and give an air of predictability to a person. In common parlance there is little difficulty in understanding a person's personality in these terms. It follows that over time people have given certain personality styles names, and that scientists have attempted to quantify various attributes of personality. A popular concept for example has been that of the axis of introversion–extroversion, and use of the Eysenk Personality Inventory (EPI) for measurement. Another well-validated scale has been the Minnesota Multiphasic Personality Inventory (MMPI). There are many others; some attend to specific aspects of personality, such as obsessionality, while others, like the MMPI, are broad in scope. An additional approach has been the scheme developed by Robert Cloninger, where personality is defined on three axes, which loosely relate to neuropharmacology. The axes are impulsivity and risk-taking, interpersonal reactivity and harm avoidance. They were originally thought to relate to the major monoamine systems, with dopamine levels correlating with risk-taking, 5-HT with interpersonal reactivity and noradrenaline with harm avoidance (Cloninger, 1987; Cloninger *et al.*, 1993, 1996a, 1996b; Svrakic *et al.*, 1993).

With such assessments, it should be possible to define normality within a population, and hence reflect on abnormality. Thus, in psychopathology, two ways of defining an abnormal personality, a statistical method and one based on ideal types, have arisen. Jaspers preferred the former, as did Kurt Schneider (1959), who defined abnormal personalities as those who '...suffer from their abnormality or through whose abnormality society suffers'

(p. 4). The alternative, invoking a kind of Platonic reality, suggests that ideal Pygmalion creations exist in nature; this is the way of DSM IV-TR.

The diagnostic criteria for the personality disorders, and other psychopathologies discussed in this book, can be found in DSM IV-TR, ICD 10 and the Structured Clinical Interview for DSM III-R Personality Disorders SCID-IIP (for personality). Caution about the use of such manuals has already been given. The types discussed in this chapter cover the following:

Psychopathic personality is a term used by Schneider to embrace several differing abnormal personality patterns, but generally now implies antisocial personality traits. In the ICD it is referred to as the dissocial personality, and in DSM IV-TR as antisocial personality disorder (ASPD). It manifests mainly as sociopathy. Sociopathic personality or antisocial personality are alternative terms. It is characterized by 'disregard for and violation of the right of others' (DSM IV-TR). It usually becomes apparent in early life, often with conduct disorder at school, a continuing history of poor interpersonal relationships, a poor work record and continuing marital difficulties. Drug abuse, alcoholism, pathological lying and prison convictions may be recorded, and sociopaths tend to display more than accepted sexual deviation, somatization and outbursts of physical violence. A characteristic feature is the tendency to remit over the years, either in early or mid adulthood.

Obsessional personality, also referred to as the anankastic personality disorder in ICD 10, and obsessive–compulsive personality disorder (OCPD) in DSM IVTR is characterized by a lifelong tendency to meticulousness and punctuality, and feelings of doubt leading to excessive caution. Patients have a reluctance to delegate tasks to others, and insist on tasks being carried out only in certain ways. It is better referred to as the anankastic personality disorder, as this saves confusion with obsessive–compulsive disorder (OCD) (see Chapter 6).

Histrionic personality has links to the antisocial personality disorder, and in many ways is contrasted with the anankastic. Jaspers (1963) defined the type thus: 'hysterical personalities crave to appear, both to themselves and others, as more than they are and to experience more than they are ever capable of' (p. 443). The characteristic traits are excessive dependence; suggestibility; shallow, labile affects; impulsiveness; verbal exaggeration and excessive gestural display; seductiveness in the presence of relative frigidity; and self-dramatization. Patients prefer to be the centre of attention, and long for appreciation. There is a tendency to take overdoses of medication or make other attempts at self-harm, and there is some association with somatization. The validity of this category has been established by factor analysis (Lazare *et al.*, 1970), from which studies its traits are clearly distinguished from the anankastic personality. In particular, the impulsivity and the tendency to approximate and exaggerate of the histrionic personality stand in contrast to the calculations and deliberations of the anankast. In contrast to sociopaths, who tend to be male, histrionic personalities are commoner in females. There are clear overlaps with both dissocial and borderline personalities.

Borderline personality was first introduced in DSM III. In the ICD 10 it is a subcategory of the emotionally unstable personality disorders. The essential feature is 'a pervasive pattern of instability of interpersonal relationships, self-image, and affects and marked impulsivity...' (DSM IV TR, p. 710). There is marked identity disturbance, impulsivity and recurrent attempts at self-harm. Patients display transient episodes of paranoid ideation, and may have dissociative symptoms.

Paranoid personality is distinguished by continued suspiciousness, mistrust and excessive sensitivity. Jealousy, transient ideas of reference, litigiousness and a tendency to avoid intimacy are all features, and individuals often take up minor concerns or causes with tenacious vigour, collecting vast amounts of documentary evidence to support them.

Schizoid personality features describe people who have little affective or social contact, with a tendency to detachment and eccentricity. While well recognized, the DSM IV-TR has split this into three groups, the schizoid, the schizotypal and the avoidant. The schizotypal appears to include oddities of behaviour, thinking, perception and speech with unusual beliefs and ideas of reference, and the avoidant emphasizes hypersensitivity and social withdrawal in spite of yearning for acceptance. The schizoid personality disorder defines those who appear cold, seem to experience no pleasure and are solitary. They seem insensitive to praise or criticism, and to social norms.

Other Personality Types

In addition to the above groupings, which find some concordance in the different systems, various other types are described, although the criteria are often less than clear. *Anxious personality* (ICD 10) defines those who display lifelong anxiety, and under stress readily develop anxiety or panic disorder. *Narcissistic personality* refers to those with a grandiose sense of self-importance or uniqueness; preoccupation with fantasies of unlimited success; exhibitionistic need for constant attention and admiration; characteristic responses to threats of self-esteem; and characteristic disturbances in interpersonal relationships. Also noted are frequent depressed moods and transient psychotic states.

DSM III included the category of the *passive aggressive personality*, those who habitually express covert aggression. Both ICD 10 and DSM IV-TR describe the *dependent personality disorder*. These individuals have a pervasive need to be taken care of that leads to submissive and clinging behaviour and fears of separation. ICD 10 refers to the *explosive personality*, in which liability to intemperate outbursts of anger are seen in people otherwise not prone to antisocial behaviour, under the emotionally unstable personality disorders.

Links between Personality and Psychiatric Illness

A form of depression less severe than major affective disorder is now referred to as dysthymic disorder, involving prolonged and persistent lowness of mood beginning early in life. This is associated with chronic psychosocial stresses and 'personality disorder ... merges imperceptibly into this condition' (American Psychiatric Association, 1987, p. 221). Patients with personality styles referred to as avoidant or dependent personalities display lifelong anxiety with bouts of panic and exacerbation under stress.

Thus, in these typologies there is not always a clear separation between personality style and certain categories of psychiatric illness that used to be referred to as neurotic, a word removed from DSM IV, but which has longstanding psychiatric understanding. If the quantitative approach to personality disorders is taken, separation between individuals takes on less clear boundaries, personality disorder relating to a statistical deviation from the norm. Schneider's model blurs the distinction between the neuroses (anxiety disorders in particular) and personality disorders, defining personality disorders as dispositions through which either the individual themself or society suffers. Some other models of psychopathology confuse boundaries even further. For example, the Meyerian reaction types, which minimized endogenous variables at the expense of 'reactions' to environmental events, drew no clear distinctions between personality idiomorphs, neurosis and psychosis. Freudian psychoanalysis also failed in this regard, the pathogenesis of all forms of psychopathology being similar in that they represent deviant childhood developments with libidinous fixations and later regressions.

In contrast, Jaspers' model emphasizes clear distinctions between personality and illness, not only phenomenologically, but also developmentally. Illness is a new feature, either skewing the development of personality or altering the matured individual, leading to phenomena that cannot be understood in terms of that individual's normal development. As Slater and Roth (1969) pointed out, this was an extremely useful clinical distinction, enabling clearer delineation of such illnesses as schizophrenia, and their distinction from the excessive reactions of various personalities. Further, it led to success in distinguishing various primary mood disorders from secondary mood changes; the endogenous from other forms. This breakdown into primary and secondary is useful. Secondary depression is that which occurs in the presence of pre-existing psychiatric disorders or chronic medical illnesses (Feighner *et al.*, 1972; Goodwin and Guze, 1984), amongst which are to be included personality disorders.

Thus, concepts of personality and neurosis seem to have been historically intertwined by several groups of authors, often writing from different perspectives. The blurred boundary has had many consequences. For one, terminology became a labyrinth of confusion. Neurotic depression and its distinction from endogenous depression became an area of intense research, the outcome of which is not clear to this day. Variants of terms such as depressive reaction, psychogenic reaction, depressive personality and dysthymia added to the confusion, and people with abnormal personalities were wrongly classified as having psychiatric illnesses.

This last point is more fundamental than is often appreciated, and itself has had consequences for biological psychiatry. First, if the illness represents the outcome of a process then it may be possible to identify that process biologically. Hence the search for biological markers in psychiatry. In some cases these markers will be identifiable as abnormal tissue pathogens, for example as in an encephalitis. In others, the neurochemical constituents alone may be at variance, and detection of the change rests in identifying variation from the normal expected range. If patients with personality disorders are confused in a group with those having a particular illness then the sought abnormality or biomarker will be diluted and not found. This problem sometimes arises with research into depressive illness, where patients with personality disorders are wrongly categorized as having a major affective disorder or dysthymia. A similar problem arises in drug trials, where heterogeneous populations masquerade for homogeneous ones, and real differences between active drugs and placebos may be minimized. Attempts, such as the DSM III and its successors, to more rigidly define categories and provide exclusions as well as inclusions are helpful for some areas of psychiatric research, but are still quite imperfect.

A second consequence relates to the image of psychiatry with nonmedical people. Patients with personality disorders often develop depressive symptoms in the setting of social stress, and may be thought, by the uninitiated, to have what psychiatrists refer to as major affective disorder. As many such people respond, albeit temporarily, to manipulation of their social environment, it is assumed that all psychopathology can likewise be remedied. This thinking, combined with lay confidence in the nonbiological therapies that characterized psychiatry a generation ago, has led to marked distractions in attempts to understand the biological bases of psychopathology.

DSM IV-TR recognizes clusters of personalities which have some identifiable overlapping features. Cluster A embraces the schizoid, paranoid and schizotypal – the odd and the eccentric; cluster B the antisocial and impulsive, the flamboyant and the erratic; and cluster C the dependent, the anxious and fearful. This line of thinking leads on to consideration of personality traits and their relationship to states. Traits are persistent underlying attitudes, while states are temporary or permanent manifestations, and will take two forms. Trait exaggeration is one form, in which a flowering of the premorbid personality is seen. The other is symptoms that arise *de novo*. Thus, traits and states do not always go hand in hand; the development of OCD or a conversion disorder (somatoform disorder) is not necessarily dependent on the premorbid personality, as predicted by some theories.

With regard to depressive symptoms, some authors described so-called depressive personalities (Schneider's (1959) depressive psychopaths) as people who are continually pessimistic, with constant anxiety about themselves and their world. This style, however, is not found in DSM IV-TR. Cyclothymic disorder, appearing with affective disorders, replaces both depressive and cyclothymic personality disorder, emphasizing the illness rather than the personality. There is some literature supporting the link between cyclothymic personality and manic–depressive illness, notably the finding of an excess of cyclothymic personalities among the relatives of manic–depressive patients (Kallmann, 1954), and evidence of cyclothymic behaviour in between illness episodes in manic–depressive patients (Winokur and Tanna, 1969) (see Chapter 8).

The strongest associations between personality traits and psychopathology are encountered between types of OCPD and OCD. In Kringlen's (1965) study, over 70% of patients with OCD had such a personality style. Another postulated relationship is between the symptoms of conversion (somatoform disorder) and the hysterical personality. However, clinical estimates note that only 18–21% of patients with conversion symptoms conform to this style (Merskey and Trimble, 1979), supported in studies of similar populations using standardized rating scales to assess personality (Wilson-Barnett and Trimble, 1985). There is an association between schizotypal personality disorder and OCD (Sobin *et al.*, 2000). Dependent personality disorder has links with panic disorder and agoraphobia (Hoffart *et al.*, 1995), and avoidant personality disorder links with social phobia.

In a study of 660 patients, axis 1 and 2 diagnoses were assessed and associations between personality disorder and psychosis were examined with logistic regression analysis. Among the associations noted were schizotypal and schizoid personalities with schizophrenia, paranoid personality with delusional disorder, histrionic personality with brief reactive psychosis and OCPD with major depression (Cuesta *et al.*, 1999; Peralta and Cuesta, 1999).

In summary, the links between personality styles and psychiatric illnesses are not so clear and much is clinical lore. In some clinical settings, notably the anxiety and affective disorders, disentangling the constitutional elements in the clinical picture is difficult, especially with limited patient contact. It is often only with time that the personality vulnerabilities of patients become exposed and the nature of the co-morbid psychopathology becomes clearer. The links however are of profound importance clinically and conceptually. For example, cluster A melds with the concept of a schizophrenia spectrum of

disorders, the latter falling at the more extreme end of the former, and broaches the subject of endophenotypes related to cognitive and emotional styles. Certain cognitive and behavioural dispositions may increase the risk for axis 1 disorders, such as substance abuse, or neurological disorders, such as head injuries, which then impact further on personality dimensions. It is unclear when some personality attributes become axis 1 disorders, what may be the genetic links, and to what extent treatment of an axis 1 profile leads to changes which alter the axis 2 designation (e.g. treating an anxiety disorder and the effects on the comorbid anxious personality disorder).

Personality Styles

The above distinctions of different personality constellations lead to consideration of the different styles of thinking and perceiving of emotion by different individuals. Shapiro, in a book titled *Neurotic Styles*, outlined the differences between four different ways of responding to the world as seen in obsessive–compulsive, paranoid, hysterical and impulsive personalities (Shapiro, 1999). The theme was that each style was characteristic, and although the book was written from a psychoanalytic era, the implication was that the styles of thinking related to underlying psychological structures, the mode of thinking itself being interlinked with the psychopathology. An act carried out by say an obsessional personality guarantees their next act, which will seem to them the most rational way of proceeding. 'The paranoid person is not simply visited by apprehensions and defensive suspicions; he searches actively and does not rest until he has located clues to new dangers' (Shapiro, 1999, p. 20). Shapiro draws attention for example to the rigid thinking of the obsessional, which can also emerge after cerebral trauma, with a narrowed focused attention which implies a lack of cognitive flexibility. Paranoid personalities have an acuteness of attention; this is continuous and always a searching for something. 'Significant' cues are seized from their context, a subjective world emerges which is endowed with special significance and reality is distorted.

The hysterical style is one of impressions and superlatives ('Wow! It's wonderful.'), with lack of factual detail, and poor concentration skills. 'Hysterical attention is easily captured ... their line of thought is easily interrupted by transient influences' (Shapiro, 1999, p. 115). This leads to an inadequate memory and a poverty of knowledge. Their cognitive style is thus impressionistic, immediate and global. Their emotional life is one of lability, emotional outbursts being a feature, but outbursts which they almost disown as something which has been visited on them. Psychopathic traits include insincerity and a proclivity to lying, impulsivity, and cognitively a lack of planning, concentration and logical objectivity.

This line of thinking is an elaboration on Jaspers, in that it suggests different cognitive anlages which define behaviour, underlying not intelligence, but the way the world and its contingencies are reflected upon and responded to. In the context of biological psychiatry, the underpinnings of this would be related to neurobiological principles, and hence the relevance of examining personality changes in neurological disorders and looking for neuroanatomical and neurophysiological profiles that relate to different personality styles. Unfortunately this has not been well researched, in part because of a reluctance on behalf of many even within the psychiatric community to accept concepts of personality disorder, or if they are accepted, to attribute the personality disorder entirely to sociological variables.

Of the many attempts to quantitatively examine the structure of personality by the use of rating scales and statistical analysis and interpretation, the rating scales of Eysenk are still most widely used. Of all the personality disorders, antisocial personality disorder has been the most researched, and Hare's Psychopathology Checklist is widely used. With factor analysis, two main factors are identified, the first relating to charm, glibness, pathological lying, lack of guilt, lack of empathy and the like, the second to a need for stimulation, easy boredom, poor behaviour control, impulsivity and irresponsibility (Guay *et al.*, 2007; Hare, 1999; Neumann *et al.*, 2007). Using Cloninger's

method, antisocial personality has been shown to be associated with somatization disorder and substance abuse (Battaglia *et al.*, 1996; Cloninger *et al.*, 1993; Svrakic *et al.*, 1993).

GENETICS

General Findings

There is considerable evidence that genetic factors are of importance in personality disorders. The early studies are well reviewed by Slater and Roth (1969) and McGuffin (1984). Animal studies have permitted the selective breeding of anxiety-prone rats (Broadhurst, 1975). These show greater corticosterone, ACTH and prolactin responses to stress, and lower ^{3}H-diazepam binding in various cortical structures and the hippocampus than non-anxious counterparts (Gentsch *et al.*, 1981).

In humans, the familial prevalence of anxiety is high, over 50% of first-degree relatives suffering from the same disorder. The clinical ratings of personality are more similar in monozygous (MZ) twins than in dizygous (DZ) pairs, even in MZ twin pairs reared apart from an early age. In the study of Shields (1962), MZ twins reared apart were more alike than MZ twins raised together, leading to the suggestion that the common environment of the twins is less relevant for this aspect of personality development than genetic factors. Shields (1954) showed that MZ twin schoolchildren resembled one another with regards to the pattern of what was then referred to as neurosis, the mean concordance rate taken from several studies of neurotic identical twins being given as 61% by Tienari (1963). In the latter's own study of 21 identical twin pairs classified as neurosis cases, only 5 had a normal co-twin, 13 pairs having a co-twin with either neurotic personality, a neurosis or an immature personality. With regards to the clinical picture, the tendency towards concordance was clearest with phobic and obsessional cases (91%).

One problem with many of these clinical studies is the vagueness of classification of the index disorders, and in many instances the diagnoses were purely given on a retrospective analysis, case notes being relied on for the historical data. Further information comes from studies using rating scales of psychopathology to quantify symptomatology. Gottesman (1962) gave the MMPI to twins and derived a hereditability index for the scales. The highest values were for Si (social introversion) and Pd (psychopathic deviation), while only low values were reported for Hy (hysteria). Likewise there is evidence for genetic factors in the personality dimensions extraversion–introversion using the EPI, estimates of hereditability values being 50%.

Torgersen *et al.* (2000), using twin and patient registries, interviewed 92 MZ and 129 DZ twin pairs using the SCID-IIP. The best-fitting models had a heritability of 0.60 for personality disorders generally, with 0.37 for cluster A, 0.60 for cluster B and 0.62 for cluster C. Among the specific disorders, the heritability given was 0.79 for narcissistic, 0.78 for obsessive–compulsive, 0.69 for borderline, 0.67 for histrionic, 0.61 for schizotypal, 0.57 for dependent, 0.54 for self-defeating, 0.29 for schizoid, 0.28 for paranoid and 0.28 for avoidant personality disorders. Family environmental influences were very limited, and the results were more strongly influenced by genetic effects – more than almost any axis 1 disorder.

One of the more interesting and controversial areas of personality and genetics in the recent literature has revolved around whether certain variants of the dopamine receptor, specifically the D4 variant, are associated with increased novelty-seeking or impulsivity. Initial studies found such an association (Cloninger, 2008), which has more recently been challenged (Paterson *et al.*, 1999; Soyka *et al.*, 2002; Thome *et al.*, 1999). More studies are needed.

Genetics of Specific Personality Disorders

There is good evidence that genetic factors contribute to individual personality disorders. Most investigated has been antisocial personality disorder (sociopathy). Concordance between MZ twins with regards to criminality has been reported by several groups (Christiansen, 1974; Lange, 1929), supported by adoption studies which show higher rates of offences in adopted

children in cases where the natural father is known to the police (Hutchings and Mednick, 1975). Baker *et al.* (2007) reported in a large socioeconomically and ethnically diverse sample of 605 families of twins or triplets that measures of antisocial behaviour such as conduct disorder, ratings of aggression, delinquency and psychopathic traits obtained through child self-reports and teacher and caregiver ratings revealed a common antisocial behaviour factor that was strongly heritable (heritability at 0.96). Family studies confirm associations between antisocial personality disorder and somatization disorder and substance abuse, linked by heritable personality traits of high novelty seeking and low self-directedness (Cloninger, 2005).

Torgersen (2000) reviewed the literature on the genetics of borderline personality disorder (BPD) and concluded that it was too early to say to what extent BPD is influenced by genes. However, since traits similar to it, such as novelty seeking, are found in BPD and are themselves influenced by genes, and because personality traits generally show a strong genetic influence, this should also be true for BPD. He opined that the effect of genes on the development of BPD is likely substantial while the effect of common family environment may be close to zero (Torgersen, 2000). Molecular genetic studies have linked BPD with a monoamine oxidase allele and with 5-HT transporter polymorphisms (Ni *et al.*, 2009).

Histrionic personality disorder overlaps with BPD, but is over-represented in females. Some imply that this is gender stereotyping, or that it is merely the feminine counterpart of male antisocial personality disorder. There are no adequate studies of the genetics, but using the Dissociative Experiences Scale (DES) Jang *et al.* (1998) reported additive genetic influences accounting for 48% and 55% of the variance measuring pathological and nonpathological dissociative experiences respectively. Heritability estimates did not differ by gender. The genetic correlation between these measures was estimated at 0.91, suggesting common genetic factors underlying pathological and nonpathological dissociative states. Genetic and environmental correlations between the DES scales and measures of personality disorder traits (Dimensional Assessment of Personality Pathology: Basic Questionnaire) were also estimated (Livesley and Jang, 2008). Significant genetic correlations were found between the DES scales and cognitive dysregulation, affective lability and suspiciousness, suggesting that the genetic factors underlying particular aspects of personality disorder also influence dissociative capacity. This same group reported that 45% of the variance for the trait narcissism could be explained genetically, an even higher figure being given by Torgersen (2000).

Chromosomal Abnormalities

Some further evidence for a contribution of genetic factors to personality development derives from patients with chromosomal abnormalities. The contention that patients with trisomy 21 (mongolism) or a translocation variant are friendly and jovial is hard to evaluate, especially in the presence of learning disability.

People with Y chromosome abnormalities, notably XYY males, tend to be taller than normals, are overrepresented in prison populations and show poor impulse control and aggressivity. They have difficulty interpreting emotional expressions of others. Neither height nor socioeconomic class explained such observations (Dorus, 1980). Other studies, of patients with variability in length of the Y chromosome, although supportive of an association with excessive criminality and aggression, are not conclusive (Dorus, 1980). XYY males show an excess of neurological problems, including EEG abnormalities, mild to moderate ventricular enlargement on pneumoencephalography, a tendency to clumsiness, incoordination and hyperacrivity, and occasionally epilepsy (Hakola and Iivanainen, 1978).

In comparison, disorders of the X chromosome present different behavioural profiles. Klinefelter's syndrome (XXY) is linked with hyposexuality, sexual deviancy, lack of self-assertiveness and immaturity. Puberty is often delayed and developmental language defects are common (Money, 1975; Walzer *et al.*, 1978). There are smaller amygdala volumes on MRI.

In contrast, lack of one X chromosome in Turner's syndrome (XO) leads to a specific vulnerability for visuoconstructive cognitive deficits, and patients are reported to be phlegmatic, showing an inertia of emotional arousal (Money, 1975). Recent studies have shown that Turner's syndrome females have difficulty processing emotional information and identifying emotional expressions, but mainly from the eye regions of the face. They have been reported to have increased amygdala and orbitofrontal cortical size bilaterally, and loss of the normal correlation between the fusiform (face recognition) cortex and the left amygdala when presented with facial expressions of fear and anger (Skuse, 2006, 2007). The clinical findings and the more recent brain-imaging studies thus suggest that different chromosomal aberrations lead to differing personality profiles; the amygdala seems especially involved in this research. Some authors have implied a specific link between the development of this structure and the X chromosome; loosely, the volume of the amygdala is inverse to the number of X chromosomes (Aleman *et al.*, 2008; van Rijin *et al.*, 2008).

Genetic Alleles

The new genetic studies have looked at associations between specific gene alleles and temperament. Early studies suggesting links between the short version of the 5-HT transporter promotor (5-HTTLPR) and anxiety have not been well replicated, although it has been associated with suicidality. Several studies point to a role of 5-HT transporter promoter polymorphism (s allele carriers) in amygdala activation during emotion perception, accounting for up to 10% of the phenotypic variance (Aleman *et al.*, 2008). Other relevant findings include reduced anterior cingulate–amygdala coupling (s allele) (Pezawas *et al.*, 2005) and altered amygdala–ventromedial prefrontal cortex coupling, which might imply genetic liabilities in s allele carriers to emotional dysregulation in settings of stress. Rhodes *et al.* (2007) have recently reported in a combined PET/MRI investigation a negative correlation between 5-HTT (transporter) availability and amygdala activity, further implicating 5-HT in amygdala reactivity. Other polymorphisms (e.g. the COMT val/met polymorphism, and variants of the tryptophan hydroxylase gene) may also be implicated, although as yet results are inconsistent (Aleman *et al.*, 2008). Meyer-Lindenberg *et al.* (2006) reported that low activity of a variant of the MAOA gene (associated with antisocial, including aggressive, behaviour) was correlated with increased amygdala arousal to emotional stimuli. As noted above, novelty seeking has been associated with dopamine-related genes (transporter: DAT 1; receptor: DRD4) (Sabol *et al.*, 1999). Some investigators have reported complex interactions between personality types, such as novelty seeking, and several polymorphisms, such as the dopamine receptor (DRD4), the 5-HT transporter promotor region 5-HTTLPR and catechol O-methyltransferase (Sabol *et al.*, 1999). Such studies are in their infancy, but are seeking to find associations between genetic polymorphisms, certain personality variables and eventually activation of cerebral circuitry.

Another interesting area of current research involves CLOCK genes, which are involved in circadian rhythm regulation and sleep needs (von Schantz, 2008). Different polymorphisms are associated with different needs for sleep and the amount that people 'fidget'. Most interestingly, they may be linked to, or moderate, bipolar disorder (Benedetti *et al.*, 2008; Imbesi *et al.*, 2009).

It may be concluded, as it was by Slater and Roth (1969), that 'heredity factors play an important role in the development of personality' (p. 68).

SOMATIC VARIABLES

In the past, measurement of bodily features relating to personality types was fashionable. An early enthusiast was Cesare Lombroso (1836–1909), who identified types, notably criminals, by their physiognomy. To our knowledge this interesting line of investigation petered out, but perhaps it has found renewed initiative, albeit in a far more sophisticated fashion, with brain imaging – looking at brains instead of scalps and facial features. Weinstein *et al.* (1999) reported that schizotypal personality-disorder patients showed more minor physical anomalies and dermatoglyphic asymmetries than a normal group, raising comparisons with similar findings in schizophrenia (see Chapter 7). Yang *et al.* (2008) have reported an increase in minor physical abnormalities in sociopathy. 'Minor physical anomalies' refers to dysmorphic features such as subtle deviations of facial structure, finger length and minor earlobe changes such as a Darwin's tubercle.

METABOLIC AND BIOCHEMICAL FINDINGS

Platelet MAO Activity

One of the peripheral markers that has been studied in personality disorders is platelet MAO activity. This is thought to reflect central brain MAO activity, to some degree, and is readily studied. The enzyme MAOB is present in human platelets, and its activity, and that of central MAO, is thought to be under genetic control, although the mechanism of the inheritance is not clear. Levels are relatively stable over time, with a tendency to increase with advancing age.

It has been suggested that reduced platelet MAO may represent a marker of genetic vulnerability for psychopathology (Murphy *et al.*, 1974). In non-patient studies, there is an association between platelet MAOB activity and personality variables. Murphy *et al.* (1977) noted an inverse relationship with higher MMPI scores, and higher ratings on a sensation-seeking scale in men only. Plasma amine oxidase activity held a similar relationship, while another enzyme, dopamine beta hydroxylase, showed no correlation to personality scales. Volunteers with the lowest MAO activity had elevation of most of the MMPI subscales, showing profiles similar to patients with psychiatric illness and low MAO activity. Comparable data are reported by others (Fowler *et al.*, 1980; Schooler *et al.*, 1978), emphasizing the association, in particular, between low MAO activity in platelets and sensation-seeking, the correlations to extraversion on the

EPI, for example, being much weaker (Oreland *et al.*, 1984).

Other studies indicate that children with low platelet MAO activity are more active at birth and are more likely to display neurotic traits in early childhood and that adults with low platelet MAO are more likely to be impulsive, monotony avoiders and aggressive. Buchsbaum *et al.* (1976) noted those with low platelet MAO have more psychiatric contacts, attempt suicide more frequently, have a higher family incidence of psychopathology, have a greater number of convictions and use illicit drugs more than those with high MAO activity.

In animals, a correlation between low MAO activity and brain 5-HT and its metabolites is reported, notably in a strain of mouse with high anxiety, irritability and aggression (Oreland *et al.*, 1984), and in primates, low MAO platelet activity relates to exploratory sensation-seeking activity. Biochemically, the relationship to 5-HT activity in the brain, confirmed in human autopsy material (Adolfsson *et al.*, 1978), suggests that, while in no way being a specific marker for any personality type, platelet MAO activity, especially MAOB, may indicate vulnerabilities to certain personality attributes and psychiatric illness. In one follow-up study of low-MAO subjects, Coursey *et al.* (1982) reported that they had more psychopathology and job instability than high-MAO counterparts, and Perris *et al.* (1984) noted that low-MAO subjects reported less life events prior to the development of depressive disorders than others.

CSF 5-HIAA

There are several studies showing relationships between aggressive, violent or impulsive behaviour and lower levels of 5-HIAA in the CSF. In patients, aggression scores are correlated negatively with the metabolite level, and a less significant but positive correlation has been noted for MHPG (Brown *et al.*, 1979). Low 5-HIAA seems to be associated with a history of suicide attempts, especially by violent means (Brown *et al.*, 1982), and to be lower in incarcerated murderers and those convicted of homicide compared with controls (Linnoila and Martin, 1983). The literature on links between 5-HT and depression (see Chapter 8) is paralleled by these studies linking suicide to low 5-HT turnover. Indeed, this relationship has been observed many times, and is one of the most replicated in the whole of biological psychiatry. Patients with low 5-HT turnover are more likely to die from suicide at follow-up, and similar biochemical findings are noted in impulsive alcoholic offenders and people with aggressive personality disorders without depression. In post mortem samples of brains from those who have committed violent suicide, 5-HT levels are interpreted as low (Stanley and Mann, 1983). Thus, the low 5-HT release relates not only to depressed affect but also to aggression, impulsivity and suicidal behaviours. Stanley *et al.* (2000) have reconfirmed the link between hostility, aggression and low 5-HT concentrations, to the extent of noting an inverse relationship between the 5-HT levels and measures taken of aggression (Sher *et al.*, 2006; Stanley *et al.*, 2000). These clinical data receive substantial support from investigations of rodents which link low 5-HT with enhanced aggression, and of nonhuman primates, in which reduced amounts of 5-HT are associated with severe forms of aggression and a greater frequency of high-risk behaviour (Mehlman *et al.*, 1994). One hypothesis put forward to explain this suggests that the 5-HT link to aggression is mediated via neuronal excitability in the amygdala. In this model, 5-HT is viewed as an activating system for inhibiting behaviour, which is impaired when 5-HT levels are low (Keele, 2005).

Impulsivity is one feature shown by many of these patients, suggesting an association with the personality attributes noted with low MAO levels reported above. A further link between the studies is that alcoholism itself is associated with low platelet MAO levels (Oreland *et al.*, 1984) and abstinent alcoholics also have low 5-HIAA CSF levels (Ballenger *et al.*, 1979; Linnoila and Martin, 1983); impulsive aggression and lifetime aggression in such subjects are related to the low 5-HIAA.

More recent work on this association has confirmed the link between hostility, aggression and low 5-HT concentrations, to the extent of noting an inverse relationship between 5-HIAA levels and the measures taken of aggression (Stanley *et al.*, 2000).

Coccaro *et al.* (1994) have investigated familial relationships. Thus, reduced 5-HIAA in the CSF is associated with a family history of depression in healthy probands and a family history of alcoholism in depressed patients. They reported that the prolactin response to a fenfluramine challenge (which releases 5-HT and prolactin) was blunted in association with an increased risk of impulsive personality disorder traits in first-degree relatives of patients with a DSM III diagnosis of personality disorder.

These data are compatible with some of the animal data, and emphasize the relationship of 5-HT and its metabolites to certain aspects of human behaviour. The genetic evidence and the links to MAO activity suggest that some personality variables, notably impulsivity, sensation-seeking, aggressiveness and proneness to alcoholism, have biochemical correlates, notably with the serotonergic system and its regulation through MAO.

NEUROPHYSIOLOGICAL AND NEUROLOGICAL DATA

Psychophysiological (autonomic) underarousal, as indicated by reduced resting heart rate and skin conductance levels and poor classical conditioning, is one of the most replicated findings in antisocial populations (Glenn and Raine, 2008; Raine *et al.*, 1994). Autonomic underarousal can be shown in infants and young children with a disinhibited temperament that suggests a predisposition to juvenile delinquency and adult aggressive behaviour. Psychophysiological measures, taken at the age of 15 years, have been related to criminality assessed at a later age (24 years). Thus criminality is somehow associated with autonomic underarousal, and the differences are not mediated by social, demographic or educational factors (Baker *et al.*, 2007, 2008; Yang *et al.*, 2008).

EEG

The frequency of EEG abnormalities in patients referred to as aggressive or psychopathic was established long ago (Hill, 1952). In particular, bilateral theta activity in temporal and central regions was reported. These data were reinforced by Williams (1969), whose studies revealed a far higher incidence of abnormal EEGs in aggressive psychopaths than in individuals selected for stability, such as flying personnel, and by Stafford-Clarke and Taylor (1949), who found over 70% of motiveless murderers to have abnormalities. Monroe (1970), reporting on 70 psychiatric patients, noted, with activation, that those who demonstrated high-amplitude paroxysmal slow waves were more likely to be seriously aggressive to themselves or others. Patients diagnosed as suffering from episodic dyscontrol frequently have EEG abnormalities, again the majority being temporal lobe in origin (Bach *et al.*, 1971), and higher levels of violence have been reported with left-focal abnormalities (Pillmann *et al.*, 1999; Shelley *et al.*, 2008). One interesting feature of these studies is that a normal EEG reflected on good personality structure, with a suggestion that cerebral dysrythmias may impede the natural process of psychological maturation (Shelley *et al.*, 2008).

These data are supplemented by observations that psychiatric patients with no history of epilepsy but a temporal lobe focus on the EEG are more likely to be aggressive (Treffert, 1964; Tucker *et al.*, 1965), and by depth-electrode studies, which indicate that feelings of dyscontrol and rage are primarily associated with discharges in the amygdala and hippocampus in both epileptic and non-epileptic patients (Heath, 1982).

In a more systematic study of the behavioural correlates of rhythmic midtemporal discharge, an abnormality frequently associated with psychopathology, Hughes and Hermann (1984) noted a relationship between the frequency of such discharges and abnormal MMPI profiles. Further, patients with BPD have a high frequency (46%) of EEG abnormalities, including nonfocal spike- or sharp-wave activity, diffuse slowing and, on occasions, posterior temporal spike-wave discharges (Cowdry *et al.*, 1986).

These data suggest links between cerebral dysrhythmia and certain personality features, and the emphasis is on impulsive aggressive behaviour. The association is particularly with posterior, often bilateral, temporal paroxysmal discharges. The aetiology of the dysrhythmias is unclear, but may reflect maturational factors, possibly genetically determined, earlier brain damage or a functional disturbance of brainstem–limbic system structures.

Evoked potential studies have also been carried out, although attempts to correlate changes to personality variables have not been reliably reproduced (Shagass, 1972). The CNV has been shown to be of higher amplitude in two studies of psychopathic patients (Howard *et al.*, 1984), although the meaning of this is unclear. In 'go'/'no-go' tasks indicating response inhibition, the differential frontal negative potential recorded at 400 ms between the two trials is diminished in psychopaths (Kiehl *et al.*, 2000; Shane *et al.*, 2008). In odd-ball stimulus detection tasks, psychopaths show larger fronto-central negative waves (N550) during target detection than nonpsychopaths.

Early childhood abuse, stress and lifetime assaultative violence have been linked to electrophysiological abnormalities. Thus an increase in fronto-temporal EEG abnormalities with an emphasis on the left side has been reported in abused children, and dysrhythmic abnormalities have been noted in 77% of those with incestuous relationships (Ito *et al.*, 1998).

Neurological Disorders

Substantial evidence that personality and the brain are closely entwined stems from observations of patients with various neurological conditions or who have suffered trauma to selected regions of the brain. Generally, any brain lesion may disrupt personality, and some authors refer to an 'organic personality change' (Lishman, 1987). This includes irritability and restlessness, lassitude, poor concentration, loss of initiative and excessive emotionality. There may be poor tolerance for change, withdrawal, insecurity and

anxiety. With more severe damage, extremes of this picture are seen, with social disorganization, loss of interest in the self, explosive irritability, shallowness of affect and a blunting of emotional responses. In such situations, an exacerbation of pre-existing personality traits is seen, for example aggressive people exhibiting outbursts of anger, and perhaps violence, with minimal provocation. While many of these features are nonspecific, their recognition is important.

The most direct evidence that the brain is intimately involved in the structure of the personality comes from the observations on patients with frontal-lobe damage. This has been discussed in Chapter 3, where the main elements of the frontal-lobe syndromes have been presented. These include reduced activity, lack of drive, loss of appropriate affect with indifference and blunting, inability to plan appropriately, impulsivity with irritability and aggression, and marked impairment of relationships with others. One recognized form of this has been termed 'pseudopsychopathic', reflecting the similarity of the behaviour to that form of personality disorder.

In contrast, changes of personality related to temporal-lobe pathology are different. The relationship between temporal-lobe pathology and personality change is noted in Chapter 3, and the subject of personality disorders in relation to epilepsy is discussed in Chapter 10, where the arguments in favour of a 'temporal-lobe syndrome' and the relation to aggression are rehearsed. The noted association between personality disorders and epilepsy crystallized with the introduction of the EEG, which led to a fuller understanding and identification of temporal-lobe epilepsy. It was suggested that patients with such an origin of their seizures were more likely to show personality changes. Such clinical information seemed in keeping with the growing literature on the role of the temporal lobes in animal behaviour, in particular the description of the Klüver–Bucy syndrome. Alterations of aggressive potential, affective tone and motoric life were a part of the syndrome, and have been described in association with other limbic-system conditions where the burden of the pathology is in the temporal lobes, such as encephalitis.

The interictal behaviour syndrome of temporal-lobe epilepsy emphasizes alterations in sexual behaviour, hyperreligiosity and hypergraphia, namely the tendency towards extensive and often compulsive writing (Waxman and Geschwind, 1975). In some patients the syndrome appeared before any seizures, and when present, even in the absence of further evidence, might suggest dysfunction at this specific anatomical site. They contrasted this picture both with the frontal-lobe syndrome and with the Klüver–Bucy syndrome, having some characteristics almost opposite to the latter. The religiosity, the excessive interest in the cosmic and supernatural, the conviction that the person has some special significance in the world or some messianic mission, the meticulous attention to detail, the hypergraphia (with detailed accounts of events being recorded, often with a moral or religious theme), the disturbed sexuality, are all features of the full syndrome. Waxman and Geschwind suggested this related to ongoing interictal abnormal electrical activity in the limbic system, a theme taken up by Bear and Fedio (1977). In their studies of patients with temporal-lobe epilepsy, using a behavioural rating scale constructed from literature descriptions of abnormalities recorded in association with the condition, they reported that many items correlated with the length of seizure history. Their interpretation of the findings was that the epileptic focus somehow led to enhanced associations between affect and stimuli, a so-called 'functional hyperconnection' (p. 465) between neocortical and limbic structures, possibly inhibiting events that normally prevent fortuitous sensory and affective connections. This can be seen as the opposite of the Klüver–Bucy syndrome. In the latter the limbic dysfunction leads to failure to attribute stimuli their appropriate emotional significance, with hypermetamorphosis, emotional blunting, diminished fear and aggression, and inappropriate sexual behaviour (limbic agnosia).

The above data reinforce the crucial importance of temporal-lobe epilepsy in unravelling the neurological basis of personality, with a pivotal role of the limbic system and related structures in determining personality dispositions.

Radiological Studies

Brain-imaging studies have contributed significantly to studies of personality disorders, although most of the data has been carried out in antisocial and borderline personality disorder.

With regards to BPD, initial CT studies yielded no useful information. Driessen *et al.* (2000) studied 21 female patients with BPD and a similar group of healthy controls using the Childhood Trauma Questionnaire and MRI volumetric measurements. They reported that in comparison with controls, the personality disorders had bilaterally smaller amygdala and hippocampal volumes. The volumes of the hippocampus were negatively correlated with the extent and the duration of self-reported early trauma (Brunner *et al.*, 2009; Tajima *et al.*, 2009; Whittle *et al.*, 2009; Zanetti *et al.*, 2007). Herpertz *et al.* (2001) have shown with fMRI that the amygdala of females with borderline personality is more reactive when viewing aversive emotional pictures (increased BOLD signal bilaterally). There is also increased signal from the fusiform gyrus. One study using proton spectroscopy has shown reduced NAA levels in the left dorsolateral prefrontal cortex in borderline patients (Tebartz van Elste, 2003).

Functional imaging with PET has not shown consistent results, although the most frequently reported finding is decreased activity in dorsolateral prefrontal cortex. Examining the hypothesis that impulsivity and aggressivity are linked with the borderline profile, Soloff *et al.* (2000) gave fenfluramine challenge (5-HT-releasing compound) and compared the results to placebo (Soloff *et al.*, 2000). Uptake of FDG with fenfluramine was greater in controls compared with patients in prefrontal cortex, including medial and orbital regions bilaterally (BA 10–11), left superior temporal gyrus and right insular cortex. In a later study, again with PET but with a 5-HT receptor ligand (18F-altanserin), Soloff *et al.* (2007) reported increased binding in the hippocampus in BPD.

Most recently investigators have used fMRI, with a variety of innovative activation tasks, to try and understand the brain deficits in BPD. To date, investigators have asked BPD patients to remember painful life events (Buchheim *et al.*, 2008; Völlm *et al.*, 2007), react to emotional faces (Minzenberg *et al.*, 2007; Wingenfeld *et al.*, 2008) or attempt to bond or self-sooth (Driessen *et al.*, 2008; Silbersweig *et al.*, 2007; Völlm *et al.*, 2007).

Interpreting these data is difficult. The studies are done on small numbers, and several have used only female patients. However, there is evidence of fronto-limbic dysfunction with alteration of amygdala size and function in borderline patients. The increased amygdala and associated fusiform gyrus activation, the latter of which processes complex facial stimuli, might imply an increased reactivity to emotional events, and the smaller hippocampi could link with similar findings in some disorders, including depression and post-traumatic stress disorder (see Chapters 6 and 8).

With regards to antisocial personality disorder, Raine *et al.* (1994) have reported a series of studies examining functional and structural brain correlates. In an early PET study they reported that murderers have reduced metabolism in the lateral and medial prefrontal cortex compared with controls, and then showed that the findings applied to murderers who had no early psychosocial deprivation (i.e. no childhood abuse, family neglect). This group have also shown an 11% reduction in prefrontal grey-matter volume in the absence of observed brain lesions in psychopathic antisocial individuals compared with controls (Raine *et al.*, 2000). They also observed in antisocial subjects a 23% increase in estimated callosal white-matter volume, a 7% increase in callosal length, a 15% reduction in callosal thickness, and increased functional inter-hemispheric connectivity. These deficits predicted group membership independent of psychosocial risk factors. Unsuccessful psychopaths (ones who get caught!) in their studies have a 22% reduction in prefrontal grey-matter volume compared with those deemed successful, but on ratings, higher total as well as subfactor psychopathy scores (arrogant/deceptive, affective

and impulsive/unstable) were all associated with low prefrontal grey volume (Yang *et al.*, 2008, 2009). In a recent meta-analysis of imaging data and other variables found in psychopathy, Raine has reported decreased frontal cortical size (especially orbital and middle prefrontal gyrus) (Figure 5.1), greatest in violent psychopaths, higher rates of cavum septum pellucidum, and a decreased amygdala size of 17% (Yang *et al.*, 2008).

These studies seem concordant with other evidence from neurological patients, EEG studies and neuropsychology (see below) that brain

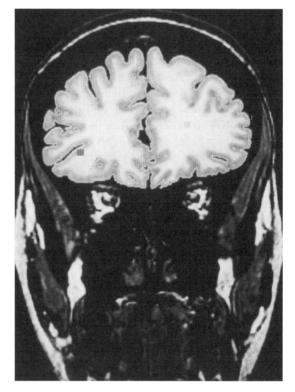

Figure 5.1 Coronal MRI scan showing the seeding points in a study by Raine and colleagues, who examined MRI-defined prefrontal white and grey matter in subjects with antisocial personality disorder, healthy age- and gender-matched controls, and controls with matched substance abuse. The antisocial-personality-disorder group had markedly smaller prefrontal grey-matter volumes (Raine and Yang, 2006; Yang *et al.*, 2005a, 2005b, 2007) (reproduced with permission from Raine *et al.*, 2000). A coloured version of this figure can be found on the colour plate

structural deficits are found in those referred to as psychopaths or who have antisocial behaviour disorders, and that the burden of the abnormalitiy is largely prefrontal. The corpus-callosal findings suggest this may be developmental. Raine suggests that these brain structural abnormalities may underlie the low arousal, poor fear conditioning, lack of conscience and decision-making deficits that have been found to characterize antisocial, psychopathic behaviour. Although these differences emerge in many group studies of antisocial personality subjects, it is unclear how they should be used in forensics or whether they might represent endophenotypes or biological markers (Raine *et al.*, 1994; Raine and Yang, 2006). It is also particularly unclear whether brain-imaging studies help establish an individual diagnosis.

There are few studies of cerebral imaging in other personality types. Raine *et al.* (2002) looked at patients with schizotypal/paranoid personalities and reported reduced prefrontal grey volumes and poorer frontal functioning on frontal neuropsychological tasks compared to controls, although they discussed this more in the context of the findings in schizophrenia than in the context of personality disorders. There are some imaging findings in schizotypal personality disorder, discussed in Chapter 7.

Neuropsychological Findings

Ruocco (2005) carried out a meta-analysis of the neuropsychological data of patients with borderline personalities and reported that, in comparison with healthy comparison groups, on selected neuropsychological tests of attention, cognitive flexibility, learning and memory, planning, speed of processing, and visuospatial abilities, the borderline patients did worse across all neuropsychological domains. There was a suggestion that these deficits were more strongly lateralized to the right hemisphere.

There are several studies of neuropsychological performance in psychopaths, who also show quite diffuse neuropsychological deficits. Meta-analysis particularly implicates deficits of frontal tasks. Impairments on dorsolateral prefrontal executive function tasks of planning

ability and set shifting have been shown, as well as on tasks such as the 'go'/'no go', which suggest ventromedial prefrontal deficits (Yang *et al.*, 2008).

SOME OUTSTANDING ISSUES

It seems to be the case that in comparison with the affective disorders or the schizophrenias, investigation of the personality disorders has been relatively neglected, certainly from a neurobiological perspective. There are several reasons for this, including difficulty with the overall concept, problems with definitions of any subtypes, a debate about the statistical as opposed to the unitary nature of individual types, and disagreement about when a personality disposition becomes a disorder. For example, why is psychopathy diagnosed more in males and histrionic personality identified more in females? Is it simply a matter of cultural bias, or is it related to hormonal, genetic and other biological variables? Added to these are the lines that are drawn between personality disorder (DSM IV axis 2) and any comorbid isomorph (axis 1). It may be that with the next editions of the diagnostic manuals some of these issues will be resolved, especially if biological markers can be identified which help differentiation. In view of the distress which certain personality types bring to themselves, and also to society, much more work with personality disorders of all dimensions would seem a priority (Hiller and Fichter, 2004; Soeteman *et al.*, 2008; van Asselt *et al.*, 2007).

There are other reasons why research in these areas lags behind the volume of work in the rest of biological psychiatry. First, it is most difficult to parse out whether a biological change (e.g. lack of regional brain volume) is fundamental to a personality disorder or arises from living a life with the behaviour flowing from the personality disorder. For example, an antisocial personality patient engages in impulsive behaviour, which leads to a head injury, which damages the orbitofrontal or prefrontal cortex, which then results in even more impulsive behaviour. And the cycle continues.

Second, some researchers and funding organizations are concerned about asking about the genetic underpinnings of personality as this gets uncomfortably close to issues of genetic determinism and even eugenics. Nevertheless, the search for genetic, epigenetic and endophenotypic variables underlying behaviour and its disorders is a central aspect of modern biological psychiatry research.

There seem to be clear associations, and perhaps similar neurobiological underpinnings, between some cluster A variables (especially schizotypal personality disorder) and schizophrenia, but the true nature of this relationship is unknown. Nonetheless, this is of more than theoretical significance: it has preventative and treatment implications. It is not known at what age schizotypal personality disorder begins to reveal itself, or what might be the potential factors that aid or protect against the glide of the mental state to psychosis. The same may be said for other associations, such as anankastic tendencies and OCD, or even the personality profiles that increase the risk for major depressive disorder.

In classical descriptions of personality there is a tendency to imply that personalities (as opposed to illnesses) are stable over time. A person's personality is biologically derived through genetic and epigenetic factors, but matures sometime in the mid to late teens, although any parent will note personality features in their children from a much younger age (even within the uterus before birth?). There are few long-term follow-ups of personality disorders, but many individuals with antisocial personality disorder seem to 'mature' with age, usually by about 40. It is not clear whether this relates to myelination of cerebral pathways (unlikely), or to some enrichment of lifestyle that may accrue with some social success, or simply to a 'burn out' and a wish to spend less time in prison or alone. However, some forms of psychopathic behaviour seem to be integrated within an individual's biological and neurological makeup, and the neurophysiological and brain-imaging data reviewed above seem crucial to understanding the pervasive and persistent nature of the behaviours. Recall above how the opposite sometimes occurs, when mild personality traits seen throughout a lifetime become more florid later in life, associated with a dementia or other disease process.

There is much evidence that personality and its variants have a strong genetic basis, and yet this has hardly been a subject of much discussion outside of small interested groups, and the implications are carefully avoided. Interactions between genetic endowment and environmental influences need parsing out much more carefully than has been the case up until now, especially with the vast improvement that has occurred with the new genetic studies. Measuring the sociological variables lags far behind the modern precision of measuring genetic markers. A good example is the difficulty in adult patients of determining accurately the amount of childhood physical or sexual abuse. Nevertheless, much behaviour which has been assumed to be environmentally driven seems to have a stronger genetic basis than is generally credited (witness the data for antisocial personality disorder). This entire area becomes more complicated because an individual with a genetic bias for a personality type will then often grow up in an environment with parents who also express these tendencies; the dysfunctional family will interact with the genetics, further changing behaviour (Hewitt *et al.*, 1997; Moffitt *et al.*, 2005; Rutter, 1994; Rutter and McGuffin, 2004). These are referred to as gene–environment interactions and they become enormously complex with respect to behaviours that can persist through several generations. Meaney and colleagues have developed animal models of parenting in rats, selecting for mothers who lick and groom their pups. One can select for good mothers, and then subject the pups to early life stressors by temporarily taking them away from the mother (separation). This early separation can then make the adult rat have a lifelong 'anxiety disorder.' However, when the pup is returned from the separation the mother tends to lick and groom it, and a good mother can almost undo the stress of the separation, which is then transmitted in a protective way to the next generation. Postweaning isolation or separation reduced exploratory behaviour in the offspring of high-licking and grooming mothers, whereas social enrichment enhanced exploration of low-licking and grooming offspring (Cameron *et al.*, 2008; Champagne and Meaney, 2007; Champagne *et al.*, 2008; Szyf *et al.*, 2008). Interestingly, these effects were also transmitted to the next generation of offspring. Thus, maternal licking and grooming exhibited a high degree of plasticity in response to changes in environment beyond the postnatal period, which then transmitted a behavioural response to novelty and maternal care across generations.

Many features that we subsume under the term 'personality' would seem to be more closely associated with non-isocortical structures, because affective tone is set more by the limbic lobe and its connectivity than by the isocortex. However, cortical structures modulate and interact with limbic regions to regulate behaviour and personality. The studies combining brain imaging and genetics are beginning to show close associations between some personality variables and monamine levels, especially 5-HT regulation and neuroanatomy, notably the amygdala and its intimate connectivity. Will, as a behavioural domain, and its relationship to behavioural dispositions and to tendencies to act (motion) in one direction or another, derive from extraconscious limbic and subcortical activity. These ideas link to such fundamental social behaviours as empathy (being moved), and how close it is possible to get to another (moving). The frontal–subcortical axis is not only central to many behavioural disorders but determines these personality propensities, just as the temporal–subcortical axis reflects on our emotional harmonies (emotion), and together they allow for not only fear and despondency but also creativity and joy.

6
Anxiety Disorders

INTRODUCTION

Historically, and from a clinical point of view, there are close links between the anxiety disorders and personality disorders (see Chapter 5). The term 'neurosis', originally introduced as a synonym for nervous diseases, was abandoned by DSM III and its successors, and terms such as 'reactive' and 'neurotic depression' have fallen out of fashion. The blurred boundary between the personality disorders and the neuroses was cleaved by DSM III and the divisions between axis 1 and axis 2 disorders.

In anxiety disorders, the predominant symptom is anxiety not associated with another psychiatric disorder. In DSM IV-TR, the following subcategories are given, with their ICD equivalents in brackets: agoraphobia without panic disorder (agoraphobia), social phobia (social phobia), specific phobias (isolated phobia), panic attack, panic disorder with or without agoraphobia (panic disorder) and generalized anxiety disorder (generalized anxiety disorder). ICD 10 has also mixed anxiety and depressive disorder as subcategories, while DSM IV-TR has anxiety disorder due to a general medical condition, substance-induced anxiety disorder and anxiety disorder not otherwise specified (NOS).

Obsessive–compulsive disorder (obsessive–compulsive disorder, OCD), and reactions to severe stress and adjustment disorders are the other two main groupings. Post-traumatic stress disorder (post-traumatic stress disorder, PTSD) is included under the latter. ICD 10 has a subcategory of acute stress reaction, with symptoms lasting only a few days. The equivalent in DSM IV, acute stress disorder, with symptoms very similar to post-traumatic stress disorder, can last up to four weeks.

This listing and lumping of the different disorders is somewhat confusing and unsatisfying. Recall the review of the anatomy of fear and anxiety in Chapter 3.

Both the amygdala and the hippocampus are involved, and there may be a distinction between the neuroanatomy of fear and anxiety. Fear relates more to interactions between primary sensory processing areas such as the thalamus and the amygdala. Hippocampal inputs to the amygdala contribute cognitive information as well as a link to cortical structures and memory, leading to anticipatory and more global anxiety (see Figures 2.16 and 6.1). Flowing from this anatomy, it thus makes sense to categorize generalized anxiety disorder and panic disorder as conditions that arise from hardwired fear and anxiety circuitry. Fear of potentially harmful events or stimuli obviously has important survival value. The specific phobias, including social phobia, also belong within this grouping of fear and anxiety. PTSD can be seen as an overreaction of this circuitry, in a pathological manner which then feeds forward in a destructive way, leading to avoidance

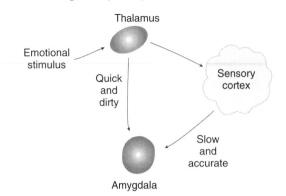

Figure 6.1 Diagram of fear circuitry. In contrast to general anxiety, fear neuroanatomy arises in response to an external threat (shown as an emotional stimulus). This information goes through the LGN of the thalamus for visual information. There are then two pathways: a slow and accurate pathway, which involves normal cortical evaluation of the threat, and a quick and dirty pathway, which sends information directly to the amygdala for certain threats that have likely had evolutionary importance, such as fearful or threatening human faces, or snakes and large predators (reproduced with permission from Higgins and George, 2007)

behaviours and social withdrawal. But like the other anxiety disorders, PTSD likely arises from a common neural substrate involving fear and anxiety regulation. The one condition that does not appear to belong in this category, reasoning from the underlying anatomy as well as from the clinical descriptions and symptoms, is OCD. In OCD, anxiety is secondary to the persistent thoughts (obsessions) or an inability to perform compulsions, or both. The anxiety is not a primary motivator. Moreover, the underlying neuroanatomy is distinct, as is discussed below. OCD will therefore be discussed separately, but within this chapter, as is PTSD, on account of its conceptual importance but also the controversy it has occasioned.

The *phobic disorders* reflect persistent and irrational fears resulting in avoidance behaviour. Phobias as such are extremely common, although in the majority they are not disabling.

Simple phobias include fear of spiders, snakes, thunderstorms, flying, subways, needles and animals. These are usually less socially incapacitating than agoraphobia, which is characterized by a fear of going into crowded places, often combined with a fear of being alone. In this condition, individuals gradually restrict their activities, until, in its most florid form, they become housebound. They use many techniques to avoid going out, and if they have to venture outside it is invariably with a friend, a spouse or a dog. In one form of the disorder, panic attacks occur. These may be only on going out, or occur in places such as the supermarket (the agora), or they may arise spontaneously at home. This may be in relationship to the thought of going out, or on going near the front door, or may suddenly come on out of the blue. Associated with the agoraphobia there is often a history of an anxious personality and a tendency to develop affective disorder. It should be noted that agoraphobic symptoms often arise in the setting of a major affective disorder, and in these cases the diagnosis is with the affective disorders. Social withdrawal and isolation are hallmarks of depression, and should be differentiated from agoraphobia in the absence of other depression symptoms.

Social phobia is a fear of embarrassment or humiliation in social situations, which thus become avoided as the individual restricts social contacts. There is anticipatory anxiety at the thought of social encounters, often confined to certain situations only, such as eating or speaking in public.

Generally, simple phobias have a better prognosis than others, especially if they start in childhood. Agoraphobia, which is commoner in women, tends to come on in the third or fourth decade of life, and may be very resistant to treatment, not the least problem being the patient's reluctance to leave home to attend the clinic for consultation.

In *generalized anxiety disorder* the patient has anxiety of at least one month's duration without phobic symptoms or panic attacks. The manifestations of anxiety are multiple, and affect every bodily system. Further, since anxiety is such a common symptom, and many of the symptoms are somatic, many patients with anxiety disorders are misdiagnosed and inappropriately treated, sometimes for many years. Common symptoms include palpitations, sometimes associated with anterior chest pain over the heart; dyspnea and a sense of choking or a feeling that the patient will not be able to take in a sufficient breath; and dry mouth, with unpleasant, often metallic tastes and abdominal tension, sometimes associated with nausea or actual vomiting. Other symptoms are constipation or diarrhoea; retention of urine or frequency of urination; poor concentration and memory difficulties; dizziness, vertigo, faint feelings and, on occasions, blackouts which resemble epileptic seizures; increased muscle tone with pain; tremor; fatigue and loss of energy; and sensory symptoms such as tingling, especially of the hands, diminished vision or a generalized hyperacusis in which sounds are distorted and magnified, sometimes accompanied by photophobia. On examination, patients with anxiety show sweating, often have cold extremities, and may show flushing. The resting pulse, respiration rate and blood pressure may be elevated and increased central body movement or restless hand movements with a tremor may be noted.

Panic attacks are frequent episodes, of a discrete nature, of panic associated with apprehension and fear. Their paroxysmal nature, their sudden onset and the absence often of any obvious precipitating factor may readily lead to a diagnosis of epilepsy. They often resemble one form of complex partial seizure (see Chapter 10).

A variant of this is the *phobic-anxiety depersonalization syndrome* (omitted from the diagnostic manuals), in which depersonalization or derealization forms a prominent part of the picture. This is a much more pervasive disorder, with generalized anxiety, affective symptoms and a danger of death by suicide. In some patients, between the more extreme manifestations, the depersonalization may persist. When severe it may lead patients to feel like automata, or as if they have left their bodies, sometimes with autoscopy. Autoscopy is when a person, while believing themselves to be awake, sees their body and the world from a location outside their self.

Post-traumatic stress disorder has a long and distinguished history, and in the past was referred to as accident neurosis, compensation neurosis or some other variant (Trimble, 1981b). Many physicians come across this in a medicolegal setting and are familiar with the arguments over the role of financial gain in the production or prolongation of the symptoms. The characteristic symptoms involve combinations of psychological re-experiencing of a traumatic event with or without physical accompaniments, avoidance phenomena and persistent symptoms of arousal.

The essential features of *OCD* are the obsessions – persistent ideas, thoughts or images that invade conscious experience against the wishes of the patient – and compulsions – repetitive semipurposeful motor acts. Both the obsessions and the compulsions are somehow alien to the individual (ego-dystonic) and are resisted. Often the thoughts are offensive and repugnant, and the compulsions are senseless stereotyped actions, from which no pleasure is derived, although there is often relief of tension. OCD implies the persistence of obsessions and compulsions, in the absence of another psychiatric disorder. The contents of the rituals most commonly found are cleaning, avoiding, repeating and checking, and some authors note that the recognition of the senselessness of the phenomena is more relevant than resistance to them (Stern and Cobb, 1978). Variants include the intrusion of vivid imaginary, scenes of unacceptable events, ruminations on trivia, convictions of a magical nature (for example, that to carry out one act will prevent another), fears of dirt, disease and contamination, and rituals of counting or performing certain acts in specific ways or in a special order. Although depressive symptoms are common, it is essential to distinguish whether the depression is secondary, or whether the obsessional symptoms derive from a primary affective disorder in an anankastic personality.

GENETICS

Modern genetics in this area is tending to identify endophenotypes and there is some overlap with the genetics underlying the depressions (Merikangas and Low, 2005). Controlled family studies reveal that all of these anxiety subtypes are familial, and twin studies suggest that the familial aggregation is attributable in part to genetic factors. Panic disorder and its spectrum have the strongest magnitude of familial clustering and genetic underpinnings. Children of parents with anxiety disorders are at an increased risk of developing mood and anxiety disorders, but there is far less specificity

of the manifestations of anxiety in children and young adolescents. Although there have been many studies designed to identify genes underlying these conditions, to date no specific genetic loci have been identified and replicated in independent samples. Several family studies have detected a higher rate of panic disorder in the relatives of affected probands than in relatives of control subjects. The relative risk to first-degree relatives of panic-disorder probands ranges between 2.6- and 20-fold, with one meta-analysis finding an eightfold increase in risk (Middeldorp, 2005). Twin studies have shown a heritability of 30–60%. There are two studies suggesting, but not proving, susceptibility loci (markers D4S413 (Kaabi *et al.*, 2006), which also harbours the neuropeptide gene, and D9S271 (Thorgeirsson *et al.*, 2003)). For OCD, the twin studies have found a higher heritability

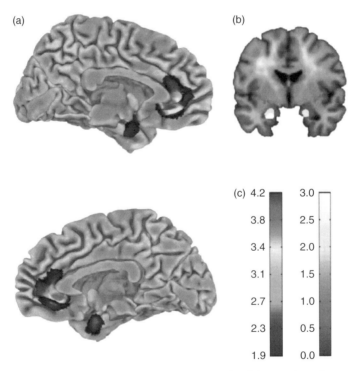

Figure 6.2 Genetic variation impacts key brain regions involved in anxiety, increasing vulnerability to dysregulation. Shown are thresholded maps ($p < 0.05$) reflecting differences in grey-matter volume in 5-HTTLPR s-allele carriers compared to the l/l genotype, with medial sagital views (a) and coronal images (b) and (c) representing the statistical thresholds for the colour on the images. Note the volume reductions in the allele carriers in the bilateral perigenual anterior cingulate cortex and amygdala (reproduced from Pezawas *et al.*, 2005). A colour version of this figure can be found on the colour plate

than panic, at 80% (Carey *et al.*, 1980), with a shared genetic diathesis involving Gilles de la Tourette's syndrome. Hu *et al.* (2006) found a genetic linkage of OCD to the short variant of the 5-HT transporter gene. Twin studies for the other anxiety disorders again show heritability (20–40% for agoraphobia and social phobia).

As discussed above, another approach to understanding the genetics of a disorder is to find an endophenotype for the behaviour and examine whether genetic differences correlate with differences in behavioural tendencies. Figure 6.2 shows that subjects with differences in the 5-HT transporter (5-HTT LPR) have differences in grey-matter volume in the anterior cingulate and amygdala (Pezawas, 2005). Moreover, an individual's genotype for the 5-HT transporter may also affect how they process fearful stimuli and respond to stress. That is, individuals with the s genotype for the 5-HT transporter may be more vulnerable to stress than those with the l genotype.

SOMATIC VARIABLES

Psychophysical variables associated with generalized anxiety have been investigated, notably monitoring autonomic activity (Lader, 1969). Lower skin conductance, more spontaneous fluctuations, increased sweating and diminished habituation of autonomic indices to stimulation, monitoring such variables as blood pressure, the EMG and forearm blood flow, have been reported. The galvanic skin response (GSR) is the sudden increase in skin conductance that can be observed with appropriate stimuli, and, since it can be abolished by atropine, it is thought to be dependent on the activity of sweat glands. Its habituation is delayed in those with anxiety states, the habituation being negatively correlated with ratings of anxiety (Lader, 1969). Tsunoda *et al.* (2008) explored whether social anxiety is associated with preattentive emotional responses to facial expressions. Skin conductance responses differed between a group with high social anxiety and one with low social anxiety. The former showed significantly greater differences in their responses between masked fearful and

happy faces than the latter. These findings suggest that the predisposition to social anxiety relates to the hard fear wiring in the 'quick and dirty' amygdala circuit.

Abnormalities of psychophysiological responses have been shown in PTSD. Traumatized patients show increased autonomic reactions to specific stimuli related to earlier psychological trauma. They also show failure of habituation to an acoustic startle response and delayed extinction of fear conditioning (Blechert *et al.*, 2007; van der Kolk, 1994).

There has been interest in an association between panic disorder and mitral valve prolapse. The latter may present with symptoms similar to anxiety, although the emphasis is on palpitations and chest pain. Whether the occurrence of the two conditions when seen together is coincidence, genetic or reflects some underlying autonomic dysfunction associated with both is not clear.

METABOLIC AND BIOCHEMICAL FINDINGS

In contrast to the affective disorders and the psychoses, there is a dearth of information regarding metabolic and biochemical links with the anxiety disorders. As suggested with the above findings, the autonomic system, and in particular adrenaline, was a focus of interest. Normals show increased stress-related increases in plasma catecholamines. Adrenaline infusions provoke somatic symptoms of anxiety or exacerbate anxiety in anxious patients (Breggin, 1964). Further, noradrenaline stimulates the production of lactic acid and free fatty acids, both of which are raised in anxiety states. Isoprenaline, a beta-receptor agonist, when infused provokes tachycardia more readily in the anxious (Frolich *et al.*, 1969).

Several groups have noted increased urinary or plasma catecholamines in anxious subjects. The difficulty with the plasma assessments from earlier studies was the insensitivity of the assay procedures, and thus more studies have been done on urine. Excretion of both adrenaline and noradrenaline are noted in anxiety-provoking situations, increased adrenaline relating to threatening or uncertain situations and noradrenaline to states of challenge, including those leading to anger or aggression (Schildkraut and Kety, 1967). Mathew et al. (1980a) have reported that both noradrenaline and adrenaline are increased in patients with generalized anxiety disorder compared with controls, decreasing after a course of biofeedback. Raised urinary catecholamines are found on PTSD (Young and Breslau, 2004).

The lactic acid link was followed by Pitts and McClure (1967) on the grounds that lactate was responsible for the anxiety. In their studies they gave anxious patients and normals intravenous sodium lactate, and nearly all the former (93%) developed severe anxiety, starting within a few minutes of the infusion. This was not seen to the same extent in the normals (20%), or following glucose–saline infusions. Since lactate combined with calcium chloride was much less effective in provoking anxiety they suggested that the lactate bound with calcium, which lowered calcium levels and thus interfered with neurotransmission.

These observations have been replicated by several groups, the main clinical conclusion being that lactate provokes anxiety, and more specifically panic in susceptible patients. It was earlier thought that the effect of lactate was a peripheral one, and that infused lactate did not penetrate the CNS. However, it has been shown using MRS that panic patients responding to lactate show higher brain lactate levels before, during and after infusion compared with nonresponders. This raises the possibility of direct CNS effects of lactate. In humans, hyperventilation with subsequent hypocapnia, which is typically seen in lactate-induced panic, may either enhance peripheral uptake or lead to endogenous increases of brain lactate (Dager et al., 1994). These data fit with the replicated observation that giving panic patients 5% CO_2 to breath will also provoke panic attacks. Since infusions of sodium bicarbonate also induce panic in the prone, theories have been developed to explain why CO_2, bicarbonate and lactic acid should all be so provocative. Since CO_2 is a common metabolite of lactate and bicarbonate, it has been suggested that CO_2 leads to cerebral hypercapnia, which leads to hyperventilation and panic (Papp et al., 1993). Patients with specific phobias do not exhibit this sensitivity to CO_2 (Anthony et al., 1997), while lactate (and yohimbine) activates flashbacks in PTSD (Southwick et al., 1997).

There are reports that platelet MAO is increased in patients with panic disorder (Gorman et al., 1985). In animals, a correlation between low MAO activity and brain 5-HT and its metabolites is reported, notably in a strain of mouse with high anxiety, irritability and aggression (Oreland et al., 1984); in primates, low MAO platelet activity relates to exploratory sensation-seeking activity. Tryptophan depletion caused increased anxiety and CO_2-induced panic in patients with panic disorder, but not controls. A blunted prolactin response to fenfluramine has been reported in PTSD, suggestive of 5-HT dysrregulation, which receives some support from the response of this condition to SSRIs and the sensitivity to tryptophan depletion.

There are few hormonal investigations of patients with anxiety disorders. Clinically, phaeochromocytomas, which secrete catecholamines, can present with intermittent episodes of anxiety. The absence of thyroid hormone at crucial stages of early life is known to markedly alter development. The clinical picture of thyrotoxicosis has long been recognized to simulate anxiety states, and assessment of thyroid function is still required in the evaluation of anxiety states. In view of the overlap, the reports of blunted TSH responses to TRH in panic-disorder patients are of interest (Roy-Byrne et al., 1985a). Basal levels of TSH seem only slightly diminished and routine thyroid-function tests are within normal limits in panic-disorder patients.

There is one report of a blunted growth-hormone response to intravenous clonidine in OCD patients, who also displayed higher MHPG and noradrenaline plasma levels than controls (Siever et al., 1983). The similarity of the clonidine response to that seen in affective disorders (see Chapter 8) suggests a biological affinity between the two, the authors suggesting an association with increased presynaptic and decreased postsynaptic noradrenergic responsiveness. In PTSD, studies have revealed elevated urinary catecholamines in comparison to patients with other psychiatric disorders (van der Kolk, 1994).

Generally patients with anxiety or panic disorder show normal cortisol suppression with the DST (Roy-Byrne *et al.*, 1985b), and suppression does not relate to anxiety symptoms in depressed patients (Saleem, 1984). Similarly, patients with PTSD and OCD show normal DST suppression (Lieberman *et al.*, 1985). In chronic PTSD, low-baseline, normal-range and elevated-baseline cortisol have all been reported, which may reflect on the heterogeneity of patients or differences between trait and state. Low cortisol has been observed in normal individuals under chronic stress as well as with chronic medical conditions, which may reflect on neuroanatomical (hypothalamic) or genetic influences.

Some of these data have led to specific examination of the HPA axis in PTSD (Shalev *et al.*, 2008; Yehuda and Golier, 2009; Yehuda *et al.*, 2007). Stress initiates autonomic changes and alters activity in the hypothalamo–pituitary–adrenal (HPA) axis. The neurone of the paraventricular nucleus of the hypothalamus contain releasing hormones such as corticotrophin factor (CRF), which increases the pituitary release of ACTH (corticotrophin), stimulating adrenal cortisol secretion. Blunted ACTH responses to CRF and elevated CSF corticotrophin are reported in PTSD (Bremner *et al.*, 1997). Plasma CRF levels are also high (de Kloet *et al.*, 2008). These data, along with the low cortisol levels, are thought to relate to an HPA axis oversensitivity to the feedback of cortisol, the low cortisol levels thus reflecting chronic changes to the HPA axis. This is secondary to an increased sensitivity of glucocorticoid receptors in target tissues. Such feedback is initiated via the hypothalamus, amygdala, hippocampus and pituitary, all areas with high concentrations of cortisol receptors (Rodrigues *et al.*, 2009; Ruby *et al.*, 2008). However, the hippocampus is central to this concept, the acute hormonal changes occurring with psychological trauma relating to abnormal memory consolidation in PTSD, supported by the hippocampal imaging data reported below. CRF receptor antagonists are currently under investigation for the treatment of anxiety disorders, although results from early clinical trials have been disappointing.

NEUROCHEMICAL INVESTIGATIONS

The three main areas of neurochemical investigation relating to the anxiety disorders are the association of anxiety with abnormal adrenergic or 5 H-T activity and the link with benzodiazepine receptors.

The interest in adrenergic mechanisms relates to the early observations that drugs such as the beta stimulants provoked many of the peripheral effects of anxiety and the finding that these were blocked by specific beta-receptor antagonists. In particular, drugs such as propranolol diminish the heart rate, inhibit palpitations, decrease tremor and inhibit the release of free fatty acids. In addition, the beta blockers have a long and respectable clinical use in anxiety. One hypothesis to emerge is that in anxiety there is an increased sensitivity of adrenergic, specifically beta receptors. Some suggest this is a peripheral phenomenon supporting the James–Lange hypothesis (Chapter 2), but this is not supported by several findings. First, in general, catecholamine-related compounds used to stimulate and block the anxiety symptoms cross the blood–brain barrier, and may thus be exerting their effects centrally. Second, the available evidence with regards to panic disorder does not show increased responsiveness. Thus, Gorman *et al.* (1983) have shown that propranolol pretreatment fails to prevent lactate-induced panic attacks, and Nesse *et al.* (1984) report that panic patients actually decrease their heart rate after an infusion of the beta-stimulant isoproteranol. Third, panic disorder responds better to imipramine than propanolol (Kathol *et al.*, 1981). Fourth, many of the infusion investigations were not carried out under double-blind conditions, and it is uncertain to what extent the infusions themselves acted as a nonspecific stressor.

In contrast, alternative theories emphasize the primacy of central mechanisms in anxiety and panic, and sometimes are seen as rivals to the peripheral theory. The origins of this go back to Cannon (1927). He acknowledged the work of others who previously had shown that decorticate animals could still experience anxiety; his own investigations showed that emotions could be generated by stimulation of CNS structures, and the experience of anxiety was not dependent on peripheral changes. The extended amygdala is one of the macrosystems considered important for these behaviours. For this theory, the somatic manifestations experienced in anxiety are an effect, not the cause, and it follows that the biochemical changes such as those of the catecholamines are also secondary.

In panic disorder there is evidence of down-regulation of beta adrenergic receptors, and increased sensitivity to the hypotensive response to clonidine, suggesting increased sensitivity of presynaptic alpha-2 receptors, but blunted clonidine growth hormone responses, suggesting subsensitive postsynaptic alpha-2 receptors (Nutt and Lawson, 1992). These data implicate brain noradrenergic systems in panic disorder.

Gorman et al. (1989) postulated a neuroanatomical basis of panic disorder involving the locus coeruleus, chemosensitive areas of the medulla, the limbic system and the frontal cortex. Patients with generalized anxiety disorder also show blunted growth-hormone responses.

Central monoamine activity in anxiety-panic disorder has been studied, with particular reference to noradrenaline and the locus coeruleus, which when stimulated provokes anxiety in animals. Drugs that increase locus-coeruleus firing, and thus release of noradrenaline, such as yohimbine, provoke anxiety in humans (Helmberg and Gershon, 1961), while the alpha-2 agonist clonidine, which reduces locus coeruleus activity, is anxiolytic, albeit modestly (Hoehn-Saric, 1982; Uhde et al., 1985). Similar down-regulation of activity is seen with tricyclic antidepressants, also effective in some anxiety patients (Nyback et al., 1975), propranolol and benzodiazepines.

A possible estimate of central catecholaminergic activity is measurement of the MHPG in urine and plasma. Ko et al. (1983) reported that plasma levels of this metabolite correlated highly with rated anxiety in patients with the phobic anxiety syndrome, and both clonidine and imipramine inhibited a panic-induced MHPG increase. In a more extensive investigation of alpha-2-receptor function in anxiety, Charney et al. (1984a) gave yohimbine to healthy subjects and drug-free patients with agoraphobia or panic attacks. In the patients the rise of plasma MHPG levels correlated with patient-rated anxiety, nervousness and the frequency of reported panic attacks; this was interpreted as evidence for impaired presynaptic noradrenergic regulation in the patients. This is supported by the observation of diminished yohimbine platelet binding in panic-disorder patients (Cameron et al., 1984).

Patients with PTSD show decreased alpha adrenergic platelet receptors (Perry et al., 1990) and increases in MHPG to yohimbine challenge (Southwick et al., 1993). Bremner et al. (1993) hypothesized that PTSD is associated with an increased responsiveness of the locus coeruleus, and increased release of noradrenaline in limbic and other areas innervated by that nuclear group in response to stressful stimuli.

Another putative neurotransmitter group of interest in anxiety is the purinergic system. Thus caffeine is anxiogenic, even provoking anxiety in normal controls at high levels (Uhde et al., 1985). Caffeine is an inhibitor of adenosine, itself a potent neuromodulator which has anticonvulsant effects, and antagonists are proconvulsant.

Buspirone, a 5-HT$_{1A}$ agonist has been shown to be effective in treating generalized anxiety disorder, suggesting involvement of the 5-HT system, supported by the observations that the SSRIs are helpful for this condition and panic disorder (see Chapter 12).

Understanding of the benzodiazepine receptor has been of importance. There are hints of an association between central benzodiazepine-receptor binding and anxious traits in animals, and in patients the benzodiazepines are most successful in the treatment of anxiety disorders. The discovery of the benzodiazepine receptor was a landmark in our understanding of the anxiety disorders, and is of great significance for biological psychiatry. Thus, the possibility of discovering abnormalities of brain structure and function in patients with major psychopathology has been a continuous endeavour, but the anxiety disorders have been somewhat excluded. Indeed, the concept of biological therapies for anxiety disorders has been criticized, and use of medications such as the benzodiazepines has been discouraged. The concept of endogenous anxiety has been ignored, and the essentially biological nature of the anxiety disorders has been sacrificed on the Cartesian shrine. In other words, many still suggest that anxiety is 'mind-based' rather than biologically 'brain-based'. That is, compared to the schizophrenias or the depressions, which are now readily treated with psychotropic medications, many anxiety-disorder patients, their families and even their physicians still fail to acknowledge the neurobiological basis of anxiety disorders.

It has to be of interest therefore that benzodiazepine receptors exist in profusion in the human brain; that in animal models, anxiety levels can be related to such receptors; and that in humans, benzodiazepines are anxiolytic. Further, benzodiazepine receptors are found in high concentration in such structures as the temporal, frontal and visual cortices, and the cerebellum and their antagonists provoke anxiety in animals and humans. These antagonists displace radioactively labelled benzodiazepines from their binding sites and reverse their behavioural and physiological effects. Two commonly used compounds are beta-carboline-3-carboxylate (beta-CCE) and Ro 15–1788, which appear anxiogenic when given alone. A derivative of beta-CCE has been given to humans and shown to provoke severe anxiety (Dorrow *et al.*, 1983). These data raise the possibility that an 'endogenous anxiolytic' exists within the brain, and Sandler (1983) proposed the name 'tribulin' for this. There are other endogenous anxiogenic compounds, most notably the gut protein, CCK; this is also found in the brain and can provoke panic attacks when given intravenously (Eser *et al.*, 2008a, 2008b).

The search is still on for a truly active 'endogenous benzodiazapine'. In many instances, the discovery of a receptor that interacts with external medications preceded the discovery of the internal endogenous ligand. For example, opiate receptors were found long before the endorphins were uncovered. It is unclear if there are endogenous benzodiazapine compounds or whether the receptor's activity involves other compounds and the modification of the receptor by, for example, CCK.

Among the disorders that are classified under the 'anxiety' moniker the role of 5-HT has been most clearly established in obsessive–compulsive behaviours. This stems from the observations that patients with obsessive–compulsive disorder responded preferentially to clomipramine, a tricyclic drug with a high selectivity for 5-HT, compared with other tricyclics, even in the absence of an associated depression (Thoren *et al.*, 1980a). It has now been shown that the response is better in patients with higher pretreatment levels of CSF 5-HIAA and HVA (Thoren *et al.*, 1980b), in those whose 5-HIAA levels fall the most during treatment and in those whose blood 5-HT decreases (Hanna *et al.*, 1993). Further, several of the selective 5-HT reuptake inhibitors (SSRI) have been shown to be efficacious in OCD (see Chapter 12).

CSF 5-HIAA, although relating to response in some studies, with higher levels before treatment being indicative of a better response (Swedo *et al.*, 1992; Thoren *et al.*, 1980b), has not been reliably different at baseline compared with controls. CSF MHPG does not relate to OCD symptoms (Swedo *et al.*, 1992). Symptoms of OCD can be exacerbated by the 5-HT partial agonist m-chlorophenylpiperazine (m-CPP), but symptoms are not exacerbated by tryptophan depletion (Berney *et al.*, 2006). The critical role of 5-HT in modulating OCD symptoms (as well as trichotillomania) was demonstrated by Rapoport *et al.* (1992) in both human studies and dogs with canine acral lick dermatitis. These double-blind crossover studies compared clomipramine with desipramine, and fluoxetine with fenfluramine against placebo. Only the

5-HT-uptake-blocking drugs were effective. The authors proposed that canine acral lick dermatitis was an animal model for OCD (Rapoport, 1992; Rapoport *et al.*, 1992).

Other findings associated with OCD include a normal prolactin response to TRH, normal alpha-2 noradrenergic responsivity, normal dexamethasone suppression, reduced prolactin release with fenfluramine, and an elevated growth-hormone response to the acetylcholinesterase inhibitor pyridostigmine (Lucey *et al.*, 1993), the latter finding suggesting cholinergic supersensitivity.

CSF studies have revealed elevated vasopressin and oxytocin in some OCD patients, especially those with no personal or family history of tics (Altemus *et al.*, 1992; Leckman *et al.*, 1994). These findings are of particular interest, since the limbic forebrain contains many sites rich in vasopressin and oxytocin receptors, and in animal models vasopressin has been shown to be associated with grooming behaviours and with maintaining conditioned responses to aversive stimuli (Insel, 1992).

There arises from these data good evidence that the serotonergic system is important in OCD, although other systems are also involved. An attempt has been made to examine receptor subtypes that may be involved by using selective agonists. The effect of mCPP on increasing obsessional symptoms can be blocked by metergoline, an antagonist of the 5-HT_{1a}, 5-HT_{1c}, 5-HT_{1d} and 5-HT_2 receptors. MK-212, a selective agonist of the 5-HT_{1b}, 5-HT_{1c} and 5-HT_2 receptor, provokes a blunted prolactin response in patients with OCD, but does not increase symptomatology (Bastini *et al.*, 1990). The 5-HT_{1a} receptor agonist isapirone seems to have no such effects (Lesch *et al.*, 1991), and there seems to be no alteration of platelet 5-HT_2 receptors (Pandey *et al.*, 1993). A working hypothesis therefore is that further examination of the 5-HT_{1d} subsystem may be worthwhile.

NEUROPHYSIOLOGICAL AND NEUROLOGICAL DATA

The Klüver–Bucy syndrome, with diminished anxiety as a central feature, has already

been described. It might be anticipated that stimulation of medial temporal structures leads to anxiety. Such is indeed the case. Heath (1982) correlated changes in various brain sites with emotions using intracerebral EEG recordings, and noted, in some patients, how the affect fear related to subcortical discharges. This has been replicated by several other groups, including Gloor *et al.* (1982) and Wieser (1983). The former recorded from, and stimulated, electrodes implanted in neocortical and allocortical sites in patients awaiting neurosurgery. Of 35 patients, 50% exhibited some kind of experiental phenomenon with recorded activity, fear being the commonest. The responses required limbic-system discharges and could not be evoked by purely cortical discharges. Particularly involved was the amygdala, a structure also identified in the studies of Wieser, who stimulated various brain regions, again using implanted electrodes, and reported fear on activation of the amygdala and periamygdaloid area.

The evidence from patients with epilepsy points in a similar direction. Williams (1956) recorded the ictal emotional experiences of 100 patients with epilepsy, and noted fear in 61. It was seen mainly with an anterior or midtemporal location of the seizure origin. Cases of partial-status epilepticus, with an origin in the temporal lobes and fear as a clinical manifestation, are described (Henriksen, 1973), and clinically on occasion it can be very difficult to distinguish a panic attack from an epileptic aura of fear.

There are several single case reports of patients with focal right-temporal lesions presenting with panic attacks (Drubach and Kelly, 1989), and Fontaine *et al.* (1990) reported significantly more temporal-lobe abnormalities compared with controls on MRI.

IMAGING

Structural Studies

As mentioned above in the imaging studies of the SERT transporter, the anatomical studies in panic, PTSD and GAD have largely focused on hippocampal or amygdala volumes. This area is problematic in that these disorders involve stress, repeated over time, and we know that stress hormones feed back in health and can actually change hippocampal size. This has been shown in studies of Cushing's disease (Belanoff *et al.*, 2001; Dubrovsky, 1993; Starkman *et al.*, 1999). Thus, there is a chicken-and-egg paradox as to what came first, small volumes or normal volumes which have then changed while subjects live a life of repeated stress (Maheu *et al.*, 2008; Sapolsky, 1996; Yehuda, 1997).

Structural imaging in OCD has failed to find consistent differences between controls. Luxenberg *et al.* (1988) noted decreased volume of the caudate nuclei, a finding replicated by Robinson *et al.* (1995). These data were not supported by the study of Kellner *et al.* (1991). Garber *et al.* (1989) reported increased T_1 values of right-frontal white matter.

In the realm of PTSD, some studies have found focal areas of abnormal signal activity in the medial temporal and parahippocampal areas on the right side. Bremner *et al.* (1995) have compared hippocampal volumes in Vietnam combat veterans with PTSD and controls, and reported smaller right hippocampal volumes in the PTSD group. A most interesting recent study examined the subject in reverse: Grafman and colleagues (Koenigs and Grafman, 2009; Koenigs *et al.*, 2008) built on work showing that PTSD is associated with hypoactivity in the ventromedial prefrontal cortex (vmPFC), hyperactivity in the amygdala and reduced volume in the hippocampus (discussed below). It is unknown whether these functional neuroimaging findings reflect the underlying cause or a secondary effect of the disorder. To investigate the causal contribution of specific brain areas to PTSD symptoms, Grafman and colleagues studied a unique sample of Vietnam War veterans who suffered brain injury and emotionally traumatic events. They found a substantially reduced occurrence of PTSD among those individuals with damage to one of two regions of the brain: the ventromedial prefrontal cortex (vmPFC) and an anterior temporal area that included the amygdala. These results suggest that the vmPFC and amygdala are critically involved in the pathogenesis of PTSD (Koenigs *et al.*, 2008).

Functional Studies

A large body of functional imaging literature now confirms our ideas about the neural circuitry of the anxiety disorders. Researchers have typically taken either control subjects or anxiety patients and then exposed them to situations that provoke their anxiety, and compare brain activity during the anxiety to brain activity at rest. These studies have been enormously helpful in destigmatizing the illnesses and in elucidating the relevant neuroanatomy.

In OCD patients, Baxter *et al.* (1988) initially found increased metabolism in the left orbital frontal region and caudate nuclei. These findings have received some replication, although others implicate more widespread frontal involvement (Swedo *et al.*, 1989b). Treatment with either selective 5-HT agents or behaviour therapy tends to decrease levels of metabolism in fronto-basal ganglia circuits (Benkelfat *et al.*, 1990; Baxter *et al.*, 1992).

Provocation studies, in which obsessive–compulsive behaviours are invoked during scanning, also show increases of CBF in fronto-basal ganglia, thalamic and cingulate areas during activated behaviours (McGuire *et al.*, 1994; Rauch *et al.*, 1994).

These data seem consistent with the hypothesis that the underlying neuroanatomy of obsessive–compulsive behaviours involves the fronto-basal ganglia–thalamic circuits discussed in Chapter 3. Frontal or caudate overactivity will lead to increased inhibition of the globus pallidus–thalamic pathway, thus releasing activity in thalamic outflow back to the cortex. Another way to achieve the same effect would be by a lesion in the globus pallidus or the anterior limb of the internal capsule, or the anterior cingulate. These approaches are being using therapeutically with gamma-knife and deep-brain stimulation. The 5-HT effects may be mediated by the substantial serotoninergic afferents to the basal ganglia.

Two early PET studies of lactate-induced panic disorder suggested that there was right parahippocampal and bitemporal activation respectively, and that similar bilateral abnormalities were also seen in patients with anticipatory anxiety (Reiman *et al.*, 1989). These findings were later attributed to increased tension in extracranial muscles associated with the anxiety (Drevets *et al.*, 1992). It does appear however that intense anxiety and panic do activate fear and anxiety circuits involving the amygdala and hippocampus.

Studies using PET in generalized anxiety patients suggest differences from controls with higher occipital-lobe, right posterior temporal-lobe, right precentral frontal-lobe and left inferior frontal-lobe metabolism, and decreased activity in the basal ganglia. Treatment with benzodiazepines resulted in decreased metabolic rates in cortical, limbic and basal ganglia areas (Wu *et al.*, 1991).

In simple phobia there have been negative studies as well as positive activation data. Fredrikson *et al.* (1993), in patients with snake phobias, showed activation of visual association cortex and thalamus, while Rauch *et al.* (1995), in patients with small-animal phobia, demonstrated activation of anterior cingulate, insular, anterior temporal, posterior medial orbitofrontal, somatosensory cortex and thalamus. The latter study was careful to exclude teeth-clenching as an artefact (Rauch *et al.*, 1995).

These data do suggest widespread involvement of limbic and somatosensory cortex in various anxiety conditions, with an emphasis on the right, especially for panic disorder.

OBSESSIVE–COMPULSIVE DISORDER

Clinically this syndrome would seem the 'most neurological' of the conditions discussed in this chapter, and in some patients the quality of the thoughts and compulsions are of psychotic intensity. The syndrome seems rather arbitrarily in the past to have been labelled a neurosis, with the supposed assumption that in doing so its pathogenesis was understood in psychodynamic terms.

Tuke (1894) was one of the earliest writers to recognize the cerebral underpinnings of the condition and since then the evidence for the neurological associations of OCD has stemmed from the clinical associations with such disorders as encephalitis lethargica, Parkinson's disease, Gilles de la Tourette's syndrome and the remarkable response of some patients to selective neurosurgical lesions.

The encephalitis pandemics of the early part of this century led to the rich variety of neuropsychiatric symptomatology described by von Economo (1931). These included obsessive and compulsive behaviours (Neal, 1942). Many patients had postencephalitic Parkinson's disease, and in some the compulsive behaviour was 'awakened' by L-dopa therapy (Sacks, 1973). The association between Parkinson's disease and obsessive–compulsive traits has been frequently mentioned, in terms of either rigid, moralistic and inhibited premorbid personality profiles or the development of obsessive–compulsive symptoms in association with the motor manifestations of the disease (Todes and Lees, 1985). Obsessional slowness – the extreme time required by some patients to carry out acts – may be likened to failure of executive motor planning, similar to that which must underlie Parkinson's disease.

Swedo *et al.* (1989a) have drawn attention to the high prevalence of obsessive–compulsive symptoms in patients with Sydenham's chorea, a known disorder of the basal ganglia. Gilles de la Tourette's syndrome is characterized by multiple tics, including vocal tics, which usually manifest before the age of 15 years (Trimble, 1981a). Although these wax and wane with time, the condition once established seems lifelong. Some of its manifestations are responsive to drugs that block dopamine receptors such as haloperidol, pimozide and sulpiride. The richness of the condition, however, extends far beyond the tics, and the motor symptoms include a great variety of complicated movements, many of which have a compulsive quality. Further, some 30–50% of patients have obsessive–compulsive phenomena, equivalent in severity to OCD as defined by the DSM III (Trimble and Robertson, 1986). These symptoms are closely interlinked with some of the central features of the syndrome, such as coprolalia and echophenomena, suggesting close biological links between the motoric and psychological phenomena.

'PANDAS' refers to paediatric autoimmune neuropsychiatric disorders associated with streptococcal infections and represents a group of disorders somehow linked with basal ganglia autoantibodies. The latter cross-react with human brain tissue, with high binding specificity to caudate and putamen, and seem associated with a spectrum of post-streptococcal movement and related psychiatric disorders, Sydenham's chorea being a paradigm. The streptococci are thought to activate antigen-specific T- and B-cells, which cross the blood–brain barrier and lead to focal cytotoxicity basal ganglia disorders. Such antibodies can be identified in up to 40% of patients with OCD.

Follow-up studies of patients with OCD reveal that about 10% go on to develop Gilles de la Tourette's syndrome, and that those who do have an earlier onset of OCD. The prognosis of OCD is worse if there is a lifetime history of tic disorder (Leonard *et al.*, 1993).

The evidence that gamma-knife surgery is influential in the relief of obsessive–compulsive phenomena is reviewed in Chapter 12, and points to anterior cingulate lesions as being an important target area. The observations of Talairach *et al.* (1973), in which patients' brains were stimulated electrically, showed that excitation of the cingulate area provoked forced integrated motor behaviour, similar in nature to compulsive movements. Such observations, combined with the known anatomical connections of the cingulate gyrus to the frontal cortex, and the role of the latter in the regulation of sensory–motor integration and motor planning (Stuss and Benson, 1984), imply a potential neuroanatomical circuit involved in OCD.

Other evidence for a neurological involvement in OCD comes from observations of increased birth abnormalities (Capstick and Seldrup, 1977), especially in patients with more bizarre rituals, and case reports of the condition developing after a head injury (Hillbom, 1960; McKeon *et al.*, 1984). There is a long history of an association between epilepsy and forms of obsessional thinking, sometimes reflected in hypergraphia, associated mainly with temporal-lobe epilepsy (see Chapter 10), and EEG studies of obsessive–compulsive patients reveal significant abnormalities in 6–60% (Flor-Henry, 1983). Evoked potential investigations show shorter latencies and reduced amplitude of the N200 component of the visual evoked response (Ciesielski *et al.*, 1981) to patterned stimulation, similar to that seen in psychotic patients. Shagass *et al.* (1984) reported high-amplitude somatosensory N60 waves in the disorder, again found in schizophrenic patients, and a lower-amplitude P90. These data were taken to support notions of excessive arousal in these patients, but, in addition, implicate and support a suggestion of Flor-Henry that there is a deficit of left-frontal inhibition, leading to an inability to inhibit verbal ideational representations and their motor counterparts.

Insel *et al.* (1982) report that patients with OCD have abnormal sleep patterns and shortened REM latencies, similar to patients with affective disorder, reinforcing the clinical and biochemical links between the two. There are several case reports of patients with lesions in the basal ganglia developing OCD, the pallidum being particularly involved (Laplane *et al.*, 1989).

Neuropsychological studies consistently suggest problems with executive function, implying frontal involvement and related deficits can be found in Gilles de la Tourette's syndrome (Flor-Henry, 1983). Set-shifting problems and impaired inhibition rather than planning and decision-making ones are reported. Patients with OCD also show problems with learning and memory. These psychological profiles are thought to relate to attentional deficits with aberrant fronto-cingulate basal-ganglia function, and are likely to be trait- rather than state-linked. (de Geus *et al.*, 2007a, b; van 't Ent *et al.*, 2007).

POST-TRAUMATIC STRESS DISORDER

This disorder also has a rather special place in the anxiety-disorder pantheon. In DSM IV-TR it is virtually the only disorder defined by its cause (post-concussional disorder being another), and there is considerable controversy over its validity, the relevance of the pretraumatic personality and the role of the trauma itself. Since it is post-traumatic, since trauma often implies accidents and since the latter usually imply that someone is responsible, there is a considerable social dimension to its presence. These arguments are rehearsed elsewhere (Trimble, 2004), but they serve to emphasize the social nature of syndrome construction, and the importance of moving to endophenotypes and biological markers as a basis for classification. The imaging studies are noted above.

There are some neuropsychological investigations of patients with PTSD, but the data are confounded by co-morbidities such as substance abuse, head injury and depression. Memory is central to the condition, traumatic memories being so vividly re-experienced. However, psychogenic amnesia is also a diagnostic feature, but one which can easily be confused with a post-traumatic amnesia of a head injury. There have been studies combining hippocampal imaging with learning tasks, but with inconclusive results.

SOME OUTSTANDING ISSUES

The anxiety disorders discussed in this chapter represent a heterogeneous group of conditions, but underling the majority, the affect of anxiety is central. This does not apply to OCD, which clinically and biologically reveals a different profile. The genetics, neuroanatomy, disease course and treatments of OCD are different from say those of panic disorder. From a neuro-chemical perspective, the links to 5-HT seem the greater with OCD, while the anatomical underpinning is the fronto-basal ganglia circuitry. Further, in a different treatment area, severe OCD was amenable to neurosurgery, which today has been replaced by the successes of DBS (Cecconi *et al.*, 2008; Greenberg *et al.*, 2008). The various targets have involved this neuronal network.

There is a more common basis for generalized anxiety disorder, the phobic states and panic disorder, although some differential may be suggested. In these, increased autonomic arousal can be shown, and the anxious-prone show increased adrenergic activity when provoked. GABA systems seem to be more relevant for generalized anxiety, but less involved in panic attacks. Panic disorder shows a closer affinity with the biochemistry of lactic acid and CO_2 provocation, and there is more evidence of 5-HT involvement in panic than with phobias.

These distinctions have been supported by the neuroanatomical findings. Reflecting recent trends in biological psychiatry, since the last edition of this book there has been much less interest in studying urine, CSF and blood hormonal profiles following chemical provocation studies, and a shift towards genetics and imaging. In contrast to OCD, the anatomical basis of the other classified anxiety disorders hinges on the temporal–limbic axis, especially involving the hippocampus and amygdala. Not only do anxious people show increased amygdala reactivity to emotionally arousing stimuli, but this structure is involved in the aetiology of social phobia and panic disorder. Other anatomical sites of primary relevance (revealed from animal studies) include the locus coeruleus. While there is also amygdala reactivity in PTSD, this disorder seems to have a different profile of biological markers. The hippocampus seems more relevant to the pathogenesis of this disorder, although it is unclear whether these anatomical findings relate to a state or a trait. The findings relating to the HPA axis would also seem unique amongst the anxiety disorders. How relevant these findings are for explaining co-morbidities and, as with all the disorders discussed in this chapter, for trying to unravel the close links between the personality dispositions and disorders and the axis 1 disorders is far from clear. The advance of combining genetics with brain imaging is likely to throw more light on these questions in the coming years. One major difficulty for research in the area of the anxiety disorders is the substantial clinical co-morbidities and overlap. Even pure samples of PD or GAD, if followed long enough, will often eventually have overlapping co-morbidites. The key concepts for future research will likely involve identification of anxiety-disorder endophenotypes.

The past trend to ignore the genetic, biological and neuroanatomical bases of the anxiety disorders, especially amongst those with little inclination towards neuroscience, is reflective of the same situation with regards to the addictions (see Chapter 9). This has retarded research in this area and hindered the development of more effective biological therapies.

7
The Schizophrenias

INTRODUCTION

Definition and Classification

Many of the illnesses referred to in the past as 'neuroses' have melted away into more clearly defined neurological conditions with a recognizable structural basis. So it is with Kraepelin's concept of dementia praecox. Although for him it represented a disease, whose origins may often be found in early life, its pathogenesis and physiological accompaniments largely eluded him. Bleuler, recognizing the heterogeneity of the condition, used the term 'disease group ... about analogous with the group of the organic dementias' (Bleuler, 1924, p. 373), while Slater and Roth (1960) refer to schizophrenia as a term 'for a group of mental illnesses characterized by specific psychological symptoms' (p. 237). Gradually over time some aetiological factors have become clarified.

Schizophrenia therefore should be considered not as a single disease, but, like epilepsy (or the epilepsies), as a group of syndromes, recognized by a collection of signs and symptoms, which have diverse pathogeneses. It is suggested that the symptoms represent the outcome of abnormal cerebral functioning, itself provoked by disease processes, some of which we readily recognize. However, it is important to understand that, as time passes, and as the cerebral basis of schizophrenic symptoms becomes clearer, the clinical diagnostic category will get whittled down, and

preferred pathological diagnoses will be given. This is one process whereby medicine advances, and the principle is as important in psychiatry as in other areas. Thus, Parkinson's disease, dementia (the dementias) and epilepsy (the epilepsies) are no longer thought of as clearly defined entities with a common cerebral pathology, but as recognizable conditions on clinical grounds, perhaps with common underlying functional changes that help explain the symptom pattern, but with several pathological antecedents.

The concept that schizophrenia (or more aptly the schizophrenias) is a single disease entity has caused much confusion in psychiatry, even leading some authors to the fanciful conclusion that it does not exist (Szasz, 1976). There remain arguments over the precise definitions, if only because they are operational and clinical, but this is common with many conditions. How to define epilepsy is likewise an elusive problem (see Chapter 10). The use of the plural in the chapter title and intermittently in the text however emphasizes that the schizophrenias should properly be viewed as a collection of disorders with differing pathogeneses.

This view is not that developed by Kraepelin, who, while acknowledging the differing clinical pictures that may arise, noted the same basic disturbances suggestive of a common underlying process. Bleuler (1911), who introduced the term schizophrenia 'to show that the split of the several psychic functions is one of its most important characteristics' (p. 5), extended the range of the observed psychopathology, referred to the group of schizoprenias and introduced Freudian psychodynamics into his ideas. He suggested that many of the typical symptoms were determined by 'psychic' causes and distinguished various types, including primary, secondary and basic. The symptoms delineated by Kraepelin were mainly secondary, derived by a reaction of the sick mind to the illness, primary ones being directly caused by the disease process. Basic symptoms, present at all times, were alteration of affect and volition, ambivalence and autism. The theory was elaborated further, particularly by Jung, to include the idea that the psychic cause could set an organic process in motion, thus being aetiological. In addition, Bleuler considerably widened the boundaries of the disorder to include personality changes and other subtle changes of mental function, atypical manias and melancholias, anergia, obstinacy and moodiness. Simple schizophrenia was added to the classification, which included many of these marginal cases, and the idea of latent schizophrenia was accepted. Bleuler's influence was profound, not only in central Europe, but also in the USA through the writings of Adolf Meyer.

An important step was taken by Kurt Schneider. Influenced by both Kraepelin and Jaspers, he was especially concerned with symptoms, and was dissatisfied with the way that Bleuler defined such concepts as primary and basic ones. He introduced the terms 'first rank' and 'second rank', quite different from the divisions of other, previous writers. The first-rank symptoms, shown in Table 7.1, were introduced for pragmatic diagnostic use, and 'if this symptom is present in a non-organic psychosis, then we call that psychosis schizophrenia ... the presence of first rank symptoms always signifies schizophrenia, but first rank symptoms need not always be present in schizophrenia' (Schneider, 1957, p. 44).

Schneider had no presumption of a common structure for these phenomena, although he discussed them in terms of the lowering of a 'barrier' between the self and the surrounding

Table 7.1 The first-rank symptoms of Schneider (after Schneider, 1957, p. 43)

The hearing of one's thoughts spoken aloud in one's head
The hearing of voices commenting on what one is doing at the time
Voices arguing in the third person
Experiences of bodily influence
Thought withdrawal and other forms of thought interference
Thought diffusion
Delusional perception[a]
Everything in the spheres of feeling, drive and volition which the patient experiences as imposed on them or influenced by others

[a] An abnormal significance attached to a real perception without any cause that is understandable in rational or emotional terms.

world. Other symptoms were termed second-rank, and were considered much less important for diagnosis.

The first-rank symptoms assumed importance for the diagnosis of schizophrenia, especially in the UK, and were employed widely in research, for example the Present State Examination (PSE) being biased to detect them for that diagnostic category. Their influence on the DSM III and its successors is clear.

The International Pilot Study of Schizophrenia was a transcultural investigation of 1202 patients in nine countries: Colombia, Czechoslovakia, Denmark, India, Nigeria, China, the USSR, the USA and the UK (World Health Organization, 1973). The main rating instrument was the PSE. The symptom profiles and the rank order of the most frequent symptoms were similar across countries, and while no single symptom was present in all patients from all cultures, the conclusion was that when psychiatrists diagnose schizophrenia they have the same condition in mind. Lack of insight, delusional mood, ideas of reference, flatness of affect, auditory hallucinations and passivity experiences were commonly recorded and although first-rank symptoms were present in only one-third, when recorded they almost inevitably led to a diagnosis of schizophrenia. The Americans and Russians differed the most, having a broader concept of the condition than the others. This difference in part led to the tightening up of the diagnostic criteria in the DSM III.

The ICD 10 refers to schizophrenic disorders as a group in which there is a disturbance of the personality, distortion of thinking, delusions, a sense of outside influence, disturbed perception, an abnormal affect out of keeping with reality, and autism. Thought, perception, mood, conduct and personality are all affected by the same illness, but the diagnosis is not restricted to one with a deteriorating course. The main types recognized are undifferentiated, hebephrenic, catatonic and paranoid, but residual and simple types were also included.

It is necessary for symptoms to have been present for a month or more for a diagnosis of schizophrenia to be given. For a more acute episode, the term *acute schizophrenia-like psychotic disorder* is used.

DSM IV-TR includes characteristic symptoms, such as hallucinations, delusions and thought disorder, but emphasizes also social and occupational dysfunction. The problems must have been present for at least six months. Illnesses lasting for a shorter time are referred to as *schizophreniform disorder*. Such Schneiderian symptoms as voices keeping a running commentary on the patient's behaviour, or two or more voices conversing with each other, are specifically associated with a diagnosis of schizophrenia.

DSM IV-TR gives the following subtypes: disorganized, catatonic, paranoid, undifferentiated and residual. The disorganized type is characterized by incoherence, an inappropriate blunted affect associated with mannerisms, social withdrawal and odd behaviour, and by an absence of well-systematized delusions. This is equated with the hebephrenia of the ICD 10. In the catatonic type there is marked motor disturbance, sometimes fluctuating between the extremes of excitement and stupor. The paranoid type emphasizes preoccupation with delusions or hallucinations. The undifferentiated type is for those not classified in these groups, and the residual is for patients who have a history of at least one past episode but have minimal psychotic symptoms in the presence of continued evidence of the illness.

Missing from the DSM IV-TR criteria are the motor disorders seen in schizophrenia (other than the catatonia), which form an integral part of the syndrome. These include stereotypies, negativisms, automatic behaviours, posturing and catalepsy. In addition, tremors, tics and choreoathetosis have all been identified – not as a consequence of treatment but as a part of the disorder (Trimble, 1981a). Further, the emphasis on current or recent symptoms detracts from the essential nature of schizophrenia, which, in the majority of cases, pursues a chronic course.

The history, typically, is of a patient, who may well have demonstrated early developmental language and behaviour problems, who manifests bizarre behaviour in late teens and early adulthood with a loss of academic potential. Initially, a bewildering variety of psychopathological states, including anxiety states, manias and depressions, may be recorded, but eventually the longitudinal course becomes apparent and the cognitive and psychotic symptoms outlined above manifest.

DSM IV-TR notes that *psychotic disorder* can be due to a wide variety of general medical conditions. This excludes disorders that only present as delirium, and is subdivided dependent on whether the predominant symptoms are delusions or hallucinations.

Both the DSM IV-TR and the ICD 10 have the category *schizoaffective*, a term that is a source of considerable controversy. It was first introduced to refer to a psychosis with an admixture of affective and schizophrenic symptoms that is precipitated by emotional stress. Sitting between the two Kraepelinian pillars of psychosis, this diagnostic category is not accepted by many, its very existence suggesting a return to a unitary psychosis theory (see below). However, family and genetic data support the concept that some form of schizoaffective subtype exists, though its prognosis is related more to the affective disorders (Procci, 1976). Some use the terms 'schizodepressive' and 'schizomanic' to reflect this; DSM IV-TR refers to the bipolar and the depressive types. It is diagnosed only when definite schizophrenic and definite affective symptoms are present simultaneously.

It must be distinguished from post-treatment schizophrenic depression.

The schizoaffective subtype may describe the same patients referred to as having *cycloid psychosis* (Leonhard, 1957). The features are psychotic episodes which resolve completely and are associated with confusion and perplexity, mood and motor changes, pan-anxiety and delusions.

Kraepelin's original concept, of a dementia praecox, embedded the idea of a progression. There have now been several follow-up studies, particularly with brain imaging (see below), that rather support his views. Thus it is estimated that some 50–70% of cases take a progressive course, which includes not only the psychotic symptoms but also the cognitive changes and loss of the ability to function independently at a high level in society.

Paranoid Disorders

The word 'paranoid' has been used in psychiatry for many years, but its meaning has shifted from a general term for madness to a more precise technical expression (Lewis, 1970). Kraepelin initially classified paranoia as a separate entity from dementia praecox; it represented the insidious development of a delusional system in the presence of an intact personality. He used the term 'paraphrenia' to refer to those who have a paranoid illness developing later than dementia praecox. Lewis (1970), after a careful consideration of the world literature, gave the following definition: 'A paranoid syndrome is one in which there are delusions of self reference which may be concerned with persecution, grandeur, litigation, jealousy, love, envy, hate, honour, or the supernatural, and which cannot be immediately derived from a prevailing morbid mood such as mania or depression' (p. 11). He felt that the adjective 'paranoid' could be applied to a personality disorder with similar features, except that dominant ideas should replace delusions.

ICD 10 uses the term 'persistent delusional disorders', and DSM IV-TR 'delusional disorder' for these syndromes. Patients develop a single delusion or a related set of delusions, not necessarily so bizarre in content, in the absence of criteria for schizophrenia. Such delusions often arise in middle age, can contain ideas about the individual's body and should last at least one month. In many patients, these disorders are persistent, but psychosocial functioning may remain adaptable. DSM IV-TR recognizes several types, namely erotomanic, grandiose, jealous, persecutory, somatic and mixed. The litigious variant is also well known to lawyers.

An important addition to this group is the psychotic disorder due to a general medical condition. Prominent symptoms are hallucinations and delusions not due to delirium or dementia.

Endophenotypes

The term 'endophenotypes' refers to a marker of an illness that might be closer to the underlying genetic mechanisms than the actual phenotype, as for example specified by DSM IV-TR and ICD 10. It was introduced in 1972 by Gottesman and Shields and represents a neurobiological trait that is related to the illness in question. The concept has assumed particular prominence in the genetics of schizophrenia and is one way to deconstruct the phenotype into component parts for a potentially more powerful genetic analysis. Most studies have highlighted cognitive and brain-imaging variables.

GENETICS

The contribution of genetics to schizophrenia has been long recognized, but is often curiously neglected in some pathogenic explanations of the disorder. It has been reviewed in detail by many authors (McGuffin, 1984; Slater and Roth, 1960; and more recently Gur *et al.*, 2007; Norton *et al.*, 2006; Porteous, 2008; Riley and Kendler, 2006; Tandon *et al.*, 2008; van Winkel *et al.*, 2008). In brief, the twin studies show impressive differences in rates of concordance between monozygous (MZ) and dizygous (DZ) pairs, and the adoption data indicate that there is a greater incidence of schizophrenia and schizophrenic spectrum disorders in those who,

Table 7.2 Classic twin studies in schizophrenia

Study	Concordance	
	Monozygous (%)	*Dizygous (%)*
Kringlen (1967)	45	15
Pollin *et al.* (1969)	43	9
Tienari (1971)	35	13
Fischer (1973)	56	26
Gottesman and Shields (1972)	58	12
Kendler and Robinette (1983)	40	6
Mean	46.1	13.5

adopted to normal parents, have a biological parent with the condition. Table 7.2 summarizes the data, indicating concordance rates from 35 to 58% in MZ and from 6 to 26% in DZ pairs.

While there were several criticisms of the early data, for example the method of ascertainment of the zygosity and the clinical diagnostic criteria for the schizophrenia, later studies have attempted to overcome these. Some authors (Gottesman and Shields, 1972; Kendler and Robinette, 1983) noted that the more severe the illness, the more likely the concordance in MZ pairs, and Kallmann (1946), whose own series noted a 91.5% concordance for MZ twins living together, reported a rising familial incidence of the condition as subjects approach a genetic relationship with index cases. Thus, compared to a percentage expectation of 0.9% for the general population, the equivalent figure for half-sibs was 7.1%, for parents 9.2%, for full-sibs 14.2%, for children 16.4%, for DZ co-twins 14.5% and for children of two schizophrenic parents 39.2%. After a review of the data, Slater concluded 'the evidence is very strong that the genetical constitution of an individual contributes a large part of his total potentiality of becoming schizophrenic' (Slater and Roth, 1969, p. 246). McGuffin (1984) calculated that the heritability of the condition was 0.66, genetic factors thus accounting for two-thirds of the variance in vulnerability to the disorder. A similar figure (68%) has been given by Kendler (1983), who notes that this is similar to that for diabetes and hypertension, and rather in excess of that for epilepsy, peptic ulcer and coronary artery disease.

There is some suggestion that schizophrenic probands resemble their affected relatives with regards to subtype, although there is much overlap, and twin and adoption studies which might clarify this issue have not been conducted. Leonhard (1980) has suggested, on the basis of family studies, that periodic catatonia has a high genetic loading, and Perris (1974) noted the same for cycloid psychosis. Winokur (1977) reported that paranoia may also be genetically separate.

McGuffin *et al.* (1984) examined the heritabilities of a twin population using six different sets of operational criteria for schizophrenia. Those of Feighner and the RDC criteria gave the highest heritability, while the Schneiderian criteria had a heritability value of zero. Dworkin and Lenzenweger (1984) examined the case histories of MZ twins in whom at least one had schizophrenia and assessed concordance for positive and negative symptoms. Their results suggested that negative symptoms may have the greater genetic component. Similar conclusions have emerged from the studies of Tsaung (1993).

With regards to interpretation, the contention that environmental factors are so important, in that the environments of MZ twins are said to be more alike than those of DZ pairs, has been discounted by the adoption studies. Heston (1966) showed that the adopted children of schizophrenic mothers, removed from them shortly after birth, had a higher incidence of the illness than the adopted children of non-schizophrenic mothers. These findings have been replicated and extended by a series of studies on Danish patients, including investigation of the relatives of adopted children who later became schizophrenic (Kety, 1983;

Kety *et al.*, 1994). These studies have not only shown the higher incidence of schizophrenia among the biological relatives but also an overrepresentation of the schizophrenia spectrum of disorders. Further, there was an overrepresentation of schizophrenia or schizophrenia-spectrum disorders in the biological relatives of adopted schizophrenic patients, significantly greater than among the relatives of nonschizophrenic adopted controls. In addition, in investigations of paternal half-siblings of schizophrenic probands, the incidence of schizophrenia was higher than in control cases, ruling out intrauterine contributions to the congenital effects.

Replication studies (Kendler *et al.*, 1981), particularly improving the criteria for schizophrenia-spectrum disorders, have been conducted. The prevalence of schizotypal personality disorder was significantly higher in the biological relatives of schizophrenic adoptees than controls, but this was not the case for delusional disorder of the nonschizophrenic type or for anxiety disorder. These adoption studies, particularly the careful analysis of the Danish patients, have confirmed the genetic contribution to schizophrenia and identified the concept of the schizophrenia spectrum more clearly.

Gottesman and Bertelsen (1989) observed that the risk for schizophrenia and related disorders was similar in the offspring of schizophrenic MZ twins and those of their nonschizophrenic co-twins, suggesting that the discordance rate in MZ twins may in part be explained by an unexpressed genetic diathesis.

With regards to the mode of inheritance, several authors favour polygenic as opposed to monogenic transmission (Kendler, 1983), mathematical models failing to provide evidence for the latter. To date, no consistent traditional genetic markers linking to schizophrenia have been identified. However, the identification of such markers will only be successful if there is a major gene effect (either single or a small number) or if there is a subgroup with such a component. HLA markers have been claimed, but the results of different studies are variable. McGuffin *et al.* (1981), after review of the available literature, noted that the most persistent genetic marker to date was HLA A9 with paranoid schizophrenia, and the more consistent associations (found by more than one group) relate to HLA A9 and B5.

There are several important negative-linkage studies to regions of chromosomes 2, 5, 9, 11, 12 and 22 and to the D_2, D_3, D_4, 5-HT$_2$ and GABA$_a$ subunits (Macciardi *et al.*, 1994; Waddington *et al.*, 1992; Su *et al.*, 1993). No mutation of the D_1 receptor gene has been found.

Crow (1988) suggested that the pseudoautosomal locus of the X or Y chromosomes is important. This is a region of the distal segment of the short arm of the Y chromosome that in meiosis exchanges genetic material with the short arm of the X chromosome. Genes there are therefore transmitted in an autosomal rather than sex-linked way. Further, genes of the pseudoautosomal locus do not seem subject to X inactivation. His theory is based on a number of observations, notably that the age of onset of schizophrenia is earlier in males, that pairs of first-degree relatives with psychosis are more likely to be the same sex, that in parent–child pairs with psychosis the mother is twice as likely to be affected than the father and that concordance by sex is paternally rather than maternally inherited. Further, sex-chromosome aneuploides such as XXY, XX, but not XO, are associated with an increased incidence of schizophrenia. No direct evidence of such linkage has yet been found (Crow *et al.*, 1994), but Crow's theory has developed to include a search for the gene responsible for handedness and cerebral dominance, which may be located at the pseudoautosomal region (Crow, 1991).

The substantial evidence for genetic influences on the development of schizophrenia has led to several studies of high-risk people. These include the Edinburgh group (Lawrie *et al.*, 2008a, 2008b; Owens and Johnstone, 2006), NAPLS (the North America Prodrome Longitudinal Study) (Addington *et al.*, 2007) and the EPOS (the European Prediction of Psychosis Study). Each of these studies has taken subjects with at least one parent with schizophrenia and followed them longitudinally, gathering data at inception before there was any diagnosis of the disorder. They are assessed at various intervals, and those who develop the disorder are then compared with those who do not on many different variables. The studies have included psychological and behavioural variables, neurocognitive profiles and imaging, although each study has varied with regards to entry criteria and measurements selected. Some have included healthy normal controls and some alternative high-risk groups such as those with learning disability (or mental handicap). Assessments have included such ratings as the Structured Interview for Schizophrenia (SIS), the Structured Interview for Prodromal Syndromes (SIPS) and tasks of verbal abilities and working memory. The results of these studies are awaited with interest. These massive projects offer some promise, but caution is needed in light of the amount of genetic work done to date that has not shown real progress. One problem is that as sample sizes have increased, the signals heralded from earlier studies seem to have weakened rather than getting stronger (Weinberger, 2009). The genome-wide studies are in fact revealing overlaps in the revealed genetics of schizophrenia and bipolar disorder. At present, if differences can be suggested, it is between susceptibility for bipolar disorder and genes involved in calcium ion-channel function, and the zinc-finger transcription factor in schizophrenia. Two promising position candidates in schizophrenia are NRG1 (neuregulin) and DTNBP1 (protein-coding dystrobrevin-binding protein 1). The deletions of the neurexin gene (involved in the development of synapses) may represent a discontinuity with bipolar disorder and the potential genetic links between the latter and the genes coding for the $GABA_a$ receptor and calcium channels may turn out to be significant (Kirov *et al.*, 2009).

It needs to be emphasized however that the genetic variations noted so far in these disorders explain only a small amount of the variability of the phenotype, and the limitations of the technique with regards to the statistics involved and the definition of phenotypes as discussed in Chapter 4 need to be taken into account.

Landis and Insel (2008) described only cautious optimism toward the results in this area at present.

SOMATIC VARIABLES

Abnormalities in muscle endplates in schizophrenic patients have been reported. Using muscle biopsies stained for motor neurones and terminals, Crayton and Meltzer (1976) reported the size and dispersion of terminal bulbs to be abnormal in psychotic patients, with larger and more variable endplate arborization and low density of endplate neural structures. Although similar findings were seen in some manic–depressive patients and no association was noted with type or length of illness, the authors felt the findings might indicate regenerative processes of previously denervated fibres, reflecting perhaps altered CNS physiology. These data are in keeping with other evidence of disturbed muscle pathology in psychotic patients. A number of authors have noted an increase in serum creatine phosphokinase in acute psychoses. This does not simply reflect the use of intramuscular injections or methods of restraint since elevations are found in a proportion of first-degree relatives and there is some correlation with the alpha-motor neurone abnormalities noted on biopsy. Further, mean creatine kinase levels during a hospital admission are also elevated (Meltzer 1980).

Schizophrenics have been shown in several studies to present with an excess of major physical abnormalities, but the contribution of mental handicap to the ensuing clinical picture is unclear. Minor physical and dermatoglyphic abnormalities are overrepresented and a number of these abnormalities are linked to the first trimester of foetal development (Guy *et al.*, 1983; Weinberg *et al.*, 2007). These seem unrelated to symptomatology or to the presence or absence of neurological soft signs. Dysmorphic craniofacial features are also increased in schizophrenia, including brachycephaly (McGrath *et al.*, 2002).

The velo-cardiofacial syndrome (DiGeorge syndrome or chromosome 22q11.2 deletion syndrome) is associated with an increased risk for schizophrenia and with alterations of cerebral structure, especially temporal-lobe size (Debbane *et al.*, 2009; Eliez, 2007; Green *et al.*, 2009; Schaer and Eliez, 2007).

METABOLIC AND BIOCHEMICAL FINDINGS

One early finding that has been replicated was of abnormal nitrogen balance in patients with periodic catatonia (Gjessing, 1947). Thus, phases of stupor and excitement were associated with nitrogen retention, with later compensatory increased excretion. In such patients it was claimed that alteration of nitrogen input, by reducing protein intake, altered the course of the illness.

The concept that endogenous neurotoxins exist, derived from the abnormal metabolism of various chemicals, was encouraged by observations of psychoses resembling schizophrenia that could be provoked by the ingestion of various psychotropic drugs, such as LSD, mescaline and amphetamine. Attempts were made to identify abnormal compounds in the blood and urine of schizophrenics, with some authors reporting success, although much of the early data was not replicated. From these ideas arose the transmethylation hypothesis (Smythies, 1976). Several hallucinogenic compounds were seen to be closely related chemically to the endogenous catecholamines and indolamines, which were notably methylated derivates. It was suggested that abnormal transmethylation of these compounds might produce hallucinogenic methylated monoamines related to the pathogenesis of at least some forms of schizophrenia. Administration of methyl donors such as methionine to schizophrenics gave variable results but, especially when combined with a monoamine oxidase inhibitor, led to the exacerbation of symptoms in some 40% of patients. These studies did not, however, distinguish between an acute organic brain syndrome and true exacerbation of schizophrenic symptoms (Wyatt *et al.*, 1971).

A related theme is the possibility that 5-HT is involved in schizophrenia. Thus, methionine may inhibit the uptake of tryptophan into the brain by competitive blockade (Smythies, 1976) and schizophrenia may in part reflect defective tryptophan metabolism. However, supplementary tryptophan loading in patients has provided only equivocal results, and to date the role of indolamines in the psychoses remains to be clarified.

Administration of the 5-HT agonist metachlorophenylpiperazine (MCPP) to schizophrenic patients increases positive symptoms (Krystal *et al.*, 1993). In controls there is no effect, suggesting a propsychotic rather than a psychotogenic effect. These data suggest a role for serotonergic mechanisms in schizophrenia. This has been supported by observations that pipamperone, a selective $5-HT_2$ antagonist, is antipsychotic, and some newer antipsychotics such as risperidone are selective $5-HT_2$ receptor antagonists (see Chapter 12).

Platelet MAO activity in schizophrenia has been studied by many authors. In general, the values are low, although, since similar data are noted in some other psychiatric conditions, it is not specific for schizophrenia (Delisi *et al.*, 1982; Siever and Coursey, 1985). Patients with paranoid symptoms probably have the lower levels, and in studies of normal adults an inverse correlation between the paranoia score on the MMPI and MAO levels has been noted. Several authors link low values to hallucinations and delusions, others to poor outcome. Baron *et al.* (1980) identified students with abnormally high or low levels of MAO and found that 70% of those with low levels and none with high levels had a diagnosis of borderline schizophrenia. This same group also reported that schizophrenic patients with a high genetic load have reduced levels in contrast to those with nonfamilial schizophrenia, and relatives with low MAO are more often affected with schizophrenia-spectrum disorders than high-MAO relatives (Baron *et al.*, 1984).

Reveley *et al.* (1983) examined MAO in MZ twins discordant for schizophrenia, normal MZ and DZ twins, and controls. The MZ pair with a schizophrenic co-twin had significantly lower values than did the healthy MZ twins and the other controls, the MZ schizophrenics having only slightly lower values than their healthy co-twins.

Although some authors have failed to find low MAO in schizophrenic patients, and further show that neuroleptic treatment may itself lower MAO (Owen *et al.*, 1981), the consistency of the data and the findings in twins, relatives and volunteers suggests some association, genetically determined, between MAO and vulnerabilities to these behaviour patterns, and are in agreement with the adoption studies that both schizophrenia and related spectrum disorders need to be considered together.

Low-platelet MAO has been implicated in both the transmethylation and the dopamine (see below) hypotheses of schizophrenia in the sense that reduced MAO activity may reflect an impaired capacity to degrade monoamines or their abnormal metabolites, thus increasing the load of these substances in the brain.

The Dopamine Hypothesis

The predominant biochemical hypothesis of schizophrenia has been the dopamine hypothesis, and a considerable amount of research work has been carried out investigating dopamine and its metabolites in patients. The hypothesis emerged in the wake of the introduction of the phenothiazines in the 1960s, stemming from recognition of the similarity of a psychosis induced by amphetamine to schizophrenia, and that in small doses they can activate symptoms in patients, and the discovery that the principal mode of action of the phenothiazines is to block dopamine receptors. The ability of neuroleptic drugs to block dopamine receptors correlated better than other biochemical effects with their efficacy in the control of psychotic symptoms (Snyder *et al.*, 1974). The dopamine hypothesis which emerged thus suggested that schizophrenia was the result of overactivity of dopamine neurotransmission in the CNS and that neuroleptics acted by reducing this. However, the evidence was largely circumstantial, and over time modifications have had to be made.

In animal models, behavioural disturbances provoked by dopamine agonists given systemically or by injection into the limbic forebrain were reversed by neuroleptic drugs (Anden, 1975), and the ability of these compounds to inhibit dopamine-sensitive adenylcyclase stimulation is proportional to their clinical potency, with notable exceptions, namely the butyrophenones. However, the recognition of different classes of dopamine receptors and the fact that the main receptor linked to adenylcyclase activity is the D_1 have helped explain this apparent discrepancy.

Generally the evidence that neuroleptics act at dopamine receptors in the limbic system is strong (Scatton and Zivkovic, 1984). Electrophysiologically their iontophoretic application antagonizes the depression of cellular activity induced by the application of dopamine agonists, and binding studies show that a variety of neuroleptics specifically bind to dopamine sites within the limbic system. Further, they increase the metabolism and turnover of dopamine, an effect related to the feedback activation of neurones following the postsynaptic receptor blockade.

Early on it was noted that some neuroleptic drugs were less frequently associated with extrapyramidal side effects. The latter were thought to occur with the blockade of dopamine receptors in the striatum, and the reason why some drugs, notably thioridazine, clozapine and sulpiride, did not do this required explanation. Some evidence pointed to differential effects at limbic and nonlimbic sites (ventral and dorsal striatum, respectively), either due to anticholinergic properties (strong with thioridazine and clozapine, anticholinergic effects being greater in nonlimbic striatal areas) or due to preferential action on different receptor subpopulations at the two sites (Scatton and Zivkovic, 1984; see also Chapter 12), drugs such as sulpiride acting mainly at the limbic receptors. It seems that the effects of neuroleptic drugs on psychotic symptoms relate to changes of dopamine turnover in the limbic forebrain at least, while the development of extrapyramidal symptoms is related to the dorsal striatum (Crow *et al.*, 1979a). Further, the antipsychotic effect most likely relates to blockade of selective dopamine receptors, especially D_2, D_3 and D_4.

An effective demonstration of the antipsychotic effect of dopamine antagonism has been provided by Crow *et al.* (1979a). Patients with acute schizophrenia took part in a double-blind trial of treatment with flupenthixol, comparing the alpha isomer, which blocks the dopamine receptor, to the beta isomer, which does not. The former had a significant effect compared to placebo, although this was confined to only certain symptoms, referred to by the authors as 'positive'. Thus, using the Krawiecka scale, the improvements were seen on scores for delusions, hallucinations and speech incoherence, but not on poverty of speech or affective flattening.

One problem for the dopamine theory relates to the time course of the clinical effect. Prolactin, which is elevated by blocking dopamine receptors (the prolactin inhibitory factor probably being dopamine), rises much faster than the noted clinical improvements, which do not become manifest for two or three weeks after commencing treatment. In contrast, the extrapyramidal effects often arise within 48 hours. This paradox has some explanation in terms of adaptive effects to the acute blockade in dopamine systems. Thus, cerebrospinal fluid (CSF) studies indicate that the initial rise of dopamine turnover diminishes after time (van Praag, 1977b), as does the plasma level of HVA (Pickar *et al.*, 1984), and similar tolerance of the biochemical effects has been observed in animals. However, it seems that the tolerance relates more to dopamine receptors in the caudate areas, less to those in the limbic forebrain and not at all to those in the frontal cortex (Scatton and Zivkovic, 1984). The latter finding may relate to the lack of autoreceptors in frontal areas. Reuptake of dopamine in frontal cortex is via the NA transporter.

Another line of evidence has been to observe the effects of drugs known to increase dopamine activity on the symptoms of schizophrenia. Paradoxically, administration of the dopamine agonists L-dopa and apomorphine seems to improve symptoms in some patients (Buchanan *et al.*, 1975; Tamminga *et al.*, 1977). In some reports the effect is on such symptoms as apathy, isolation and blunted affect (Gerlach and Luhdorf, 1975); in others it is on hallucinations and delusions (Tamminga *et al.*, 1977). However, several carefully conducted trials have failed to replicate these findings (Ferrier *et al.*, 1984b; Syvalahti *et al.*, 1986). It is suggested that any observed effect is due to inhibition of dopamine release by interaction with presynaptic receptors.

More direct evidence of abnormal dopamine activity in schizophrenia has been hard to demonstrate. If dopamine is overactive in the CNS then low basal levels of prolactin may be expected, but studies have generally been negative. In contrast, provocation tests using apomorphine and measurements of either growth hormone (raised by dopamine agonists) or prolactin have been more successful. Growth-hormone responses have been reported to be greater in patients with first-rank symptoms (Whalley *et al.*, 1984), with delusions, hallucinations and thought disorder (Meltzer *et al.*, 1984), and to be both increased (Meltzer *et al.*, 1984) and blunted in association with negative symptoms and in chronic schizophrenia (Ferrier *et al.*, 1986). Prolactin baseline levels and apomorphine-induced prolactin suppression have been shown to correlate inversely with the presence of positive symptoms (Johnstone *et al.*, 1977; Ferrier *et al.*, 1984b), especially in patients with normal ventricular size on CT scans (Kleinman *et al.*, 1982b). Although the interpretation of such findings may be easily blurred by the effects of medication on hormonal release, these studies were on drug-free patients, and the results tend to support the hypothesis that at least some symptoms in schizophrenia are related to dopaminergic mechanisms, notably hallucinations, delusions and thought disorder, similar to the ones shown to respond preferentially to dopamine-antagonist drugs.

Other estimates of dopamine activity have related to peripheral markers. Plasma dopamine has been reported to be elevated in some studies (Bondy *et al.*, 1984). Measurement of dopamine beta-hydrolase, the enzyme that converts dopamine to noradrenaline, has provided inconsistent results (Castellani *et al.*, 1982), as have measurements of plasma HVA.

Other markers have included the reporting of reduced platelet cyclic-AMP production (Kafka *et al.*, 1979) and elevated spiperone binding to lymphocytes apparently unrelated to treatment (Bondy *et al.*, 1984). Further evidence that links dopamine to schizophrenia comes from CSF and post-mortem studies, and is discussed below (see Table 7.3).

PET ligand-binding studies have mainly used tracers that bind to one or more of the dopamine receptors. There is discrepancy of results, partly based on technical factors such as the ligand used. There are more negative findings with normal D_2 densities in schizophrenia (Martinot, 1990; Farde *et al.*, 1990; Pilowsky *et al.*, 1995) than positive ones (Tune *et al.*, 1992), failing to provide direct evidence for increased dopamine-receptor activity in schizophrenia. Fletcher *et al.* (1996) have used apomorphine as a dopamine agonist to show that in schizophrenia, using a verbal fluency activation task, there is impaired activation in the cingulate cortex, which is enhanced by apomorphine. Their data suggest a regional functional deficit in schizophrenia, which can be modulated by dopamine. Research continues with dopamine PET imaging, with some studies suggesting an important role for dopamine in schizophrenia (Howes *et al.*, 2009; Howes and Kapur, 2009) and others not (Valli *et al.*, 2008).

Catechol-O-methyl-Transferase (COMT) is one of several enzymes that degrade the catecholamines, such as dopamine or noradrenaline. A series of studies have now fairly consistently found that individuals with certain COMT gene variants (specifically the val variant) carry an increased risk of developing schizophrenia, and the val variant of the COMT gene is associated with both structural and functional brain changes within patients with schizophrenia (van Haren *et al.*, 2008; Lawrie *et al.*, 2008a; Ross *et al.*, 2006; Roffman *et al.*, 2006). These findings raise suspicion that an abnormality in catecholamine metabolism is fundamental to schizophrenia pathogenesis, at least in some subjects (Gur *et al.*, 2007; Benes, 2007; Keshavan *et al.*, 2007; van Haren *et al.*, 2008).

The Noradrenergic Hypothesis

An alternative to the dopamine hypothesis is the noradrenergic hypothesis, suggested by Stein and Wise (1971) and revived recently by Yamamoto and Hornykiewicz (2004). This was based on the idea that the central noradrenergic pathways, then shown to be related to a central reward system, might degenerate and lead to at least some of the symptoms of schizophrenia. Generally the data are less favourable for this hypothesis, although several studies indicate a role of noradrenergic mechanisms in some symptoms of schizophrenia. This has been reviewed in detail (Kleinman *et al.*, 1985). No noradrenergic abnormalities have been reported in urine of schizophrenic patients, although there is one report of increased levels in the plasma of drug-free patients (Ackenheil *et al.*, 1979). Neither plasma nor urine 3-methoxy-4-hydroxyphenylglycol (MHPG) or vanillylmandelic acid (VMA) levels have been consistently abnormal in schizophrenia, most studies showing no difference from controls. CSF and neurochemical data are discussed below. Attempts to assess the functions of alpha-2 adrenergic receptors have been done

Table 7.3 Main arguments for and against the dopamine hypothesis

For:

1. Amphetamine-induced psychosis produces a schizophrenia-like illness
2. Amphetamine exacerbates schizophrenia
3. Drugs that block dopamine receptors are antipsychotic in relationship to their blocking potential
4. Post-mortem and endocrine studies
5. Animal models of dopamine agonism resemble psychosis, and are reversed by dopamine-blocking agents

Against:

1. Time course between administration of a dopamine blocker and clinical response
2. Dopamine agonists have an inconsistent effect on psychosis
3. Direct evidence of increased dopamine activity is poor

either by direct measurement of platelet binding or by changes of metabolites after challenge with clonidine. Alpha-2 receptors have been reported as increased in platelets in only a minority of subjects, probably those who are schizoaffective (Kafka *et al.*, 1980), while others have noted decreased binding in a group with negative symptoms and poor response to treatment (Rosen *et al.*, 1985), with subsensitivity of MHPG release to a clonidine challenge (Sternberg *et al.*, 1982).

The Glutamate Hypothesis

It has been known for some time that phencyclidine and ketamine, drugs which are antagonists at the NMDA receptor, increase symptoms in schizophrenia. Glutamate is ubiquitous in cerebral cortex, and is the main excitatory neurotransmitter regulating activity in the cortical-basal ganglia thalamic re-entrant circuits. This relates not only to motor control but also to sensory gating. The NMDA receptors are therefore hypothesized to be hypofunctional in schizophrenia. Serum glutamate levels are low at the onset of the disorder (Palomino *et al.*, 2007), as are serine levels in serum and CSF, serine being modulatory at the NMDA receptor. Attempts to use this hypothesis to develop new treatment strategies include trials of the glutamate agonist D-serine, which is released by glutamate from astrocytes. Pathological studies in support of this hypothesis are discussed below.

Other Studies

Early investigations of endocrine function in schizophrenia yielded inconsistent results and were aimed in particular at examination of the thyroid and adrenal glands. Schizophrenia-like psychoses have been described in association with several endocrinopathies, including hypo- and hyperthyroidism and hypoparathyroidism (Lishman, 1987). The prolactin and growth-hormone data, utilized more as a method of challenging hypothalamic–pituitary (HPA axis) function than to implicate the hormonal

changes themselves as pathogenic, have been discussed. Few other studies of endocrine function in schizophrenia have been carried out recently, although there are reports of lower LH and FSH levels in chronic schizophrenia, with an inverse relationship to positive symptoms, while negative symptoms have been inversely related to testosterone levels (Alias, 2008). There seems to be loss of normal episodic secretion of LH, possibly reflecting disturbed hypothalamic or limbic-system function (Ferrier *et al.*, 1982). Further evidence for this is the finding of blunted FSH and prolactin responses to thyrotropin-releasing hormone in similar patients (Ferrier *et al.*, 1983).

In contrast to what is seen in the affective disorders, the number of schizophrenic patients showing abnormal dexamethasone suppression is low, unless there is coexistent depression (Munro *et al.*, 1984).

Finally, following the discovery of enkephalins, attempts have been made to examine peptide function in schizophrenia, largely by giving peptides to patients and estimating clinical changes. Table 7.4 lists some of the substances tried to date, but the results have been disappointing.

Of growing importance has been the cannabinoid group of compounds, especially the social use of cannabis. It is acknowledged that the strength and the availability of cannabis preparations has increased, and it is known that patients with psychotic disorders are more likely to abuse illicit drugs. Schizophrenic patients are often heavy cannabis users, and

Table 7.4 Some peptides used as treatments in schizophrenia

Peptide	Author
CCK	Lostra *et al.* (1984)
	Albus *et al.* (1984)
Des-tyrosine gamma-endorphin	van Praag *et al.* (1982)
Des-enkephalin gamma-endorphin	van Praag *et al.* (1982)
Beta-endorphin	Berger *et al.* (1980b)
Thyroid-releasing hormone	Prange *et al.* (1979)

the administration of tetrahydrocannabinol increases the reporting of psychotic symptoms in healthy volunteers and schizophrenic patients in remission (Henquet *et al.*, 2008; Tandon *et al.*, 2008; d'Souza *et al.*, 2005).

Several long-term follow-up studies have been reported in which populations have been examined over several years and their drug usage noticed or monitored. A Swedish cohort of over 50 000 conscripts noted that cannabis use by the age of 18 was associated with a 2.4-fold increase in a diagnosis of schizophrenia (Andreasson *et al.*, 1987). A longer follow-up of the same population (27 years) reported a dose relationship between the amount of cannabis use at entrance and the later risk of developing the disorder (Zammit *et al.*, 2002). A Netherlands study (three-year follow-up of nearly 5000 people) confirmed these findings and noted that those who had reported any psychotic symptoms at baseline were more likely to go on to develop schizophrenia if they were cannabis users (van Os *et al.*, 2002). Arseneault *et al.* (2002) followed 759 people in a cohort from birth to young adulthood. Cannabis use by age 15 increased the risk of developing psychosis. In a meta-analysis of the data, the increased risk of developing a psychosis with cannabis use was given as 1.4 (odds ratio), and the dose response was confirmed (odds ratio 2.84). Most studies in this area had adjusted for confounding factors such as the use of other drugs and psychotic symptoms at baseline (Moore *et al.*, 2007). One problem with interpreting these results in a causal way is that evidence that the incidence of schizophrenia is increasing *pari passu* is not yet reliably available. However, elevated anandamide (a cannabinoid agonist) has been reported in CSF (Leweke *et al.*, 2007), as has increased density of CB1 receptors in prefrontal cortex (Dean *et al.*, 2001).

NEUROCHEMICAL INVESTIGATIONS

In order to explore further the dopamine and related neurochemical hypotheses in schizophrenia, many neurochemical investigations have been conducted. The CSF data will be discussed first, followed by neurochemical pathological data.

CSF

The main metabolite assessed in CSF to test the dopamine hypothesis is HVA, although it is suggested that the main source of this is nigrostriatal dopamine and not mesolimbic and mesocortical dopamine. Nonetheless, the anatomical proximity and the overlap between these systems suggests that at least some of it reflects limbic-system dopamine function. In general, either the baseline CSF values or the accumulation of metabolite after probenecid administration have been sampled. The latter technique inhibits the exit of HVA and related compounds from the CSF, diminishing the gradient that exists between ventricular and spinal CSF values. Theoretically this should provide a more accurate determination of metabolite turnover and concentration, but it too has methodological difficulties. Not the least is that the results are related to the CSF probenecid levels.

One of the early baseline studies of HVA was that of Rimon *et al.* (1971), who reported normal values, except that patients with paranoid symptoms had elevated levels. Generally, however, the baseline data have failed to show differences between schizophrenics and controls, although Sedvall and Wode-Helgodt (1980) reported that high HVA levels were associated with a family history of schizophrenia. The probenecid studies likewise have tended to be negative with singular exceptions. There are reports of decreased accumulation in patients with Schneiderian first-rank symptoms (Bowers, 1973; Post *et al.*, 1975) and a suggestion that those with low values have poorer prognosis (Bowers, 1974). These data are compatible with increased dopamine-receptor sensitivity, which subsequently decreases dopamine turnover. Some support for this comes from a study in which the relationship between apomorphine-induced growth-hormone release and CSF–HVA levels was assessed in drug-free schizophrenic patients. An inverse relationship was found, those patients with low HVA having a higher release of hormone (Zemlan *et al.*, 1985). Thus low HVA was associated with higher dopamine-receptor activity, and in addition with first-rank symptoms and thought disorder. Pickar *et al.* (1990) also reported negative correlations between HVA ratings of psychosis and positive symptoms.

Both CSF levels of DOPAC and dopamine itself are reported as normal in schizophrenia (Berger *et al.*, 1980a; Gattaz *et al.*, 1983b), as are prolactin levels (Rimon *et al.*, 1981).

With regard to the noradrenergic hypothesis, MHPG levels are consistently reported as normal (Kleinman *et al.*, 1985), although there are reports of increased levels of noradrenaline (Gomes *et al.*, 1980; Lake *et al.*, 1980), especially in paranoid subtypes, and of MHPG correlating with negative symptoms (Pickar *et al.*, 1990).

A variety of other substances have been measured in the CSF of schizophrenic patients, some of the more important ones being shown in Table 7.5.

Brain Neurochemistry

Most studies in this area relate to testing the dopamine hypothesis. Studies on post-mortem brains are difficult to interpret. Not only are they derived from patients that have usually been on medication or have used a large dose of psychotropic drugs to kill themselves, but also rapid post-mortem biochemical changes occur. Several groups have set up centres designed specifically for collection of brains and appropriate storage after death, control specimens being treated in the same manner. It seems likely that peptides and receptors are much more stable than monoamines and their metabolites. Generally the areas of brain examined have been those with a high level of the neurotransmitter under investigation, and studies have mainly concentrated on the limbic system and related structures. For all of these reasons, ligand PET imaging is somewhat better, although it also has problems, primarily that not all substances, particularly peptides, can be measured with PET.

The majority of post-mortem neurochemistry studies show normal values for both dopamine concentrations and HVA, notably in the caudate nucleus, putamen and nucleus accumbens. However, Bird *et al.* (1979) reported increased concentrations of dopamine in the nucleus accumbens and the anterior perforated substance. In an extended study on over 50 schizophrenic brains, with controls, Mackay *et al.* (1982) confirmed the significant elevations, especially in patients with early onset of illness. Owen *et al.* (1978) reported increases in dopamine in the caudate nucleus, but not in the putamen or nucleus accumbens,

Table 7.5   Some CSF studies in schizophrenia

Compound	Result	Reference
Dopamine beta-hydrolase	Normal	Lerner *et al.* (1978)
Dopamine sulphate	Increased: negative symptoms	Risby *et al.* (1993)
5-HIAA	Normal	Post *et al.* (1975)
		Gomes *et al.* (1980)
		Roy *et al.* (1985)
Cyclic-AMP	Decreased	Biedermann *et al.* (1977)
	Increased	Gomes *et al.* (1980)
Cyclic-GMP	Decreased	Gattaz *et al.* (1983a)
GABA	Normal (↓ young females)	van Kammen *et al.* (1982)
Angiotensin-converting enzyme	Decreased	Beckmann *et al.* (1984)
Neurotensin	Decreased (subgroup only)	Widerlov *et al.* (1982)
Glutathione	Decreased: also in prefrontal cortex (MRS)	Do *et al.* (2000)
Kynurenic acid	Decreased, correlated with grey-matter densities	Schroeder *et al.* (2008)
Copper	Decreased	Tyrer *et al.* (1979)
D-serine	Decreased	Bebdikov *et al.* (2007)

and a significant decrease in HVA in the caudate. Farley *et al.* (1977) reported increases in dopamine only in the septal region of chronic paranoid patients. The cingulate has been rarely examined, but Wyatt *et al.* (1995) have reported decreased DOPAC levels in anterior cingulate cortex.

Reynolds (1983, 1987) has attempted to assess laterality effects in relation to neurochemistry in schizophrenia. Comparing patient brains to controls, dopamine was increased in the amygdala of the schizophrenics, selective for the left side. In one study, the increase of dopamine in the amygdala was found to correlate with decreasing levels of GABA binding in the hippocampus (Reynolds *et al.*, 1990).

Dopamine-receptor binding, with such compounds as haloperidol, spiperone, flupenthixol and apomorphine, has also been investigated. Studies of the dopamine receptor *in vivo* with PET imaging have shown high interindividual variability, which links to personality variables (Farde *et al.*, 1990; Karlsson *et al.*, 1995; Karlsson *et al.*, 2002) and to cognition (Cervenka *et al.*, 2008). Most of the studies in schizophrenia show increased binding in some areas, although the interpretation of this has led to much debate. In summary, most studies of D_2 receptors show increases of caudate binding (13 of 16) (Clardy *et al.*, 1994), others show increases in the putamen and/or nucleus accumbens. The contribution of prescribed neuroleptic drugs to these findings continues to be an important controversy, although some authors examined groups of drug-naive patients (Owen *et al.*, 1978) or patients drug-free for a long time (Lee and Seeman, 1980). However, these very same changes can be observed in rat brains given long-term neuroleptics (Clow *et al.*, 1979).

Other dopamine receptors have been less studied. D_1 receptors seem normal (Seeman *et al.*, 1987), similar to data from animals receiving neuroleptic drugs. However, D_4 binding in the striatum has been reported as increased (Seeman *et al.*, 1993).

It remains unclear what it is that drives the increase in dopamine activity. Early work had suggested a link through GABA. Decreased terminals of GABA in the hippocampus correlate with increased dopamine levels and are linked to the observation of increased $GABA_a$-receptor activity. Attention has now centred on a subgroup of GABA neurones, the parvalbumin-containing cells. Parvalbumin, along with calretinin and calbindin, is a calcium-binding protein, which develops at between three and six months of foetal development. Decreased parvalbumin cells are found in the frontal cortex and hippocampus in schizophrenia. This all suggests GABAergic deficits, which it is postulated lead to disturbed neuronal rhythmic (oscillatory) expression in key structures (the hippocampus, but also areas of frontal cortex), and to altered dopamine release.

Glutamate is also linked with this story. Glutamate input to dopamine-releasing cells (from, for example, the hippocampus and the pedunculopontine areas) normally induces bursts of spikes within the VTA, which are disrupted by a deficit of glutamate. Glutamate can be identified within neurones by looking at transporters (EAAT3 or VGluT1 – the neuronal and vesicular transporter respectively), and recent studies have shown decreases of these in post-mortem material, especially in the left-temporal area (Nudmamud-Thanoi *et al.*, 2007; Reynolds and Harte, 2007). These are associated behaviourally to novelty detection, which under normal circumstances activates the VTA and accumbens, interlinked with behavioural reward, and which in schizophrenia is thought to become disrupted (Lodge *et al.*, 2009; Sohal *et al.*, 2009).

Glutamic acid decarboxylase levels are reported as decreased in prefrontal cortx (Volk *et al.*, 2000). The changes in GABA are supported by decreases in reelin mRNA, reelin being a protein released by GABAergic neurones, and decreased GABA transporters in DLPFC neurone (Costa *et al.*, 2001; Akbarian *et al.*, 1995).

Several studies of glutamate binding have been carried out. Measurement of glutamate levels in CSF had earlier yielded conflicting results, but the psychotomimetic agent phencyclidine (PCP) was known to be an NMDA-receptor antagonist, leading to the hypothesis that glutamate transmission may be reduced in schizophrenia. Decreased kainate and glutamate binding have been reported (Kerwin *et al.*, 1988; Deakin *et al.*, 1989), especially in the left temporal lobes, as has reduced release of both glutamate and GABA from synaptosomes from temporal cortex following application of the agonists kainic acid or NMDA (Sherman *et al.*, 1991). Data from frontal areas are equivocal, especially for GABA$_a$ receptors, although they suggest, if anything, increased glutamate binding in orbitofrontal areas. These data argue for decreased cortical excitatory transmission in some areas of the limbic system in schizophrenia.

Noradrenaline and its metabolites have also been examined. Decreased levels of noradrenaline have been reported in the putamen (Crow *et al.*, 1979b); others have reported no differences (Bird *et al.*, 1979; Winblad *et al.*, 1979) and others selective increases (Farley *et al.*, 1977). MHPG is reported to be elevated in the hypothalamus and nucleus accumbens by one group (Kleinman *et al.*, 1982a). Dopamine beta-hydrolase and monoamine oxidase appear normal.

Binding of 5-HT receptors to various brain regions has been variable. Low 5-HT$_2$ binding to frontal cortex has been noted by some groups, especially if patients who commit suicide are excluded from the sample (Laurelle *et al.*, 1993),

although the contribution of chronic neuroleptic treatment to these effects remains unclear.

Peptides have also been studied. Levels of angiotensin-converting enzyme were reduced in the substantia nigra and globus pallidus (Arregui *et al.*, 1980). Opioid and naloxone binding is probably normal (Owen *et al.*, 1985). Ferrier *et al.* (1984a), in an extensive study of peptide distribution in limbic structures in schizophrenic and control brains, reported that CCK was reduced in temporal cortex, especially in the hippocampus and amygdala of patients with negative symptoms (type 2 of Crow); somatostatin was likewise decreased in hippocampus in the same group, while VIP was increased in the amygdala of those with positive symptoms (type 1 of Crow). No changes were seen for neurotensin, while substance P was increased in the hippocampus. A fuller review of the post-mortem findings of peptides in schizophrenia is given by Caceda *et al.* (2006, 2007).

Several other compounds have been assessed in various brain regions, and many of these are summarized in Table 7.6.

Neuropathological Data

A related area of research has been neuropathological studies of the brains of patients who had

Table 7.6   Some post-mortem biochemical findings

Chemical	Result	Author
Dopamine	Increased D$_2$, D$_3$, D$_4$/ transporter normal	Review, see Guillin *et al.* (2007)
GABA	Probably normal	Cross *et al.* (1979)
Glutamic acid decarboxylase	Normal	Bird *et al.* (1979)
5-HT	Increased: Putamen	Crow *et al.* (1979a)
	5-HT$_{1a}$ frontal cortex	Gurevich and Joyce (1997)
		Abi-dargham (2007)
	5-HT$_2$ probably normal Lower:	
	Hypothalamus	Winblad *et al.* (1979)
	Medulla oblongata	
	Hippocampus	
	Frontal cortex	Bennett *et al.* (1979)
Tryptophan	Normal	Crow *et al.* (1979b)
Cathechol-O-methyl transferase	Normal	Crow *et al.* (1979b)
Tyrosine hydrolase	Normal	Crow *et al.* (1979b)
Choline acetyl transferase	Normal	Bird *et al.* (1979)
Muscarinic receptors	Decreased	Dean *et al.* (2002)
Neurotrophins BDNF	Variable results	Buckley *et al.* (2007)

'the schizophrenias'. Although many studies over the years have been carried out, all of them detecting changes in some brains examined, such data are often criticized on account of the lack of consistency of the findings. However, similar criticisms would apply to pathological studies of such disorders as the dementias or the epilepsies if it were supposed that they represented the outcome of only a single process.

Earlier studies had shown abnormalities in thalamic, hypothalamic, periventricular, periaqueductal and basal forebrain areas (Nieto and Escobar, 1972; Stevens, 1982). Since that time other investigators have examined post-mortem collections of brains and while most detect some abnormalities, there are differences between types of pathology and areas affected. The most consistent abnormalities have been noted in hippocampal and related structures.

Overall, the volumes of schizophrenic brains are reduced (Pakkenberg, 1987). This is associated with negative symptoms (Johnstone *et al.*, 1994), and an excess of nonspecific focal pathology can be seen, often in basal-ganglia structures (Bruton *et al.*, 1990). The length of the sylvian fissure on the left is decreased (Falkai, 1992).

There are reports of abnormal gyral patterns, especially in the frontotemporal areas, with associated cytoarchitectural abnormalities (Jacob and Beckman, 1989) confirmed with MRI structural imaging.

Structural disorganization of hippocampal pyramidal cells (Kovelman and Scheibel, 1984; Bogerts *et al.*, 1985), reduced hippocampal mossy cell-fibre staining (Goldsmith and Joyce, 1995), decreased hippocampal volumes and cell loss (Falkai and Bogerts, 1986) and abnormalities or reduced volumes of the subiculum and hippocampal CA regions have all been reported (Arnold *et al.*, 1995). In the entorhinal cortex, smaller neurones, displaced pre-alpha and pre-beta cells, and reduced neuronal number and density have been noted (Arnold *et al.*, 1991). The changes reported are in both the left (Kovelman and Scheibel, 1984; Bogerts *et al.*, 1985) and the right hemispheres (Conrad *et al.*, 1991).

Crow and colleagues (Brown *et al.*, 1986), in a comparison of brains from patients meeting strict criteria for affective disorder and schizophrenia, noted that the latter had larger temporal horns of the lateral ventricle and thinner parahippocampal gyri. The greater differences were noted in the left hemisphere.

Some of these reports suggested that gliosis was a typical pathological reaction in schizophrenic brains. However, most studies fail to find gliosis, supporting the suggestions of Kovelman and Scheibel (1984) that the pathological changes instead represent developmental anomalies.

Other neuropathological findings include diminished neuronal density in some layers of the frontal, cingulate and motor cortices (Benes *et al.*, 1986), higher numbers of long vertical axones in cingulate cortex, possibly representing increased input of associative axones (Benes *et al.*, 1987), and abnormal arrangement of cells and decreases of small interneurones (possibly inhibitory) in cingulate cortex (Benes and Bird, 1987; Benes *et al.*, 1991). Increased neuronal density has been reported in hippocampus and prefrontal cortex (Selemon *et al.*, 1995), while reduced dendritic spine density of pyramidal neurone in the DLPFC has been found. These findings add evidence to the growing appreciation that the schizophrenias may be neurodevelopmental disorders, and that abnormalities in cortical cytoarchitexture and connectivity may be key facets of the underlying pathophysiology.

Akbarian *et al.* (1993) reported reduced numbers of NADPH-diaphorase-stained cells in superficial and increased numbers in deep layers of the dorsolateral prefrontal cortex. The stain specifically identifies cells of the embryological subplate area, the findings suggesting anomalous migration of cells. In another study, decreased gene expression for glutamic acid decarboxylase in prefrontal cortical neurones was found. This occurred in the absence of any cell loss, suggesting a functional down-regulation of neurotransmitter gene expression (Akbarian *et al.*, 1995). This may relate to the reported decrease in glutamic acid decarboxylase levels in prefrontal cortex and decreased GABA axon terminals. The changes in GABA are supported by decreases in reelin mRNA. As with many studies, the contribution of medication to these effects is unknown.

There are reported decreases of neurones in medial dorsal nucleus of the thalamus and nucleus accumbens (Pakkenberg, 1990), substantia innominata (Stevens, 1982) and cerebellum (Jeste *et al.*, 1985). The thalamic findings are of interest in view of the increasing evidence from imaging studies of thalamic abnormalities in schizophrenia. Some evidence has emerged for abnormalities of glutamate receptors (NMDA) and transporters in this structure, but also in other areas such as the caudate, hippocampus, DLPFC and cingulate gyrus (Watis *et al.*, 2008).

A selective reduction in glial cells in cingulate cortex (Brodmann's area 24) has been shown in schizophrenia patients relative to comparison subjects, calling into question whether cingulate changes are specific only for affective disorders (Stark *et al.*, 2004).

Recently, direct measurement of protein expression in brain areas has been carried out (proteomic studies) using electrophoresis or specialized mass-spectrometry techniques. These can identify the profile of many hundreds of proteins, but to date have not yielded useful clinical information. Likewise there are a growing number of studies in which gene expression in various cortical areas has been looked at, again with heterogenous results. The frontal cortex and genes that link with neurotransmitter function have been most studied. Genes related to myelin-forming oligodendrocytes and metabolic enzymes, as well as synaptic marker proteins such as synaptophysin, spinophilin (markers at pre- and post-synapyic terminals, respectively) and dysbindin, have all been reported to be reduced in some areas, notably hippocampus (Weickert *et al.*, 2007). The mRNA that encodes GAD 67 (glutamic acid decarboxylase), an enzyme that synthesizes GABA, is reduced in the DLPFC. This is reported particularly for the parvalbumin-expressing neurones, which have been shown in several studies to be reduced

in schizophrenia in the hippocampus and prefrontal cortex.

While the pathological studies achieve some degree of agreement, there is also quite a bit of confusion. This relates to several factors. Agonal changes, prior drug prescriptions and statistical analysis of such databases are problematic. It is also necessary to take into account the methods selected for analysis and the heterogenous population. There seems to be evidence for cell loss or disarray, or both, in frontal and temporal areas, but also for alterations of cell density, which may better reflect cell size rather than loss. However, the abnormalities are related to the structures implicated in the anatomy of schizophrenia, especially the prefrontal areas, medial temporal (especially hippocampal structures) and thalamus. Glutamate and GABA systems are becoming very relevant as attention has been directed to underlying anatomical circuitry. The enthusiasm for post-mortem studies has waned in recent years, overtaken particularly by the advances in brain imaging, but newer methods of protein and gene analysis are also ascendant and may lead to important findings, especially if they can be coordinated with imaging and genetic data.

NEUROPHYSIOLOGICAL AND NEUROLOGICAL DATA

EEG

Soon after the introduction of the electroencephalogram, reports of abnormalities in schizophrenia appeared. Hill (1950) reviewed these as follows: EEGs suggestive of epilepsy were most often seen in catatonia, although generalized nonparoxysmal dysrhythmias and other paroxysmal phenomena were also found. Since then, there have been many reports of EEG abnormalities in schizophrenic patients. In a comparison with patients suffering from affective disorder, Abrahams and Taylor (1979) noted that the proportion of EEG abnormalities was twice as great in the schizophrenics, who had more temporal abnormalities. Slow-wave asymmetries, slow bursts, spikes and sharp waves were the recorded changes, and they tended to be more frequent on the left side. In patients with temporal-lobe EEG changes this laterality was associated with formal thought disorder and emotional blunting, but not first-rank symptoms. Although patients were on medications, this did not correlate with the EEG findings.

Investigations of patients using electrodes implanted within the brain have clearly demonstrated abnormalities in schizophrenics, again notably within the limbic system. In a series of studies, Heath (1982) investigated 63 patients with psychosis, 38 being diagnosed as schizophrenic. Spiking was seen in the septal region. This is defined by Heath as an area bordered dorsally by the base of the anterior horn of the lateral ventricle and the head of the caudate nucleus, and ventrally by the free surface of the gyrus rectus of the frontal lobe. It includes septal nuclei, the accumbens, olfactory tubercle and the diagonal band, as well as parts of the gyrus rectus. It has extensive frontal and temporal connections. The abnormalities occurred when, and only when, the patients were actively psychotic. In many cases changes were not observed on surface recordings, and neither were similar findings noted in chronic-pain control patients. Violence and aggression were associated with hippocampal and amygdala discharges. Some patients showed activation in sensory-relay nuclei in association with hallucinations (for example, medial geniculate recordings) and often cerebellar discharges. Similar findings, especially with regards to the septal region, have been reported by others (Rickles, 1969).

Examination of the spectral power of EEG frequencies in schizophrenia reveals more fast beta activity, more theta and delta, and less alpha than normals (Itil, 1975). Psychotic children and those with a high risk for schizophrenia show a similar pattern of changes. Generally these patterns are 'normalized' by antipsychotic medication.

Fenton *et al.* (1980) noted the changes to be maximal over temporal derivations in acute schizophrenic patients, while chronic patients showed more diffuse slow-wave power, notably theta and delta, diffusely or maximally frontoparietally.

Stevens and Livermore (1982) used telemetered EEG recordings during psychotic behaviour of schizophrenic patients. They identified so-called 'ramp patterns', characterized by a monotonic decline in power from lowest to highest frequencies, which can be seen in epileptic patients during subcortical spike activity. These were seen only in recordings from schizophrenic patients in their sample, and not in controls. Patients with catatonic episodes showed them in the right temporal region, while 50% of paranoid patients with auditory hallucinations had left-sided ramps, with increased slow activity. Psychotic events recorded clinically were associated with suppression of left temporal alpha frequencies.

Evoked-potential studies in schizophrenia are numerous, and the results complicated to interpret. Several reviews are available (Shagass, 1972; Flor-Henry, 1983). Generally, evoked potentials show greater variability and amplitudes are decreased; a subgroup of patients show a 'reducing' pattern of decreasing amplitude with increasing stimulus intensity. Flor-Henry (1983) summarized a review by stating 'the evoked potential characteristics in schizophrenia consistently implicate the left hemisphere, and particularly the left temporal region' (p. 215). The contingent negative variation (CNV) also tends to be reduced, maximally over frontal areas.

Studies using brain electrical activity mapping (BEAM) EEG have shown increased frontal delta and diminished left temporal P300 amplitudes (Morihisa *et al.*, 1983; Morstyn *et al.*, 1983).

More recent studies have investigated rhythmic oscillations and synchronizations between neural networks. Such oscillations undergo changes during development and are closely related to GABA and glutamate activity. As noted, there are suggestions of decreased GABA neurones in cortical structures in schizophrenia, especially those neurone which express parvalbumin (chandelier neurones) with thalamic afferents. Alteration of this input can disrupt inhibition and hence oscillatory patterns (Lodge *et al.*, 2009; Sohal *et al.*, 2009).

Using MEG it has been shown that responses recorded from auditory cortex in schizophrenia to rhythmic auditory trains or to visual stimuli are different from controls, with decreases of higher frequencies (40 Hz, gamma) and excess of lower ones (20 Hz, beta). Gamma and beta oscillations have different source generators, the latter coming from deeper cerebral areas. This disruption of gamma oscillations in schizophrenia is in keeping with theories of disruption of GABA/glutamate activity, and with disturbed cognition, especially with working memory (Rotarka-Jagiela *et al.*, 2009; Haenschel *et al.*, 2009; Haenschel *et al.*, 2007).

Radiological Studies

A common saying throughout the 1900s was that 'schizophrenia was the graveyard of neuropathologists'. That is, numerous neuropathologists had worked for many years to find neuropathological evidence correlating with the behavioural changes observed by patients and clinicians, all to no avail. A modern update of that saying might be that 'schizophrenia is the graveyard of neuroimagers'. However, what is different with the modern methods is that many, in fact most, published imaging studies do in fact find differences between patients with schizophrenia and controls. Nonetheless, often the studies are methodologically flawed or are of small sample size and the results do not replicate.

MRI

The earlier findings with CT are reviewed in previous editions of this book, but remain both interesting and valid. MRI has become the predominant research method. There are well over 1000 studies, and they have served to confirm much of the earlier CT data, but in addition have provided new findings. A summary is given in Table 7.8.

With MRI it has been possible to confirm that the cerebral cortex is smaller than in controls

Table 7.7 Some features of ventricular enlargement of schizophrenia

Early brain damage or birth complication
Poorer premorbid adjustment
More negative symptoms
Less positive symptoms
Cognitive decline
Poorer response to treatment
More minor neurological signs
Decreased CSF–HVA
Decreased frontal CBF

(Zipursky *et al.*, 1992), even at the onset of the illness (Degreef *et al.*, 1991). The degree of loss correlates with the severity (Young *et al.*, 1991) and duration of the schizophrenic symptoms (Waddington *et al.*, 1991). Ventricular enlargement has been confirmed in many reports, again at the onset of the illness (Degreef *et al.*, 1991). The relationship of this to positive and negative symptoms is unclear (Table 7.7).

One of the significant advantages of MRI is the production of high-resolution images of temporal-lobe structures. Reduced temporal-lobe volume and increased size of the temporal horn of the lateral ventricle is a well-replicated finding (Suddath *et al.*, 1989; Kawasaki *et al.*, 1993). Smaller superior temporal-lobe gyri on the left have been noted by several authors, with correlations to clinical phenomena, namely auditory hallucinations (Barta *et al.*, 1990), thought disorder (Shenton *et al.*, 1992) and reduced P300 amplitude (McCarley *et al.*, 1993). These findings are of particular interest since the superior temporal gyrus contains the planum temporale and Heschl's gyrus (primary auditory cortex) and merges into Wernicke's area, and is therefore intimately involved with language and the manipulation of symbolic knowledge.

Suddath *et al.* (1990) studied 15 MZ twins discordant for schizophrenia, and found the affected twin to show larger lateral and third ventricles, and smaller hippocampi with decreased grey-matter volume, an effect greater on the left. No such differences were found in normal twin pairs. In a further study of twin pairs, they noted a significant relationship between the left hippocampal volume, and rCBF activation

Table 7.8 Summary of MRI findings in schizophrenia

Region of interest	Findings
Cerebrum	Volume loss in cerebral cortex and abnormal relaxation times
Cerebellum	Inconclusive
Ventricles	Enlarged lateral and third ventricles
Temporal lobes	Abnormal relaxation times and volume loss in grey matter
Superior temporal gyrus	Smaller – especially on the left
Mesial temporal structures	Abnormal relaxation times and smaller amygdala–hippocampus–parahippocampus in particular the left side; associations between hippocampal size and prefrontal cortex activity; reduced NAA in left hippocampus with MRS
Frontal lobes	Smaller and abnormal relaxation times; decreased phospholipid turnover
Caudate nucleus	Various reports, smaller and larger
Thalamus	Smaller
Septum pellucidum	Enlarged and higher incidence of cavum septum pellucidum
Corpus callosum	Thinner/thicker/longer/shape distortion or normal
Cingulate gyrus	Smaller on both sides
Gender effects	Brain abnormalities more in males
Progression	Ventricular enlargement – nonprogressive > progressive Brain volume loss – cortical thinning
Clinical correlation	Positive symptoms: mesial temporal structures and superior temporal gyrus Negative symptoms: ventricular enlargement and frontal lobe abnormalities

in the prefrontal cortex with the Wisconsin card-sorting test with differences between healthy and affected twins. In the affected twins, prefrontal activation was correlated to both right and left hippocampal volumes.

Individual structures in the temporal lobe have also been examined. The hippocampi have been reported smaller, a finding that is more robust on the left (Breier *et al.*, 1992; Weinberger *et al.*, 1992; Bogerts *et al.*, 1993), and in one study correlated with the severity of positive symptoms (Bogerts *et al.*, 1993). The amygdala, a much more difficult structure to measure than the hippocampus, is also probably reduced in size on the left (Barta *et al.*, 1990; Shenton *et al.*, 1992) or bilaterally (Breier *et al.*, 1992). The parahippocampal gyrus is also smaller on the left (Shenton *et al.*, 1992; Kawasaki *et al.*, 1993) or bilaterally (McCarley *et al.*, 1993).

The frontal cortex has also been investigated. Abnormal relaxation times of both T_1 and T_2 have been reported, in some studies correlated with the severity of negative symptoms (Besson *et al.*, 1987; Williamson *et al.*, 1992). The prefrontal cortex is also smaller (Breier *et al.*, 1992), the size correlating with reduction of prefrontal activation during the Wisconsin card-sorting

test (Weinberger *et al.*, 1992), but also with non-deficit symptoms (Buchanan *et al.*, 1993). However, unlike the findings with the temporal lobes, many of the investigations of frontal areas are negative (Suddath *et al.*, 1990).

Other MRI findings include increased third ventricular enlargement, which is correlated with the degree of cognitive deficit (Bornstein *et al.*, 1992); variable abnormalities of the corpus callosum in thickness, length or shape (Casanova *et al.*, 1990), which findings cannot yet be resolved; smaller cingulate gyri (Blackwood *et al.*, 1991); and less grey-matter volume in areas of heteromodal association cortex such as the dorsolateral prefrontal cortex, the inferior parietal area and the superior temporal gyrus (Schlaepfer *et al.*, 1994).

Several of the MRI studies have noted greater effects in male patients (Waddington *et al.*, 1991; O'Callaghan *et al.*, 1992). Most now agree that the bulk of ventricular enlargement is early in the disease course and reaches a plateau (Borgwardt *et al.*, 2009; Delisi, 2008).

A particularly interesting MRI method involves diffusion tensor imaging (DTI), which allows one to test white-matter fibre integrity and potential anatomic connectiveness. DTI studies in schizophrenia have repeatedly found abnormalities in white-matter fibre tracts. Included are the uncinate fasciculus. As with most findings in schizophrenia, it is not clear if these changes are primary, or simply reflect problems elsewhere in the brain and are 'Wallerian degeneration-like' (Delisi *et al.*, 2006a)

A summary of the morphological MRI findings is that nearly all reported studies have found abnormalities of morphology in schizophrenia (Tables 7.7 and 7.8). Smaller brain size, third and lateral ventricular atrophy and increased size of the temporal horns are robust findings. Abnormalities of the left temporal lobe seem to be reported more than findings on the right, especially with decreases in size of the superior temporal gyrus and hippocampus, which seem inversely correlated with the presence of positive symptoms. The frontal lobes are also abnormal. These data substantially support the neuropathological data presented above, and emphasize the relevance of abnormalities of the limbic system, especially on the left, in the pathology of schizophrenia.

Unfortunately, contemporary meetings of the American Psychiatric Association or the US Society of Biological Psychiatry, or other forums related to schizophrenia research, are filled with poster after poster of imaging studies, but often without an ability to extrapolate the findings into a comprehensive understanding of the illness. The vast and ever-growing literature however can be distilled down into a few key findings that appear to be replicated and tend to transcend the different methods (CT, MRI):

1. Enlargement of the lateral ventricles, particularly the left, and the temporal horn.
2. Diffuse grey-matter reductions and thinning bilaterally.
3. Reduced white-matter integrity (particularly now as seen with DTI).
4. Reduced size of the entire temporal cortex, superior temporal gyrus and hippocampus.

There are also multiple reports of increased brain asymmetries, abnormalities of the cavum septum pellucidum and corpus callosum, and enlargement of the caudates with medications, particularly the antipsychotic medications.

Studies of individuals at first onset of psychosis and then following them through the first phases of the illness have shown that with time there is a decrease in size of the left parahippocampal gyrus, bilateral cingulate gyri and left fusiform and orbitofrontal gyri.

Recent longitudinal studies have shown that many of the abnormalities are progressive, with left ventricular expansion, bilateral hemispheric volume decreases, changes in the cerebellum and corpus-callosum thinning. Relatives from high-risk families who may be exhibiting prodromal symptoms also have measurable brain changes as a group. The high-risk individuals had reduced apparent diffusion coefficient (ACD) DTI values in the left parahippocampal gyrus, lingual gyrus and superior and middle frontal gyri compared to controls (Delisi *et al.*, 2006a).

The interested reader is referred to several recent reviews of this massively expanding and complex area (Abi-Dargham and Guillin, 2007; Delisi *et al.*, 2004, 2006a, 2006b). A recent summit of the experts in this area concluded '(1) that progressive brain change associated with schizophrenia is a real phenomenon, (2) that it is widespread in the brain, but that (3) it varies among individuals in how widespread or severe it is and it varies in the timing. (4) It was generally agreed that there is much evidence to suggest that in the majority of patients it occurs early in the illness and levels off. (5) Although the underlying cause is not known, it could be partly genetic and cannot wholly be accounted for by pharmacological treatment. (6) It clearly has clinical implications; and (7) its unknown cause is a likely future target for pharmaceutical intervention' (Borgwardt *et al.*, 2009).

CBF and PET Studies

Ingvar and Franzen (1974) initially reported that schizophrenic patients had normal mean hemisphere blood flows, but demonstrated a shift in distribution such that higher levels were less common in frontal structures and more common in postcentral structures when compared with controls. This 'hypofrontality' has become a well-replicated finding using several different imaging techniques. However, like most areas with functional brain imaging, there is a problem with causality. Does the hypofrontality occur because the patients with schizophrenia are not activating the prefrontal cortex as well – that is, they are not doing the task as well – as controls? Or is it primary? We still do not understand this basic problem, which continues to plaque the early PET studies and the more recent fMRI BOLD-activation studies.

Several early studies used xenon inhalation to measure CBF and used brain-activation paradigms. For example, Gur *et al.* (1983a, 1983b), in medicated patients, assessed cerebral activity during verbal and spatial tasks. No hypofrontality was seen, but schizophrenic patients, unlike controls, showed no changes in hemisphere activation during the verbal task, and a greater increase than expected in left hemisphere activity when carrying out the spatial task. Further investigations on unmedicated patients (Gur *et al.*, 1985) showed higher resting left hemisphere flow. Further, more severely affected patients showed decreases of anterior left hemisphere activity during spatial tasks, a pattern rarely found in normals. Their data, they suggested, supported a hypothesis of left-hemisphere overactivation in schizophrenia, and the differences between medicated and unmedicated patients suggested that medication helps restore symmetrical blood flow, the main effect being on the left hemisphere.

Weinberger *et al.* (1986) have specifically tested frontal-lobe function by administering patients the Wisconsin card-sorting test during xenon-133 inhalation. Controlled cognitive tasks, such as a number-matching test, were also used, patients being drug-free for a minimum of four weeks. During the number-matching task no differences were noted between patients and controls, but with the frontal-lobe task the clear increases seen in controls were not seen in frontal regions in the schizophrenic patients. The changes were regionally specific, in particular involving the dorsolateral aspect of the prefrontal association cortex. These data, they suggested, indicate that patients with schizophrenia have a specific physiological dysfunction of prefrontal cortex. In later studies (Berman *et al.*, 1986), similar results have been obtained in patients off medication and in twin studies, only the affected MZ twin shows hypofrontality on activation (Berman *et al.*, 1992). Further, since schizophrenic patients and controls did not differ on a continuous-performance task with regards to CBF, the abnormalities recorded were thought to be independent of medication status and of state factors such as attention and mental effort.

There have been many SPECT- and PET-activation studies in schizophrenia. The earlier PET investigations were largely with glucose, but more recently oxygen and ligand studies have yielded the more interesting results. A caveat to most of these studies is that they invariably use patients that have been on neuroleptic medications, even if they were free from medication at the time of testing. Generally, hypofrontality has been reported (Buchsbaum *et al.*, 1990; Siegel *et al.*, 1993), although there is considerable overlap with control values, and there are several negative studies, especially in acute-onset medication-free patients (Sheppard *et al.*, 1983). Hypofrontality does not seem to correlate with ventricular dilatation and is increased by neuroleptic medication (Delisi and Buchsbaum, 1986). The hypofrontality is in part a reflection of hyperoccipitality, and is more prominent in medial rather than lateral frontal cortex (Siegel *et al.*, 1993).

Increased anterior temporal-lobe activity has been shown with deoxyglucose PET (Delisi *et al.*, 1989) and oxygen (Liddle *et al.*, 1992).

Hallucinations have been associated with increased blood flow in Broca's area with SPECT (McGuire *et al.*, 1993) and PET (Cleghorn *et al.*, 1992), and with lower metabolism in the region of Wernicke's area and increased activity in the anterior cingulate regions and striatum with fluorodeoxyglucose PET (Cleghorn *et al.*, 1992).

Based on factor analysis of patients' symptoms in schizophrenia, Liddle (1987) proposed three clusters, respectively referred to as psychomotor poverty, reality distortion and disorganization syndromes. The former involves poverty of speech, affect and movement; reality distortion comprises hallucinations and delusions; and the disorganization syndrome refers to formal thought disorder and inappropriate affect. While each syndrome can coexist in the same individual, they were postulated to represent independent functional systems, corresponding to limbic and subcortical distributed brain systems.

Using $^{15}O_2$-PET and SPM, Liddle *et al.* (1992) identified separate neuroanatomical profiles for the three clusters shown in Table 7.9 (Liddle *et al.*, 1992). These data, especially for the reality-distortion factor, have received partial replication (Kaplan *et al.*, 1993). Friston *et al.* (1992) have identified the left parahippocampal region as being the central neuroanatomical substrate of schizophrenia, abnormalities here being associated with dysfunction in distributed limbic-association areas, the pattern of distribution dependent on the presenting behavioural syndrome. The primacy of the hippocampus and cingulate region has also been discussed by Tamminga *et al.* (1992).

Friston *et al.* (1992) point out a resolution to the conflicting data with regards to hypofrontality. Thus, a patient can have regional hypofrontality (associated with psychomotor poverty in the psychomotor-poverty syndrome) and hyperfrontality (in the anterior cingulate in the disorganisation syndrome).

There is little conformity of data with regards to basal ganglia findings in psychotic patients, high, normal and low values being noted (Volkow *et al.*, 1985; Gur, 1986; Buchsbaum *et al.*, 1992). Increased values in basal ganglia regions following neuroleptic treatment are reported from several PET studies (DeLisi and Buchsbaum, 1986; Gur, 1986; Cleghorn *et al.*, 1992). These data are in keeping with the known high dopamine content of these regions of the brain and their possible abnormalities in patients with psychosis.

Following an analysis of 50 male schizophrenics and controls using SPM, Andreasen (1995) has highlighted the thalamus and white matter connecting to the frontal lobes as possible key areas of abnormality. More recently the role of the thalamus has been emphasized by Buchsbaum and colleagues (Hazlett *et al.*, 2008; Byne *et al.*, 2009).

Examination of the dopamine hypothesis has been further enhanced by the development of selective radioactive dopamine ligands (e.g. fallypride and 11c NPA for the D_2/D_3 receptor), although none are selective for just the D_2 receptor. In the past much attention was given to striatal activity, but with these ligands linked to higher-resolution scanners (as low as 2 mm), extrastiatal dopamine has been examined. The thalamus has become a centrepiece, especially the dorso-medial nucleus. There are several studies suggesting a decreased size and/or activity of this nucleus (Byne *et al.*, 2006) and decreased dopamine binding (Buchsbaum *et al.*,2006). Interestingly, the majority of studies, but not all, report

Table 7.9   PET findings in the syndromes of schizophrenia (Liddle *et al.*, 1992)

Syndrome cluster	*Clinical features*	*PET*
Psychomotor poverty	Poverty of speech, affect, movement	Decreased: prefrontal L parietal Increased: caudate
Reality distortion	Hallucinations and delusions	Increased: L – parahippocampal; ventral striatum Decreased: R – post-cingulate; post-temporal
Disorganization	Thought disorder; inappropriate affect	Increased: ant cingulate, mediodorsal thalamus Decreased: R frontotemporal, Broca's area; R, L angular gyrus

Increased/decreased refers to cerebral blood flow compared with controls.

that the left side is the more affected (Kessler *et al.*, 2009). The thalamus is looped with the basal ganglia and with frontal cortex, the medio-dorsal nucleus being a relay between sensory and cognitive systems representing an additional way in which dopamine may be involved in the pathogenesis of schizophrenia. There is in normals usually a tight correlation between frontal and medio-dorsal thalamic activity, which is lost in schizophrenia (Hazlett *et al.*, 2008).

The Viral Hypothesis

As noted in earlier chapters, the possibility that viral infections of the limbic system are associated with some cases of psychosis has had a long history. There are several reasons to search for viruses, including the known excess of winter births in schizophrenia (Fuller Torrey *et al.*, 1977), the schizophrenia-like presentations of some patients with known encephalitis, the discovery of slow viruses which affect the nervous system, but whose effects are delayed for many years (Fuller Torrey and Peterson, 1973), and the reporting by some authors of evidence for viral activity in schizophrenic patients.

A second line of evidence has been to examine serum and CSF for abnormal antibody titres, or to seek impaired immunological function in schizophrenic patients. Scattered early reports of decreased delayed hypersensitivity, prior to the introduction of neuroleptic drugs, are of interest, implying possible immunological dysfunction which cannot be attributed to these agents (Delisi, 1984). Estimations of lymphocyte characteristics, including the percentages of B- and T-cells, have produced variable data, as has the quantitative assessment of various immunoglobulin classes. Oligoclonal IgG bands appear normal (Roos *et al.*, 1985). Reports of raised cytomegalovirus antibody levels in CSF in up to 70% of patients (Albrecht *et al.*, 1980) have not consistently been replicated (Shrikhande *et al.*, 1985; Alexander *et al.*, 1992) and post-mortem brain studies using staining for these viruses have also been negative (Stevens *et al.*, 1984).

There is thus minimal evidence that viral illness is aetiologically related to schizophrenia, and the variable findings, in particular the abnormal features of the immunological system, may reflect immunosuppression related to medications.

The search for a viral aetiology has turned into a quest to implicate prenatal infection, and the influenza virus has attracted most attention. As noted above, there is good evidence that there is an excess of winter births in schizophrenia. From over 50 studies, the number that confirm this effect outways negative results. The effect may be more robust in females and those without a family history, and exposure to the A2 influenza virus has been most strongly implicated (Mednick *et al.*, 1988; O'Callaghan, 1991; Adams *et al.*, 1993; Takei *et al.*, 1994). Infants in their second trimester of foetal development were said to be vulnerable to later developing schizophrenia, timing which fits well with some of the neuronal development abnormalities discussed above (Jacob and Beckman, 1989) and the observed excess of minor physical abnormalities noted in schizophrenics.

This view has its detractors, however. They claim that the largest cohorts do not reveal the effect, that there are statistical objections to the handling of the data and that prospective studies are negative (Crow, 1994). In the National Child Development Study in the UK, in which all children born in a specified week in 1958 were followed at regular intervals, no excess of schizophrenia was noted in children of mothers who suffered influenza in the 1957 epidemic (Crow, 1994). A further problem seems to be that the influenza virus fails to cross the placental barrier.

Another way to examine this theory, or at least the theory that chronic infection has something to do with the slow progression of schizophrenia, has been to examine the inflammatory cytokine profiles. The implication is that there is a mild but chronic immune process that alters certain brain structures and may alter neurochemical expression. Thus the proinflammatory cytokines (INF, TNF) shift the balance of the metabolism of tryptophan from 5-HT towards kynurenine, a compound which has been shown elevated in CSF in schizophrenia and is a NMDA-receptor antagonist.

Associations with Neurological Disease

The most comprehensive survey of the relationship of schizophrenia-like psychoses to neurological conditions is that of Davison and Bagley (1969). It has already been pointed out (in Chapter 3) that a variety of pathologies that affect the limbic system may lead to a

disorder with a phenomenological appearance of a schizophreniform psychosis, the most convincing data so far being collected for epilepsy, in particular temporal-lobe epilepsy (see Chapter 10).

Table 7.10 lists the neurological conditions that have been associated with a schizophreniform psychosis, giving the expected number and the actual number in the early published literature. Taken from Davison and Bagley's review, it indicates a higher than expected frequency, in particular for Huntington's chorea, narcolepsy,

Table 7.10   Comparison of the relative proportions of CNS disorders with psychosis in the 1958–1967 literature and their prevalence in the general population (from Davison and Bagley, 1969, p. 149)

CNS disorder	Prevalence in general population (per 100 000)[a]	Distribution of psychotic cases in 1958–1967 literature	
		Expected number	Actual number
Trauma	–	–	532
Epilepsy	548	211	276
Huntington's chorea	4	2	86[b]
Cerebrovascular disease	450	173	42[b]
Parkinsonism	114	44	20[b]
Narcolepsy	–	–	19[b]
Choreoathetosis	–	–	19[b]
Cerebral glioma	8.3	3	19[b]
Benign cerebral tumour	30	12	17
Pituitary adenoma	5.4	2	17[b]
Postmeningitis/encephalitis	–	–	16
Multiple sclerosis	80	30	11[b]
Congenital disorders	–	–	8
General paresis	24	9	5
Hepatic encephalopathy	–	–	5
Wilson's disease	–	–	4
Cerebellar degeneration	7	3	3
Other cerebral degeneration	–	–	3
Cerebral lipoidosis	–	–	3
Hypoglycaemia	–	–	3
Motor neurone disease	11	4	2
Cerebral reticulosis	–	–	2
Torsion spasm	–	–	2
Leber's optic atrophy	–	–	1
Phenylketonuria	–	–	1
Schilder's disease	–	–	1
Friedreich's ataxia	–	–	1
Myotonia congenital	–	–	1

[a]Prevalence figures taken from Brewis *et al.* (1966).
[b]Indicates probable significant difference.

cerebrovascular disease, cerebral gliomas and pituitary adenomata. A lower than expected incidence occurs with Parkinson's disease and multiple sclerosis.

The conclusion with regards to tumours in particular emphasizes temporal-lobe and diencephalic locations. A survey of the world literature on psychiatric symptomatology in Huntington's chorea reveals an excess of schizophrenia-like and paranoid conditions, the psychopathology often emerging before the onset of the movement disorder (Trimble, 1981a). It is of interest that this condition is associated with relative overactivity of dopamine function, in contrast to Parkinson's disease, in which the incidence of psychosis is said to be rare, unless provoked by dopaminergic medications such as L-dopa or bromocriptine. Wilson's disease, in which condition the main pathological findings are multilobular cirrhosis of the liver and cerebral changes maximal in the putamen, caudate nucleus and globus pallidus, is also not associated with an excess of schizophrenia-like symptoms. Sydenham's chorea and idiopathic basal ganglia calcification (Cummings, 1985) are sporadically reported to be associated with a schizophreniform psychosis.

In contrast to some of the other conditions mentioned, multiple sclerosis is a white-matter disease affecting in particular periventricular structures, and its psychopathology, which includes emotional lability, affective disorder and a characteristic euphoria (Trimble, 1981a), is markedly different. On the other hand, metachromatic leucodystrophy is an autosomal recessive disorder due to a deficiency of aryl-sulphatase A which leads to an accumulation of sulphated sphingolipids. In the juvenile and adult-onset forms metachromatic leucodystrophy presents with behavioural symptoms, which include personality changes, dementia and a schizophrenia-like illness (Hyde *et al.*, 1992).

Davison and Bagley (1969) particularly emphasized diencephalic, brainstem and temporal lobe locations of pathology. Midline cerebral malformations, especially cavum septum pellucidum, agenesis of the corpus callosum and aqueduct stenosis, are also overrepresented in patients presenting with schizophrenia (Scott *et al.*, 1993).

There is additional literature emphasizing neurological impairments and signs which may be found in patients at risk for schizophrenia or those with the condition. Offspring of schizophrenic parents, thus representing a high-risk group for the later development of the disorder, have an increased number of pregnancy and birth complications. The high-risk subjects who have a psychiatric breakdown have the greatest number of such complications, and show abnormal electrodermal galvanic skin responses with shorter latency, slower habituation and greater resistance to extinction (Parnas *et al.*, 1981). Further, infants at risk for schizophrenia show increased evidence of neurological dysfunction, with neurological soft signs, poor motor coordination and perceptual deficits (Marcus *et al.*, 1985). Schizophrenic patients have lower birth weights than expected (Parnas *et al.*, 1981), and cerebral dysfunction, as shown by neurological signs, EEG abnormalities or a history of seizures, is overreported in patients with infantile psychosis (Kolvin *et al.*, 1971).

Data from the National Child Development Study showed children who later developed schizophrenia to have early language, reading and motoric disturbances, and these abnormalities are seen earlier and more frequently in males (Crow, 1994). Similar findings are being reported in more recent studies of high-risk people which emphasize neuromotor development and cognition, especially memory/learning. Interestingly, such studies suggest that family and environmental variables are largely secondary or indirect associations. Nonspecific affective symptomatology prior to the onset of the disorder seems to be of more importance than most psychotic phenomena (Owens and Johnstone, 2006).

Patients diagnosed as schizophrenic frequently show neurological abnormalities on routine testing. These affect up to 60% of patients and cannot be solely ascribed to medication or undiagnosed neurological illness (Woods and Short, 1985); they may also be detected in a high proportion of relatives (Kinney *et al.*, 1986). Potential frontal-lobe signs, such as the grasp reflex, and perseveration are especially reported (Cox and Ludwig, 1979), while Fuller Torrey (1980) reported abnormal face–hand tests (particularly pronounced in the right hand, suggesting left-hemisphere involvement) and graphesthesia. Minor motor and sensory disturbances, more recognizable choreoathetotic, dystonic and tic-like presentations, gait disturbances, difficulties with coordination and smooth performance of motor activities, reflex changes (increased or decreased) and the presence of infantile reflexes such as palmomental reflexes, mirror movements and variable Babinski responses, have all been reported (Claude and Bourguignon, 1927; Quitkin *et al.*, 1976; Tucker and Silberfarb, 1978; Keshavan *et al.*, 1979). These have an inverse relationship to IQ levels (Quitkin *et al.*, 1976), but no apparent association to prognosis.

Abnormalities of eye blinking (Stevens, 1978), either decreased or increased, or episodic rapid paroxysms of blinking, have been noted in schizophrenia, the paroxysms being associated with psychotic episodes. Disturbed eye tracking, including abnormal smooth-pursuit eye movements and saccadic eye movements, are also reported. These movements are made as the fovea tracks a moving object. Saccades are fast but ballistic movements that bring the fovea and the target together, while the smooth-pursuit eye movements are responsible for fixation of slower-moving targets, and thus are continuous with the fovea sited on the target. Saccadic movements can be voluntarily executed, whereas smooth-pursuit movements require stimulus activation and are maintained by attention to the target. Up to 85% of schizophrenic patients are reported to show abnormal smooth-pursuit tracking, similar abnormalities being noted in 34% of relatives (Holzman *et al.*, 1984). This does not appear to be related to inattention, motivation or drug effects, and higher concordance for the abnormality is shown for MZ as opposed to DZ twins. Saccadic abnormalities have also been described in schizophrenia (Mialet and Pichot, 1981).

Neuropsychological Disturbances in Schizophrenia

That patients with schizophrenia have altered neuropsychological performance on a variety of tests has been known for many years and the findings have been reviewed by several authors (Flor-Henry, 1983; Cutting, 1990). The Cognitive Neuroscience Treatment Research to Improve Cognition in Schizophrenia (CNTRICS) group has summarized the literature in specific domains and has issued recommendations about standardized tests or measures of attention, social cognition and working memory (Barch *et al.*, 2009a, 2009b; Carter *et al.*, 2009; Nuechterlein *et al.*, 2009). In general, all who have looked for it have noted intellectual decline of some sort in schizophrenic patients, reflecting Kraepelin's (1919) summary that profound dementia occurs in 75% of patients with hebephrenia and 59% of those with catatonia. The Halstead–Reitan test battery, designed to identify patients with brain damage, fails to discriminate between schizophrenic patients and those with known neurological damage (Heaton and Crowley, 1981), and decrements are more likely to be found in those with longer hospitalizations and chronic illness (Goldstein and Halperin, 1977). The decline does not appear to be related to neuroleptic medication; in fact, cognitive testing is often seen to improve in patients receiving these drugs (Heaton and Crowley, 1981).

Patients with simple schizophrenia show the most markedly dilapidated cognition, while those with a delusional form of the disorder may be least impaired (Robertson and Taylor, 1985). Schizophrenic patients demonstrate average reading and spelling abilities in the setting of lower IQ and memory scores, the former tasks reflecting premorbid ability; similar patterns are noted in the dementias (Dalby and Williams, 1986).

Other studies emphasize altered attention, psychomotor speed and problem-solving (Goldberg *et al.*, 1993), and the concept of deterioration of working memory has become important. This involves the memory capacity to hold information for short periods of time, usually seconds. It is required for guiding future behaviour from representations of the outside world, rather than for responding to immediate stimuli (Goldman-Rakik, 1994). It provides temporal and spatial continuity between past experience and present actions. In animal studies it is impaired by frontal lesions, which produce decrements on delayed response tasks. During such delays, increased neuronal firing is found in Brodmann's area 46 of primate brains. This is equivalent to part of the middle frontal gyrus in humans, and in primates is anterior to area 8, lesions of which produce smooth-pursuit eye deficits, similar to those reported in schizophrenia. Since patients with schizophrenia can also be shown to be impaired on delayed-response tasks, it has been suggested that these frontal impairments are central to the psychology of schizophrenia.

Liddle and Morris (1991) presented cognitive data on their patients, separated into the three syndromes discussed above. Psychomotor poverty was associated with impairment of abstract thinking and long-term memory; disorganization syndrome with impaired concentration and new learning; while reality distortion was associated only with impairment of figure ground perception. Frontal-lobe tasks were performed badly by those in the psychomotor-poverty and disorganization groups, but were done better by patients in the reality-distortion group. The disorganization syndrome was associated with impaired verbal fluency.

Johnstone *et al.* (1978) have drawn attention to age disorientation in chronic schizophrenic patients, affecting approximately 25%, in which they usually underestimate their age. Those with this problem are more likely to have had a younger first admission to hospital and a longer duration of stay. This same group has drawn attention to the 'dementia' of dementia praecox. They thus note that there appears to be a subgroup of patients with schizophrenia who not only show intellectual impairment but on CT scan demonstrate evidence of structural brain damage. These patients often display 'negative features' such as poverty of speech, retardation and affective changes, while patients with 'positive features' such as hallucinations, delusions and thought disorder are less likely to show a cognitive decline.

Laterality effects have also been examined. Schizophrenic patients perform abnormally on tests of aphasia. On a battery of neuropsychological tasks including subsets from the Halstead–Reitan and the Luria–Nebraska batteries, schizophrenic patients (the majority drug-free) not only displayed marked impairments but had maximal abnormalities on tests related to frontotemporal functions bilaterally (Taylor and Abrams, 1984). In a more comprehensive evaluation, Flor-Henry (1983) compared large numbers of schizophrenic and affective-disorder patients and noted asymmetric frontotemporal dysfunction, the left side being more impaired than the right in the schizophrenic sample. When an analysis of covariance was carried out, looking at depression, mania, schizophrenia and control patients, a continuum of increasing cerebral disorganization was seen, depression showing minimal changes, while schizophrenia showed maximal.

Recently much attention has been paid to the potential for cognitive abnormalities to be endophenotypic variants, and deficits of executive function and working memory have been the focus of attention (Gur *et al.*, 2007). The latter is capacity-limited; in other words, there is an inverted U-shaped curve of efficiency in normals, closely linked to increased activation of the dorsolateral prefrontal cortex. Abnormalities of working memory have been well recorded, schizophrenic patients operating at or beyond efficiency being unable to maintain performance within their expected capacity. During working-memory tasks and imaging they show either hyperfrontality or hypofrontality in a complex relationship with task difficulty and performance (Karlsgodt *et al.*, 2009). Unaffected sibs of patients also show difficulties with working memory, including unaffected MZ twins (Prata *et al.*, 2008a, 2008b; Filbey *et al.*, 2008; Toulopoulou *et al.*, 2006) and genetic links have been probed. The latter have included an association with the disrupted-in-schizophrenia 1

(DISC1) gene (Matsuzaki and Tohyama, 2007; Ishizuka *et al.*, 2006; Callicott *et al.*, 2005).

Another strategy has been to use high-risk subjects. Neuropsychological impairments have been shown in those who later develop the disorder, more severe than that seen in those who go on to develop bipolar disorders, and working memory again is highlighted. Performance abnormalities on verbal tasks, including verbal learning and fluency, are most often reported in those who later convert to schizophrenia. However, these early cognitive problems do not clearly correlate with later psychotic symptoms, except weakly with negative features. What is more relevant is the identification of abnormal thinking, reflecting abnormal cognitive structure in these high-risk people. In addition to these cognitive variables, other strong predictors are high scores on the SIPS and SIS, bizarre thinking, schizotypal personality disorder, suspiciousness, poor social functioning and poor social skills. These findings link with others such as deficits of facial recognition and emotional discrimination of faces in schizophrenia, correlated with abnormal early evoked potentials, suggesting processing problems occur at an early stage of sensory processing.

Of particular interest is the potential link and overlap with findings from patients with autism, who show many similarities to and differences from schizophrenia. The largest similarities are in the problems with social cues, face processing, empathy and understanding the actions of others, called 'theory of mind' (Anckarsater, 2006; Rapoport *et al.*, 2009; Völlm *et al.*, 2006).

SOME OUTSTANDING ISSUES

The evidence reviewed clearly indicates a significant genetic contribution towards the development of schizophrenia. However, it is clear that this contribution to schizophrenia does not explain all the variance, and environmental variables have been persistently sought. Individually, these environmental factors are of unknown effect size and several have been suggested, although exactly how they interact with the genetic liability is unclear.

Further, the consensus that what is inherited is a schizophrenia spectrum, as opposed to schizophrenia per se, has gained ground, and certain biological markers, for example platelet MAO activity or dysfunction of eye movements, may reflect upon underlying genetically determined biochemical or neurocircuitry propensities to develop psychosis under certain conditions. The search for the gene(s) responsible for the schizophrenias continues. Some obvious candidates, especially relating to dopamine regulation, seem to have been ruled out. The consensus has been to look for co-acting loci, and there have been many reports of linkage findings or results from genome-wide scans, with quite heterogenous results; some 30–40 susceptibility genes have been identified at threshold significance. In part this may reflect the fact that genetic markers are themselves only proxies for the risk variant. But there are other confounding factors, including the problem of the quality of genotype analysis, the statistical requirements of such potentially large data sets and the delineation of the phenotype. What are the features of a subset of cases that show an enhanced genetic signal? The strategy of looking at endophenotypes, and away from DSM IV-TR-defined categories, seems a promising way forward, but to date no endophenotypes related to schizophrenia have yielded any secrets to genetics. However, recent attempts to combine genetics with brain imaging are proving interesting, examining the genetic contributions to the cerebral structural, functional changes and endophenotypic variance.

There was hope that the newer generation of genome-wide studies might prove more powerful than linkage and candidate gene strategies. That promise has not been fulfilled as yet. The latest genome-wide studies if anything tend to suggest similarities, rather than differences, between bipolar affective disorders and the schizophrenias (Esslinger *et al.*, 2009; Keshavan *et al.*, 2007; Tan *et al.*, 2008; van Haren *et al.*, 2008; Lin and Mitchell, 2008; Thaker, 2008; van Os *et al.*, 2008) (see Chapter 8).

To date, and so many years after Slater's studies, the picture remains that there may be several or many genes of small effect contributing to the schizophrenia spectrum. Essentially we may be learning that, with only a few exceptions such as Huntington's disease, there are no genes for mental illness per se, but rather genetic effects that relate to information processing in the brain and subsequent cognitive and behavioural strategies, the endophenotypes, which provide a substrate for the later development of the phenotype. No longer is a statistical relationship between genes and a DSM IV-TR diagnosis being looked for, but rather the relationship between the neurobiological effects of genes and the processes that lead to any particular phenotype.

With regards to environmental agents, there is evidence that some schizophrenic patients demonstrate increased early brain damage, either through perinatal or uterine insults. Murray *et al.* (1985) advocate it would be useful to divide schizophrenia into familial and sporadic cases. The sporadic cases are thus associated with increased ventricular size (highly replicated) and environmental traumas reflective of perinatal damage or early head injury. The genetic predisposition, if strong, will promote the disorder, while, in the presence of a lesser genetic vulnerability, the environmental insult becomes necessary for the full expression of the illness. Where there is no genetic vulnerability, as in, for example, some cases of epilepsy, the cerebral pathology itself directly provokes the schizophrenia-like symptoms.

More recent discussion of environmental effects has concerned epigenetic and pharmacological influences. The former should include uterine and neonatal events on cerebral development, synaptogenesis and synaptic pruning, as well as early psychosocial stressors (Parent and Meaney, 2008). Alternative environmental insults have been sought, in particular neurological conditions, head injury or infection, for example with viruses. However, recent research has centred on the use of psychoactive drugs, especially cannabis. The emphasis from CNS disorders is on those which affect temporal-lobe, basal-ganglia and diencephalic function. Temporal-lobe disorders, in particular such conditions as epilepsy affecting limbic structures, seem to be more associated with hallucinations, while basal-ganglia disorders lead more to disturbances of motoric activity, motivation and cognition via the fronto-striatal re-entrant networks.

The pathological and MRI studies reviewed reinforce a neuroanatomical approach, emphasizing medial temporal structures in association with hallucinations, paranoia and thought disorder, and the basal-ganglia frontal axis with negativism and motor signs. Such findings emphasize that the 'anatomy of schizophrenia' (Stevens, 1973) is predominantly related to allocortical and subcortical structures, particularly those of the limbic lobe (entorhinal cortex: hippocampus), the thalamus and the related basal ganglia.

In cerebral development, neuronal migration is from the ventricular zone outwards to the cortical plate. Younger neurones thus migrate through more mature ones, and the migration is directed by previously formed radial glial fibres. In the human entorhinal cortex, these migrations are complete by six months of gestation; the hippocampus and temporal neocortex are somewhat later, the hippocampus not reaching adult volume until about the age of two years, and continuing to myelinate well into adult life (Benes *et al.*, 1994).

The upper layers of the entorhinal cortex, especially layer 2, containing pre-alpha cells, are sites of origin of the glutamate projections to the hippocampus, and receive a dopaminergic input. It is important to note that during normal development, the ventricular volume is reduced, and so abnormal development will lead to increased volumes. Further, the development of the left hemisphere is later than the right, and any damage that influences early development of these structures is therefore more likely to impact on the left.

The parts of the entorhinal cortex involved in pathological studies of schizophrenia are intimately connected with the insula and the orbitofrontal cortex, and it is of interest that these entorhinal areas are not found in other animals, including other primates.

Some authors have drawn attention to the likeness of some schizophrenic symptoms to frontal-lobe disorders. In particular this involves the dorsolateral prefrontal cortex, and the symptoms include those seen following frontal injury, such as affective changes, impaired motivation, poor insight and other 'defect' symptoms frequently seen in schizophrenia. Indeed, the evidence for frontal-lobe dysfunction in schizophrenic patients is clear, and has been noted not only in the neuropathological studies but also in EEG, evoked-potential data, neuropsychological studies (especially those of working memory), testing for soft neurological signs, and more recently imaging techniques such as PET and MRI.

The pathological studies of frontal cortical areas are more limited, but do suggest some changes, which either represent evidence of more generalized pathology in schizophrenic brains or are a localized contribution to the development of the psychopathology.

The orbitofrontal and temporal pole areas are connected by the uncinate fasciculus, and lesions at such sites may impair higher-order cognitive processes and lead to disordered social communication. Recent data clearly suggest that abnormal hippocampal structure is associated with functional impairment of frontal-lobe activity, supporting a suggestion that the temporal/limbic changes may be primary. Alternatively, disturbances of frontal projections to the parietal and temporal association areas may impair sensory representations in these areas, explaining positive symptoms, setting the frontal lobes as crucial for the development of both positive and negative symptoms. More recent imaging studies have concerned changes in white-matter tracts and have identified alterations in white matter, including the corpus callosum, the uncinate fasciculus and the anterior limb of the internal capsule. It is quite unclear whether these are part of the structural alterations that relate to schizophrenia or are secondary to other neuronal loss. It does seem to be the case that many of the structural (and functional) changes occur early on in the disorder, are not secondary to antipsychotic drug prescriptions and may be seen in the high-risk group before diagnosis.

The evidence for two distinct syndromes in schizophrenia has been pursued by Crow and colleagues (Crow, 1980). The suggestion is that there is both a neurochemical and a neuropathological contribution to schizophrenia, with two syndromes. Thus, the type I syndrome (equivalent to acute schizophrenia) is characterized by positive symptoms (delusions, hallucinations and thought disorder) and is related to change in dopaminergic transmission. The type II syndrome (equivalent to the defect state) is characterized by negative symptoms (affective flattening and poverty of speech) and is associated with intellectual impairment and structural changes in the brain. Current thought also involves a continuum model and includes consideration of the schizophrenia spectrum. It is established that abnormalities of cognition and thinking are present well before the onset of the actual psychosis. The high-risk studies all come to similar conclusions, namely that a prodromal state can be identified linked to unusual thinking and cognitive problems, especially with working memory and verbal tasks, which, if identified early, may be more amenable to treatment strategies than the fully-developed syndrome. However, the studies beg the question as to whether the identified pattern should be seen as part of the schizophrenia, especially as it also includes those who achieve a diagnosis of schizotypal personality disorder. In other words, should the syndrome schizophrenia(s) not include such preludes? The role of environmental factors in the actual descent into psychosis remains unclear, although neurochemical invasions, especially from psychoactive drugs such as cannabis, are clearly implicated.

There is certainly considerable evidence that structural changes are likely to be found in some schizophrenic brains and that cerebral atrophy on the whole is related to more negative symptoms. Positive symptoms, in particular the first-rank symptoms of Schneider, have been related to abnormal dopaminergic transmission. The dopamine hypothesis has in part stood the test of time. Dopamine is closely linked to disorders of motivation (see Chapter 9), a prominent part of the schizophrenia clinical picture, and the known interactions between brain areas such as the frontal cortex, the accumbens and the midbrain dopamine areas (VTA) as part of the underlying anatomy of schizophrenia are supported by pathological and MRI findings. Patients with positive symptoms show increased growth-hormone responses to apomorphine, decreased baseline prolactin, low CSF–HVA accumulation and minimal heritability (first-rank symptoms), and tend to have less cerebral atrophy. Further, the pathological and PET data reviewed suggest that temporal-lobe, including parahippocampal gyrus, abnormalities may be more related to such symptoms. These data certainly support a particular relationship between positive symptoms, relatively normal brain structure, abnormalities of dopamine and possibly temporal-lobe dysfunction.

In contrast, negative symptoms appear more related to periventricular abnormalities, cerebral atrophy and environmental insults, and are perhaps related to dopamine dysfunction, but in a different way (as the disorder progresses and disorder of motivation becomes more apparent). Experimental support for defining two subtypes has derived from intercorrelations of patients' symptoms, which indicate generally that positive symptoms correlate positively, as do negative symptoms, although the internal consistency is much greater for negative symptoms (Andreasen and Olsen, 1982).

The important contribution of abnormalities of dopamine to schizophrenia has been persistently argued. But it is well known that the antipsychotic effects of neuroleptic drugs are not confined to schizophrenia, and they ameliorate psychotic symptoms in mania and acute organic brain syndromes. Further, because such medications alleviate some symptoms of schizophrenia does not mean that dopamine itself has the primary role in pathogenesis. While it has been noted that the dopamine-blocking effect of these drugs is the most important for helping the psychosis, it should be remembered that anticholinergic drugs alleviate the symptoms of Parkinson's disease, even though the primary pathology in that condition relates to dopamine and not acetylcholine. Other neurochemical hypotheses have obviously been entertained, and as noted involve serotonergic, other catecholaminergic, peptidergic and glutaminergic abnormalities. Mackay (1980) has argued that a chronic dopamine deficit is related to schizophrenia, rather than overactivity, highlighting the reported low CSF–HVA levels. This reduced dopamine turnover leads not only to reduced presynaptic dopamine accumulation but also to a compensatory postsynaptic dopamine-receptor proliferation. In his theory, both positive and negative symptoms thus relate to a defect of dopaminergic function, the positive symptoms emerging as a result of a switch from a deficit to an increase in presynaptic release of dopamine, the latter interacting with the excessive number of postsynaptic dopamine receptors and leading to the florid positive symptoms.

An alternative is that abnormally low prefrontal dopamine activity is related to deficit symptoms and excess dopamine activity in subcortical structures relates to positive symptoms. The mainly negative PET dopamine ligand-binding studies to date were disappointing for those in favour of the dopamine hypothesis, although attention is now being directed to alternative dopamine receptors, especially D_2, D_3 and D_4. The importance of frontal dopamine activity is highlighted by the data that relate it to working memory, and the links to COMT alleles, genes associated with an enzyme closely linked with dopamine metabolism and shown to be associated with cognitive performance (Lawrie *et al.*, 2008a Roffman *et al.*, 2006; van Haren *et al.*, 2008).

Decreased D_2 and D_3 receptor occupancy is well replicated in several brain areas. These findings have been enhanced by the development of selective radioactive dopamine ligands (e.g. fallypride and 11c NPA for the D_2/D_3 receptor, although none are selective for just the D_2 receptor). In the past much attention was given to striatal activity, but with these ligands, extrastiatal dopamine can be estimated. The thalamus, especially the dorso-medial nucleus is important (Andreasen *et al.*, 1994). Several studies suggesting a decreased size and/or activity of this nucleus (Siegel *et al.*, 1993; Shihabuddin *et al.*, 2001), along with decreased dopamine binding are reported. Lower prefrontal cortical dopamine has been shown to correlate with increased striatal release. This may be mediated by the reduced excitatory feedback from frontal cortex (glutamate) to the inhibitory GABA neurones in the VTA, thus increasing firing and hence output of dopamine from the VTA to striatal structures such as the accumbens.

While dopamine remains a key transmitter in the schizophrenia story, it is obviously involved in a variety of psychopathologies, and a question remains as to its biological function in regulating behaviour aside from its role in motor programming. The findings related to disorders of motivation (Chapter 9) suggest it is related to novel reward detection in the environment and is interlinked with hedonia. It somehow attributes motivational salience to neural events, influencing attention and the subsequent behavioural repertoires. This in itself does not lead to psychotic symptoms, but the abnormal attribution of salience to environmental and somatic representations may lead over time to cognitive restructuring (Kapur, 2006). This may vary with pre-existing or consequent structural neuronal and circuitry changes, and such hypotheses need to be integrated with the accumulating knowledge of brain morphological changes.

The current status of the dopamine hypothesis suggests that D_2/D_3 receptors are still central to the theories, decreased receptor occupancy being well replicated in several brain areas. Attention has moved to extrastriate regions and their involvement not only with the anatomy of the cortical–striatal–thalamic re-entrant circuits, but with reciprocal relationships between GABA and dopamine, and the link through glutamate.

It remains unclear what it is that drives the increase in dopamine activity. Early work had suggested a link through GABA, especially with a subgroup of GABA neurones, the parvalbumin-containing cells. Disturbed neuronal rhythmic expression in key structures is a developing story.

The known importance of the balance between GABA and glutamate within the CNS for coordinating neuronal firing and oscillations, and the importance of glutamate in the regulation of the cortical–subcortical re-entrant circuits, has led to looking at GABA

as well as glutamate as possible substrates. Thus, glutamate input to dopamine-releasing cells (from, for example, the hippocampus and the pedunculopontine areas) normally induces bursts of spikes within the VTA, which are disrupted by a deficit of glutamate. These theories put more emphasis on the possible relevance of cortical changes as primary in the disorder.

Crow (1993) has persistently argued against the Kraepelinian dichotomy, pointing out that overlaps of schizophrenia and affective disorders occur phenomenologically and genetically (the proportion of relatives of schizophrenics that have an affective disorder is increased). In his continuum (see Figure 7.1), which extends from unipolar depression at one end to schizophrenia with a defect state at the other, variations of sociability and emotionality are expressed.

Murray *et al.* (1992) on the other hand argue that there is a congenital schizophrenia, with a primary genetic defect and/or a primary environmental insult such as a viral infection, and abnormal neuronal maturation in crucial CNS sites. These patients show personality and social impairments in childhood, and develop the more severe cognitive impairments and negative symptoms. In contrast, patients with adult-onset schizophrenia, which includes several syndromes, do not have the classic dementia

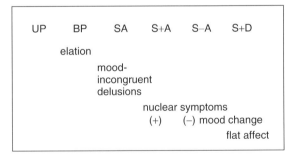

Figure 7.1 The continuum concept of psychotic illness. UP, unipolar affective illness; BP, bipolar; SA, schizoaffective psychosis; S, schizophrenia with and without significant mood disturbance (+ and – A), and with defect state (S+D) (reproduced with permission from Crow, 1993; *Biol Psych*, 2 Ed, p. 223)

Table 7.11   Evidence for laterality in schizophrenia

Neurological examination	Increased abnormalities in right-side sensory testing; increased left-handedness
Neuropsychology	Association with poor performance on language tasks
EEG	Dominant hemisphere abnormalities on routine testing, power spectra, with telemetry, evoked potentials and BEAM studies
CT studies	Density changes; new onset cases
MRI studies	Especially positive symptoms: left superior temporal gyrus changes
PET studies	Variable: recent thalamic findings
Neurochemistry	Increased dopamine, left amygdala; decreased GABA and glutamate, left hippocampus
Neuropathology	Parahippocampal gyrus abnormalities in some studies only
Neurology	Epilepsy and head-injury studies

praecox and are more likely to have relapsing, remitting psychosis with positive and affective symptoms.

The search for virus infections has not been rewarding and the evidence that intrauterine infection with the influenza virus is important is at present quite unclear. However, one importance of the infective theory relates to some historical considerations of schizophrenia: it has been suggested that schizophrenia was uncommon in the medical literature prior to the 19th century, implying, rather like AIDS encephalitis, that it may have been a new disease, and that an environmental agent, such as a virus, must have become prevalent around that time. The alternative is that it is an old condition which has been ubiquitous and always present. The problem then is to explain its persistence in view of the low fecundity of schizophrenic patients (Hare, 1979). This paradox remains unresolved.

Finally, substantial evidence has accumulated suggesting that at least in some forms of schizophrenia, the major disturbance is in the dominant hemisphere (see Table 7.11). Because one of the cardinal features of schizophrenia is a disturbance of thought and language and the dominant hemisphere is known to be involved in modulating such activities, it is hardly surprising that the weight of evidence suggests that the dominant hemisphere is primarily involved, and this continues to be the case. It is clear that to implicate the left hemisphere alone would be nonsensical. In fact, Cutting (1990) made a strong case for the nondominant hemisphere having a primary role in the symptomatology, a view recently supported by Crow and his colleagues (Crow *et al.*, 2007, 2009; Crow 2009). Nonetheless, the role of the dominant hemisphere is of outstanding importance, perhaps early on in the disorder, or in providing the key harmonic that reverberates through the developing phenomenology. The findings from pathology, and the progressive nature of the imaging data, have initiated a discussion as to whether schizophrenia should be viewed as a progressive disorder, as Kraepelin originally envisaged, or even as a degenerative disorder: a 'dementia' in our current-day terminology. Although at first sight the degenerative hypothesis seems possible (schizophrenia being viewed as a dementia praecox), this is an unlikely hypothesis. The early age of onset vis-à-vis the dementias, the subtle nature of the pathological changes and the eventual defect state as opposed to a continued progressive decline argue against it.

In summary, the current perspective on schizophrenia is to view it as a neurodevelopmental disorder, with a clear genetic component. The final clinical picture however must be viewed as a spectrum, reflecting alterations in the structure of the cognitive and perceptual abilities of those who become patients, these being yoked with aberrant neuroanatomy and neurophysiology.

8
Affective Disorders

INTRODUCTION

A difficulty in reviewing the literature on affective disorders is the various classifications that have been used by investigators. Although for the present the DSM IV-TR seems likely to be influential, much biological information had been accumulated prior to its introduction, and in some areas the lack of consistency of results reflects the lack of similarity of patients. A recurring theme is the confusion between depression as an illness and a reaction or an ordinary state of misery or grief. Lewis (1934) gave as a definition of the depressive state 'a condition in which the clinical picture is dominated by an unpleasant affect, not transitory, without evidence of schizophrenic disorder or organic disorder of the brain, and in which, moreover, the affective change appears primary...' (p. 277). This concept, the essential criterion being the disturbance of mood, continues to be embodied in DSM IV-TR, the mood being referred to as a prolonged emotion (American Psychiatric Association, 1987). Episodes of more transient mood change or chronic minor changes of mood are referred to as dysthymic disorder, which replaces depressive neurosis, depressive personality and similar categories. The issue of 'reaction', which has so long pervaded this area, is not discussed.

Winokur (1982), whose own classification distinguishes a primary (bipolar/unipolar) from a secondary depression, has given support for the concept of neurotic depression, citing positive criteria for its diagnosis. These include younger age, poorer response to treatment, family history of alcoholism and personality problems. These then are patients with lifelong personality disorders who recurrently display depressive symptoms, more often than not DSM TR IV dysthymic disorder. They represent an entirely different problem from those in whom the depressive process is referred to as endogenous depression.

A more widely accepted distinction, adopted by the DSM III and originally made by Leonhard (1957), is that between unipolar and bipolar forms of affective illness. While the latter are readily identifiable, biological differences between the two are emerging, and the failure to identify manic episodes in a patient's history may provide a further source of error.

In summary, there is still much confusion regarding the nosological status of subtypes of depressive illness, although the entity referred to as endogenous depression seems well recognized and more homogeneous than others. The DSM III and successors have disbanded the concept of neurotic depression, the evidence for which emphasizes the importance of personality vulnerabilities for its expression, but confusion with the endogenous form still abounds in clinical practice and research. This confounds attempts to expose the biological substrates of the depressive process, and often leads to inappropriate treatments. This is not to say that patients with other forms of depressive symptoms do not require treatment, or are not meaningful subjects for research. In fact, so numerous are these patients, and so chronic often are their disorders, that more effective remedies urgently need to be sought for them, particularly psychotropic agents.

The nosologic confusion can be seen in the current attempts to describe bipolar disorder. While there is little debate concerning bipolar 1, where patients must have had a clear manic episode, controversy begins with attempts to define 'softer' bipolar disorder. Akiskal and Benazzi (2006) have argued for a bipolar 2 disorder, where recurrent depressions alternate with periods of hypomania or cyclothymia. They have also proposed a bipolar 3 diagnosis, where depressions exist alongside a volatile temperament or a strong family history of bipolar mood swings (Akiskal, 2007; Benazzi and Akiskal, 2008; Fountoulakis and Akiskal, 2008; Gonda *et al.*, 2009; Rihmer *et al.*, 2007). Even more confusing is the 'unipolar' patient who develops mania or hypomania while being treated with an antidepressant, a form of iatrogenic bipolar disorder. Clearly, the nosology continues to evolve.

Unipolar major depression is a surprisingly common disorder, with many studies finding a 20% lifetime incidence and a 5% point prevalence. Bipolar disorder is less common in its purer form (i.e. not the spectrum extensions discussed above), with many studies estimating a 1% lifetime incidence. Because the affective disorders are so common, often developing into chronic forms with associated other illnesses such as diabetes and pain syndromes, major depression is currently the leading cause of disease burden in North America and other high-income countries, and the fourth-leading cause worldwide. In the year 2030 it is predicted to be the second-leading cause of disease burden worldwide after HIV, according to the World Health Organization (Mathers and Loncar, 2006).

GENETICS

As with most other conditions reviewed in this book, the affective disorders have an important genetic component to their pathogenesis. This is particularly so for bipolar illness.

Family studies reveal that the risk for affective illness is increased severalfold in first-degree relatives of probands over that expected by chance (Gershon, 1983). Further, while bipolar patients often have relatives with unipolar illness, the converse is uncommon. Estimates, based on combined data from several studies, put the risk at 20% for first-degree relatives of bipolar probands and 7% for first-degree relatives of unipolar patients (McGuffin, 1984).

Winokur (1982) has identified three types of unipolar illness based on familial patterns: familial pure depression disease (FPDD), with a family history of depression; depressive spectrum disease (DSD), with a familial history of alcoholism or antisocial personality; and sporadic depressive disease (SDD), with negative family history.

The concept of a genetic spectrum for bipolar disorders emerges with the reporting of an increased frequency of schizoaffective disorder and cyclothymic personality in relatives of probands (Gershon, 1983). Studies of schizoaffective patients tend to show both affective illness and schizophrenia in the relatives (Angst *et al.*, 1979), greater for affective illness, and Perris (1974) reported that in cycloid psychosis an increased frequency of the same condition was seen in relatives.

Twin data give a concordance rate, by combining studies, of 69% for monozygotic (MZ) and 13% for dizygotic (DZ) pairs (McGuffin, 1984). Most of the investigations were carried out prior to the acceptance of the unipolar/bipolar distinction, but Bertelsen *et al.* (1977) calculated the pairwise concordance rates for MZ twins to be 0.43 for unipolar and 0.74 for bipolar illness, the corresponding figures for DZ pairs being 0.19 and 0.17. The concordance was particularly noted for females, and the differences between the unipolar and bipolar rates were significant, supporting the familial data that the bipolar form carries the greatest heritability.

Price (1968) reported 67% concordance in 12 pairs of MZ twins raised apart. This and the adoption study of Mendlewicz and Rainer (1977), in which the rate of affective illness was significantly greater in biological (28%) as opposed to adoptive (7%) parents of probands separated in early life, further support the genetic contribution to the illnesses.

A single autosomal dominant gene with reduced penetrance and variable expressivity was supported by Slater (Slater and Roth, 1969), while others have suggested X-linked (Winokur and Tanna, 1969) and multifactorial models, implying underlying quantitative liability to an affective disorder, greater for bipolar illness (Gershon, 1983). The X-linked hypothesis seems unlikely, in that father–son transmission of affective disorder is frequently seen, although it received initial support from linkage studies with colour blindness and glucose-6-phosphate dehydrogenase deficiency (Mendlewicz *et al.*, 1980), known to be sex-linked. These data have not been consistently replicated (Gershon, 1983) and no X-linkage has been demonstrated.

Linkage studies of bipolar disorder to date have not revealed reliable markers. The early studies in Old Order Amish pedigrees identifying the short arm of chromosome 11 have not been replicated. The gene for tyrosine hydrolase is located at this site, but reports of a positive association between tyrosine hydrolase RFLPs and bipolar illness have been mainly negative. Lack of association has also been reported for the D_1, D_2, D_4 and $5-HT_{1A}$ receptor genes, for dopamine beta-hydrolase, and for sites on chromosome 5 in the region of the glucocorticoid and beta-2 adrenergic receptors (Curtis *et al.*, 1993; Debruyn *et al.*, 1994; Mirow *et al.*, 1994; Nothen *et al.*, 1992). No mutations have been found on the D_1 receptor gene.

One study of the tryptophan hydrolase gene demonstrated a significant association between that genotype and low CSF 5-HIAA levels. The clinical associations were with suicide attempts but not impulsivity (Nielsen *et al.*, 1994).

In the last decade more than 15 different candidate genes have been identified for mood disorders with at least partial replication, using genome-wide approaches and single-nucleotide polymorphisms (SNPs) (for review see Hayden and Nurnberger, 2006). Those of interest include brain-derived neurotropic factor (BDNF), COMT and DISC1, a candidate gene involved in cortical development which is also associated with schizophrenia.

Particular interest has recently focused on the gene for the 5-HT transporter, called the SERT gene. The protein re-takes 5-HT into the synaptic cleft and terminates its function. The gene, found on chromosome 17, can have several variations – either in length, or with SNPs. The promotor region for this gene can also have variations with short or long repeats (5-HTTLPR). Studies on the 5-HT transporter have combined neuroimaging and genetic methods. For example, a voxel-based morphometry study found less grey matter in perigenual anterior cingulate cortex and amygdala for short allele carriers of the 5-HTTLPR polymorphism than for subjects with the long/long genotype (Munafo *et al.*, 2008; Pezawas *et al.*, 2005).

Other recent interest involves a new family of genes called circadian locomotor output cycles kaput, or CLOCK, genes. These genes encode proteins regulating circadian rhythm. The CLOCK protein, found in all animals, even fruit flies, affects both the persistence and length of the circadian cycle. Recent studies have suggested that CLOCK-gene abnormalities may predispose to developing bipolar disorder, or determine its age of onset (Kishi *et al.*, 2009; Severino *et al.*, 2009; Shi *et al.*, 2008). Many have long suspected that bipolar disorder is a disease of circadian cycles, as sleep–wake disturbances sometimes trigger cycles and the mood state responds to circadian manipulations. Not only might these findings explain this commonality, they would suggest that treatment may involve aggressively re-regulating sleep–wake cycles (McClung, 2007a, 2007b; Wood *et al.*, 2009).

In addition to findings of high rates of familial incidence of mood disorders, some studies have also found that family member risk and overall population risk have increased in those born in more recent decades. This ominous trend, referred to as an age-period-cohort effect, may reflect sampling and reporting biases, but may also be caused by other factors such as increasing prevalences of prior comorbid disorders (Kessler and Walters, 1998).

There is a great deal of interest in using the new power of genetics to potentially better parse our diagnoses and provide better disease classifications. However, several recent large-scale genome-wide analyses suggest that even bipolar disorder and schizophrenia share common genetic linkages, calling into question our clearest distinction, in effect challenging the Kraepelinean dichotomy (Czeizel, 2009; Lichtenstein *et al.*, 2009; Maher *et al.*, 2008; O'Donovan *et al.*, 2008). These studies tend not to support the distinction of bipolar disorder from schizophrenia, at least in terms of genetic predisposition.

METABOLIC AND BIOCHEMICAL FINDINGS

Early metabolic studies found abnormalities of electrolyte distribution in affective disorder, in particular retention of sodium intracellularly (including bone) during depressive episodes (Coppen and Shaw, 1963), with increased loss during recovery. In mania even more marked changes were reported (Coppen *et al.*, 1965). Some interpreted these data as a reflection of dietary changes consequent to the change of mood. No evidence has shown that the brain is also involved, or that the changes somehow lead to an alteration of cell membrane excitability.

Naylor *et al.* (1970) examined erythrocyte electrolytes in affective disorder and reported falling sodium levels with recovery. The activity of sodium/potassium-activated ATPase, thought to reflect sodium pump behaviour, is lower in the depressive phase of a manic–depressive psychosis, and possibly in the manic phase as well, with increased activity on recovery. These data do suggest impaired handling of electrolytes in association with affective disorder, reflected in part by alteration of membrane transport (El-Mallakh and Wyatt, 1995). Studies of calcium suggest this is not influenced by the illness, and data on magnesium are inconsistent.

The essential trace element vanadium has been studied in relation to the electrolyte changes. It is an inhibitor of Na^+/K^+ ATPase. It is reported to be raised in hair but not blood, in mania, and in blood and serum in depression, with a fall on recovery. Substances that lower vanadium concentration, such as ascorbic acid and EDTA, are therapeutic in mania and depression (Naylor *et al.*, 1984). Lithium responders are reported to have lower erythrocyte Na^+/K^+ ATPase and to show the greatest increases in activity when on lithium compared with nonresponders (Naylor *et al.*, 1976).

Platelet MAO activity has been reported in affective disorders, although results show variability. It is of interest, however, that several groups have reported increased values, particularly in unipolar (Reveley *et al.*, 1981) as opposed to bipolar patients, in which reduced values are more frequently reported. This seems a trait as opposed to a state finding, and low levels are also noted in first-degree relatives of bipolar patients (Leckman *et al.*, 1977). However, there are reports of significant positive correlations between scores on depressive rating scales and MAO activity (Mann, 1979). Some authors report an increase in MAO activity with age and link this to the increasing incidence of depressive disorders in later life. MAOI drugs lower MAO activity, the effect of lithium treatment is unclear, whilst ECT has no effect (Mann, 1979). The variability of results, especially with bipolar patients, presumably reflects different patient populations and different techniques of measurement of MAO with differing substrates.

Sandler *et al.* (1975) gave a tyramine conjugation test to untreated patients with severe depression. Following an oral load, most tyramine is degraded by MAO to its main metabolite *p*-hydroxyphenylacetic acid, but some 15% is conjugated. In the patients the secretion of conjugated tyramine was significantly low, suggesting increased MAO activity. Sandler *et al.* have since gone on to suggest that the tyramine test may be a possible biological marker of depressive illness, useful in diagnosis and in predicting response to tricyclic drugs (Hale *et al.*, 1989). This deficit persists after recovery from illness, and is noted in both bipolar and unipolar patients (Harrison *et al.*, 1984).

With regards to central monoamines, in contrast to the literature on schizophrenia, that on the affective disorders has been dominated not by dopamine, but by noradrenaline and 5-HT.

The 5-HT (Serotonin) Hypothesis

The main biochemical hypotheses relating to the affective disorders were inspired by the revolution in psychopharmacology of the 1960s. Early observations were that reserpine, a drug that depletes monoamines, led to a depressive illness in some 20% of patients taking it (mainly hypertensives); that MAOI drugs, initially used to treat tuberculosis, were mood-elevating and increased monoamine levels; and that the other class of antidepressants, the tricyclic drugs, also, by a different mechanism, elevated functional levels especially of noradrenaline and 5-HT. One emerging hypothesis was therefore that depletion of monoamine levels related to depressive illness. While investigators in the United States provided many data on catecholamines, in Europe the serotonin (5-HT) hypothesis was more vigorously pursued.

Pharmacological Evidence

In order to test the 5-HT hypothesis, patients were treated with amine precursors, notably tryptophan and 5-hydroxytryptophan (5-HTP). In normals, both compounds led to elevation of mood, minimal with the former and more dramatic with the latter (Wirz-Justice, 1977). In depressed patients, L-tryptophan had a limited antidepressant effect, enhancing that of either clomipramine (a relatively selective inhibitor of 5-HT uptake) (Walinder *et al.*, 1976) or an MAOI (Coppen *et al.*, 1963) when given together. 5-HTP has antidepressant properties alone, or when given with clomipramine (van Praag *et al.*, 1974) or an MAOI. In contrast, parachlorophenylalanine, a drug that selectively depletes 5-HT, reverses the antidepressant effect of both tricyclic and MAOI antidepressants, but such an effect was not observed with the catecholamine depleter alpha-methyl-paratyrosine (Shopsin *et al.*, 1976).

Tryptophan in the plasma has been measured by several groups. It exists in a free and bound form (unlike other amino acids that are not bound to plasma protein), and entry across the blood–brain barrier is competitive with other amino acids. Since the rate-limiting enzyme for 5-HT formation, tryptophan-5-hydrolase, is not saturated under ordinary conditions, the level of tryptophan in the plasma can influence central 5-HT synthesis. Results of plasma tryptophan studies are not consistent, with reports of decreased total (Riley and Shaw, 1976) or normal total but reduced free (Coppen and Wood, 1978) and normal free levels (Møller *et al.*, 1979), even when unipolar and bipolar patients were examined separately (Møller *et al.*, 1979). A seasonal variation exists, possibly related to the seasonal variations of depressive illness. Studying the ratio of plasma tryptophan to those of five other amino acids, Meyer *et al.* (1981) reported lower ratios, but mainly in samples taken within 72 hours of hospital admission in unipolar depressed patients. Improvements in depression, rated on the Hamilton scale, correlated significantly with an increasing ratio, suggesting lowered brain availability of tryptophan in the depressive phase. In a later study they reported normal platelet and whole-blood 5-HT in depressed patients, but lower platelet levels in patients who made a suicide attempt (Mann *et al.*, 1992).

In summary, there is a suggestion that lower plasma tryptophan levels are associated with some aspect of depressive illness, but further investigations are required to establish their significance.

Delgado and colleagues pioneered the development of the tryptophan depletion technique, where subjects drink an amino-acid drink that leads to around an 80% depletion of plasma total and free tryptophan (TRP), resulting in a moderate but significant reduction of central 5-HT metabolism (Delgado *et al.*, 1991, 1994; Miller *et al.*, 1992). If subjects tolerate the procedure (it induces nausea and vomiting in many), healthy controls often experience mood shifts and many of the behaviours of a depressive episode (Delgado *et al.*, 1994). As would be predicted, patients with prior episodes of depression are more likely to report a transient 'depression' following this technique, as are first-degree relatives of patients with mood disorders (Allen *et al.*, 2009; Delgado *et al.*, 1991). Some researchers have used this as an acute treatment for mania (Applebaum *et al.*, 2007) or the antidepressant discontinuation syndrome, where patients continue to have vertigo, sensory dyskinesias and headaches after stopping SSRIs (Delgado, 2006).

Another way to examine this issue is the use of platelet-binding studies. Platelets take up and store 5-HT in a manner thought similar to synaptosomes, and have therefore been used as a model for central 5-HT terminals. Early reports found decreased V_{max} (maximum transport rate) through the platelet membrane in manic–depressive, depressive, unipolar, bipolar and schizoaffective patients (Meltzer *et al.*, 1981). It is unclear from the data whether values return to normal with recovery or the relationship to response with tricyclic drugs. Imipramine and related compounds are potent inhibitors of the active transport of 5-HT into platelets (Todrick and Tait, 1969), although the site of this action may not be identical to that of the 5-HT transporter under all conditions. Thus imipramine labels a low-affinity site that is unrelated to the 5-HT transporter, but paroxetine binding is more specific. Other compounds used include labelled ketanserin and LSD. Decreased imipramine binding sites (B_{max}) have also been reported in several studies in a variety of depressive subgroups (Briley *et al.*, 1980; Lewis and McChesney, 1985), including unipolar, bipolar and FPDD patients, although considerable overlap with control values is seen, and it is unclear whether this is a state- or trait-dependent marker.

Brusov *et al.* (1985) have identified plasma low-molecular-weight compounds that inhibit both the imipramine binding and 5-HT uptake of platelets, suggesting possible endogenous compounds that may regulate 5-HT platelet and synaptosome activity and play a role in affective illness. The issue is more complex, however, since seasonal variations of both 5-HT uptake and platelet binding have been reported, with lower levels in the winter and spring, accounting for some of the variability in the results (Egrise *et al.*, 1986). The results of paroxetine-binding studies in depression and seasonal affective disorder are negative (Ozaki *et al.*, 1994), and results with LSD binding are inconclusive (McBride *et al.*, 1994). However, a meta-analysis of platelet imipramine binding concluded that B_{max} for binding is significantly decreased in depressed patients, an effect not related to the taking of antidepressant drugs (Ellis and Salmond, 1994).

Another haematological marker is red-blood-cell choline. This is reported elevated in some unipolar patients, possibly those that do not show altered imipramine binding (Wood *et al.*, 1983).

Attempts to identify changes in urinary metabolites of 5-HT in depression have not been consistent. Only about 5% of urinary amine metabolites are of central origin, with the exception of the catecholamine derivative MHPG, the urine being too remote from CNS activity to provide meaningful data. Further evidence for the 5-HT hypothesis from CSF and brain-binding studies is discussed below.

The Noradrenaline Hypothesis

Pharmacological Evidence

Although most antidepressant drugs influence catecholamine uptake (there are exceptions, for example iprindole, mianserin and the selective 5-HT agents), the evidence that precursor loading with, for example, dihydroxyphenylalanine and L-dopa in depression improves the response of other drugs, or is antidepressant, is poor. Further, alpha-methylparatyrosine does not reverse the antidepressant effect of imipramine (Shopsin *et al.*, 1976). However, L-dopa may switch a patient from the depressive to the manic phase of a bipolar illness, and alpha-paramethyltyrosine does the opposite (Murphy *et al.*, 1971). Some antidepressants are reported to be selective for noradrenergic systems (for example maprotiline), although this does not necessarily reflect on their mode of antidepressant action.

Biochemical Evidence

Tyrosine levels in blood have been evaluated, but there is little consistency between studies.

Plasma noradrenaline levels have been reported as increased in affective disorder by several groups (Lake *et al.*, 1982; Roy *et al.*, 1985), notably in those with major affective disorder, especially those unipolar patients with melancholia (Roy *et al.*, 1985). The increased levels fall with ECT (Cooper *et al.*, 1985). Esler *et al.* (1982) measured the rate of entry of noradrenaline to plasma from sympathetic nerves ('noradrenaline spillover') with tritiated noradrenaline and showed higher levels and spillover in patients with endogenous depression characterized by retardation or agitation. This suggested increased sympathetic tone, although interestingly, in this and some of the other studies, the raised levels were not accompanied by elevated blood pressure. In a small number of patients, tricyclic drugs led to a drop in both noradrenaline levels and spillover. Plasma adrenaline (Esler *et al.*, 1982) and dopamine beta-hydrolase (Friedman *et al.*, 1984) tended to be normal.

Various strategies have been adopted to test catecholamine-receptor function. These include the tyramine pressor test, clonidine challenge, and estimation of the alpha adrenergic receptors on platelets and the beta receptors on lymphocytes. Some of these assess both presynaptic autoreceptor and postsynaptic autoreceptor function (e.g. the effect of clonidine on blood pressure), others are postsynaptic (e.g. yohimbine on sedation or blood pressure, or the effects of clonidine on growth hormone release).

The tyramine test involves assessing changes in blood pressure after a tyramine load. The blood pressure is elevated in depressed patients in some studies (Ghose *et al.*, 1975) but not others. Clonidine, an α-2 adrenergic agonist, leads to a fall in blood pressure by acting on central α-2 receptors, and also lowers plasma noradrenaline and MHPG. Results in depressed patients are variable, although one group (Siever and Uhde, 1984) has reported decreased response to the MHPG decrement in major depressive disorder. This is compatible with other evidence of blunted postsynaptic alpha-receptor activity reported in clonidine studies (see below). Tricyclic antidepressants attenuate the physiological responses of clonidine on MHPG and blood pressure (Charney *et al.*, 1981), one postulated mechanism being that the increased synaptic neurotransmitter levels after treatment lead to negative feedback and reduction of neuronal firing and autoreceptor subsensitivity. Interestingly, similar effects were not observed with mianserin, indicating that not all antidepressants act in this way (Charney *et al.*, 1984b).

Platelet alpha-2 receptors have been examined using agonist ligands such as clonidine and antagonists such as dihydroergocryptine or yohimbine. Of the studies to date, some show a difference, with increased binding (Garcia-Sevilla *et al.*, 1981; Healy *et al.*, 1983), but the majority are negative. Using an alternative technique, that of examining the functional response of platelets, Garcia-Sevilla *et al.* (1986) studied platelet aggregation to adrenaline hydrochloride and found it increased in patients with major affective disorder, the effect being diminished by lithium. In contrast, Siever and Coursey (1985) reported decreased prostaglandin-E_1-stimulated cyclic AMP production in platelets, an indication of subsensitivity, while others have reported no change.

Antidepressants (long-term), lithium and ECT reduce the sensitivity of the α-2 autoreceptor in both animal models and patient studies (Healy *et al.*, 1983). These attempts to find alteration of α-2-receptor function in depressive illness and changes with treatment stem from hypotheses that implicate the receptor in the aetiology of depression, at least in a subgroup of patients, enhanced α-2-autoreceptor activity being associated with reduced noradrenaline output. However, while there is some evidence to support these ideas, results are not reliably consistent. Further, the platelet data presuppose that the platelet α-2 receptor replicates the CNS receptor. This is unlikely, as centrally the α-2 receptor is both pre- and postsynaptic.

Studies of the β receptor, using lymphocyte binding, are also inconclusive, although decreased responsiveness of cyclic AMP or adenylate cyclase to isoprenaline challenges have been reported in manic and depressed patients (Extein *et al.*, 1979; Pandey *et al.*, 1979). This effect is observed in both major depressive disorders and dysthymia (Mazzola-Pomietto *et al.*, 1994). These data suggest downregulation of the receptor, possibly a response to high circulating noradrenaline levels.

Increased urinary noradrenaline and normetadrenaline and lower dihydroxyphenylacetic acid (DOPAC) levels have been reported in unipolar depressed patients (Roy *et al.*, 1986a). However, the main urinary metabolite studied has been MHPG, some 20–60% deriving from central sources. The earlier studies, particularly from Schildkraut *et al.* (1984), found low levels, especially in a subgroup of patients with the depressed phase of a bipolar illness, and higher levels in manic or hypomanic episodes. Similar findings were not found with VMA, adrenaline or normetadrenaline. Estimates of MHPG levels in unipolar depression have been variable, some authors reporting low levels (Maas *et al.*, 1972), others finding no change, but a wide variation suggesting subtypes with both high and low levels (Schildkraut *et al.*, 1984). Patients with low excretion rates have been found to be particularly responsive to treatment with tricyclic drugs (Maas *et al.*, 1972; Hollister *et al.*, 1980). This is more consistent for imipramine, nortryptiline and desipramine than for amitryptiline, for which higher excretion rates are reported in responders (Modai *et al.*, 1979), possibly reflecting pharmacological differences between the drugs, especially on noradrenergic systems.

Wiesel *et al.* (1982) reported on urinary excretion values of MHPG, HVA, 5-HIAA and DOPAC in healthy volunteers. Those with a family history of psychiatric morbidity had increased variance of MHPG levels. This correlated positively with CSF levels and suggested that altered noradrenergic metabolism might be related to vulnerability to psychopathology.

Other Biochemical Hypotheses

In addition to the above hypotheses, which have dominated depression research in recent years, both dopamine and choline hypotheses have had supporters. Further, biochemical findings relating to other systems have been reported and are of interest.

The dopamine hypothesis has been strongly supported by Randrup *et al.* (1975). It is based on pharmacological evidence that neuroleptic drugs block dopamine receptors and are effective antimanic agents; that a 'depression' is not infrequently seen in patients on these drugs; that some neuroleptics, especially in small doses, may be antidepressant; on the facts that many antidepressants act, at least to some extent, on dopamine uptake systems and that L-dopa, in some patients, may be antidepressant or may precipitate a manic phase; and on animal pharmacology that links certain behaviours (especially stereotypy) to increased central dopamine activity.

Some support for this derives from CSF data and the association of depressive illness with Parkinson's disease (see below), although there is, to date, relatively little direct evidence to implicate dopamine in the primary pathogenesis of affective disorders.

Cholinergic mechanisms have been implicated by Janowsky *et al.* (1980). In particular they discuss the relative balance between cholinergic and adrenergic tone, with depression representing a cholinergic and mania an adrenergic excess. The evidence is as follows: animal data show that cholinergic agents inhibit self-stimulation; many, especially of the older, first-generation, antidepressants, have considerable anticholinergic properties; cholinomimetics such as physostigmine produce an 'inhibitory syndrome' of lethargy and psychomotor retardation and may reverse mania, sometimes provoking a switch to a depressed phase; and precursors such as deanol and choline may provoke depressive symptoms (Tammingar *et al.*, 1976). Patients with affective disorder are reported to be more sensitive to the behavioural effects of physostigmine (Janowsky *et al.*, 1980), and some show elevated levels of red-cell choline (Wood *et al.*, 1983) or reduced acetylcholinesterase levels (Mathew *et al.*, 1982).

GABA has recently been implicated following observations that the anticonvulsant sodium valproate may have antimanic properties (Emrich *et al.*, 1984) and that some precursor drugs, such as progabide, may possess antidepressant properties (Morselli *et al.*, 1980). However, other anticonvulsants that act at the benzodiazepine-GABA receptor, such as phenobarbitone, clonazepam, tiagabine and vigabatrin may be associated with depression. Plasma GABA has been reported low in euthymic bipolar patients and CSF data offer some support for these findings (Berrettini *et al.*, 1983). Several groups have found abnormal brain GABA levels in patients with depression using MR spectroscopy (Sanacora *et al.*, 2002, 2006). To date it has not been possible to reconcile these findings, but the possibility that low trait GABA reflects a susceptibility for the development of depression, which then becomes manifest with an increase of GABA and subsequent alteration of monoamine status, has been suggested.

Urinary cyclic AMP has been reported to be decreased in depression and increased in mania (Paul *et al.*, 1971b), and in rapid-cycling patients there appears to be an increase in cyclic AMP levels during the switch from depression to mania (Paul *et al.*, 1971a). With treatment, values tend to return to normal (Abdulla and Hamadah, 1970). It is difficult to interpret these data since some 50% of urinary cyclic AMP derives from the kidneys. However, they may reflect altered receptor function in affective disorders, a suggestion supported by observations that antidepressant drugs and lithium decrease noradrenaline-stimulated cyclic AMP. The inhibition of ADH-activated cyclic AMP is a possible explanation for one of the side effects of lithium, namely polyuria.

The phenylethylamine hypothesis states that this compound, structurally related to amphetamine and the catecholamines, is a neuromodulator that is deficient in depressive illness. It is excitatory in animals, and is degraded by MAOB to phenylacetate. The latter and beta-phenylethylamine are reported low in patients with major depressive disorders (Sabelli *et al.*, 1983).

Peptides have also been implicated. Initial observations that some, for example TRH or beta-endorphin (Kline *et al.*, 1977), may possess antidepressant properties have not led as yet to any therapeutic advances. Marangell and colleagues (1997) demonstrated rather convincingly that administering TRH intrathecally could induce almost complete symptom remission in a group of highly treatment-resistant depressed patients. Unfortunately, the effects of a single intrathecal injection lasted only 24 hours and then the depression returned. Plasma beta-endorphin levels have been reported as normal in patients with unipolar major affective disorder (Alexopolous *et al.*, 1983).

Low levels of folic acid have been reported in association with a variety of neuropsychiatric conditions, especially in patients with epilepsy. There are several reports of depressive illness being associated with low levels (Trimble *et al.*, 1980), not explained away in terms of diet or institutionalization, in outpatients and in community studies (Edeh and Toone, 1985). Reynolds *et al.* (1984) have drawn attention to the fact that the methyl donor SAM is antidepressant, that folate megaloblastic anaemia is more frequently associated with affective disorder than is B_{12} deficiency, and that folic acid is reported to improve mood, notably in patients with folate deficiency. The fact that SAM and folate are intimately connected with monoamine metabolism may mean that CNS methylation is intimately involved with the regulation of mood.

As in other psychiatric disorders like schizophrenia, researchers have recently begun focusing on the glutamate system in mood disorders (Kugaya and Sanacora, 2005; Sanacora *et al.*, 2008). Animal models of depression transiently respond to glutamatergic manipulation (Banasr *et al.*, 2008; Engin *et al.*, 2009). Small open-label trials of the N-methyl-d-aspartate (NMDA) glutamate-receptor antagonist ketamine, used in general anaesthesia, have produced rapid, albeit transient, antidepressant effects. Double-blind studies are underway to test this novel hypothesis, and to devise ways of extending the effect beyond the acute stage (24–48 hours).

BDNF has been a compound of interest recently. The brain is more dynamic than previously thought and contains undeveloped stem cells that can migrate and mature into neurone or glial cells. There is evidence that this process is disrupted in depression and corrected with successful treatment. Structural imaging studies and post-mortem analysis of depressed patients have documented subtle volumetric loss in several important structures such as the hippocampi, prefrontal and orbitofrontal cortex, cingulate gyrus and cerebellum (Lenze *et al.*, 1999; Sheline *et al.*, 1999). Additionally, microscopic examinations have shown decreased cortical thickness as well as diminished neural size in similar regions. One possible explanation is that HPA axis activation is neurotoxic to the brain. Another possibility involves a disruption of normal nerve growth. The prospect that depression is related to problems with nerve-growth factors has opened up a new way of conceptualizing its pathophysiology. That is, a failure of neurogenesis and growth-factor proteins such as BDNF may cause subtle shrinkage of the brain, which is a part of the neurobiology of depression.

BDNF is one of a family of neurotrophins that regulate the differentiation and survival of neurone. There are a multitude of growth-factor proteins maintaining and stimulating nerve growth, but at this point BDNF is the most widely studied in depression. Figure 8.1 shows an example of the effects of BDNF on serotonergic neurone in the rat cortex. Saline or BDNF was infused directly into the rat frontal cortex for 21 days. Then the animals were sacrificed and the cortex at the site of the infusion was stained for 5-HT neurone. Note the profound arborization of the 5-HT axons in the cortex of the rat exposed to BDNF.

Thus, growth-factor proteins such as BDNF provide ongoing maintenance of neurone in the brain. Disruption of these nerve-growth factors results in reduced size of neurone as well as some cell loss. It is difficult to assess the quantity and quality of BDNF in living humans, so the evidence connecting BDNF and depression is indirect. In rats almost all effective antidepressants have been shown to increase BDNF, including lithium. Many of the brain-stimulation techniques (ECT, TMS, VNS), oestrogen and even exercise also raise BDNF levels. A post-mortem analysis of suicide subjects found a marked decrease in BDNF in the prefrontal cortex and hippocampus in

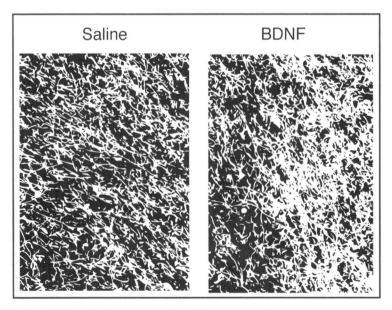

Figure 8.1   BDNF infused directly into the rat frontal cortex results in a supranormal branching of 5-HT axons (adapted from Mamounas *et al.*, (1995); from Higgins and George, 2007)

suicide subjects compared to controls (Dwivedi *et al.*, 2003). Serum BDNF levels in depressed patients prior to treatment are significantly less than in healthy subjects. After eight weeks of antidepressant treatment, serum BDNF levels increased significantly and were no longer different from controls (Gonul *et al.*, 2005). Studies in rats have demonstrated that fluoxetine stimulates neurogenesis in about the same amount of time as it takes for humans to respond to the treatment. The rats given fluoxetine did not generate new neurone at a rate any different from placebo after five days, but did separate from placebo by 28 days. Of particular interest, it also took 28 days for the rats to change their behaviour, demonstrating a greater willingness to move into open, lighted areas to eat (Santarelli *et al.*, 2003). At this point it is still unclear whether BDNF changes in depression are causal or secondary.

Hormonal Data

With the development of new techniques for the accurate measurement of small quantities of hormones, a plethora of data appeared assessing neurohormonal function in affective disorders. Raised plasma cortisol levels and corticosteroid excretion rates have been observed in patients with depression. Most interest has centred around cortisol and the dexamethasone suppression test (DST). Reviews are readily available (Arana and Baldessarini, 1985; Braddock, 1986; Dahl *et al.*, 1992).

Following investigation of over 400 patients, Carroll *et al.* (1981) defined a standardized protocol and suggested that the test may be 'a specific laboratory test for the diagnosis of melancholia'. The object of the test is to suppress ACTH with a dose of dexamethasone, and most laboratories have adopted a schedule as shown in Table 8.1, or a variant of it. Normal subjects show a diurnal rhythm of secretion of cortisol, with inhibition during the nocturnal hours. They suppress cortisol for 24–48 hours after dexamethasone.

The use of 1 mg of dexamethasone gives the most sensitivity, although doses up to 8 mg have been used in some studies. The most

Table 8.1 Schedule for the dexamethasone suppression test

Day 1	Day 2		
2300	0800	1600	2300
↑	↑	↑	↑
Dex 1 mg oral	Cortisol determinations		

Nonsuppression: cortisol >5 mg per 100 ml (157 nmol/l)

practical time to take the sample for cortisol measurement is at 1600 hours, although the use of additional times may increase the rate of positivity. Using a plasma cortisol criterion value of >5 mg per 100 ml, Carroll *et al.* (1981) gave an overall test sensitivity (true-positive rate) of 43% and a specificity (true-negative rate; that is, 100% minus false-positive rate) of 96%. The diagnostic confidence for a diagnosis of melancholia with values above this level was 96%, although that for ruling out melancholia at levels below this was only 54%. In other words, a positive result had much more significance than a negative result.

In a review of over 5000 cases, Arana and Baldessarini (1985) found the sensitivity to be 44% and the specificity 93% when distinguishing major depression from normal controls, but the latter fell to 76.5% in comparison to all other psychiatric disorders. However, DST specificity remained high when major depression was compared with bereavement (90.5%), anxiety and panic (88.2%), schizophrenia (86.9%) and alcoholism not active or in acute withdrawal (80.0%).

In contrast to these data, other authors have been more critical, and in particular have noted high levels of positivity in other psychiatric conditions. Some of these are shown in Table 8.2.

Age and gender do not seem related to the results, although higher levels of positivity are reported in older patients. The DST response is not affected by the use of antidepressant or neuroleptic medications or lithium. There are a number of conditions that give false-positive results, shown in Table 8.3.

The data with some psychiatric populations other than depression are often confused by the inclusion of patients with associated affective symptoms, which increases the rate of positivity. The results in schizophrenia are influenced by

Table 8.2   Abnormal DST results and psychiatric diagnoses

Psychiatric condition	Result (%)	Reference
Melancholia	45	Carroll *et al.* (1981), Arana and Baldessarini (1985)
Mania	0–40	Rabkin *et al.* (1985)
Schizophrenia	0–20	Coppen *et al.* (1983), Munro *et al.* (1984)
Panic disorder	25	Roy-Byrne *et al.* (1985b)
Obsessive–compulsive	2	Checkley (1985)
Anorexia nervosa	36–100	Rabkin *et al.* (1985)
Bulimia	35–67	Lindy *et al.* (1985)
Borderline personality	8	Krishnan *et al.* (1984)
Normals	4–27	Carroll *et al.* (1981), Braddock (1986)

Table 8.3   False-positive DST

Medications	Benzodiazepines
	Anticonvulsants
	Barbiturates
	Reserpine
	Alpha-methyl dopa
	Methadone
	Morphine
	Spironolactone
	Indomethacin
	Cyproheptadine
Drugs	Alcohol; excess caffeine
Diseases	Diabetes mellitus
	Dementia
	Cerebral tumour
	Cardiac failure
	Cushing's disease
Metabolic	Dehydration
Other	Pregnancy
	Acute medical illness or trauma

acute psychosis and hospital admission, both of which increase the nonsuppression rate. False-negative results are seen in Addison's disease and hypopituitarism.

Although no specific clinical features of the melancholia have been associated with the positive result, some findings are clinically relevant. There are several reports that the DST reverts to normal after treatment, and that failure to do so, or reversion back to a positive response after normalization, is a bad prognostic factor (Arana and Baldessarini, 1985) and may signal an increased risk of suicide (Targum *et al.*, 1983a). In a meta-analysis of the DST as a predictor of outcome, Ribeiro *et al.* (1993) noted that while baseline DST did not predict response to antidepressant treatment, or outcome after hospital discharge, persistent nonsuppression after treatment was associated with a high risk of early relapse and poor outcome after discharge. Coppen *et al.* (1985) have suggested that if higher cutoff points (for example 10 mg per 100 ml) are taken then prediction of response may be improved. In addition, endogenicity, as assessed by the Newcastle scale, may be relevant (Coppen *et al.*, 1983), as may severity of depression as measured by the Hamilton rating scale (Meador-Woodruff *et al.*, 1986). Patients with psychotic depression and bipolar illness have higher levels of nonsuppression (Arana and Baldessarini, 1985), as shown in Table 8.4.

Some have reported that abnormal DSTs are associated with a family history of depression (Mendlewicz *et al.*, 1982), although others do not find this (Rudorfer *et al.*, 1982). There are several reports suggesting that patients with secondary depression have lower rates of suppression than

Table 8.4   Nonsuppression in DST and affective state (from Arana and Baldessarini, 1985)

	Nonsuppression (%)
Normal control	7.2
Acute grief	9.5
Dysthymic disorder	22.9
Major depressive disorder	43.1
Melancholia	50.2
Psychotic affective, includes bipolar disorder	68.6
With suicide intent	77.8

those with primary depressive illness, and in a smaller number of studies, psychotic depressives yield a higher rate than nonpsychotics (Rabkin *et al.*, 1985).

The abnormal responses are not due to an unusually rapid clearance of the dexamethasone by patients with melancholia (Carroll *et al.*, 1981) and the circulating half-life of the cortisol is normal (Butler and Besser, 1968). Depressed patients seem to have an increased number of cortisol secretory episodes with an increased time per day of release (Sachar *et al.*, 1973).

ACTH levels are higher and dexamethasone plasma levels lower in DST-positive patients, in spite of the normal dexamethasone clearance (Arana and Baldessarini, 1985). One explanation of the raised ACTH levels is that the hypothalamic–pituitary–adrenal axis is 'set' at a higher level in the nonsuppressors. Holsboer *et al.* (1985) have given corticotrophin releasing factor (CRF) to nonsuppressing depressed patients, and repeated the investigation on recovery when suppression was normal. No differences in the profiles of ACTH, cortisol or corticosterone output were noted in the two conditions. This implies that the hypersecretion of steroids in depression is not the result of excessive hormonal reserves in the pituitary or adrenal glands. However, blunted ACTH responses to CRF in depressed patients are reported by a number of authors (Gold *et al.*, 1988), suggesting downregulation of pituitary CRF receptors (Dinan, 1994), with an abnormality above the pituitary. Hypersecretion of CRF leads to downregulation of pituitary CRF receptors and decreased ACTH in response to CRF. Whalley *et al.* (1986) measured the number of glucocorticoid receptors on lymphocytes in patients with depression, schizophrenia and controls. The number of receptors was significantly lower in the depressed patients, even in those who had not received psychotropic medication. This suggests that in depression there may be changes in steroid-receptor sensitivity, which if they also occurred in the brain would lead to dexamethasone nonsuppression.

Other studies support the concept of reduced glucocorticoid-receptor activity, helping to explain why patients with affective disorders

do not become cushingoid in the presence of raised glucocorticoid levels (Dinan, 1994).

Although studies of these peripheral markers may not reflect central receptor activity, one hypothesis is that there are reduced central glucocorticoid receptors. In animal models, Sapolsky *et al.* (1985) showed that excessive exposure to steroids reduces the number of hippocampal neurones, suggestive of a direct toxic effect.

Others have assessed adrenal hyperresponsiveness, showing increased cortisol response to ACTH. This may be related to adrenal hypertrophy, since there are several studies showing an increased size of the adrenal gland in patients with affective disorder (Nemeroff *et al.*, 1992; Szigethy *et al.*, 1994).

In relation to other biological markers, patients with dexamethasone nonsuppression have higher platelet MAO activity (Schatzberg *et al.*, 1985) and higher plasma MHPG (Jimerson *et al.*, 1983).

Among the factors that may influence the DST must be included the method of cortisol analysis and patient compliance. Thus part of the variation in the data may reflect the use of radioimmunoassay as opposed to a competitive protein-binding assay, the latter appearing to be more reliable (Meltzer and Fang, 1983). HPLC and mass spectrometry are rarely used, but will be even more accurate. Poor compliance may be one reason why inpatient studies show higher rates of nonsuppression than outpatient investigations, although severity of the illness is a more likely explanation. Some authors have suggested that weight loss is a critical variable, although others have failed to replicate this (Keitner *et al.*, 1985).

A summary of the abnormal glucocorticosteroid responses in patients with depression is shown in Table 8.5. The abnormal suppression has been interpreted in terms of a simple response to stress, although an alternative is that it reflects abnormal limbic–hypothalamic function. The lower levels of abnormality in association with anxiety disorders and bereavement are against this being a nonspecific stress response. Further, an abnormal DST does not relate to an excess of life events as assessed by the Bedford College Life Events and Difficulties

Table 8.5 Abnormalities of the hypothalamic–pituitary–adrenal axis in patients with depression (glucocorticoids)

Cortisol hypersecretion
Increased urinary free cortisol
Increased CSF corticotrophin-releasing factor
Increased circulating ACTH
Abnormal circadian rhythms of cortisol
Abnormal dexamethasone suppression
Decreased glucocorticoid-receptor sensitivity
Decreased release of ACTH to CRH
Increased adrenal-gland size

Schedule, although patients with severe life events in a six-month period prior to the onset of depression have higher urinary-free cortisol levels than those without (Dolan *et al.*, 1985a) and acute stress will elevate postdexamethasone cortisol levels (Baumgartner *et al.*, 1985). It is unlikely that the raised cortisol levels have a causative role in the depressive illness since cortisol itself tends to provoke euphoria or mood elevation when given to patients, and in Cushing's disease, although depression is common, it is not universal, being severe in less than 20% of patients (Cohen, 1980). However, Dinan (1994) has argued that activation of the hypothalamic–pituitary–adrenal axis in biologically predisposed individuals is central to depression, altering monoamine responses, which are therefore secondary.

A more attractive hypothesis is that the abnormal DST reflects altered CNS function, especially neurotransmitter action in hypothalamic and related limbic pathways, and is thus a marker of some more fundamental biological change. This has been explored by Carroll *et al.* (1980), whose data suggest a cholinergic mechanism. They noted that physostigmine, an inhibitor of anticholinesterase, allowed normal subjects to escape from suppression, an effect that could be blocked by atropine.

Patients with organic mental disorders have been investigated, and generally high levels of nonsuppression are reported. In particular, the DST does not seem to differentiate reliably between depressive illness and dementia (Spar and Gerner, 1982). It is abnormal in patients after the acute phase of a cerebrovascular accident,

and this relates both to the presence of major depression and to greater lesion volume on CT examination (Lipsey *et al.*, 1985).

Cortisol plasma levels may also be stimulated by amphetamine and methylamphetamine. As this can be blocked by alpha adrenergic antagonists, the effect is thought to be mediated noradrenergically. This response seems blunted in depressed patients (Checkley, 1979). Clonidine appears to normalize the hypercortisolaemia of depression (Siever and Uhde, 1984), providing support for a role of adrenergic mechanisms.

Some conclusions regarding the ever-accumulating information on the DST are given in Table 8.6. In recent years this area has again become prominent as researchers have developed potential antidepressant compounds which directly alter ACTH activity (Gomez *et al.*, 2006; Keller *et al.*, 2008; Schatzberg and Lindley, 2008).

Other Neurohormonal Data

Several other neuroendocrine responses in depression have been assessed. These include the thyroid-stimulating-hormone (TSH) response to thyroid-releasing hormone (TRH), growth-hormone responses to dopamine agonists, insulin, L 5-HTP and clonidine, and prolactin response to tryptophan, D-fenfluramine and buspirone.

In the TRH test, 200–500 mg of IV-TRH are given, and blood samples are taken over the

Table 8.6 Some conclusions regarding the DST in psychiatry

1. An abnormal DST is found in some patients
2. This suggests hypothalamic–pituitary axis dysfunction
3. It is most abnormal in anorexia nervosa
4. It is often abnormal in depression, especially endogenous, melancholic and psychotic subtypes
5. It is state- rather than trait-dependent
6. It may help differentiate anxiety disorders from depression
7. It may predict relapse after treatment

next hour for the assessment of TSH values. Some 40–50% of patients with depression show blunted responses (Extein *et al.*, 1981; Calloway *et al.*, 1984). One group, studying 145 medication-free depressed patients, gave the specificity of the test as 93% with a sensitivity of 56%, and predictive value of a maximum TSH response (the peak level after infusion–baseline) of <7 m IU/ml as 91% for major unipolar depression (Extein *et al.*, 1981). The response tends to normalize with treatment (Extein *et al.*, 1982). Claims that this test may distinguish different subgroups of affective disorder have not been upheld. Further, although cortisol excess itself leads to impaired TSH release, not all patients with blunting on this test are dexamethasone nonsuppressors. About 30–40% of patients are abnormal on both dexamethasone and TRH tests, although this does not identify any particular diagnostic group. Interestingly, a subgroup of patients with blunted responses have an elevated free-thyroxine index (FTI), some, while not being clinically hyperthyroid, having values in the hyperthyroid range (Calloway *et al.*, 1984). Abnormal responses are also reported in alcoholism, anorexia nervosa and acute starvation. In depression, it is thought that the blunted responses reflect decreased TRH-receptor sensitivity.

Because of the observed endocrine changes in depressed patients, other investigators have given multiple neuroendocrine challenges to look for a more generalized hypothalamic–pituitary defect in the disorder. Brambilla *et al.* (1978) gave TRH and LHRH to 16 patients with primary affective disorder, and 79% had some demonstrable abnormality. Winokur *et al.* (1982), using TRH, LHRH, DST and insulin challenge tests in patients with primary unipolar depression and controls, reported abnormalities in 96.2% of patients and only 29% of controls.

Both growth hormone and prolactin have been studied because of the relationship of their release to underlying neurotransmitters. Growth hormone is affected by a number of factors including stress, fasting and diet, but is thought to be released under the influence of growth-hormone releasing factor (GHRF, somatostatin) from the hypothalamus. Release of growth hormone is altered by drugs that act on the adrenoceptor, being stimulated by clonidine, methoxamine and phenyephrine (alpha agonists), an effect potentiated by propranolol. This suggests that alpha receptors are excitatory and beta receptors inhibitory. The growth-hormone response to apomorphine is related to dopamine-receptor stimulation, and it can be blocked by dopamine antagonists such as chlorpromazine. Other neurotransmitters also probably involved in growth-hormone release include 5-HT and GABA, although their influence is weaker.

Growth-hormone responses have been studied in depression. Impaired release is reported after metamphetamine (Checkley, 1979), insulin hypoglycaemia (Mueller *et al.*, 1969), clonidine (Checkley, 1985; Siever and Uhde, 1984) and desmethylimipramine (Glass *et al.*, 1982), a tricyclic drug that selectively blocks the re-uptake of noradrenaline. Responses to apomorphine are not reliably altered, supporting a major role for alpha-adrenergic mechanisms in affective disorder with decreased alpha-2-receptor responsiveness, probably at the hypothalamus. GHRF itself has provided mixed results (Skare *et al.*, 1994). Katona *et al.* (1985) have reported that patients with blunted growth-hormone responses to clonidine are more likely to be DST nonsuppressors, suggesting a common underlying mechanism for these changes.

Wieck *et al.* (1991) gave women with a history of affective psychosis the apomorphine challenge test four days post partum. Growth-hormone responses were significantly greater in those that developed a recurrent psychotic illness, suggesting that in this group at least, hypothalamic dopamine receptors had increased sensitivity.

Prolactin release, regulated by prolactin-inhibitory factor (PIF), itself thought to be dopamine, is stimulated by dopamine antagonists and inhibited by dopamine agonists. Tryptophan, 5-HTP, 5-HT and GABA also stimulate its release. The response to tryptophan is thought to result from activation of postsynaptic $5-HT_{1A}$ receptors and the $5-HT_2$ receptor.

More selective 5-HT receptor agonists include gepirone and buspirone for the 5-HT$_{1A}$ site. Stimulation leads to a rise in GH and ACTH.

Baseline prolactin levels are consistently normal in depressed populations. In one study, the degree of suppression following apomorphine has been reported impaired in major depression and schizoaffective disorder, the degree of depression as rated on the Hamilton scale correlating with the degree of suppression (Meltzer *et al.*, 1984), although in this investigation baseline levels were elevated. While this may suggest a role of dopaminergic systems, blunted prolactin responses have also been reported after methadone (Judd *et al.*, 1982) and tryptophan (Heninger *et al.*, 1984), suggesting both peptide and serotonergic abnormalities.

Studies with buspirone (a 5-HT$_{1A}$ agonist) in depressed patients failed to reveal altered GH, cortisol or prolactin (postsynaptic 5-HT$_{1A}$) release compared with controls (Cowen, 1994; Meltzer and Maes, 1994), but did attenuate hypothermic responses (presynaptic 5-HT$_{1A}$ effect) (Cowen, 1994). One conclusion of these data is that there is decreased 5-HT$_{1A}$ autoreceptor function in depression (Cowen, 1994). This may reflect decreased release of 5-HT and compensatory downregulation of the autoreceptor.

In contrast to the many studies in depression, neuroendocrine challenges in mania are few. Prolactin responses to buspirone seem normal (Yatham, 1994).

A summary of some of these neurohormonal findings in affective disorder is found in Table 8.7. In general, taking into consideration the methodological problems associated with

Table 8.7   Summary of neurohormonal data

Hypersecretion of cortisol
Loss of normal circadian cortisol cycle
Increased urinary excretion of cortisol and
   metabolites
Abnormal response to dexamethasone
Blunting of growth hormone output to
   alpha-adrenergic stimulants
Blunting of TSH responses to TRH
Blunted prolactin responses to several agents
Blunted ACTH responses to CRF

Table 8.8   Some important methodological considerations

Influence of age and sex
Influence of circadian, monthly and annual
   cycle of hormone activity
Influence of stress, diet and associated illness
Many hormones are released in a pulsatile
   fashion
Influence of nicotine and alcohol intake
Influence of psychotropic drugs
Variability of assay procedures
Lack of specificity for receptors of drugs

these data (see Table 8.8), they offer support for adrenergic and serotoninergic involvement in major affective disorders, the most robust findings relating to studies of the α adrenergic receptor in depressive disorders.

NEUROCHEMICAL INVESTIGATIONS

There have been a considerable number of investigations of CSF in the affective disorders, the majority examining the noradrenergic, 5-HT and BDNF hypotheses. In contrast to the studies in schizophrenia, the neuropathological studies are few in number.

CSF

The main metabolites investigated, in studies with or without the probenecid technique, have been 5-HIAA and MHPG. Overall, more studies report lower levels of 5-HIAA than no differences compared with controls. Many of the early studies did not use the probenecid method, and were dismissed on account of methodological problems. First, much 5-HIAA released from the brain is removed from the CSF by an active transport system, giving a 3:1 gradient from ventricular to lumbar fluid. Second, factors such as diet, time of day and patient height and posture were often not taken into account. Third, the spinal cord was known to contribute to the 5-HIAA pool, further diminishing the relevance of lumbar-fluid findings.

Using the probenecid technique, several groups have shown diminished accumulation of 5-HIAA, further lessened by the administration of antidepressants (Post and Goodwin, 1978) but elevated by L-tryptophan and 5-HTP (Takahashi *et al.*, 1975). In addition, the low levels seem to persist on clinical recovery in both baseline (Coppen *et al.*, 1972) and probenecid (van Praag, 1980a) studies. In a series of investigations, van Praag (1980a), using the probenecid method, reported low levels of 5-HIAA to characterize some 40% of cases, although he did not report any psychopathological differences between these and other patients. In contrast, Banki *et al.* (1981) reported anxiety, insomnia, retardation, fatigability and suicide to be more prevalent in a subpopulation of patients with low 5-HIAA. The low levels are noted in patients with an absence of significant adverse life events in the six months prior to onset of their illness (Roy *et al.*, 1986b).

A relationship between suicide and low 5-HIAA has been replicated by most studies that have examined it. Åsberg and colleagues (Åsberg *et al.*, 1976; Lidberg *et al.*, 1985) reported 5-HIAA as lower in those who attempt suicide, even in nondepressed subjects, and in those who have murdered sexual or familial partners or their children. They have also reported in a follow-up study of depressed patients that those with low values are more likely to die from suicide in the ensuing 12 months. Since similar findings are reported in schizophrenics who attempt suicide (Ninan *et al.*, 1984), in alcoholic impulsive violent offenders (Linnoila *et al.*, 1983b) and in patients with aggression who have borderline personality disorders without depressive illness (Brown *et al.*, 1982), one interpretation is that the low 5-HT turnover is related to impulse control and aggression, rather than to depression per se. Of related interest is the study of Higley *et al.* (1992) in rhesus monkeys, where high rankings for aggression were negatively correlated with CSF 5-HIAA, and positively with CSF noradrenaline.

There has been one investigation of ventricular fluid metabolites in depression. Bridges *et al.* (1976), in a study of patients with chronic or persistently resistant depression having resective brain surgery, reported severely depressed patients to have the lowest and agitated patients to have the highest 5-HIAA levels.

In contrast, results of 5-HIAA levels in mania have been contradictory, some studies reporting increased and others decreased values.

CSF catecholamine or catecholamine metabolite levels have been studied with less consistent results. In keeping with the urine investigations, some authors report low levels of MHPG (Post *et al.*, 1973) and others show normal results (Post *et al.*, 1985) and no relationship to suicide. Low HVA levels have been reported in subgroups of patients, notably those with retardation (van Praag, 1977a) or who attempt suicide (Roy *et al.*, 1992). This observation is consistently reported in probenecid studies and seems robust. In contrast, agitation and psychosis are reported to be related to increased HVA levels (Banki *et al.*, 1981).

Estimates of noradrenaline levels have produced inconsistencies, although there are two reports of elevations in mania (Gerner *et al.*, 1984; Post *et al.*, 1985) associated with paradoxically decreased dopamine beta-hydroxylase levels (Post *et al.*, 1985). Lower adrenaline levels have also been reported in depressed patients, returning to normal with recovery (Christensen *et al.*, 1980).

There are several reports of CSF data combining with other biological markers. In particular, DST nonsuppressors show lower HVA and a poor association with adverse life events (Roy *et al.*, 1986b).

Lower CSF GABA has been noted in several studies (Berrettini *et al.*, 1983; Gerner *et al.*, 1984), as has lower CSF somatostatin (Rubinow *et al.*, 1985), especially in dexamethasone nonsuppressors (Doran *et al.*, 1986). This suggests a functional interdependence of CRF on somatostatin, possibly at the level of the hypothalamus, and receives some support from observations of higher CSF cortisol in depression (Träskman *et al.*, 1980), associated with nonsuppression of the DST.

Other CSF changes reported include lower AVP (Gjerris, 1988), lower pregnenolone

(George *et al.*, 1994a) and decreased S-adenosyl methionine (Bottiglieri *et al.*, 1990).

Brain Neurochemistry

The CSF data provide limited support for changes in catecholamines in depressive illness, especially in relation to motor activity. The data from brain neurochemical studies in this area are minimal. Those reported lend weight to changes in the 5-HT system, and are largely derived from studies of brains of patients who have committed suicide. These data are difficult to interpret methodologically, especially since psychotropic drugs are often the main cause of death in such patients, and there are difficulties with controlling for post-mortem degradation.

Most studies of cortical 5-HT and 5-HIAA in post-mortem brains reveal no changes, findings from the brainstem being more consistent in showing lower levels than controls (Lloyd *et al.*, 1974; Shaw *et al.*, 1967). In a study of bipolar patients, Young *et al.* (1994) reported decreased 5-HIAA and HVA levels in cortex, and increased noradrenaline turnover, reflected in increased MHPG/NA ratios.

Attempts to examine binding sites have mainly used labelled imipramine, amitriptyline or paroxetine, and this use of different ligands may be important. Results are very variable (Lawrence *et al.*, 1990) and no conclusions can be drawn. There are several studies supporting the early findings of increased frontal binding of 3H-spiperone, suggesting raised 5-HT$_2$ receptors at this site (Stanley and Mann, 1983), but results using 5-HT$_{1A}$ ligands are conflicting.

It has already been noted that an important variable with regards to 5-HT function relates perhaps more to violence and impulsivity than to depression. The changes in 5-HT$_2$ binding seem more consistent in studies of violent suicides (Arora and Meltzer, 1989; Stanley and Mann, 1983). These data are interpreted as reflecting low 5-HT turnover, with compensatory increase in postsynaptic binding sites.

In other studies, brain MAO, noradrenaline levels and muscarinic cholinergic binding have been studied with negative results. One group has reported low dopamine levels in the caudate

nucleus (Birkmeyer *et al.*, 1977), and others have shown significantly increased beta-adrenergic receptor binding to frontal cortex (Mann *et al.*, 1986), increased clonidine (alpha-2) binding in suicide patients (Meana *et al.*, 1992) and increased frontal benzodiazepine binding sites (Cheetham *et al.*, 1988).

MR spectroscopy allows one to noninvasively assess brain chemistry. Using this technique some investigators have found abnormal choline metabolism in bipolar affective-disorder patients in the caudate (Moore *et al.*, 2000). As mentioned above, MRS studies have also found abnormal low GABA activity in depression (Kaufman *et al.*, 2009; Sanacora *et al.*, 2002).

NEUROPHYSIOLOGICAL AND NEUROLOGICAL DATA

Electrophysiological Studies

Some of the earliest reports of EEG traces in affective disorder found a higher than expected incidence of abnormalities. For example, Finley and Campbell (1941) found abnormalities in 33% of 137 manic–depressive patients, and similar data were given by others (Davis, 1941). As with schizophrenia, attention was drawn to the presence of abnormally high frequencies (20–50 Hz).

Abrams and Taylor (1979) analysed the records of 27 schizophrenic and 132 affective-disorder patients, noting that in contrast to the more extensive and temporal location of the abnormalities in schizophrenia, the affectives had more parieto/occipital changes (24%). In cases where the abnormalities were lateralized, 71% were right-sided. This did not relate to age, severity of illness or medication.

Two waveforms in particular have been associated with affective symptoms. The six-per-second rhythmic waves, also referred to as rhythmic midtemporal discharges (RMTD), are associated with an increased risk for psychopathology, including high hypochondriasis and depression scores on the MMPI (Hughes and Hermann, 1984) (see Figure 8.2). Small sharp spikes (SSS), brief-duration small-amplitude spikes that are sometimes

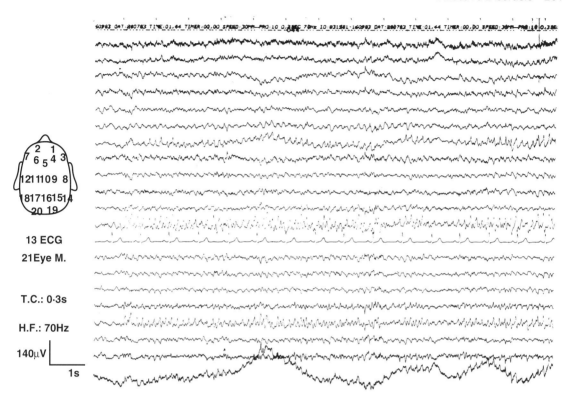

13 ECG

21Eye M.

T.C.: 0·3s

H.F.: 70Hz

140µV

1s

Figure 8.2 Rhythmic midtemporal discharges. Note trains of notched waves, maximal in the left temporal regions (leads 7 12, and 18) (courtesy of Dr Colin Binnie, Institute of Psychiatry)

exclusively temporal in location and manifest in drowsy states or light sleep, have been associated with neurovegetative symptoms, affective disorders and a tendency to suicide (Small, 1970) (see Figure 8.3). In particular, related symptoms included mood swings, anxiety, insomnia, concentration difficulties and feelings of hopelessness. Further, in patients with bipolar affective disorder, 43% show SSS, which may be significantly related to a family history of affective disorder (Small *et al.*, 1975).

Struve *et al.* (1979) reported a highly significant positive relationship between paroxysmal EEG abnormalities and suicidal ideation and acts, and assaultive/destructive acts, unrelated to medication. Both SSS and RMTD were included in the paroxysmal events that were associated with suicide. The relevance of these findings for such conditions as episodic dyscontrol and the association between epilepsy and affective disorder and suicide is not clear.

However, they do emphasize the importance of paroxysmal electrophysiological events beyond epilepsy, and that 'all that spikes is not fits' (Stevens, 1979).

Data from power spectra analyses have been reported in detail by Flor-Henry (1983). He confirms the increased amount of 20–50 Hz activity, notably bilaterally in the temporal regions for both mania and depression, and in the left parietal region in mania. In his studies there was a significant reduction of right parietal alpha energy in both states, thought to reflect abnormal activation of the nondominant hemisphere. Examining interhemispheric organization by means of an EEG measure of left/right-hemispheric energy oscillations, at rest and during certain cognitive tasks that activated one or other hemisphere, he reported that the organization is most disturbed and bilateral in schizophrenia, is intermediate and in the dominant

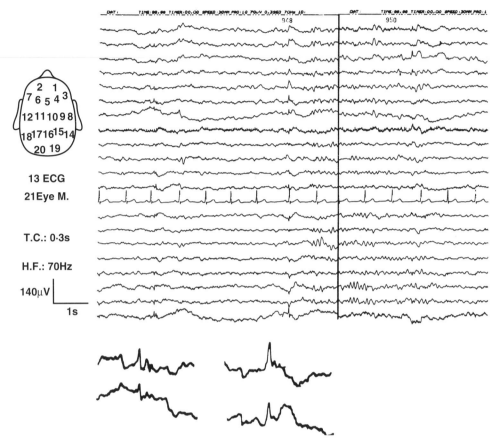

Figure 8.3 Small sharp waves (benign epileptiform transients of sleep). Note the short-duration spikes. A magnification of those from channels 6 and 7 is shown below. These are predominant in the temporal regions and seen during drowsiness or stages 1 and 2 sleep (courtesy of Dr Colin Binnie, Institute of Psychiatry)

hemisphere only in mania, and is normal in depression.

The evoked-potential literature is confusing and difficult to interpret. Shagass *et al.* (1981), in studies where potentials were evoked by four different kinds of sensory stimuli, claimed to show differences between psychotic depressives and schizophrenics. They reported that the amplitudes of earlier peaks were higher in the latter, while later peaks (P90, N130 and P185) were higher in the former. However, in both groups most amplitudes were lower than controls. The data were interpreted as suggesting some impairment of sensory processing in depression, although less than that seen in schizophrenia. Laterality differences have been reported, but the results are inconsistent, some

suggesting nondominant- (Flor-Henry, 1983) and others dominant-hemisphere (Shagass *et al.*, 1979) abnormalities.

Davidson and colleagues, working over several decades now, have suggested that prefrontal EEG laterality measures can distinguish a sad from a normal affect, melancholic disposition from controls, and depression from health (Davidson, 1995). Similarly, Korb and colleagues (2008) have proposed that a measure of laterality and prefrontal EEG power (called cordance) can distinguish depressed patients from controls. More ambitiously, they also suggest that serial measures of cordance can be used to determine who will eventually respond to a given antidepressant medication, and that EEG changes can be observed in eventual responders as early as one to two weeks after beginning to take a medication, before clinical symptoms begin to change (Cook *et al.*, 2005; Hunter *et al.*, 2006).

Sleep Studies

One biological marker of depression that has become of interest is polygraphically defined sleep changes. Some disorder of sleep has long been held to be a key symptom of depression, notably early-morning waking and nocturnal restlessness in endogenous depression. The major changes of sleep in depression are shown in Table 8.9.

One consistent observation is the shortening of the time from the onset of sleep to the first REM period (REM latency). This falls by about 30%, and is associated with an increase in the length of the first REM period and decreased stages 3 and 4 sleep. The REM period is said to be more dense, with an increased number of eye movements per minute. Patients show increased waking during the night, and will complain of both early-morning wakening and poor sleep quality.

The shortened REM latency does not seem specific for depression, and has been reported in such conditions as narcolepsy, anorexia nervosa, some schizophrenics and in normals following artificial REM deprivation (Gillin *et al.*, 1985). However, in depression it has good sensitivity (60–70%) and high specificity (80–97%), and is associated with some other biological markers. Latencies are briefer in patients who are cortisol nonsuppressors (Mendlewicz *et al.*, 1984; Rush *et al.*, 1982).

Benca *et al.* (1992) conducted a meta-analysis of sleep disorders, reviewing data from over 7000 patients. While most psychiatric groups showed reduced total sleep time, accounted for by decreases of non-REM sleep, percentage REM was increased in affective disorders. Decreased latency was seen in several disorders, but overall the findings for this and other parameters were more consistently disturbed in depressed patients.

The meaning of these changes is unclear. They seem to identify a pattern of depression referred to as endogenous, and may be presumed to be a reflection of the underlying biochemical abnormality associated with the condition. Manipulation of sleep, for example deprivation, has an antidepressant effect, and, in patients switching from depression to mania, a change in sleep pattern heralds the change in mood and motoric behaviour. Several hypotheses have been advanced (Gillin *et al.*, 1985). Since REM sleep is regulated by monoamines and is influenced by cholinergic medications (REM latency can be shortened by physostigmine), one suggestion is that it reflects a disturbed cholinergic/aminergic balance. Another is that the short latency represents a 'phase advance', a shift of diurnal rhythms. This is particularly interesting given the new data on CLOCK genes and bipolar disorder discussed above.

Radiological Studies

CT and MRI

Early CT data revealed a subgroup of patients with affective disorder that had ventricular dilatation and cerebral atrophy (Dolan *et al.*, 1985b; Nasrallah *et al.*, 1982a). Increased ventricular size has been reported in group studies of patients with manic–depressive illness (Pearlson and Verloff, 1981), psychotic depression with delusions (Targum *et al.*, 1983b), mania (Nasrallah *et al.*, 1982b), young

Table 8.9 Sleep and affective disorder

Patient symptoms	Difficulty getting off to sleep
	Poor sleep
	Early morning waking
	Increased waking
Duration	Decreased total time
Non-REM sleep	Increased stage 1
	Decreased stages 3 and 4
REM sleep	Decreased REM latency
	Increased REM time in early hours
	Decreased REM in late hours
Treatment	Sleep deprivation
	Selective REM deprivation
	Antidepressants, some of which suppress REM

manics (Nasrallah *et al.*, 1982b) and elderly depressives (Jacoby and Levy, 1980b).

MRI data have confirmed and extended these findings. There are several reports of increased subcortical white-matter intensity lesions in the elderly with depression (Coffey *et al.*, 1993) and in bipolar disorder (Strakowsi *et al.*, 1993). In the elderly, this may be related to vascular disease, and is more prominent in the frontal areas (Coffey *et al.*, 1993). It seems that the presence of atrophy in the elderly may predispose to the development of affective disorder.

Other findings in depression include decreased caudate volumes (Krishnan *et al.*, 1992), decreased temporal-lobe size (Hauser *et al.*, 1989) and decreased brainstem and cerebellar vermis volumes (Shah *et al.*, 1992). In bipolar disorder a similar reduction of temporal volumes has been reported (Altschuler *et al.*, 1991), but with increased caudate volumes (Aylward *et al.*, 1994). However, it is clear that fewer studies of MRI have been conducted in affective disorder than in schizophrenia, and some of these data await confirmation. Harvey *et al.* (1994) found no volumetric differences between bipolars and controls.

Dolan *et al.* (1990) reported increased frontal T_1 values in unipolar but not bipolar patients, possibly related to lithium treatment in the latter. Rangel-Guerra *et al.* (1983) reported that bipolar patients had higher T_1 values than controls, which decreased following lithium treatment.

Using phosphorous MRS in patients with bipolar disorder, Kato *et al.* (1993) reported increased phosphomonoester peaks in frontal cortex, which decreased when patients were euthymic. In contrast, Deicken *et al.* (1995) noted lower phosphomonoester values and higher diester values in both frontal lobes in medication-free bipolar patients.

In a combined PET/MRI study of mood disorders, Drevets and colleagues (2008) demonstrated that the mean grey-matter volume of the subgenual cingulate area (sgACC, Brodmann's area 25) cortex is reduced in subjects with major depressive disorder and bipolar disorder, irrespective of mood state. Neuropathological assessments of sgACC tissue acquired post mortem from subjects with major depressive disorder or bipolar disorder confirmed the decrement in grey-matter volume and revealed that this abnormality was likely due to reduced glia, not neurone. In PET studies the metabolic activity was elevated in this region in the depressed relative to the remitted phases of the same major-depressive-disorder subjects, and several studies have suggested that effective antidepressant treatment is associated with a reduction in sgACC activity (Mayberg *et al.*, 1997, 1999). The white-matter fibre tracts projecting to this area are now a target for deep-brain stimulation in treatment-resistant major depressive disorder (Mayberg *et al.*, 2005).

Another finding using structural imaging is increased amygdala size in patients with chronic affective disorder and bipolar disorder. Notwithstanding the difficulties of measuring amygdala size volumetrically, this has been replicated in several studies (Altshuler *et al.*, 2000; Hauser *et al.*, 2000). Whether this relates to trait or state is unclear at the present time, although the amygdala contains islands of small undifferentiated neurone, and it could be related to neuronal plasticity.

CBF and PET Studies

Early SPECT and PET findings in depression were variable, but most suggested reduced CBF maximally frontally (Baxter *et al.*, 1985; Mathew *et al.*, 1980b). There are reports that the abnormalities are maximal on the left (Baxter *et al.*, 1989; Buchsbaum *et al.*, 1986) and normalize with treatment. Other findings include decreased caudate metabolism (Buchsbaum *et al.*, 1986).

More recent studies with higher-resolution scanners have examined regional metabolism more discretely. Biver *et al.* (1994) reported decreased dorsolateral frontal and parietal cortical fluorodeoxyglucose uptake, but increased activity in orbital frontal lobe.

Similar data are reported by Bench *et al.* (1993) using oxygen PET and statistical parametric mapping (SPM). Decreased rCBF was seen in depression in the left dorsolateral prefrontal cortex, left anterior cingulate and left angular gyrus. These findings seemed unrelated to treatment conditions. Interestingly, there were region-specific correlations to symptom patterns, anxiety and agitation relating to increased activity in posterior cingulate and inferior parietal lobules bilaterally, and psychomotor retardation correlating negatively with flow in the left superior temporal gyrus and areas of the left parietal and left inferior frontal and dorsolateral prefrontal cortex. Cognitive function was correlated positively with left medial frontal flow. Following recovery from depression, maximal changes occurred in the left anterior cingulate, left angular gyrus and left dorsolateral prefrontal cortical regions.

A common abnormality of the left dorsolateral prefrontal cortex therefore emerges in studies of both schizophrenia and depression. Since in schizophrenia this is not activated by frontal tasks such as the Wisconsin card-sorting test, but in depression it can be, Berman *et al.* (1993) have argued that the pathophysiology of the abnormality differs between the two conditions. It seems to relate to a common symptom pattern shared between the diagnoses, namely psychomotor retardation.

The involvement of the cingulum is of particular interest (Drevets *et al.*, 2008). It is related to attentional mechanisms, which are disturbed in depression; to pain appreciation; and it is central to the limbic circuitry modulating emotion. In studies where sleep deprivation has been attempted to treat patients with depression, increased cingulate activation predicts a good response (Wu *et al.*, 1992). In a series of studies, Mayberg *et al.* (1997, 1999) have suggested that the subgenual anterior cingulate may represent a final common pathway involved in depression pathogenesis and treatment response.

In PET studies using SPM it has been shown that the cingulum can be activated by the STROOP test, which involves selecting appropriate responses and inhibiting others. Patients with depression fail to activate the cingulate gyrus with this task, but activate the dorsolateral prefrontal cortex (George *et al.*, 1994d). Another activation task used by George *et al.* (1994c) is a facial emotion-recognition task, separating the response for identity recognition

from that for emotional expression recognition. There is now a large literature using this form of activation to probe affective circuits in health and depression. In the original study, depressed subjects had a deficit in matching faces for emotional content, and failed to activate the right insula as seen in controls with this task. More recent work with these facial emotion-activation tasks has focused on amygdala as well as cingulate and prefrontal activation (George *et al.*, 1995c, 1998; Minzenberg *et al.*, 2007).

In an attempt to understand the role of some of these structures in emotion, investigators have imaged healthy volunteers in different emotional states using oxygen PET and more recently BOLD fMRI. George *et al.* (1994b, 1994c) reported that transient sadness activated the amygdala, the anterior temporal lobes, the cingulate gyrus and the orbital and prefrontal cortex bilaterally. These same areas are activated by intravenous procaine, a drug that activates limbic structures and causes dysphoria. In contrast, transient happiness produces decreased activity in temporoparietal cortex bilaterally and right frontal cortex. Thus, while these volunteer studies help to outline further an anatomy of mood, the direction of the changes noted requires explanation. George *et al.* speculated that perhaps a chronic increase in limbic activity overwhelms the normal regulatory role of the prefrontal cortex, and the overall circuit decreases in activity with the onset of a depression in mood-disorder patients.

Procaine-induced euphoria is associated with activation of the amygdala, basal forebrain and anterior cingulate (Ketter *et al.*, 1994). Using SPM and PET, George *et al.* (1994b) examined rCBF in mania. They reported increased activity in right temporal structures. The only other study of PET in mania was that of Baxter *et al.* (1985), which reported global hypermetabolism.

There are few receptor studies. D'haenen and Bossuyt (1994), using ketanserin and IBZM SPECT, reported frontal asymmetries with the former, and increased uptake of the latter in depression. Wong *et al.* (1985), using PET, did not initially find increased D_2 receptors using methylspiperone in bipolar patients, but more recently they have (Pearlson *et al.*, 1995); thus the findings with IBZM are difficult to interpret. However, Ebert *et al.* (1994) reported that responders to sleep deprivation showed a decrease of D_2 receptor occupancy after treatment. Newer studies have imaged 5-HT_{1A} receptors directly (Cannon *et al.*, 2006, 2007; Drevets *et al.*, 2007). Other studies do not image a receptor directly, but rather image the brain in groups where different receptor genetic variants exist (Burnet *et al.*, 1999; Munafo *et al.*, 2008; Pezawas *et al.*, 2005). Using 11^cWAY, the 5-HT_{1A} receptor has been shown to be reduced in the raphe and medial temporal cortex in depressed especially bipolar subjects (Savitz et *et al.* 2009).

Another new form of functional brain imaging involves examining the 'resting state'. Patients are placed in the MRI scanner and given no specific task. Over a period of time the scanner measures small variations in regional brain activity. These serials scans can then be analysed, looking for regional covarations, or functional connectivity at rest. Several studies have now been carried out with this technique in depressed patients, implicating disrupted cortico-limbic connectivity (Anand *et al.*, 2005a, 2005b; Greicius *et al.*, 2007).

Consistent with the structural studies mentioned above, amygdala activity has been shown to be enhanced in patients with mania or depression, or with anxiety disorders (Drevets, 2003). There do not appear to be consistent imaging differences between unipolar and bipolar depression.

Neurological Data

It is clear that depression can be associated with a wide range of somatic illnesses, including endocrine disorders (particularly adult-onset diabetes), malignancy, viral disorders, hepatic and pancreatic disease, electrolyte disorders and the collagenoses (Hall, 1980). Further, many people with chronic illness become despondent and demoralized. These states, often associated with some symptoms of a major depressive illness, are sometimes referred to as secondary depression or depressive reactions, but in most instances their phenomenology has not been well specified, and their response to conventional antidepressant treatments not evaluated. Again it is of importance to understand the definition of a depressive illness and to differentiate it from understandable reactions to adverse circumstances and human misery. Failure to do so leads to confusion over biological data collected in supposed major affective disorder and to unnecessary prescription of antidepressant drugs, which themselves carry morbidity. This said, it is important to aggressively treat comorbid depression after attempts have been made to address the underlying condition, as this can have beneficial effects on quality of life as well as the primary illness.

Secondary mania, although rarer, has been noted with several CNS conditions, including postencephalitic states, Huntington's chorea, tumours, epilepsy, following head injury and with cerebellar atrophy (Krauthammer and Klerman, 1978; Yadalam *et al.*, 1985). Euphoric mood changes were commonly described in generalized paralysis of the insane (GPI), and a 'eutonia' and 'empty' euphoria accompanies the periventricular demyelination of multiple sclerosis. Most studies reveal that the focal lesions that lead to secondary mania are right-sided and involve the orbitofrontal cortex, caudate nuclei, thalamus or basotemporal areas (Table 8.10). This is in contrast to many studies which have found that left-sided lesions predispose to depression, particularly those in the frontal cortex.

A number of drugs may precipitate, provoke or exacerbate a depressive illness, and the role of reserpine in originally providing

Table 8.10 Disorders associated with secondary mania

Cerebrovascular accidents
Epilepsy
Parkinson's disease with dopamine agonist
  therapy
Idiopathic basal ganglia calcification (Fahr's
  disease)
Huntington's disease
Traumatic brain injury
Multiple sclerosis
Frontal-lobe degenerations
Cerebral syphilis

Table 8.11 Some drugs commonly associated with affective disorders

Depression	Alcohol
	Anticonvulsants
	Barbiturates
	Benzodiazepines
	Butyrophenones
	Digitalis
	Disulfiram
	Fenfluramine and appetite suppressants
	Methyl dopa
	Metronidazole
	Nonsteroidal anti-inflammatory drugs
	Oral contraceptives
	Phenothiazines
	Propranolol and other beta blockers
	Reserpine
Mania	Amphetamine and other stimulants
	Bromocriptine
	L-dopa
	MAOI antidepressants
	Steroids
	Tricyclic antidepressants

an insight for the biochemical theories has been mentioned. A short list of commonly used drugs associated with causing or exacerbating depression is shown in Table 8.11; more extensive reviews are available (Hall, 1980; Whitlock and Evans, 1978).

Depressive illness is common with neurological disorders, and the literature has been reviewed elsewhere (Cummings, 1985; Cummings and Trimble, 1995; Trimble, 1981a). The association is more than just an accompaniment to chronic illness, and touches upon the biochemical and neuroanatomical underpinnings of affective expression. The conditions most considered are head injuries, cerebrovascular disease, epilepsy, multiple sclerosis and Parkinson's disease. Depressive symptoms in dementia are discussed in Chapter 11. It is germane to note that head injuries, often of a relatively trivial nature, may provoke depressive symptoms, often in the setting of a post-traumatic stress disorder. The contributions of neuronal, personality and psychosocial influences to the final picture have been discussed elsewhere (Trimble, 1981b).

Lesion location has been shown to be important, especially with early-onset depression. Left dorsolateral frontal and left basal ganglia lesions are particularly implicated (Jorge *et al.*, 1993).

With regard to tumours, meningiomas, especially frontal meningiomas, are notoriously liable to induce a picture of typical major depressive disorder. Both temporal- and frontal-lobe tumours are likely to present with changes of affect, including euphoria, hypomanic-like features, lability, depression and irritability, with a tendency to be commoner with dominant-hemisphere pathology (Cummings, 1985; Lishman, 1987). However, parietal and diencephalic tumours are also reported to lead to affective change, especially hypomanic swings with diencephalic lesions (Greenberg and Brown, 1985).

The association between basal-ganglia disorders and depression is of particular interest. In Parkinson's disease some 30–60% of patients have a depressive illness, not entirely due to the limitations of the chronic disability. The subject has been well reviewed by Cummings (1992). The clinical picture may be dominated by anxiety, although all typical depressive features are seen. No consistent relationship to age of onset is noted, although some suggest it is commoner with early-onset disease. There is a correlation between depressive symptoms and motor impairment, but no consistent relationship between for example Hoehn and Yahr staging and depression ratings.

Biological associations have been reported. A relationship between right-sided hemi-Parkinsonism and severity of depression has been noted (Starkstein *et al.*, 1990), as has greater depression in 'off' phases in patients displaying 'on–off' phenomena (Brown *et al.*, 1984).

The depression associated with Parkinson's disease is often reported to occur prior to the onset of the motor disorder, responds to ECT, and has been associated with decreased CSF 5-HIAA levels (Mayeux *et al.*, 1984).

PET studies have shown decreased CBF in the frontal and cingulate areas, in regions that overlap with the abnormalities shown in primary depressive illness (Ring *et al.*, 1994).

Huntington's chorea also often presents with disorders of affect, including psychotic-depressive and hypomanic pictures. Again this can be dissociated from the motor disability, and may be seen prior to the onset or diagnosis of the chorea. Further, a high frequency of suicide is reported, even in those with no knowledge of their diagnosis. In a comparison between the frequencies of major affective disorder in this condition and in Alzheimer's disease, Mindham *et al.* (1985) reported that the Huntington's disease patients showed twice the incidence, emphasizing some special relationship, as opposed to the depressive symptoms merely being a prodrome to the dementia. PET studies reveal decreased orbital and inferior prefrontal cortical metabolism related to depression in this condition (Mayberg, 1994).

Other basal-ganglia disorders associated with affective change, either depressive or euphoric, include Wilson's disease, Sydenham's chorea and the blepharospasm–oromandibular–dystonia syndrome (Bruegel's or Meige's syndrome) (Trimble, 1981a).

Cerebrovascular accidents (CVA) regularly leave neuropsychiatric sequelae, and depression is common. A controlled study in comparison with similarly disabled orthopaedic controls revealed a significantly higher level of depression in the CVA patients (50% against 13% for controls), suggesting the mood change is not a simple reaction to disability (Folstein *et al.*, 1977).

In a series of studies, Robinson and colleagues have explored this using CT evaluation of lesion extent and site (Robinson and Szetela, 1981; Robinson *et al.*, 1984; Starkstein and Robinson, 1993). In patients with CVA they noted 27% to have a major depressive disorder and 20% a dysthymic disorder. They found that in the dominant hemisphere, the nearer the lesions to the frontal pole, the more severe the depression. In the nondominant hemisphere, the further away from the frontal pole, the higher the frequency of the depression. There was no association with aphasia, although others have noted depression to be more prevalent in association with Broca's aphasia (Benson, 1979). On follow-up, the major depressive disorder persisted in 60%, and others

developed a new depressive syndrome. The correlation to the left frontal pole persisted. A similar relationship was confirmed in a series of only left-handed patients. Subcortical atrophy identified by brain imaging and a family history of depression seem predisposing risk factors.

Using PET and methylspiperone, Mayberg and colleagues (1988) reported increased binding (5-HT$_2$ receptor) in uninjured brain areas in patients with CVAs, but only for right-hemisphere strokes. In left-hemisphere lesions, the ratio of ipsilateral to contralateral binding in temporal cortex was correlated with depression scores. These data require replication, but suggest that the mechanism of post-stroke depression is different between the two hemispheres. Mayberg and colleagues speculated on the possible reasons for the association of lesion site to severity of depression, citing their own animal work. They produced experimental stroke lesions in rats and noted greater post-lesion decline in catecholamine levels with anterior as opposed to posterior cortical lesions. They suggested that a frontal lesion interrupts more arborizing monoamine projection pathways than does a posterior lesion, leading to greater destruction of axons and more catecholamine depletion.

Patients with affective disorder have been examined for clinical neurological abnormalities. Generally these are noted with a lower frequency than in schizophrenia, and no specific pattern emerges (Manschreck and Ames, 1984).

Neuropsychological Disturbances in Affective Disorder

There is no doubt that a marked cognitive impairment can accompany depressive illness, and that complaints of poor memory, impaired concentration and difficulty with planning, decision-making and abstracting abilities by patients are common. The term 'pseudodementia' has been used to specify this (Caine, 1981; Wells, 1979). It can be argued that this state is better referred to as one of 'reversible dementia', and categorized as a subcortical dementia (see Chapter 11).

The presentation can so resemble dementia that many patients are misdiagnosed as having Alzheimer's disease, and left untreated. The importance of the recognition of pseudodementia is that it is a reversible state of cognitive decline, and improves in association with improvement of the depressive illness.

Although there are other causes of pseudodementia, which include hypomania, hysteria and schizophrenia (Trimble, 1981a), that associated with depression is the commonest, and some degree of cognitive impairment is found in most cases. Important clues to help distinguish pseudodementia from dementia include: a past history of affective disorder; the relatively acute onset, with little evidence of decline prior to the development of affective symptoms; the patient's distress and complaints about cognitive function (as opposed to the lack of insight often seen in dementia); the response to questions in the mental-state examination (patients often using 'don't know' as an answer, whereas in dementia the answers are more evasive, skirting the correct but lost answer); and the performance on more structured psychological tasks, which do not reveal the focal deficits of Alzheimer's disease and produce patchy, inconsistent impairment.

Pseudodementia is one of the most common problems leading to an inappropriate diagnosis of dementia, and follow-up studies of patients with dementia often reveal a subgroup that has not declined or has even improved over time. Depressive illness is then often diagnosed retrospectively (Marsden and Harrison, 1972; Ron *et al.*, 1979).

In addition to the clinical features, CT and EEG evaluation are essential, both often being within normal limits. However, since a subgroup of patients with depressive illness has cerebral atrophy, confusion will occur if CT data are taken in isolation.

There is no clear pattern of cognitive impairment that emerges, but often the patients' subjective complaints are worse than their performance on objective tests. When patients with depressive illness are compared with controls on cognitive-test batteries they tend to show impairments of attention, lack of speed in mental processing, poor attention to detail (Caine, 1981), difficulty in abstraction and memory difficulties, especially on tasks that require effort, motivation and active processing.

There is some suggestion of more nondominant-hemisphere dysfunction, with greater impairment of performance as opposed to verbal abilities, especially for spatial information (Weingartner and Silberman, 1985). Although not entirely consistent, the literature from investigations adopting different testing strategies does suggest predominantly nondominant frontotemporal dysfunction in depressive illness (Flor-Henry, 1983; Taylor and Abrams, 1984). These impairments seem greater with more severe depression, and improve with treatment and clinical response of the depression.

SOME OUTSTANDING ISSUES

It seems clear that much biological information about the affective disorders has been accumulated in recent years. Although there are many conflicting data, there is also a growing body of consistency, and some of the earlier difficulties have been overcome by improved technology, better patient selection and clarification of hypotheses to be tested. However, new problems have arisen with the wealth of investigations now available to the investigator, and the complexities of interpreting empirically-derived data, often collected without reference to any clear underlying hypothesis.

Classification is still quite unsatisfactory, and continues to be a potential source of data conflict. Although the DSM IV and DSM IV-TR have provided a reasonable attempt to unify the researchers' ideals, this attempt fails, perhaps in the sense of being too broad for identifying truly homogeneous groups. The loss of the reactive–endogenous dichotomy is welcomed, not only because of the inconsistency and confusion surrounding the word 'reactive', but because it has falsely assumed a classification based on aetiology. Despite the original scheme of Möbius, in which 'endogenous' was contrasted with 'exogenous' on grounds of causation, the evidence that depressions are somehow either provoked by external circumstances or the result of a mysterious internal process does not stand up. There are many studies employing life-event methodology which show that antecedent life events do not predict clinical pattern (Paykel and Hollyman, 1984), although the fact that human adversity may lead to depressive symptoms hardly requires scientific validation. The important questions are, why do some people develop a depressive illness, and what are the constitutional, neurophysiological and neurochemical correlates of vulnerability, resilience and presentation? The confusion that continually arises when mood changes based primarily on underlying personality disorders are mistaken for depressive illness has already been discussed, but cannot be overemphasized.

Most authors seem to identify a core of patients that suggests a biological syndrome, and in the past the term 'endogenous' has been used to describe them. In DSM IV-TR 'major depressive episode' is a substitute. The relationship to bipolar-disorder depression still requires clarification, and to date neurobiological differences between them have not been identified. While clinically they are identical in phenomenology, there may be important biological differences. Further, the affiliation with dysthymic disorder should be questioned.

The genetic studies have so far not revealed any specific genes of major effect, and there are considerable problems with phenotypic identification. Depressive disorder and the depressive phase of a bipolar disorder may be confused clinically, and the introduction of the bipolar spectrum throws up additional confusions. The profile of the prospective candidates in some studies suggests differences from those of schizophrenia, and if this turns out to be the case it raises problems for those who might support a continuum hypothesis for the psychoses.

With regards to the similarities and differences between patients with bipolar disorder and schizophrenia, it has become clear that the long-term prognosis of bipolar disorder can also be poor, and that many patients remain unwell (subclinically with cognitive problems and mood instability) in between their episodes of depression or hypomania. Their neurocognitive deficits seem different from those identified in schizophrenia. Further, for bipolar disorder, an identifiable prodrome has not been identified and endophenotypes have hardly been investigated.

The differences between the schizophrenias and those bipolar disorders which may be identified at the present are shown in Table 8.12.

The relative lack of data in mania is immediately obvious. This stems in part from the fact that it is less common, and manic patients, because of their clinical state, are often poor research subjects. Much information is hidden under the term 'bipolar disorder', patients occasionally being examined in both a depressed and a manic phase. The main hypotheses tested, as in depressive illness, relate to the various monoamine hypotheses.

The initial monoamine theories were simple, depression relating to a deficit of catecholamine or 5-HT activity or turnover. In the United Kingdom the data have concentrated more on the latter, while in the United States it is the former which became predominant. More recently discussions have shifted to GABA, BDNF and growth factors, as well as G-protein-coupled receptors (Mathew *et al.*, 2008; Sanacora *et al.*, 2008). As shown in Table 8.13, evidence reviewed in this chapter provides support for the involvement of both transmitters, but this is hardly surprising. Few would uphold any suggestion that neurotransmitters act in isolation, and the various feedback and regulatory events that exist between them, now including the neuromodulators, are gradually being unravelled.

Schildkraut and Kety's (1967) original hypothesis was that some or all depression was associated with 'a relative deficiency of noradrenaline at functionally important adrenergic receptor sites in the brain, whereas elations may be associated with any excess of such amines' (p. 8). Maas went on to suggest two types of depression, A and B, the former having disordered noradrenaline and the latter abnormal 5-HT systems. Another catecholamine, dopamine, has also been involved,

Table 8.12 Some putative differences between the schizophrenias and the affective disorders

	Schizophrenias	*Affective disorders*
Birth/obstetric problems	Positive	Negative
Neurocognitive changes	Widespread/working memory	Subtle/not widespread/attentional deficits
Anatomy	Volume loss/amydala decreased	Less volume loss/amygdala increased/area 25 involved
Neurochemistry	Dopamine/glutamate	GABA/5-HT
Treatments	Dopamine antagonists	5-HT/noradrenalin uptake inhibitors
Course	Slowly progressive	Progressive in a small number
Risk for cardio-vascular disease	Greatly increased (1–5×)	Increased ??
Life expectancy	Reduced up to 20 years	Reduced

Table 8.13 Evidence for the 5-HT and catecholamine hypotheses

	5-HT	Noradrenaline
Precursor drug studies	+	–
Reversal by inhibitors	+	×
Chemistry of antidepressants	+	+
Selective uptake inhibitors	+	+
SSRI	+	–
Plasma precursors	?	+
Platelet studies	+	?
Urine studies	×	+
Hormone release studies	×	+
CSF data	+	–
Post-mortem studies	+	–
Association with neurology	+	+

+, reasonable supportive evidence; –, little supportive evidence; ×, inadequate or no data.

although there has been less enthusiasm to develop a 'dopamine hypothesis', even though two antidepressant medications developed specifically on this hypothesis (nomifensine, buproprion) have good efficacy and may work through dopamine-related effects. After careful consideration of all the data, van Praag (1980b) concluded that dopamine deficiency characterizes vital depressions and is linked to the motor features of the illness. This is consistent with the observed associations with Parkinson's disease, common neurotransmitter abnormalities being implicated in both conditions. He further accepted that 'within the group of vital depressive patients with central monoamine disorders,

it is either the 5-HT system or the noradrenaline system that is predominantly disturbed' (p. 51).

Others have speculated on the role of catecholamines in relation to brain-reward systems, deficiencies leading to lack of pleasure (the clinical counterpart being anhedonia), or have invoked animal evidence that links learned helplessness (an animal model of depression) to catecholamine systems (Willner, 1983).

Van Praag (1980a) has also considered in detail the role of 5-HT. He pointed out the substantial evidence for at least a subgroup of patients having a 5-HT-deficiency syndrome that seems to persist when the depressive illness has abated. It is thus a trait factor, linked to susceptibility to develop depression and with poor control over aggression. The 5-HT deficiencies are unlikely to be secondary to increased sensitivity of the postsynaptic 5-HT receptor. First, the precursor loading studies with increased 5-HT function alleviate depressive symptoms, and second, the limited binding studies of brain or platelets do not support the hypothesis.

Other transmitter hypotheses have been put forward. The 'permissive amine hypothesis', originally suggested by Prange *et al.* (1974), stated that central 5-HT deficiency related to a vulnerability to affective illness; lowered catecholamines correlated with depression and raised values with mania. Cholinergic mechanisms have been implicated (Janowsky *et al.*, 1980), and a cholinergic–adrenergic imbalance suggested. Depression was seen as a state of cholinergic dominance, mania one of adrenergic excess. The evidence for involvement of the cholinergic system at present is very limited, being mainly of an indirect nature from the effects of drugs that influence the choline system and mood.

Recently attention has shifted from neurotransmitter levels and turnover to the role of receptors, both pre- and postsynaptic. The investigations of Sulser (1984) revealed that nearly all treatments effective in depressive illness lead to decreased activity (downregulation) of the postsynaptic noradrenergic receptor. This applies to antidepressant drugs and relates to the adenylate cyclise-linked beta receptor. This downregulation is dependent on an intact presynaptic 5-HT neuronal input, and can be reversed by 5-HT depletion. Further, the time course of these events correlates better with the known clinical effects of antidepressants, emerging over days rather than acutely. Much of the receptor-binding and neurohormonal data reviewed above have been aimed at testing hypotheses relating to alteration of monoamine-receptor activity in depressive illness. At present interpretation is difficult, but a summary is given in Table 8.14. The blunted growth-hormone responses, especially to clonidine, support decreased alpha-2 noradrenergic-receptor activity (the growth-hormone effect is probably mainly mediated by postsynaptic hypothalamic receptors), which could be accounted for by increased presynaptic noradrenergic output but decreased efficiency of the noradrenergic system. The decreased receptor sensitivity may explain some of the other neurohormonal findings, including the abnormalities of cortisol and failure to suppress with dexamethasone. However, the way in which different receptors may interact, the primacy of any changes (in other words whether a receptor modification succeeds or leads to synaptic changes of neurotransmitter activity) and the whole area of linking more traditional monoamine hypotheses to receptor theories are unresolved.

The introduction of the SSRI antidepressants has led to a renewed search for the mechanisms of action of antidepressants and the role of 5-HT and its receptors. Increased responsivity of 5-HT$_2$ receptors can lead to decreased 5-HT$_{1A}$ function, and a primary abnormality of the former can therefore explain some of the neurochemical abnormalities discussed in this chapter. However, raised cortisol can lead to a similar picture by reducing 5-HT$_{1A}$ function, leading Deakin *et al.* (1991) to suggest that the 5-HT$_{1A}$ abnormalities may be primary. Antidepressants are thought to reverse this deficit. However, the relative contribution of the 5-HT$_{1A}$ autoreceptor, as opposed to the postsynaptic receptor, is unclear. It seems that SSRIs (and MAOIs) initially lead to a flooding of the synapse with 5-HT, following which the system seems to close down. There is then, over a time course compatible with the delayed action of these drugs, a resumption of activity but a further decrease of 5-HT$_{1A}$ responsivity. This decrease of autoreceptor sensitivity enhances 5-HT release and normalizes 5-HT$_2$ receptor function.

With greater use of brain-imaging studies, the discussion has shifted to circuits and intercollated brain regions. That is, depression may involve an abnormality of a specific neuromodulator in a specific region of circuitry. Involvement of the subgenual cingulate is a good example of this thinking and much attention is now focusing on cortical–limbic regulatory circuits.

Table 8.14   Sensitivity of neuronal receptors in depression and effect of antidepressants

| | Adrenergic | | | 5-HT | | |
| | *Alpha* | | *Beta* | *1a (auto)* | *1a (postsynaptic)* | *2* |
	Presynaptic	*Postsynaptic*				
Depression	↑?	↓	↑	↓	↓	↑
Antidepressants	↓	↑?	↓	↓	↑	↓

Laterality has been discussed in relation to affective disorder, as it has for schizophrenia. Generally the evidence is less convincing, but important observations have been made. Flor-Henry (1983), starting from his own observations that patients with psychosis and epilepsy awaiting temporal lobectomy are more likely to have a manic–depressive picture if they have a nondominant-hemisphere focus, has persistently argued for a role of that hemisphere in the regulation of mood. The most persuasive data come from the EEG and psychometry studies of patients with depressive illness and patients with secondary mania. Observations of patients with CVA affecting either one or the other hemisphere (Gainotti, 1972), studies of split-brain patients and direction of gaze in response to stimuli (to the left in affective disorder and to the right in schizophrenia, the direction implying activation of the opposite hemisphere (Myslobodsky *et al.*, 1979)) have all been used to support the concept. Certainly the proposition that the nondominant hemisphere in health is concerned with emotional behaviour is convincing (Bear, 1986), and its link to affective disorders is thus a reasonable postulate. However, not all findings support this, especially the recent data from CVA, epilepsy (see Chapter 10) and imaging in primary depression. The latter emphasize frontal-basal-ganglia circuitry in the anatomy of depression, especially the prefrontal cortex (George *et al.*, 1994d). Distinctions between mania and depression are emerging, both with respect to changes of cerebral blood flow at key frontolimbic sites (increased in mania, decreased in depression) and with regards to laterality (right side in mania, left in depression).

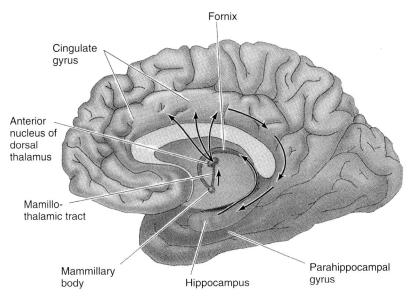

Figure 2.5   Circuit of Papez

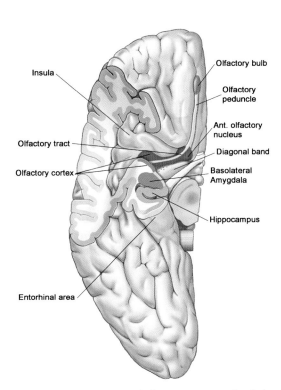

Figure 2.6   The insula, buried beneath the cortex following removal of the frontal and temporal polar opercula. The position of the amygdala, hippocampus and entorhinal cortex are shown (courtesy of Dr Gary van Hoesen)

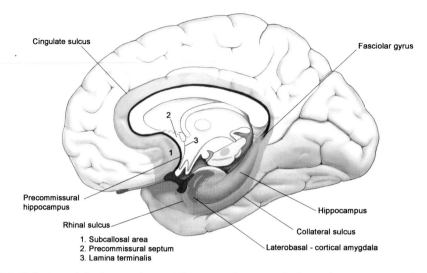

Figure 2.7 Medial view of the human brain. The areas shown in darker colours represent limbic structures (courtesy of Dr L. Heimer)

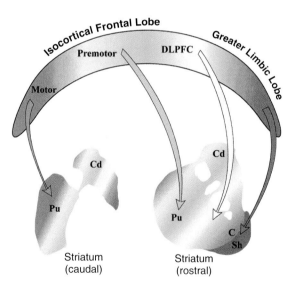

Figure 2.9 Diagram of the cortical projections (from frontal and limbic cortices), showing how the cortex projects to the basal ganglia and how this process is continuous; in essence there is no discrete break between the frontal inputs and limbic inputs. It should be noted that this figure helps to emphasize that cortico-striatal projections come from the entire cerebral cortex (courtesy of Dr L. Heimer)

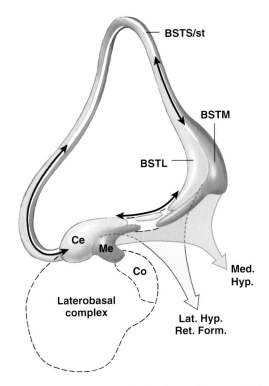

Figure 2.14 The extended amygdala shown in isolation from the rest of the brain. Ce, Central and Me, Medial amygdaloid nucli; BSTL and BSTM, lateral and medial divisions of the extended amygdale; Co, cortical amygdala nucleus; BSTS/st, supracapsula part of the bed nucleus (courtesy of Dr L. Heimer)

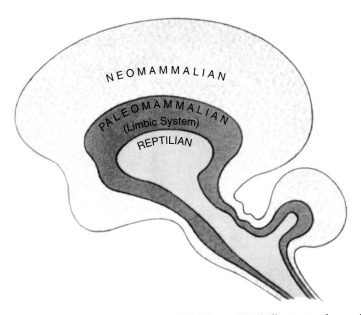

Figure 3.1 The triune brain. This diagram from Paul MacLean (1968) illustrates the evolution of the human forebrain and how it expands along the lines of three basic formations that anatomically reflect an ancestral relationship to reptiles, early mammals and late mammals (reproduced from Maclean, 1990)

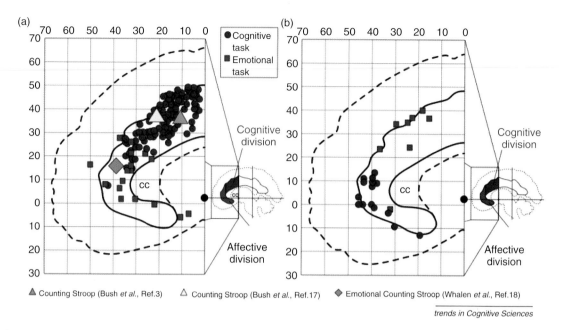

Figure 3.2 Meta-analysis of the different imaging studies carried out, highlighting the differences between the cognitive and affective divisions of the anterior cingulate. Note that the studies employing cognitive tasks, commonly employing multitasking, cause activations in the upper cingulate (in circles), while studies manipulating emotion cause activation in the lower affective division (in rectangles) (reproduced from Bush *et al.*, 2000)

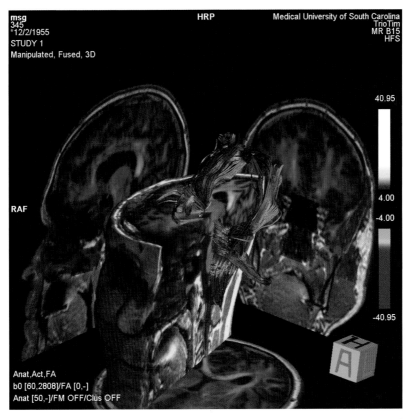

Figure 4.6 Structural MRI scan shown in 3D, with diffusion information superimposed and DTI tracts arising from brainstem (courtesy of Dr Mark George)

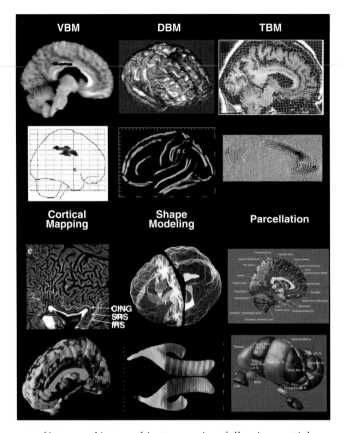

Figure 4.7 (a) The concept of inter- and intra-subject averaging, following spatial normalization. All scans are first fitted into a standard space, and subsequent comparison of pixel values is based upon standard parametric statistical techniques. Areas of significant difference between groups are illustrated as statistical maps in three formats. These are (left to right): T-maps, orthogonal projections showing areas of significant difference or surface renderings onto a standard brain template (reproduced with permission from Dr K. Friston, Wellcome Department of Cognitive Neurology, Queen Square). (b) Six major types of analysis of structural images, showing some of the main types of data used in each case. Voxel-based morphometry (VBM; top-left panels) compares anatomy voxel by voxel to find voxels (shown here in blue) where the tissue classification (grey, white matter, CSF) depends on diagnosis or other factors. Results are typically plotted in stereotaxic space (lower panel), and their significance is assessed using random field or permutation methods. Deformation-based morphometry (DBM) can be used to analyse shape differences in the cortex or brain asymmetries (coloured sulci; red colours show regions of greatest asymmetry). Tensor-based morphometry (TBM) uses 3D warping fields with millions of degrees of freedom (top) to recover and study local shape differences in anatomy across subjects or over time (red colours indicate growth rates in the corpus callosum of a young child). Other methods focus on structures such as the cerebral cortex, which can be flattened to assist the analysis (bottom left), or the lateral ventricles (shape modelling). If anatomic structures are represented as parametric surface meshes, their shapes can be compared, their variability can be visualized and they can be used to show where grey matter is lost (e.g. in Alzheimer's disease; bottom-left panel, red colours denote greatest grey-matter loss in the limbic and entorhinal areas). Fine-scale anatomical parcellation (lower right) can be used to compare structure volumes across groups, or to create hand-labelled templates that can be automatically warped onto new MRI brain datasets. This can create regions of interest in which subsequent analyses are performed (reproduced from Lawrie *et al.*, 2003, with permission of Oxford University Press)

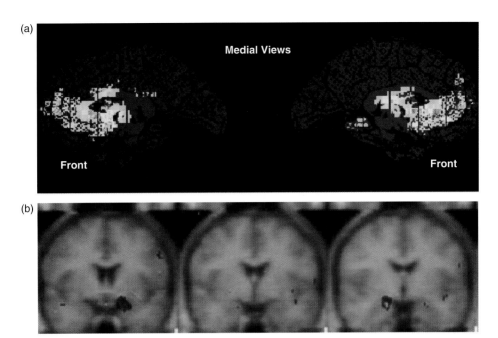

Figure 4.10 (a) Statistical parametric maps (O15 PET) of the brain regions activated during transient sadness induced by remembering sad events and viewing sad faces. The control task consisted of remembering neutral events and viewing neutral faces. Note that anterior limbic structures (septum, anterior cingulate, medial temporal (?amygdala)) and left prefrontal cortex are activated. All points in dark tone represent significant increases in activity (p < 0.01) (courtesy of Dr Mark George). (b) Three consecutive coronal slices through the brain of the group brain activation that occurs when healthy subjects are unconsciously exposed to ultra-brief (subliminal) pictures of human faces which look fearful. The subjects were unaware after the imaging study that they had even been exposed to anything unusual. Note that the 'early warning system for danger', the amygdala, bilaterally show activation during the time the subjects are exposed to the fearful faces, compared to when they are not. This was one of the first demonstrations of the rapid fear response system of the amygdala (reproduced from Whalen *et al.*, 1998)

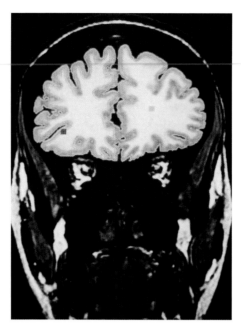

Figure 5.1 Coronal MRI scan showing the seeding points in a study by Raine and colleagues, who examined MRI-defined prefrontal white and grey matter in subjects with antisocial personality disorder, healthy age- and gender-matched controls, and controls with matched substance abuse. The antisocial-personality-disorder group had markedly smaller prefrontal grey-matter volumes (Raine and Yang, 2006; Yang *et al.*, 2005a, 2005b, 2007) (reproduced with permission from Raine *et al.*, 2000)

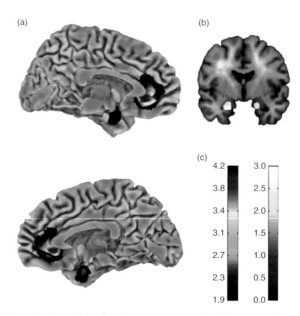

Figure 6.2 Genetic variation impacts key brain regions involved in anxiety, increasing vulnerability to dysregulation. Shown are thresholded maps ($p < 0.05$) reflecting differences in grey-matter volume in 5-HTTLPR s-allele carriers compared to the l/l genotype. Note the volume reductions in the allele carriers in the bilateral perigenual anterior cingulated cortex and amygdala (reproduced from Pezawas *et al.*, 2005)

9
The Addictions and Disorders of Motivation

INTRODUCTION

Most commentators agree that addiction to a variety of psychoactive drugs is one of the most pressing problems facing Western society at the present time. The problem embraces not only the huge cost of managing the direct consequences of substance abuse, and the criminal activity which seems to go hand-in-hand with obtaining illegal substances, but also the associated social morbidity in terms of unemployment, family breakdown and early mortality. In the United States, the National Institute on Drug Abuse (NIDA) estimates that the total cost of substance abuse is more than $484 billion per year. The World Health Organization (WHO) estimates that there are currently 2 billion alcohol abusers, 1.3 billion tobacco users and 185 million users of illicit drugs worldwide; in 2001, these three categories together contributed to 12.4% of total deaths. According to the US National Epidemiologic Survey on Alcohol and Related Conditions (NESARC), the one-year point prevalence of DSM IV substance-use disorders (excluding nicotine) is 9.35% in the United States, representing 19.4 million adults.

Such pressures call out for a coordinated approach to the addictions, and there is a desire to understand the problem from a neurobiological perspective in order to seek new avenues of treatment. Yet this area of biological psychiatry had suffered from neglect until quite recently, stemming from the almost entirely social approach to management of the addictions in times past, and to an unfortunate fragmentation of interests and funding bureaucracies. For example, those interested in alcohol abuse (funded in the USA by the National Institute on Alcohol Abuse and Alcoholism, NIAAA) have lacked interest in opiate addiction (which is funded separately and competitively through the NIDA). Both groups have historically failed to grasp how important it is to understand addiction and the processes leading to it. There needs to be a better global understanding of the more fundamental aspects of human behaviour, which are not substance-specific but interlink with substance abuse, from lethargy and apathy to drive and motivation; that is, 'what makes you tick'. Indeed, it may not be an exaggeration to state that understanding disorders of motivation lies at the heart of psychiatry in general and biological psychiatry in particular – and yet neither DSM nor ICD in any of their respective classifications recognizes disorders of motivation as an independent group of conditions. 'Substance-related disorders' are however identified in DSM IV-TR, including dependence, intoxication and withdrawal, and the various abused substances are grouped under 11 classes, from alcohol to anxiolytics and from caffeine to cannabis.

Biological Psychiatry 3e Michael R. Trimble and Mark S. George
© 2010 John Wiley & Sons, Ltd

There is also acknowledgement that abuse can occur outside of this list, and that more than one drug can be involved – polydrug abuse.

The central features of dependence are repeated compulsive self-administration, which can be associated with tolerance (needing increased quantities with diminished effect from the same amount consumed), withdrawal symptoms (physical and psychological) and craving (a strong subjective drive to use the substance). For dependence, there needs to be clinically significant impairment or distress, although abuse without any dependence but with direct harmful effects of the drug is also recognized.

Until recently, many psychiatrists, and certainly those involved in driving social policy, have viewed drug dependency simply as a social problem with social causes and social solutions in spite of the evidence from genetics, the obvious fact that the abused substances have psychoactive and hence neurochemical properties, and the developing understanding of the underlying neuroanatomy of drive and motivation, which clearly have identifiable neurobiological substrates.

DISORDERS OF MOTIVATION

Addiction is not only a brain-based disorder, it is central to an understanding of a wider spectrum of conditions referred to here as 'disorders of motivation'. These are listed in Table 9.1. In all of these disorders there is an alteration of goal-directed behaviour and a change of desire and striving. Motivation has direction and intensity, and implicates initiation of activity and persistence of such activity. In general terms, motivation can be increased or decreased. It is closely linked with

the word 'will', which is now conceptually moving from a philosophically-bound construct or a psychological faculty to a neurobiological attribute discussed in terms of frontal-lobe activity and executive functions. The word 'motivation' implies motion, moving toward or away, giving direction and change to the status quo. 'Will' expresses a desire, a subjective tone of inclination. Individual motivations are variously available to the self-reflecting consciousness. Altered motivation as a feature of hypomania and mania is manifest by increased goal-directed activity and pursuit of (high-risk) pleasurable activity; in impulsive disorders individuals fail to resist environmentally-bound directed activities (e.g. pyromania); in the obsessions and compulsions there is the persistent directing of activity to focal (pointless) goals and an inability to stop actions (or thoughts). Other disorders that have been included in this spectrum include the Klüver–Bucy syndrome (with apathy; see Chapter 5) and the Gastaut–Geschwind syndrome (with driven hypergraphia and religiosity; see Chapter 10). A pure apathy syndrome, with diminished emotional responses to goal-directed events, must not be confused with depression (although some apathy is often seen in depression), and the pure apathy syndrome does not respond to antidepressants. The right-hemisphere syndrome is seen following strokes, and emotional indifference is a central feature, with apathy or even abulia (see below) as key components. Drug-induced causes of apathy would include the obtunding sometimes seen with some psychotropic drugs, notably antipsychotics, benzodiazepines and the SSRIs. The dopamine dysregulation disorder associated with L-dopa abuse in Parkinson's disease is a disorder of increased motivation.

Table 9.1   Disorders of motivation

Decreased	*Increased*
Apathy	Addiction (substance addiction)
Abulia	Hypomania/mania
Akinetic mutism	Impulse-control disorders
Negative symptoms (depression, schizophrenia, dementias)	Obsessive–compulsive disorder
Emotional indifference/right-hemisphere syndrome	Gilles de la Tourette's syndrome
Drug-induced (antipsychotics, benzodiazapines, SSRI)	Drug-induced (L-DOPA, stimulants)

The underlying anatomy of these disorders brings the subject close to the limbic/basal-ganglia neuroanatomy discussed in Chapter 2, and lays a foundation for seeking a neurobiology of fundamental behavioural attributes which drive normal social interactions, and which become misapplied paradigmatically in disorders of motivation and, for the purposes of this chapter, in addictive behaviours.

CONDITIONING

Traditional Pavlovian conditioning involves an external stimulus, initially neutral (the conditioned stimulus (CS)), being paired with an unconditioned (biologically significant) one (unconditioned stimulus (US)); the result is the conditioned response (CR). Novel stimuli thus become paired with innate biological responses, enlarging the repertoire of an animal's behaviour. However, it is the case that such pairings are not singular, and the conditioned stimulus may attach to several associations, including an affect. With instrumental conditioning, a contingency is set up between a behaviour and a reinforcing outcome, the reward strengthening the association between the stimulus and the response, reflective of habit learning. However, the flexibility of the system is such that motivational states influence goal direction, such that both Pavlovian and instrumental conditioning are influenced by central states of 'affect'. Thus, Pavlovian-conditioned stimuli that signal an emotionally significant outcome can enhance responding: cues gain motivational significance.

In experimental psychology, stimuli that repeatedly lead to approach behaviours are considered rewarding, reflecting the positive valence of the organism to the particular circumstance. Such stimuli can either incite or reinforce actions, by invoking memories of previous reward experiences, or increasing the probability that a behaviour will be repeated. The underlying neuroanatomy, as revealed through animal investigations, involves the amygdala, the accumbens, the insula and the prefrontal cortex (orbito-frontal and medial). This underscores the importance that understanding the

new neuroanatomy of the basal forebrain has had in unravelling the biological basis of motivational behaviours generally, and addictions specifically.

All addictive drugs decrease the amount of stimulation needed in a brain-reward stimulation paradigm. The ventral striatum in particular, along with the connections to and from the basolateral amygdala, has been shown, in animal models and in human imaging studies (see below), to be the anatomical core of not only pathological addictive behaviours but also quotidian-motivated activities. Two of the main nuclear components of the amygdala (the basolateral and the central nucleus) and their afferents and efferents, at least in animal models, seem to play different roles in conditioned behaviours. The basolateral nuclei, with an important role in emotional memory, allow a conditioned stimulus (sensory inputs from the thalamus and cortex) to access the valency of an unconditioned stimulus, while the central nucleus via the extended amygdala macrosystem, the accumbens core and the medial forebrain bundle affects arousal and the overall response through downstream brainstem activation of autonomic and somatomotor outputs. There is also reverberation back to the limbic forebrain, with influence on the VTA, substantia nigra, the raphe nuclei, the locus coeruleus and the cholinergic nuclei. Cardinal *et al.* (2002c) sums this up as follows: 'we are remarkably close to this situation with the suggestion that the central nucleus of the amygdala encodes or expresses Pavlovian stimulus-response associations, while the basolateral amygdala encodes or retrieves the affective value of the predicted unconditioned stimulus' (p. 333) (see also Cardinal *et al.*, 2002a, 2002b, 2003; Robbins and Arnsten, 2009).

The accumbens and its striatal circuitry are central, being involved with stimulus-reinforcement associations and attributing motivational effects to stimuli (Cardinal *et al.*, 2002). The accumbens shell is considered most relevant, relaying information to the accumbens core to translate motivation into action, thus potentiating the behaviours, but also having outputs to the hypothalamus and brainstem.

The accumbens core then 'mediates aspects of preparatory behaviour ... not consummatory behaviour...' (Cardinal *et al.*, 2002c, p. 337). The shell is sensitive to psychoactive drugs. In addition, exposure to unconditioned stimuli or novelty causes local release of dopamine. The extended amygdala may then play a special role here, its output being directly through the medial forebrain bundle, that neuronal pleasure highway which so excited researchers in the 1950s on account of its role in self-stimulation experiments in which animals would continue to stimulate in preference to other rewards, to the limits of exhaustion. Finally, the dorsal striatum, involved in habit learning, also shows increased dopamine release during second-order reinforcement schedules, suggesting that it is related to the compulsive nature of drug-seeking. It seems that as the drug-seeking behaviour becomes established, the neuronal substrate may migrate from the accumbens shell to the core and then to the dorsal striatum: behaviourally, a shift from motivations to habits (Figures 9.1 and 9.2) (Hyman *et al.*, 2006, 2007).

Cortical influences are from the orbito-frontal cortex, with its reciprocal connections to the basolateral amygdala, its afferents from polymodal sensory cortex, and its accumbens

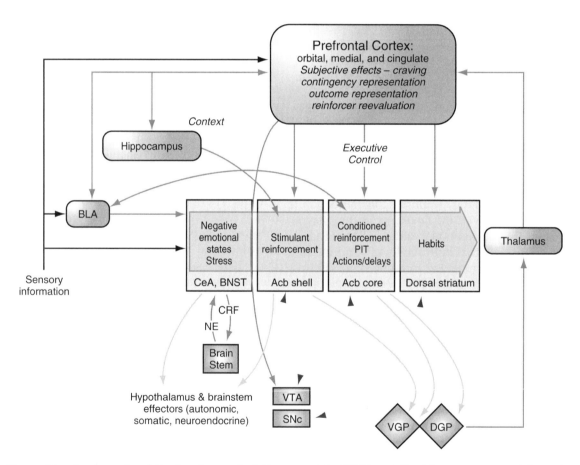

Figure 9.1 A schematic of the involvement of the amygdala (BLA) and the hippocampus, and the role of the prefrontal cortex, in the process of conditioned reinforcement, showing how habits depend on the interaction between prefrontal cortex and the dorsal striatum. Acb, accumbens; VTA, ventral tegmental area; SNc, substantianigra pars compacta; VGP, ventral pallidum; DGP, dorsal pallidum; BNST, bed nucleus of stria terminalis; NE, noradrenaline; CRF, corticotrophin-releasing factor (reproduced from Squire *et al.*, 2008)

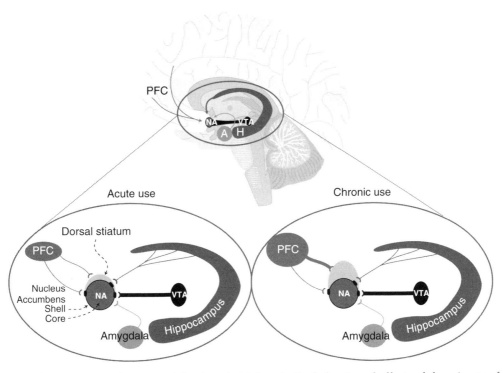

Figure 9.2   The greater involvement of the dorsal striatum in the behavioural effects of chronic use of drugs of addiction (reproduced with permission from Higgins and George 2007)

and hypothalamic influences relating to motivational state; it has been shown to contain neurones that are responsive to the reward value of stimuli such as food. The insula, as visceroreceptive cortex, is thought to be important in storing or retrieving memory of the sensory value of stimuli, and the anterior cingulate, responsive to emotionally significant stimuli, including drug-associated cues, plays some part in action selection. Dopamine has been shown to be critical for learning, and dopamine antagonists block the reinforcing properties of addictive drugs, but not the drug-seeking behaviour, supporting some of the above-noted anatomical dissociations between the different phases of the addictive process.

Social preferences, while being in part genetically determined, including drug addictions, are learned behavioural intentions, and associated social cues (such as drug-taking paraphenalia in the addictions) become conditioners for the establishment of conditioned responses. Drug cues elicit craving; the drugs, the social

surroundings and the related rituals become linked initially to intense pleasure, a learning process involving the hippocampus as well as the circuits already outlined above. Alteration of activity in these structures and their efferents with drug use leads to tolerance and craving following withdrawal of the drug. The latter intentions exert a control over future actions and become associated with dysphoria rather than euphoria, and lead on to associated mood changes and anhedonia.

GENETICS

By far the largest amount of work in genetics and addictions has been carried out on alcoholism, in part because alcohol has been a readily available substance for wide abuse over several generations. For example, it is hard to do genetic studies of ectasy, LSD or even methamphetamine addiction as these substances have only become available in recent times. There are no pedigrees of people addicted to these substances as they did not exist a couple of generations ago; it is hard to know if one's parents would have become addicted to a substance that has just been created or just become available. Moreover, many patients have polysubstance abuse, or abuse different substances in various phases of their lives, so pure pedigrees are difficult to examine by the substance of abuse (e.g. cocaine, morphine, etc). Future work in understanding the addictions will require identification of genes that either have a role in altered substance-specific vulnerabilities such as variation in drug metabolism or drug receptors, or that moderate the role of shared vulnerabilities predisposing to addiction such as variation in reward or stress resiliency, or both.

The genetic studies of alcoholism will be reviewed in this section, followed by a discussion on whether or not there are genes, or polymorphisms, that bias toward an overall addictive endophenotype. Many patients with depression or bipolar disorder also have problems with addictions. The genetic studies in those disorders have been discussed in Chapter 8. Also, there are genetic crossovers with personality disorders (see Chapter 5), particularly antisocial personality disorder (ASPD) and borderline personality disorder (BPD). Finally, the impulsivity factor in Cloninger's personality schema is associated with increased tendency to addictions.

Addictions are among the most heritable of psychiatric disorders, as shown in studies of large, carefully characterized cohorts of twins, including epidemiologically ascertained cohorts from Virginia, USA, and Australia. Heritabilities range from 0.39 (for hallucinogens) to 0.72 (for cocaine). The addiction liability of a substance generally predicts its heritability moderately well. That is, cocaine and opiates, among the most addictive of substances, are also among the most heritable. Hallucinogens are among the least addictive, and are also the least heritable. These data point toward an inheritance of variation in the core neurobiological basis of addiction discussed above, such as the pathways that mediate reward, behavioural control, obsessionality, compulsivity or stress and anxiety response.

Genetics of Alcoholism

Some individuals do not become addicted to a substance because they simply do not experience pleasure when ingesting it. For example, a human variant of the $GABA_a$ receptor has been linked to sensitivity to alcohol and benzodiazepines in relatively small datasets. Additionally, two outstanding examples of verified human 'addiction genes' encode for enzymes that catalyse consecutive steps in alcohol metabolism: alcohol dehydrogenase (ADH) and aldehyde dehydrogenase 2 (ALD). ADH metabolizes ethanol to acetaldehyde, a toxic intermediate, which is in turn converted to acetate by ALD. The most important functional loci at these genes are His47Arg in the ADH gene and Glu487Lys in the ALD gene. Either higher activity of ADH (conferred by the His47 allele) or lower activity of ALD (conferred by the Lys487 allele) leads to accumulation of acetaldehyde following an alcohol load. Acetaldehyde accumulation causes the aversive flushing reaction that discourages further alcohol intake, much like the effects of disulfiram (a drug that is used to prevent relapse) and certain antiprotozoal drugs, such as metronidazole, that inhibit ALD. In several East Asian countries, such as Japan, where both His47 and Lys487 are highly abundant, most of the population carries a heterozygous or homozygous genotype that is protective against alcoholism. The protective effect seems to vary across environments and the effects of genotypes are additive. Interestingly, each of these protective alleles apparently represents a single ancient mutation, which likely did not evolve to protect against alcoholism. Researchers think that the common gene variants might have conferred some other effect on fitness, such as protection against severe infectious diseases by protozoans, that are sensitive to inhibition of alcohol metabolism, either because of their localization in the gut or because of their lack of intrinsic aldehyde dehydrogenase (Goldman *et al.*, 2005).

In addition to genes that make it unlikely to become addicted because of a change in how the substance is metabolized, there are others that apparently predispose individuals to develop an addiction. This might be referred to as the genetics of risk-taking. Behavioural control is a name for the ability to inhibit the immediate pursuit of pleasurable stimuli and for the development of structured patterns of behaviour that produce long-term rewards. In children, deficits in developing behavioural control can lead to various problems, including substance use and abuse. For example, in the Virginia twin cohort, a common factor encompassing externalizing disorders such as ASPD and conduct disorder (CD) accounted for 71% of the genetic liability to alcoholism and 67% of the inheritance of vulnerability to illicit drug abuse or dependence. Several genes that influence impulsivity and externalization have also been found. Polymorphisms in both the DRD4 gene and the dopamine transporter have been linked to attention-deficit hyperactivity disorder (ADHD) and CD. Monoamine oxidase A (MAOA) metabolizes dopamine, and a rare stop-codon variant of this gene was linked to impulsive behaviour among males in a Dutch family. An abundant MAOA variable-number tandem-repeat locus is linked to antisocial behaviour in children. 5-HT is the neurotransmitter that is most consistently implicated in aggression and impulsivity by neurochemical and neurobehavioural studies in humans and other species. The 5-HT receptor 1B (HTR1B) gene is located at the site of several mouse alcohol quantitative trait loci (QTLs) on chromosome 9, and mice in which this gene had been knocked out were more aggressive and had a preference for alcohol. HTR1B was linked to 'antisocial alcoholism' in a Finnish family sample that was ascertained through criminal alcoholic probands, and in a south-western Native American community sample. However, replication of the association of HTR1B with impulsivity or aggression has been variable and no functional locus polymorphism is known.

There are thus genes that can protect against developing substance abuse, as well as genes that can push one to become addicted. There are also other interesting combinations: Thorgeirsson *et al.* in 2008 reported on a gene variant of the nicotinic acetylcholine receptor on chromosome 15q24 that both increases the

likelihood of becoming nicotine dependent and independently increases the risk of developing lung cancer or peripheral arterial disease. The findings provide a case study of a gene–environment interaction, highlighting the role of nicotine addiction in the pathology of other serious diseases (Stefansson *et al.*, 2009).

METABOLIC AND BIOCHEMICAL FINDINGS

Different drugs of addiction have differing neurochemical effects, but they may all lead to a similar effect on the neuroanatomical systems described above. All addictive drugs increase the activity of dopamine in the accumbens, either directly or indirectly. Some argue that this may be a final common pathway for all of the addictions. Cocaine blocks dopamine, 5-HT and noradrenaline transporters, leading to increased release of these monoamines, resulting in increased prefrontal dopamine and accumbens activity, driving motor output. On withdrawal, increased CRF release has been shown usually associated with adverse events. Amphetamine likewise potentiates monoamine activity by increasing release, also leading to motor activation. Alcohol, opiates, cannabinoids and nicotine also modulate activity in the accumbens but via different pathways. For example, opiates increase dopamine by removing the GABAergic tonic inhibitory activity on ventral tegmental dopamine cells (GABA interneurones having mu opiate receptors), while alcohol acts more directly on GABA receptors in the ventral tegmental area. Nicotine acts on nicotinic acetylcholine receptors in the ventral tegmental area, releasing dopamine. Phencyclidine antagonizes excitatory glutamate input to the accumbens, impinging on GABAergic inhibition of dopamine. Cannabinoids interact with ventral tegmental area cannabinoid receptors (Figure 9.3) (Higgins and George, 2007; Hyman *et al.*, 2006). Of the dopamine receptors, D_1, D_2 and D_3 are all involved, although D_3 receptors, found almost exclusively in the accumbens shell, are probably of most relevance since virtually all significant addictive drugs lead to increased dopamine-shell

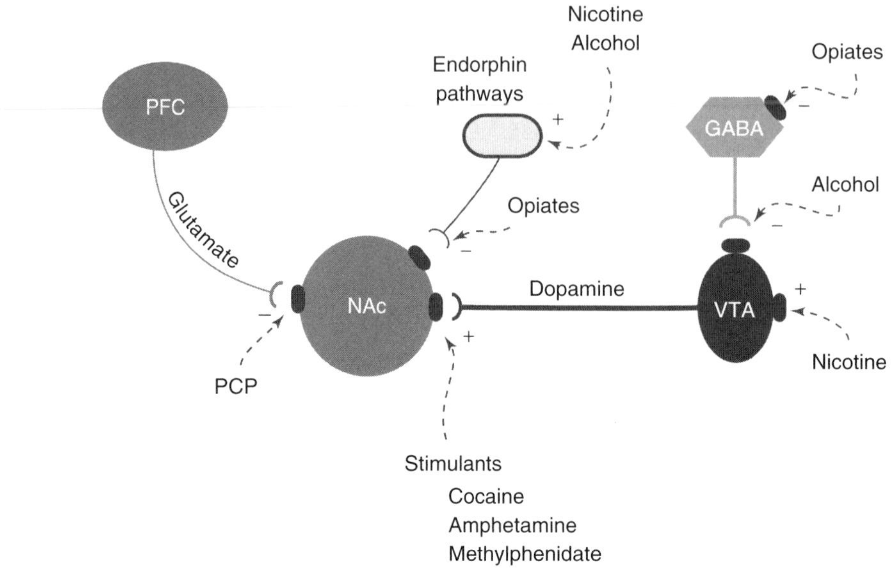

Figure 9.3 The pathways and sites of action of substance-abuse drugs on cerebral structures (reproduced with permission from Higgins and George 2007, p. 114, Figure 9.9)

activation. The precise role of dopamine remains unclear. It seems essential for reward-related learning but it does not directly relate to hedonic responses; thus it may be essential for motivation (Hyman *et al.*, 2006). However, addictive agents differ from conventional reinforcing stimuli in a lack of habituation, and repeated exposure does not lead to satiation. Natural rewards lead to brief firing of dopamine cells, whereas drugs of addiction elevate dopamine release for much longer periods of time. Abstinence with several drugs is associated with reduced dopamine transmission in the accumbens (Table 9.2). This is an anhedonic state leading to the need for the drug, satisfaction of which amplifies the incentive properties of the drug.

Other brain changes that may relate to these neurochemical intrusions of the addictive

Table 9.2 Neurotransmitters implicated in the motivational effects of withdrawal from drugs of abuse

Decreased	Increased
Dopamine	Corticotrophin-releasing factor
Opioid peptides	
5-HT	
GABA	

drugs include alteration of activity of ventral tegmental area and accumbens glutamate receptors, and morphological and molecular neuronal alterations. In animal models, an increase of the density of dendritic spines in medium spiny neurones and increased dendritic branching have been shown in the accumbens (shell and core) and medial frontal cortex with amphetamine, nicotine and cocaine, but decreases have been shown with morphine. These changes persist following drug withdrawal. More recently, research has examined intracellular mechanisms associated with learning and addiction, including the role of the transcription factors such as CREB and Fos, which bind to the promoter region of some genes and may alter the long-term activity of cells (McClung and Nestler, 2003). It is unclear whether the intracellular mechanisms that are altered in substance use are specific to addictive states, or whether they represent intrinsic natural processes that are hijacked by the drugs in the process of creating and maintaining dependency. This matters in terms of whether therapies that block or modify these processes will be specific anti-addiction therapies, or whether they are nonspecific and affect many intracellular systems, with resultant side effects.

NEUROPHYSIOLOGICAL AND NEUROLOGICAL DATA

EEG

Although the EEG has been used to investigate addictions, there are all the problems mentioned above in terms of specificity of any particular drug. There is also the confound of whether the changes predict substance abuse or arise from the use of the drug or other secondary factors associated with abuse and dependence (like delirium tremens, head injury, poor nutrition and vasculitis (cocaine)). There is EEG evidence of altered brain functional connectivity with chronic opioid abuse, with increased local and decreased remote functional connectivity in abusers (alpha and beta bands). Pathological gambling has also been shown to be associated with EEG dysfunction (Regard *et al.*, 2003). An increased P300 wave can be elicited with opiates in comparison with neutral stimuli in addicts, suggesting that drug cues acquire valence that enhances their attention. Such cue-related evoked-potential changes with drugs in addicts have also been shown for other substances (Lubman *et al.*, 2007). Cocaine craving elevates plasma cortisol levels, and with quantitative EEG it has been shown that cue exposure increases beta activity and decreases delta power in the frontal cortex.

Radiological and Brain-imaging Studies

Researchers and clinicians have used the full gamut of neuroimaging tools described in Chapter 4 to understand and characterize the addictions. To organize the discussion of this large body of studies, the imaging studies are presented as follows. There are group and even individual studies that characterize the predisposition or tendency to become addicted, or which speak to disorders of motivation or impulse control. These studies, for want of a better term, are described as imaging studies of addictive temperament or disordered motivation or impulse control. There are also imaging studies characterizing the brain changes that arise as a function of chronic substance abuse or dependence. Finally, there are newer studies attempting to actually image the brain while subjects are craving, which use the results to predict response or find new treatments.

Imaging Studies of Addictive Temperament or Disordered Motivation or Impulse Control

The above review of the neurochemical and neuroanatomical bases of addictive behaviours receives considerable support from brain-imaging studies examining individuals with an 'addictive temperament' or problems with impulse control.

Imaging studies in the amotivational state have consistently revealed problems with medial and orbito-frontal activation, similar to the changes seen in the famous orbito-frontal patient Phineas Gage. In one of the first modern studies in this area, Bench *et al.* (1993) scanned 40 depressed patients using PET. They then analysed the scans with a factor analysis. High loadings for psychomotor retardation and depressed mood correlated negatively with rCBF in the left dorsolateral prefrontal cortex and left angular gyrus. These data indicate that symptomatic specificity may be ascribed to regional functional deficits in major depressive illness. Other imaging studies focusing on the symptom of apathy or psychomotor retardation have similarly found decreased prefrontal activity (see discussion in Chapters 7 and 8).

A most interesting and controversial literature revolves around whether abnormal prefrontal or orbito-frontal structure or function predates and predisposes substance abuse, use and dependence, along with other impulsive behaviours. For example, Raine *et al.* (1994) have performed a series of imaging and psychophysiology studies in impulsive or psychopathic patients, many of whom have substance-abuse problems. In one such study, they measured MRI prefrontal grey- and white-matter volumes in 21 antisocial patients and in three control groups, comprising 34 healthy subjects (control group), 26 subjects with substance dependence (substance-dependent group) and 21 psychiatric controls. The ASPD group showed an 11.0% reduction in prefrontal grey-matter volume in the absence of ostensible brain lesions, and reduced autonomic activity during a stressor. The authors speculate that this prefrontal structural deficit may underlie the low arousal, poor fear conditioning, lack of conscience and decision-making deficits that have been found to characterize antisocial, psychopathic behaviour, and may represent a risk factor in developing substance abuse and dependence.

There is thus some brain-imaging evidence to support the idea of a functional neuroanatomy of apathy or abulia, and that disorders of prefrontal and orbito-frontal cortex might predispose patients to develop disorders of substance abuse.

There are imaging studies of hypermotivated states. Tics are involuntary, brief, stereotyped motor and vocal behaviours often associated with irresistible urges. They are states of 'hypermotivation' and are a defining symptom of the classic neuropsychiatric disorder Gilles de la Tourette's syndrome, and constitute an example of disordered human volition. Stern *et al.* (2000) used event-related [(15)O]H(2)O positron-emission tomography techniques combined with time-synchronized audio and videotaping to determine the duration of, frequency of and radiotracer input during tics in each of 72 scans from 6 patients with Gilles de la Tourette's syndrome. This permitted a voxel-by-voxel correlational analysis within statistical parametric mapping of patterns of neural activity associated with the tics. They found that tics were correlated with increased activity in the medial and lateral premotor cortices, anterior cingulate cortex, dorsolateral-rostral prefrontal cortex, inferior parietal cortex, putamen and caudate, as well as primary motor cortex, Broca's area, superior temporal gyrus, insula and claustrum. In an individual patient with prominent coprolalia, such vocal tics were associated with activity in prerolandic and postrolandic language regions, insula, caudate,

thalamus and cerebellum, while activity in sensorimotor cortex was noted with motor tics. These researchers concluded that aberrant activity in the interrelated sensorimotor, language, executive and limbic circuits might account for the initiation and execution of diverse motor and vocal behaviours that characterize tics in Gilles de la Tourette's syndrome, as well as for the urges that often accompany them (Stern *et al.*, 2000).

Imaging Studies of the Consequences of Abuse

While the studies above are somewhat theoretical, and controversial, there is a much larger and noncontroversial body of imaging studies detailing the damage that chronic substance-abuse dependence might produce in the brain. To summarize this literature, it is easiest to state that there is no real consensus on long-term brain damage associated with tobacco (except for the associated cardiovascular changes and risk of cancer), cannabis, benzodiazepines and opiates.

There are however many studies detailing the damage caused by alcohol, cocaine and to a lesser extent MDMA (ecstacy). It is very clear that chronic alcohol use causes brain damage, and that the entire brain volume shrinks. MRI studies have documented ventricular volume enlargement as well as deficits in grey- and white-matter volumes in alcoholics as compared to nonalcoholic subjects (for review see George *et al.*, 2002; Mann *et al.*, 2001). This cellular loss is greater in older alcoholics than younger alcoholics, even after the duration and amount of alcohol consumed are taken into consideration. The loss in both grey and white matter is different than that found in other neurodegenerative disorders such as Alzheimer's disease, in which the cell loss is grey matter alone. In addition, the grey- and white-matter loss in alcoholics is most pronounced in the frontal lobes. Interestingly, some but not all of the brain-volume loss associated with alcoholism has been found to reverse within a few weeks of abstinence.

While many studies have evaluated brain structure in alcoholic men, alcoholic women have received less research attention. Women may be more vulnerable to the brain effects of alcohol, given that while they develop alcoholism later in life, they often manifest adverse consequences of alcoholism sooner than do male alcoholics, a phenomenon often referred to as 'telescoping'. For example, two early studies using CT found that male and female alcoholics had a similar effect on ventricle:brain ratio despite the fact that the women had less daily alcohol consumption. This led to the hypothesis that women may be more vulnerable to the toxic effects of alcohol. Hommer and colleagues (2001) evaluated 43 alcohol-dependent men and 36 alcohol-dependent women, as well as 39 healthy control subjects. They found that the alcoholic women had greater white- and grey-volume loss as well as increased sulcal and ventricular volumes compared to control females. Furthermore, the difference in brain-volume loss, particularly in the grey matter, was greater in the females than the males. However, Pfefferbaum and colleagues (2001) performed volumetric MRI measurements on age- and length of sobriety-matched alcoholic men and women as well as age-matched healthy controls. While the alcoholic women showed no differences in brain-volume indices in comparison to healthy control women, alcoholic men showed volume deficits compared to nonalcoholic men (Mann *et al.*, 2001a). These findings are consistent with a PET study in which alcoholic men had deficits in energy utilization which were not found in alcoholic women. Thus, while some studies have supported the idea that women are more vulnerable to the detrimental brain effects of alcohol than are men, more research is needed to conclusively settle the issue. The role of diet and other comorbid conditions needs further exploration as well.

In addition to examining brain structure, neuroimaging technology has also been utilized to examine brain function in alcoholism. These studies have evaluated brain activity after immediate cessation of alcohol use, as well as after sustained abstinence. Unfortunately there are relatively few neuroimaging studies in close temporal proximity to alcohol withdrawal. Volkow and colleagues (1992) used PET scans in recently-abstinent alcoholics (6–32 days) and healthy controls and found that alcoholics had lower overall brain metabolic rates. In a follow-up study in 1994, 10 alcoholic men were serially scanned using glucose PET at 8, 16 and 30 days after their last use of alcohol. These scans were then compared over time with scans from 10 age-matched nonalcoholic healthy controls. On the scan 8 days after alcohol cessation, alcoholics showed lower brain metabolism in numerous brain regions compared to the control group; over the period of abstinence, brain metabolism improved significantly (Volkow *et al.*, 1994). Berglund and Risberg (1981) found a significant global reduction in CBF in 12 subjects in the first two days of withdrawal with the ^{133}Xe inhalation method. However, they reported relatively high temporal and low parietal flows coupled with aggravated symptoms of alcohol withdrawal. Caspari *et al.* (1993) studied 15 alcoholics with perfusion single-photon-emission-computed tomography (SPECT) during day 1 or 2 of acute alcohol withdrawal and again three weeks later. During acute alcohol withdrawal, relative perfusion was elevated in the bilateral inferior temporal regions and reduced in the bilateral superior temporal regions.

To evaluate the role of the pattern of alcohol use on regional brain activity, George *et al.* (1999) studied 14 adults with brain perfusion SPECT on days 7–9 following their last drink and 2–3 days since their last detoxification medication. Seven healthy adults were scanned as control subjects. The alcoholics, compared to controls, had widely reduced relative activity in cortical secondary-association areas and relatively increased activity in the medial temporal lobes. Thus, while functional neuroimaging studies examining the basal 'resting' state of the brain following alcohol cessation have demonstrated that chronic alcohol use globally reduces neuronal activity for several weeks, the limbic area seems to exhibit increased activity during this period.

Chronic cocaine causes selective vasoconstriction and can lead to white-matter abnormalities and strokes. Since the development of alkaloidal 'crack' cocaine in the 1980s, there has been a significant rise in the number of case reports describing both ischemic and hemorrhagic stroke associated with cocaine use. The exact mechanism of cocaine-induced stroke remains unclear but there are likely to be a number of factors involved, including vasospasm, cerebral vasculitis, enhanced platelet aggregation, cardioembolism and hypertensive surges associated with altered cerebral autoregulation. The use of MDMA (ecstasy), a popular recreational drug, has been related to ischemic and hemorrhagic cerebrovascular events, as well as atrophy.

Imaging Studies of Craving

Researchers have been able to induce craving for substances while subjects are inside the fMRI or PET scanner. Interestingly, and consistent with the neuroanatomy discussed above, there is a large convergence of these studies. Craving involves a common neurobiology regardless of the object being craved, be it chocolate, a loved one or crack cocaine. These studies are summarized in Figure 9.4. Some groups are using this craving signal induced within the fMRI scanner

Drugs

1. Cocaine
2. Alcohol
3. Amphetamines
4. Methylphenidate
5. Nicotine

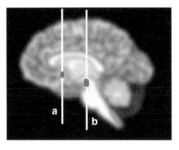

Feelings

6. Romantic love
7. Listening to music
8. Humor
9. Expectation of $$$
10. Inflicting punishment
11. Looking at beautiful faces
12. Social cooperation
13. Eating chocolate

a. Nucleus accumbens   b. Ventral tegmental area

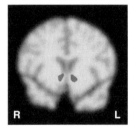 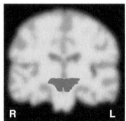

Drugs

1. Acute Effects of Cocain on Human Brain Activity and Emotion. Neuron 1997;19:591-611.
2. Alcohol Promotes Dopamine Release in the Human Nucleus Accumbens. Synapse 2003; 49: 226-31.
3. SPECT Imaging of Srtiatal Dopamine Release After Amphetamine Challenge. J Nuc Med 1995;36:1182-90.
4. Role of Dopmaine in the Therapeutic and Reinforcing Effects of Methylphenidate in Humans:Results from Imaging Studies. Eu Neuropsychophar 2002; 12:557-66.
5. Nicotine-induce Limbic Cortical Activation in the Human Brain: a Functional MRI Study. Am J Psych 1998;155:1009-15.

Feelings

6. Reward, Motivation, and Emotion Systems Associated with Early-Stage Intense Romantic Love. J Neurophysiol 2005;94:327-337.
7. Intensely Pleasurable Responses to Music Correlate with Activity in Brain Regions Implicated in Reward and Emotion. PNAS 2001;98:11818-23.
8. Humor Modulates the Mesolimbic Reward Centers. Neuron 2003;40:1041-48.
9. Functional Imaging of Neural Responses to Expectancy and Experience of Monetary Gains and Losses. Neuron 2001;30:619-39.
10. The Neural Basis of Altruistic Punishment. Science 2004;305:1254-8.
11. Beautiful Faces Have Variable Reward Value:fMRI and Behavioral Evidence. Neuron 2001;32;537-551.
12. A Neural Basis for Social Cooperation. Neuron 2002; 35:395-405.
13. Changes in Brain Activity Related to Eating Chocolate. Brain 2001;124:1720-33.

Figure 9.4   Summary of craving studies, showing how the same structures are involved in addiction and craving irrespective of the substance or object of desire (reproduced with permission from Higgins and George 2007, p. 111)

to screen potential treatments before they are used in a large-scale clinical trial (George *et al.*, 2001; Myrick *et al.*, 2008).

Associations with Neurological Disease

Patients with primary amotivational states are frequently encountered in clinical practice, and secondary disorders of motivation are noted in a wide variety of psychopathologies (Table 9.3). The latter merge with apathy and flattened affect, and with anergia (as seen in the chronic fatigue syndrome or in hypothyroidism). The paradigm of a primary motivational state is abulia, in which the patient literally has no will. Patients will sit in a chair all day long doing nothing. Whereas in apathy, patients cannot be bothered to do things, in abulia there is simply no desire. Further, when asked if they ever feel bored, patients with abulia simply say, 'no'. The latter disorder is most frequently encountered in patients with basal-ganglia disorders, especially those which damage or destroy anterior cingulate and striatal connections. Abulia may be seen in Parkinson's disease, but also following strokes to the basal ganglia and head injuries which impinge on fronto-striatal structures. Secondary disorders of decreased motivation are seen in the schizophrenias (with negative symptoms), in some depressions (with apathy and anhedonia) and in such disorders as the emotional indifference of a Klüver–Bucy syndrome. Apathy may be a feature of pituitary and hypothalamic disease (e.g. adenomas or craniopharyngiomas) and has been associated with alteration of the morphology of the accumbens in HIV patients. Bhatia *et al.* (1993) studied the behavioural and movement disorders reported in 240 patients with lesions affecting the caudate nucleus, putamen and globus

pallidus (lentiform nucleus). Dystonia was the most frequent movement disorder recorded (36%), but the most common behavioural disturbance was the syndrome of abulia (13%), mainly noted with caudate lesions (28%). Depression was a relatively nonspecific finding.

Increased states of motivation occur in association with hypomanic and mania drivenness; the intensely driven motor behaviour of Gilles de la Tourette's syndrome, which is often associated with comorbid OCD; the latter too may be viewed as another dysregulation of motivation.

The main conditions leading to alteration of motivation therefore involve frontal- or basal-ganglia function, and imply either overactivity or underactivity in the cortico–striatal–pallidal–thalamic re-entrant circuits described in Chapters 2 and 3.

Neuropsychological Disturbances

All the addictive substances or their metabolites cross the blood–brain barrier and will lead to acute toxicity, with interference with a subject's ability to perform neuropsychological tests. These effects should be short-lived and will abate as the drug is washed out from the brain. However, there is growing evidence of longer-term use leading to alterations of cognition. Unfortunately, obtaining data is very difficult. Many people are polydrug abusers; their pre-ingestion cognitive abilities will be largely unknown, and their drug histories unreliable. Some drugs such as cocaine may lead on to neurological disorders from vasculitis or seizures, which themselves alter cognition. Since the individual drugs have differing chemical profiles, some neuropsychological differences of long-term use may be expected, but are hard to identify under the generalized cognitive blunting that is often reported.

Cannabis use has been associated with memory and attentional deficits and an amotivational state. Chronic cocaine ingestion impairs executive function, psychomotor speed and manual dexterity, which effects persist after periods of abstinence. Amphetamine abuse is reported to lead to poor decision-making (akin to orbital-frontal deficits) and impaired

Table 9.3 Neuropsychiatric disorders where there is alteration of motivation

Parkinson's disease and variants
Basal-ganglia lesions
Frontal-lobe disorders
Obsessive–compulsive disorder
Gilles de la Tourette's syndrome
Encephalitis

spatial working memory, while opiate abuse leads to delayed decision-making and a similar working-memory problem. A common theme underlying these findings, especially with stimulants, is disruption of monoamine influences in association with disordered frontal-lobe function.

The increased use of ecstasy has attracted considerable interest, and it has been associated with deficits of immediate and delayed memory and attention, the former correlating with diminished 5-HT turnover as measured by CSF 5-HIAA levels, even after periods of abstinence (Quednow *et al.*, 2006, 2007).

Chronic alcohol abuse has been reported to impair cognition across several domains, with mild to moderate difficulties of executive function and visuospatial abilities, but relative sparing of episodic memory. Alcohol has been shown to inhibit neurogenesis, which may have something to do with these cognitive deficits. The neurocognitive deficits have been shown to be partially reversible with abstinence (Gilman and Hommer, 2008). Interestingly, in the serial functional imaging studies in abstinent alcoholics, which show a gradual return of function over the course of at least one month (George *et al.*, 1999), the areas most affected persistently following chronic alcohol use are not primary motor or sensory but rather multimodal association areas used in higher cognitive tasks.

The cognitive impairments identified in these studies may have profound consequences, not only making the road to rehabilitation more difficult, but also, by decreasing impulse control, unfortunately fostering the tendency to continue the illicit drug-taking.

SOME OUTSTANDING ISSUES

Drugs are not the only rewarding factors in our lives, and many social stimuli from food to gambling to sex are reinforcing. As with drugs, surrounding environmental contexts assume significance to enhance the chance of a behavioural sequence, but there are differences between addictive drugs and natural rewards from a cultural point of view. Drug rewards may seem overwhelming of other ones, narrowing the behavioural repertoire, and ultimately depriving the individual of a healthy life. However, some addictions, like that of the workaholic, have equal drive, motivation and behavioural consequences, but are channelled in a socially accepted manner.

The reviewed literature suggests that similar cerebral and neurochemical systems underlie these behaviours, whether drug-driven or not. This raises the important questions of when a behaviour becomes pathological, and what are the neurobiological correlates of the pathogenesis. Genetic influences are clearly important in the ease with which addictive behaviours are acquired, as may be the risk for comorbid psychiatric disorders such as bipolar disorder or schizophrenia. These two categories of psychopathology are frequently comorbid with substance abuse, and substance abuse is often a precursor to the later psychopathology, perhaps initially providing self-medication for developing symptoms (such as benzodiazepine, alcohol or cigarette use to calm anxiety). Also, cannabis use is often a precursor to the development of schizophrenia (see Chapter 7). The underlying neurobiology of addictive behaviours outlined in this chapter reveals circuits and neurotransmitters that cross over with major psychopathology. Not only can this enlighten the understanding of the biology of the specific psychiatric disorder, but unravelling the neurochemical and neuroanatomical associations which are common with addictive behaviours will enhance preventative and treatment possibilities.

The role of the limbic forebrain and dopamine is so important in driving behaviour that damage to such structures may be expected to have profound clinical effects. Indeed it does, but disorders of motivation find no place in such diagnostic manuals as the DSM IV-TR, and as such are poorly recognized clinically and are underdiagnosed. Understanding of the neuroanatomy of the limbic forebrain allows for a better comprehension of these behaviours, which are intimate with that prime force, referred to as the 'will', once seen as an independent psychological faculty, now viewed as tightly bound with identifiable neuroanatomical and neurochemical substrates. Such abrogation of traditional philosophy many find uncomfortable.

A reclassification scheme of psychopathology focusing on the spectrum of disorders of motivation would aid the field in numerous ways. It is difficult to educate, diagnose and treat amotivational disorders (e.g. abulia) if they are not listed in classification schemes such as DSM IV-TR. Additionally, focusing on the overarching problem of disordered motivation might also improve understanding of some other conditions, such as the eating disorders (which unfortunately, due to space issues, are not covered in this text). One might also place catatonia under the umbrella of disordered motivation, with the hypothesis being that the catatonic patient is well motivated but is unable to translate this into subsequent movement. These suggestions arise from imaging studies showing that catatonic patients have widespread and active brain metabolism, which requires inhibition (e.g. benzodiazepines) in order that normal behaviour can resume (de Tiege *et al.*, 2003).

More recent human studies, a spin-off from the direct studies of drug addiction, have combined brain imaging, notably fMRI, and social reward tasks (for money or other positive reward pairings – attractive faces as opposed to unattractive ones). Studies using fMRI have revealed how the accumbens is reliably activated in states of expectancy, in euphoria and with craving for not only drugs of addiction but also sexual cues (see Figure 9.4) (Breiter *et al.*, 1997). This line of research is leading to understanding of human motivation in a more general way, which when combined with genetics will profile the brain associations of motivations and their subsequent behaviours in some detail. Although much of the work in unravelling the

neurobiology has come from animal studies, the basics seem to hold for humans. At the present time, investigators are attempting to define an integrative model of addictive behaviours which includes the ventral tegmental area, accumbens, hippocampus and amygdala (related to salience attribution); the cingulate gyrus–prefrontal, orbitofrontal cortex and accumbens (related to craving and expectation); and loss of top-down regulation associated with frontal cortex changes (with bingeing and loss of control) (Kalivas and Volkow, 2002). Many attempts at therapy now specifically target different aspects of the complex behaviours associated with addiction, which map rather nicely on to these various circuits.

The work with drugs of addiction is also leading to an understanding of basic mechanisms of learning, the development of long-term potentiation, the role of glutamate receptors, the importance of dopamine and the links between episodic and emotional cues to learning and memory. Persistence of relapse long after stopping an addictive drug suggests long-term brain adaptations. These have been likened to the setting up of memory traces, responding to renewed presentation of past salient external and internal cues.

In view of the importance to neuroscience and to society of studying addicts and their propensities, it is disappointing that, until recently, relatively little funding has been given or directed research carried out. Since all drugs of addiction lead to a final common neurochemical and neuroanatomical pathway, it is strange that historically specialists in alcohol addiction seem to be divorced from those interested in cocaine and so on. Further, so many of those involved in treatments seem uninterested in the basic anatomy and chemistry, and still consider that the problem is one of only a social dimension, devoid of any neurobiological substrate.

10
Epilepsy

INTRODUCTION

The longstanding relationship between epilepsy and psychiatry has already been noted. The links have been explored by a number of authors (Temkin, 1971) and stem back to at least the ancient Greek tradition. It is only in the 20th century that chronic epilepsy has become more the province of neurology than psychiatry. However, there are four reasons why psychiatrists need to know about epilepsy and its complications. First, the history of its association with psychiatry emphasizes the changing nature of ideas with regards to neuropsychiatric conditions, both their supposed pathogenesis and their psychopathological manifestations. Second, in any psychiatric setting, patients with epilepsy, particularly chronic epilepsy with continuing uncontrolled seizures, are still seen. Third, some forms of epilepsy, particularly temporal-lobe epilepsy, are associated with cognitive and emotional sequelae which closely resemble psychopathology seen in non-epileptic patients. Finally, many drugs and stimulation devices used in the management of epilepsy have also been used to treat psychopathology, from the bromides and barbiturates to, more recently, lamotrigine and vagus nerve stimulation.

PREVALENCE AND CLINICAL CHARACTERISTICS

Defining epilepsy is, as with schizophrenia, difficult. The often-quoted definition of Hughlings Jackson, of 'occasional, sudden, rapid and local discharges of grey matter' (Taylor, 1958, p. 100), emphasizes the acute paroxysmal nature of the disorder, but fails to distinguish it from other similar disorders such as migraine or acute panic attacks. Further, it misses the point that the seizure is but one manifestation of the underlying anatomico/physiological disorder of the brain which leads to the potential to have seizures. Thus, while it is accepted that the cardinal clinical symptom of epilepsy is the seizure, and it is usual to accept that epilepsy requires recurrent seizures as opposed to a single seizure before the diagnosis can be made, it has to be emphasized that epilepsy refers to a heterogeneous group of conditions, and, like schizophrenia, clear evidence for organic brain dysfunction becomes evident the more it is looked for. However, in a number of cases, even with modern technology, recurrent seizures are found in the absence of identifiable neuropathology.

CLASSIFICATION

It is important to distinguish the classification of seizures from that of epilepsy. An abbreviated version of the classification of seizures is given in Table 10.1. Although this classification dates back to 1981, it is still generally accepted and no new version has yet been published.

Partial seizures are those in which the clinical and EEG changes suggest a focal onset, and the classification is based mainly on whether or

Table 10.1 Revised ILAE classification of epileptic seizures (1981)

I. Partial (focal, local) seizures
   A. Simple partial seizures (consciousness not impaired)
   B. Complex partial seizures (with impairment of consciousness; may sometimes begin with simple symptomatology)
   C. Partial seizures evolving to secondarily generalized seizures (this may be generalized tonic–clonic, tonic or clonic)
II. Generalized seizures (convulsive or nonconvulsive)
III. Unclassified epileptic seizures

not consciousness is impaired in the attack. In a simple partial seizure, consciousness is retained. Various forms are recognized, for example focal motor seizures (when accompanied by a march these are referred to as Jacksonian); seizures with somatosensory or special sensory symptoms; with autonomic symptoms; or with psychic symptoms such as dysphasia, dysmnesia (for example déjà vu), cognitive, affective, illusory or hallucinatory experiences. This last group of symptoms is usually accompanied by impairment of consciousness, and therefore is often associated with complex partial seizures. In these, the impairment of consciousness is often the first clinical sign, although simple partial seizures may evolve into the complex variety. In patients presenting to psychiatric clinics, complex partial seizures are the commonest seizure type, and they usually, but not inevitably, give a history of progression to occasional generalized motor seizures.

Generalized seizures are those in which the first clinical changes suggest bilateral abnormalities with widespread disturbances of both hemispheres. Absence seizures (petit mal) are usually associated with regular 3 Hz spike and slow-wave activity on the EEG, although variants of this with 2–3 Hz activity may be seen. Myoclonic seizures typically present with myoclonic jerking, and are sometimes associated with clearly delineated EEG changes. Tonic–clonic seizures are the classical grand mal attacks with associated EEG abnormalities.

Finally, seizures that cannot be classified into the above groupings are included as unclassified seizures.

Classic tonic–clonic seizures are unmistakable. There is sudden loss of consciousness, often without warning, and tonic muscular contractions are followed by clonic ones. Following the attack, the patient is unrousable for a time, and there follows a period of postictal confusion. If the attack has a focal origin prior to its generalization then the patient may experience an aura, namely a brief feeling or sensation immediately before the attack, which represents the origin of the epileptic activity. These auras need to be distinguished from prodomata, which occur several hours or even days before a seizure, and serve to warn the patient that one is forthcoming. Prodromal symptoms are often changes of mood, but may also be headaches or changes of appetite.

Generalized seizures that present as absence attacks impair consciousness briefly and are virtually unaccompanied by motor signs. They occur primarily in children and in many cases cease before the age of 20, although in about 50% of patients this form of seizure is replaced by generalized tonic–clonic seizures. In the generalized absence seizure there is sudden arrest of attention, some blinking and eye-fluttering and perhaps pallor with subsequent amnesia.

The symptoms of focal attacks correspond to the site of origin of abnormal electrical activity, the commonest disturbances seen in psychiatric practice relating to a temporal-lobe location. There may be disturbance of thought, perception, behaviour, affect and, in complex partial attacks, consciousness. Hallucinations may be formed and complex, as opposed to those which arise from seizures of primary sensory cortex, which are usually simple, for example a flash of light. Characteristically in epilepsy the hallucination is constant and with repeated episodes is carefully reproduced. Any recognized emotion may occur, although the commonest experience is fear, which is intense, and is often associated with a fear of death. Ictal fear may be commoner with right temporal lesions (Hermann *et al.*, 1992), and associated with the development of paranoid states (Devinsky *et al.*, 1991). The only aura that has been reliably shown to have lateralizing significance is that of déjà vu to the right temporal lobe (Palmini and Gloor, 1992). Depression is uncommon but well documented (Robertson and Trimble, 1983), although rage and outbursts of anger are rare. Cursive seizures refer to running during attacks; gelastic seizures are laughing attacks, while those associated with crying, which are rarer, are called dyscrastic seizures. In uncinate seizures, the patient experiences an unpleasant smell or taste, usually unidentifiable, and this may be accompanied by chewing movements and lip-smacking.

Automatisms, which may occur with partial or generalized seizures, refer to 'all kinds of doings after epileptic fits, from slight vagaries up to homicidal actions' (Jackson, quoted in Taylor, 1958, p. 122). Characteristically, the motor activity is automatic and occurs during a state of altered consciousness, for which time there is amnesia. During automatisms, which generally last less than 15 minutes, patients carry out complex quasi-purposeful behaviour; violence is unusual, but if the patient is interfered with during the automatism, aggression may result. The neurophysiological basis for automatisms is thought to be bilateral involvement of the amygdaloid–hippocampal region (Fenton, 1972).

Myoclonic seizures are sudden, brief jerk-like contractions which may be generalized or confined to one or more muscle groups. They may be solitary or repetitive, and may be triggered by action. They commonly occur late at night or early in the morning, and in some people herald a generalized tonic–clonic seizure.

Status epilepticus denotes recurrent epileptic seizures without return of consciousness between attacks. Persistent focal seizures are referred to as epilepsia partialis continua, and when complex partial seizures are continuous (complex partial-seizure status), prolonged states of behaviour disturbance may be seen. These occur with detectable but minimal alteration of higher cognitive function, and associated hallucinations and delusions may closely resemble those of schizophrenia. In contrast, during absence status, prolonged alteration of cognitive function occurs with intermittent prolonged stupor. Occasionally it may present as a psychotic illness, with hallucinations and delusions, intermingled with a fluctuating confusional state and associated EEG changes.

Although approximately 1 in 20 people may have a seizure during their lifetime, the prevalence of epilepsy is far less, being around 0.5% for the general population. The currently-used classification of the epilepsies is shown in Table 10.2 (ILAE, 2006).

Terms found in earlier classifications of epilepsy, such as 'primary' and 'secondary', have been omitted and the main dichotomy separates epilepsies with generalized seizures from those with partial or focal seizures, the latter being referred to as localization-related partial or focal epilepsies. The term 'cryptogenic' was introduced to reflect disorders in which the aetiology was assumed to be symptomatic but was hidden or occult. Subsequent discussions have revealed the unsatisfactory nature of the term, and indeed of the classification scheme generally, but as yet no revised version has been published (Engel, 2006a, 2006b). Of particular relevance for psychiatrists are the localization-related symptomatic seizures, further designated by the area of localization affected. For example, frontal-lobe epilepsies often present as brief episodes of behavioural change with minimal or no postictal confusion.

Table 10.2 Classification of epilepsies (ILAE, 1989)

1. Localization-related (focal, local, partial) epilepsies and syndromes
   Idiopathic with age-related onset, e.g. benign epilepsy of childhood
   Symptomatic, e.g. frontal lobe, temporal lobe
   Cryptogenic, presumed symptomatic with unknown aetiology
2. Generalized epilepsies or syndromes
   Idiopathic, e.g. juvenile myoclonic epilepsy
   Cryptogenic and/or symptomatic, e.g. West's syndrome
   Symptomatic
3. Epilepsies and syndromes undetermined as to whether they are focal or generalized
4. Special syndromes, e.g. febrile convulsions

There may be deviation of the head and eyes, sometimes referred to as an adversive seizure. The sudden onset of some frontal seizures, followed by sometimes bizarre motor movements often of the lower limbs (cycling-like), may lead these attacks to be diagnosed as pseudoseizures (they are in fact pseudopseudoseizures!).

Under temporal-lobe epilepsies there is a category with particular emphasis on hippocampal and amygdala pathology. These epilepsies characteristically present with partial seizures, alteration of consciousness and often automatisms.

Some distinctive syndromes are included in the classification of epilepsies. West's syndrome (infantile spasms) consists of a characteristic picture of infantile spasms in association with hypsarrhythmia on the EEG. The onset is in the first year of life, and the spasms are flexor or extensor, or both. Males are affected more commonly than females, and a symptomatic subgroup is recognized with clear evidence of pre-existing brain damage.

Lennox–Gastaut syndrome occurs in children up to the age of about 8 and presents with a variety of seizures, focal, myoclonic, atonic and absence, with a markedly disturbed EEG and associated learning disability.

Benign childhood epilepsy is a syndrome that affects children between 3 and 16 years of age. It has a good prognosis, and presents with simple partial seizures, which may or may not lead to secondary generalized attacks, and an EEG with characteristic centrotemporal spikes.

Juvenile myoclonic epilepsy (Janz's syndrome) presents in late childhood or early adolescence with myoclonic jerks, especially in the early mornings, which may or may not progress to generalized tonic–clonic attacks.

Landau–Kleffner syndrome (LKS) is a childhood disorder consisting of an aquired aphasia associated with paroxysmal EEG changes, usually bitemporal. The latter changes are often seen in slow-wave sleep, and for this reason this disorder may be closely linked with the syndrome of continuous spike and waves in slow-wave sleep (CSWS, also known as electrical status epilepticus of slow-wave sleep, ESES). In the latter, up to 85% of sleep may be infiltrated by the EEG changes, and severe behavioural changes follow. In LKS permanent disruption of linguistic processing may occur.

Rasmussen's encephalitis is a chronic hemispheric encephalitis, of unknown aetiology but sometimes following blunt trauma, associated with seizures.

The prognosis of epilepsy is dependent upon the aetiology, the age of onset of the condition and the setting in which outcome is examined. While in the majority of patients the outlook is favourable, and some 55–68% of patients with new-onset disorder will become seizure-free, and if children are followed into adulthood, over 60% will have gone into long-term remission (Beghi *et al.*, 2009; Hauser and Beghi, 2008). The most striking association with failure of treatment to control the attacks is the presence of additional neurological or psychiatric illness (Shorvon and Reynolds, 1982). In particular, patients with combined partial and generalized seizures and those with symptomatic epilepsy show a poorer prognosis.

Sudden unexpected death in epilepsy (SUDEP) occurs with an incidence around 0.09–2.7 per 1000 person years, and the causes are unknown.

Why patients have seizures when they do is not clear, although 'reflex epilepsy', where seizures are provoked by sensory or motor events, has been well described. Visually-evoked seizures, by photic stimulation, and musicogenic seizures, in which attacks are triggered by patterned tones, are well-known examples. 'Psychogenic seizures', where seizures are evoked by specific mental activity, also occur. Fenwick (1981) divides these into primary and secondary types. In the former, a direct act of will precipitates seizures, for example intense concentration or sudden alteration of attention. In the latter there is precipitation by a mental act without the deliberate intention of the patient. Examples include attacks brought on by mental arithmetic, or solving Rubik's cube. (The use of the term 'psychogenic' here is clearly different from its use signifying one form of non-epileptic (pseudo)seizure.)

GENETICS

The division of epilepsy into idiopathic and symptomatic groups recognizes that in many patients there is no known or suspected aetiology other than potential hereditary disposition. It has been shown that there is an increased incidence of seizures in siblings of epileptic patients (6–12%) (Andermann, 1980), and the concordance rate for MZ (12–100%) is higher than for DZ (0–35%) twins (Newmark and Penry, 1980). Further, an abnormal EEG is common in close relatives of epileptic patients, particularly showing generalized spike-and-wave discharges (Newmark and Penry, 1980).

The hereditability of epilepsy depends to a considerable extent on the seizure type of the proband, being greatest for generalized-seizure disorders and least for partial and symptomatic seizures. However, most studies suggest a slight increase in positive family histories of patients with symptomatic seizures, emphasizing an environmental–genetic interaction.

Of particular interest has been the discovery of a specific pathological lesion, namely mesial temporal sclerosis, in some patients who have simple and complex partial seizures. It is often unilateral, and specifically there is sclerosis of the hippocampus and related structures of the temporal lobe, with neuronal loss and increased glial elements. Many patients who develop this have a history of febrile convulsions in childhood, and similar lesions can be produced in primates by experimentally provoking seizures (Meldrum, 1976). It has been suggested that the pathology represents damage to the temporal lobe which occurs secondary to anoxic episodes at vulnerable periods during life. Since children with febrile convulsions are likely to have a positive family history for epilepsy (Newmark and Penry, 1980), it seems they inherit a lowered seizure threshold. This renders them prone to febrile convulsions and to the resulting structural damage. The latter then leads to an even greater chance of the development of complex partial seizures in adult life, emphasizing the complexities of environmental and genetic interactions in these conditions.

There are a number of Mendelian epilepsy syndromes such as progressive myoclonic epilepsies (e.g. Unverricht–Lundborg disease), and the association between epilepsy and for example metabolic abnormalities such as storage disorders. A number of specific epilepsy syndromes have been shown to have genetic linkage. These include juvenile myoclonic epilepsy and familial forms of frontal- and temporal-lobe syndromes. Autosomal dominant nocturnal frontal-lobe epilepsy seems a discrete syndrome linked with genes coding for subunits of the cerebral nicotinic receptor (Picard and Brodtkorb, 2007).

SYMPTOMATIC EPILEPSY

Some of the underlying pathologies and metabolic defects related to seizures and epilepsy are outlined in Table 10.3.

There is variation with age. Neonatal seizures may be caused by prenatal events such as cerebral malformations, rubella embryopathy, toxoplasmosis and perinatal birth damage from hypoxia or trauma. Postnatal events include metabolic changes such as hypoglycaemia, hypocalcaemia, hypomagnesaemia, infections such as meningitis, and a number of inborn errors of metabolism which become expressed early in life.

Early-childhood epilepsy (starting around the age of three) is more likely to be idiopathic, while in adult life, tumours and cerebrovascular disease become prominent causes. Dysembryoplastic neuroepithelial tumours (DNT) are benign tumours with mixed glial and neuronal cell types thought to be developmental in origin. They are often misdiagnosed as gliomas, and are easily treated by surgical resection.

Head injury is a common cause at any age, and is most likely to be responsible if the dura is penetrated or if the injury produces coma and a post-traumatic amnesia of more than 24 hours. Early seizures following injury increase the probability of the later development of epilepsy (Jennett, 1975), and the usual pattern is of focal or secondary generalized attacks. Fifty per cent of patients who develop post-traumatic epilepsy

Table 10.3 Some causes of seizures and epilepsy

Developmental	Heterotopias and dysplasias
Genetic	Autosomal, dominant, nocturnal, frontal-lobe epilepsy
Metabolic causes	Hypoglycaemia, hypomagnesaemia, fluid and electrolyte disturbances, acute intermittent porphyria, amino acid disorders
Trauma	Head injuries, especially penetrating wounds and birth injuries
Neurological causes	Tumours, cerebrovascular accidents, degenerative and storage disorders, demyelinating diseases, Sturge–Weber and other malformations, tuberose sclerosis, infections such as cytomegalovirus, toxoplasmosis, meningitis, cysticercosis and syphilis
Drug withdrawal	Especially alcohol and the barbiturates
Vitamin deficiency	Pyridoxine
Poisons	Lead, strychnine
Temperature	Fever

have their first attack within 12 months of injury, although in some patients onset is delayed for several years: the relative risk remains elevated for some 10 years or longer with severe injury (Annegers *et al.*, 1998). Genetic factors may be important here, but evolving neurophysiological and neurochemical events are presumably also involved. This model has relevance for schizophrenia, where the interaction of genetic and early environmental insults does not necessarily lead to the expression of the clinical condition for a number of years.

Cortical dysgenesis has been shown to have an important association with epilepsy in perhaps up to 20% of patients with intractable seizures. This can take the form of gyral abnormalities or heterotopias. The gyral pattern is shown to be disorganized with thickening of individual gyri; there is disturbance of

the white/grey boundary, and clumps of heterotopic cells may be seen. These abnormalities may not be seen with CT, but are readily apparent on MRI. Microdysgenesis, essentially microscopic islands of ectopic neurones and disturbed cortical layering, has also been shown on pathological examination of brains from some epileptic patients.

The aetiology of these dysgeneses is unclear, but some are familial, with presumed genetic basis.

BIOCHEMICAL FINDINGS

In contrast to affective disorder and schizophrenia, there have been relatively few clinical investigations relating to the biochemical underpinnings of the epileptic process. However, since epilepsy is associated with hypersynchronization of large numbers of neurones, reduced inhibition or increased excitation via neurochemical processes is considered relevant to pathogenesis. Experimental investigations have looked at alterations of monamine and acetylcholine activity, but GABA and the excitatory amino acids such as glutamate and aspartate have attracted most attention.

In general, catecholamine agonists raise the seizure threshold, while antagonists lower it (Trimble and Meldrum, 1979). In particular, drugs such as chlorpromazine may precipitate seizures, although dopamine agonists such as apomorphine are not therapeutically valuable. Experimentally, some antiepileptic drugs increase CNS 5-HT levels, while others decrease release, so 5-HT may have some effect on regulation of the seizure threshold, although data from patients are variable, reflecting either an increase, no change, or a decrease of activity (Reynolds, 1981).

The evidence for the role of GABA is substantial, although it largely derives from animal studies. Some antiepileptic agents such as sodium valproate, benzodiazepines, gabapentin tiagabine and vigabatrin are GABA agonists, and GABA antagonists such as picrotoxin and bicuculline are proconvulsant. Both glutamate and aspartate provoke excitatory neuronal activity and they can be inhibited by certain antiepileptics (Chapman *et al.*, 1983). Recent evidence has suggested that these excitatory amino acids may be endogenous neurotoxins, increased release of which may provoke neuronal damage via a calcium-dependent mechanism. Since the depolarized NMDA receptor allows the flow of calcium into the cell, a cascade of events leads to an amplification of excitation at many synapses and such excessive activation might underlie seizure generation. The relevance of the calcium influx for cell toxicity and thus progressive neuronal damage in recurrent seizures is however a considerable focus of interest, and is one model for seeking out drugs which decrease glutamate activity and which thus may be neuroprotective.

The role of voltage-gated ion channels and the regulation of calcium currents are relevant. The former determines the excitability of neurones, and sodium currents are largely responsible for the generation of action potentials. Voltage-gated currents are related to the generation of seizures, and a number of antiepileptic drugs act at the sodium channel. The influx of calcium through voltage-gated calcium channels activates calcium-dependent potassium channels and regulates a number of calcium-dependent intracellular processes, including transmitter release. Low-voltage calcium channels are referred to as T-type channels and play a role in the action of ethosuximide. Voltage-gated calcium channels are controlled by subunits, one of which, the alpha-2-delta subunit, is a binding site for the antiepileptic drugs gabapentin and pregabalin.

INVESTIGATION AND DIFFERENTIAL DIAGNOSIS

Following history-taking and neurological examination, it is customary to request routine haematology and electrolytes, also estimating calcium and, less nowadays, serology. These days the imaging technique of choice is either a CT or an MRI scan. High-resolution MRI scans, with specific sequences such as FLAIR, will yield evidence of structural lesions in a much larger proportion of patients than routine imaging, and detection of tumours, malforations

and migration defects has important treatment implications. An EEG is helpful; it may aid with diagnosis, but it also forms a baseline for any future investigations.

Any suggestion from clinical examination or the EEG that the seizures are focal should alert the clinician to the possibility of an intracranial lesion being present, and brain imaging for such patients is mandatory. The finding of intracranial pathology will obviously require further investigation under the appropriate specialist, using more sophisticated radiological techniques.

Where there is doubt about the epileptic nature of the seizures, the possibility of non-epileptic (pseudo)seizures arises. Further psychiatric exploration will become necessary to rule out psychopathology, and possibly admission to a specialized unit where prolonged observation with videotelemetry or ambulatory monitoring can be carried out.

With careful neuropsychiatric investigations it is possible to reach a diagnostic conclusion in the majority of patients who present difficulties. However, there are patients, especially among those seen at special referral centres, for whom diagnosis is difficult and a primary psychiatric diagnosis is most likely. Current estimates suggest that up to 20% of patients in a tertiary referral epilepsy clinic diagnosed as having epilepsy may suffer from alternative conditions.

PSYCHIATRIC DISORDERS IN EPILEPSY

Classification

One way to classify the psychiatric disorders of epilepsy is in relation to the seizure itself. Ictal (peri-ictal) disorders are directly related to the seizure, while interictal disorders are unrelated in time to the seizure. A third category is of disorders which, due to brain damage or disease, lead to both seizures and psychiatric illness. In this would be included many causes of learning disability (mental handicap), and some epileptic syndromes such as those of West and Lennox–Gastaut. It would also cover organic mental disorders such as autism and the disintegrative psychosis of childhood, and cerebrovascular disease and Alzheimer's disease in adults.

The international classifications of epilepsy reviewed above takes no account of psychopathology. Further, classifications such as the DSM IV and ICD 10 are inadequate when dealing with such neurally-based disorders. In response, to examine this issue, the Commission on the Psychobiology of Epilepsy of the ILAE has published guidelines for a classification of the psychiatric disorders of epilepsy (Table 10.4). This is multiaxial, takes into account comorbidities, and recognizes that the syndromes are phenomologically discrete (Krishnamoorthy *et al.*, 2007). It acknowledges comorbidity, namely that people with epilepsy can get as anxious or obsessional as anyone else,

and can be awarded a DSM IV TR category. However it also notes the disorders which seem bound in with the epilepsy, giving an organic variation to the clinical picture. The main ones are the interictal psychoses, the interictal dysphoric disorder, the Gastaut–Geschwind interictal personality disorder and the postictal psychoses. Other relevant information recorded (apart from relationship to the seizure) includes relationship to the EEG change (Forced Normalization) and relationship to antiepileptic drug prescription.

Ictally-related Psychiatric Disorders

No one doubts that acute disruption of cerebral activity, as occurs with the electrical events of the seizure, may disturb cortical function sufficiently to provoke acute psychiatric

Table 10.4 The commission on psychobiology of epilepsy classification of psychiatric disorders in epilepsy

Category	Clinical features	Key conclusions in draft classification proposal
The problem of co-morbidity	• Anxiety and phobic disorders • Minor and major depression • Obsessive compulsive disorder • Other somatoform, dissociative and neurotic disorders	No different from the range of common mental disorders prevalent in the community and in clinic/hospital populations. Classification should be as per ICD-10 and DSM-IV TR
Psychopathology as presenting symptom of epileptic seizures	Altered awareness, confusion, disorientation, memory disturbances, anxiety, dysphoria, hallucinations and paranoid syndromes	Complex partial, simple partial and absence status and other epilepsy syndromes can be diagnosed; clinically supported by EEG
Interictal psychiatric disorders that are specific to epilepsy	• Cognitive dysfunction including memory complaints • Psychoses of epilepsy • Affective/somatoform disorders • Personality disorders • Anxiety and phobias specific to epilepsy	• May be general or specific; diagnosed with standard neuropsychological tests • To be classified based on the relationship to seizure-prodromal, inter-ictal, post-ictal and alternating • Hyperethical, viscous, labile, mixed and other • Both trait accentuation and disorder to be coded • Fear of seizures recognized as a distinct and disabling entity
Other information of relevance	• Relationship to AED therapy • Relationship to EEG change	Coded as not documented; associated with institution and/or withdrawal with specified time periods for both presence or absence of associated EEG change documented

syndromes. Many of the manifestations of simple and complex partial seizures outlined above are psychological symptoms which, in other settings, would clearly be described as psychopathology. In addition, prodromal symptoms, predominantly dysphoric, and the psychiatric presentations of both generalized absence and complex partial seizure status, are included in this category.

Postictal confusion occurs immediately following the seizure, when there is usually still disruption of the EEG, mainly with diffuse slow frequencies and little normal activity. Patients present with a variety of behaviours, the underpinnings of which are clearly-defined confusional states. These are short-lived, rarely lasting more than an hour, but occasionally can persist for days or longer, especially in the learning-disabled. Recurrent seizures, which do not allow for mental-state recovery between attacks, can also lead to prolonged states of obtunding.

Typical emotional experiences include fear and depression. The severity of the latter ranges from mild to severe, and in some patients suicidal ideation is reported. Ictal depression lasts longer than other ictal epileptic experiences, and may persist for longer than 24 hours.

Ictally-driven psychoses may be schizophrenia-like, especially in complex partial-seizure status, although more often they represent an obvious organic brain syndrome with a variety of hallucinatory and delusional experiences and evidence of cognitive disruption in association with a disturbed EEG.

Postictal states such as the above should not be confused with the later-developing postictal syndromes, although the syndromes may emerge from the repeated acute states. In many cases however the postictal syndromes come on several hours or more following the seizure, when the acute confusion of the immediate postictal phase has passed.

Logsdail and Toone (1988) conducted a survey of patients with postictal psychoses. Most had complex partial seizures with secondary generalization, and the majority had an increase in seizures prior to the onset of psychosis, usually as a cluster. A lucid interval, from one to six days, was clearly described in 80% of cases. On

Table 10.5 Clinical features of postictal psychoses

Clusters of seizures
Lucid interval
Variable alteration of consciousness
Mixed affective state
Fear of impending death
Religious hallucinations and delusions
Time-limited (days to weeks)

follow-up, after several years, 21% had become chronically psychotic. These postictal psychotic states have a number of features which are hallmarks and when present lead to the diagnosis. These are shown in Table 10.5. Notable are the religious hallucinations and delusions, the fear of impending death and the relative absence of clouding of consciousness. The EEG often is not so abnormal, and may show an improved pattern on the interictal state, suggesting links between this state and Forced Normalization (see below). The level of consciousness is very important clinically since if patients have command hallucinations to commit suicide, they can plan such acts and carry them out. This is in contrast to any self-harm, which occurs in the immediate postictal phase of confusion, when such directed actions are not possible.

Kanemoto and colleagues (2002) noted 2% of all patients attending an epilepsy centre had a postictal psychosis, but that in the subgroup with temporal-lobe epilepsy, the figure was 11%. In their series, the 'lucid interval' ranged from less than 24 hours to 7 days, and the psychosis itself from 12 hours to more than 1 month. They have stressed the close link with psychic auras such as déjà vu and ictal fear.

Kanner and colleagues (2004) have studied the postictal behavioural disorders in some detail. They have noted in addition to the psychoses (7%) a spectrum which includes anxiety (45%) and dysphoric/depressive symptoms (45%) and hypomania (22%). These presentations were associated with a past history of depression and anxiety; they are often not recognized to be related to the ictus (with the time interval after the attack not being immediate) and are usually untreated, even though they can be very distressing for patients.

The pathophysiology of the postictal psychoses is unknown. Logsdail and Toone (1988) hypothesized that postictal psychosis results from increased postsynaptic dopamine sensitivity. Ring *et al.* (1992) tested this hypothesis using single-photon-emission computed tomography (SPECT) and the D_2 ligand [123I]IBZM. They noted that patients with epilepsy and psychoses had decreased binding to the ligand, suggesting that there was increased release of endogenous dopamine in the psychotic state. Others have suggested that the disorder represents a restricted limbic-status epilepticus, but limited functional imaging studies have produced contradictory results (Kannemoto *et al.*, 2002). The SPECT data with IBZM suggest increased activity in the right fronto-temporal area.

Interictal Psychiatric Disorders

There are few reliable epidemiological studies of the psychopathology of epilepsy. Many are carried out only on selected populations, and both the classifications of the epilepsy and the psychopathology may be hard to verify. Most point to a higher prevalence of interictal psychopathology with localization-related temporal-lobe epilepsy and in patients with difficult-to-control seizures. The general-practice survey of Edeh and Toone (1985) revealed 48% of patients to be classified as cases using the Clinical Interview Schedule. Patients with focal epilepsies had more psychopathology than those with generalized epilepsies; in a temporal-lobe group, 36% had an affective disorder, and 8% an affective or organic psychosis.

Jalava and Sillanpaa (1996) examined a prospective population-based cohort over a span of 35 years, and noted that patients with epilepsy, in comparison with controls, had a fourfold risk of developing psychiatric disorders.

The rates of psychopathology are greater if selected populations are examined, such as the learning-disabled or those in tertiary-referral special clinics. Further, it has recently been shown that the relationship, at least with depression, is two-way. In other words, people with depression have an increased risk for seizure disorders, and vice versa (Hesdorffer *et al.*, 2006).

Personality Disorders

This at one time was a most controversial issue. The main arguments revolved around whether any personality changes seen are secondary to an organic brain syndrome, preferentially affecting the temporal lobes and especially limbic structures, or whether they are due to secondary factors such as recurrent head injuries, social stigmatization and the long-term prescription of anticonvulsant drugs. Amidst the theorizing, several advances in the neurosciences revealed the important role of the frontal lobes in regulating behaviour, and frontal-lobe syndromes, essentially personality disorders, were described in animals and humans. Further, a temporal-lobe syndrome, namely the Klüver–Bucy syndrome, was described after bilateral damage to the temporal lobes, which presented as an alteration of personality traits, with calming of emotions, visual agnosis and alterations of sexual behaviour.

Many studies in this area have used the MMPI to detect personality change, and while some show differences between epileptic patients and a normal population, many fail to show statistical differences between temporal-lobe and generalized epilepsy subgroups (Trimble, 1991). Interestingly, several of these 'negative' results show nonsignificant but higher levels of psychopathology in a temporal-lobe group, raised paranoia or schizophrenia scales being quite common. In some studies, scores for psychotic behaviour are higher in those with combined psychomotor and generalized seizures or those with bilateral foci. In addition, in a meta-analysis of MMPI studies in the literature (Hermann and Whitman, 1984), patients with epilepsy were compared to others with chronic medical disorders. Epileptic patients who were classified as abnormal by the MMPI showed more severe psychopathology than other groups, suggesting that while chronic illness may be one variable, patients with epilepsy were more susceptible to severe problems.

To overcome the shortcomings of the MMPI, Bear and Fedio (1977) developed a rating scale of 18 behavioural features, drawn from the literature, thought to be associated with temporal-lobe epilepsy. Their scale was applied to epileptic patients with a temporal-lobe focus, neurological control patients and healthy controls. They reported that the temporal-lobe group scored significantly higher on several subscales, notably humourless sobriety, dependency, obsessionality, and religious and philosophical concerns. This study has had partial replication from other groups (Hermann and Riel, 1981; Hermann *et al.*, 1982), who also highlighted a sense of personal destiny, dependence, paranoia and philosophical interests in patients with a temporal-lobe origin of attacks when compared with those with generalized seizures. Psychopathology has been reported to be especially overrepresented in patients with auras of ictal fear, being more often classified, using Goldberg's sequential diagnostic system for the MMPI, as psychotic. An aura of ictal fear immediately suggests a periamygdaloid, and hence limbic, focus for the onset of the seizure.

Other evidence that patients with limbic-related epilepsies may be more prone to psychopathology derives from Nielsen and Kristensen (1981). They also applied the Bear–Fedio scale to patients with temporal-lobe epilepsy, and noted that those with a medio-basal EEG focus showed significantly more hypergraphia (a tendency towards extensive and compulsive writing), elation, guilt and paranoia than those with a lateral focus. Adamec (1989) applied the Bear–Fedio inventory to 114 patients with epilepsy, and to other groups with psychiatric illness and no epilepsy, normal controls and patients with chronic illness other than epilepsy. Cluster analysis revealed a cluster with psychiatric illness and seizures that was distinguished from the nonpsychiatry-seizure patient cluster by the presence of depression and metaphysical symptoms, and the reporting of 'limbic' auras such as jamais vu, time changes and formed images. Thus several studies have used a limbic marker (auras or EEG findings) to identify patients with limbic epilepsy, and noted an association between the latter and psychopathology (Trimble, 1991).

The importance of these and related findings for biological psychiatry and neuropsychiatry cannot be overemphasized. Generally, the data

suggest that patients with epilepsy do show abnormal personality profiles, although the main argument relates to whether a subgroup with temporal-lobe epilepsy may be identified. While the results do not support the concept that a specific 'epileptic personality' exists in all patients with temporal-lobe epilepsy, they do suggest that patients with temporal-lobe lesions, particularly those with medially-sited limbic lesions, are more susceptible to severe psychiatric disturbances, notably scoring high on such parameters as religiosity, emotionality and paranoia. This should be seen as representing the outcome of an organic process in the limbic system.

The view that there is a specific interictal syndrome of temporal-lobe epilepsy receives most support from clinical evidence and has been strongly made by Geschwind and colleagues (Geschwind, 1979; Waxman and Geschwind, 1975). They have drawn attention in particular to disorders of sexual function, plasticity of behaviours, religiosity, hypergraphia, philosophical concern and irritability (see Table 10.6), and disturbances of mood, often short-lived, are noted. Further, there are nascent intellectual interests, with preoccupation with religious, moral and philosophical themes. Finally, there are altered interpersonal dispositions, which include increased preoccupation with detail (obsessionality), circumstantiality of speech and a tendency to prolong social encounters, referred to as viscosity. Such diagnostic manuals as the DSM IV-TR are of no help in understanding this syndrome, since it and other well-defined syndromes of epilepsy (e.g. postictal psychosis) will not be found therein.

The hypergraphia of this syndrome frequently leads to a written output that is meticulous, obsessional and carried out with

Table 10.6 Features of the Gastaut–Geschwind syndrome

Hypergraphia
Hyposexuality
Hyperreligiosity
Increased concern with philosophical matters
Irritability
Mood lability
Viscosity

a compulsion. The content is often moral or religious. Repetition of words and sentences may be seen. Variants include excessive drawing or painting, or the hiring of a third party to write down information. There is some suggestion that hypergraphia is associated with nondominant-hemisphere temporal-lobe disturbances (Trimble, 1986c).

Rao *et al.* (1992) examined viscosity, another feature of this syndrome. This refers to a stickiness of thought processes, and to an 'interpersonal adhesiveness', or increased social adhesion. Patients display circumstantiality, have difficulty terminating conversations, and tend to prolong interpersonal encounters, for example interviews with physicians, beyond what is indicated by social cues. They reported this trait to be commoner in patients with a left or bilateral seizure foci, and suggested it represented a subtle interictal language disturbance.

Religiosity

The 'heightened religiosity' of epilepsy has been recognized since the 19th century by the French and German alienists (Trimble, 2007b). Studies have found that 'religiosity trait' scores can distinguish between patients with temporal-lobe epilepsy, normal controls and patients with other psychiatric or neurological conditions, including extra-temporal focal epilepsy and generalized epilepsy. Ecstatic ictal experiences, in some cases accompanied by visions of a religious nature, have been reported in patients with EEG evidence of temporal-lobe discharges (Saver and Rabin, 1997), and sudden religious conversions have been reported in the postictal period, noted above.

Trimble and Freeman (2006), using the Bear–Fedio scale in addition to other scales that assess aspects of individual religious experiences and behaviour, examined three experimental groups. The first consisted of 28 people with temporal-lobe epilepsy and a prominent devotion to religion, identified clinically. The second consisted of 22 people with temporal-lobe epilepsy who had no religious affiliations. In the third group were 30 regular churchgoers

without known epilepsy. The purpose of the study was to examine in more detail the psychological profile of those patients with epilepsy and religiosity, and, by comparing them with the other epilepsy sample, to examine the underlying epilepsy variables that might be related to the religious experiences.

They were able to reconfirm the original findings of Geschwind and his school, and show that the temporal-lobe religious group not only, as expected, endorsed the religiosity subscale of the Bear–Fedio scale, but also revealed other elements of the Gastaut–Geschwind syndrome (see Figure 10.1). Notably, the religious group also scored highly on the subscales of emotionality, philosophical interests, anger and sadness, dependence and hypergraphia. They were also rated by a significant other to have more paranoia and mental viscosity than the nonreligious sample. Thus, the profile that emerged in the religious patients with epilepsy was true to the original clinical descriptions of the Gastaut–Geschwind syndrome, and emphasized hypergraphia, philosophical interests and emotionality linked with the hyperreligiosity.

When the two groups of patients with temporal-lobe epilepsy were compared, those with the religiosity were noted to more often have had a history of episodes of postictal psychosis (although they were not psychotic at the time of interview) and more electroencephalogram changes that were bilateral than those without the religiosity.

The ordinary churchgoers were different in their backgrounds from the epilepsy patients (more females, of an older age, who were more likely to be married, and with a better educational level and occupational status), but they also differed in their religious behaviours. The patients with epilepsy and religiosity were more likely to belong to a religion not regarded as mainstream (i.e. Church of England or Catholic), Seventh Day Adventism being popular. The question 'How often have you felt as though you were very close to a powerful spiritual force that seemed to lift you outside?' was endorsed significantly more by those with epilepsy and religiosity than the non-epilepsy churchgoers, but interestingly, there was no significant difference

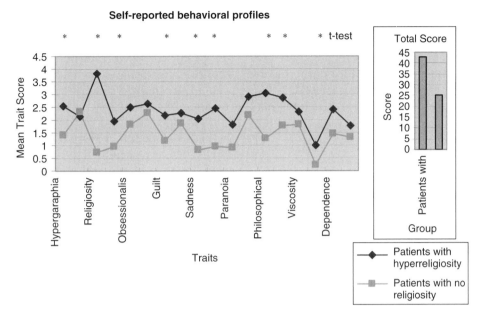

Figure 10.1   Profiles on the Bear–Fedio self-reported rating scale, comparing patients with epilepsy with and without religiosity. This confirms the original Bear–Fedio syndrome, with high ratings on religiosity, hypergraphia, emotionality and philosophical ideas * = p < 0.05

in response to the question that asked if they had had any religious experience. Neither was there any difference in responses to questions which asked about the frequency or duration of the religious experiences that they had.

With regards to the actual religious experiences, the epilepsy religious sample reported more experiences of the feeling of the presence of some external being, either of evil or of great spirituality, associated with feelings of death or dying and intense fear. The experiences were ineffable and noetic, not simply an awareness. There was identification, of and with that essence, and ecstasy and miracles were features of the descriptions.

These results lead to some relevant conclusions. First, temporal-lobe epilepsy can be associated with an identifiable constellation of behavioural dispositions, which have been identified for years, but are now better documented with rating-scale assessments. This constellation in its full form is referred to as the Gastaut–Geschwind syndrome. Second, patients with epilepsy and hyperreligiosity have often experienced postictal psychotic

states, underscoring the potential links between their psychological profile and that of an epilepsy-related psychosis.

From the neurological point of view, it was the patients with temporal-lobe epilepsy and bilateral disturbances of function (as revealed through the electroencephalogram) in their temporal lobes who reported the most intense religious experiences, especially endorsing items to do with the inner subjective nature of their experiences, their ineffability and the spatial–temporal component.

In a further investigation, in which the volumes of the hippocampus and the amygdala were measured, using MRI, in patients with epilepsy whose interictal behaviour was rated using the Bear–Fedio scale, Wuerfel *et al.* (2004) found that patients who met the criteria for hyperreligiosity had significantly lower mean right hippocampal volumes than those reported as not religious. While in itself this finding was interesting, confirmation of the anatomical association emerged when the actual scores on religiosity were correlated with hippocampal size. Thus, there was a significant negative association between religiosity scores and hippocampal size, on the right side only. Further, this correlation was found for both patient self-ratings and on the independently obtained carer ratings; the smaller the right hippocampus, the greater the expressed religiosity. These data suggest that the right-sided limbic structures may be of central importance to the development of these personality attributes.

Personality Changes in Juvenile Myoclonic Epilepsy (JME)

Although most of the discussion of the personality changes in epilepsy has revolved around the interictal syndrome of temporal-lobe epilepsy, the personality associations with one of the generalized epilepsies was described by Janz (2002). These include poor sleep habits, going to bed early and waking late, and a personality profile characterized by 'unsteadiness, lack of discipline, hedonism and indifference towards their illness'. These patients were prone to mood swings, were suggestible, and could react with undue sensitivity. These characteristics often led to poor compliance with treatment regimes, and made management difficult.

Several studies have used rating scales to assess groups of patients with JME, although little has come from them, being few in number and using standardized ratings of psychopathology, which, as with the temporal-lobe-epilepsy studies, may be inappropriate. It is however of interest that studies of cognition in patients with JME suggest that they do less well on frontal-lobe tasks than matched patients with temporal-lobe epilepsy (Trimble, 2000).

Aggression

As emphasized in Chapter 3, neurophysiological studies in aggression strongly point to alteration of the limbic system, in particular amygdala function. Since this area of the brain is frequently damaged in patients with temporal-lobe epilepsy, it may be expected that they would display more aggression than those with other forms of epilepsy. This is an area of considerable controversy. While ictal violence, recorded using videotelemetry, has been clearly described (Delgado-Escueta *et al.*, 1981), the problems of recording and quantifying interictal aggressive behaviour, almost entirely seen in an interpersonal setting, have led to considerable variability of results in clinical studies. Hermann and Whitman (1984) noted the high risk factors for aggression in epilepsy, which include organic cerebral disease, low socioeconomic status and poor environmental upbringing. Fenwick (1986) noted the evidence from intracranial implanted electrode studies, which suggests that the amygdala is involved in the mediation of aggression in man, further commenting that an amygdalectomy improves aggressive behaviour in those series where it has been tried. In addition, patients with temporal-lobe epilepsy who undergo temporal lobectomy show improvement of seizures and improvement of behaviour, most notably aggression. His conclusion was that a relationship between seizure discharges and aggressive behaviour had been shown, although the relationship was more between poor impulse control and brain damage than the seizure process itself.

In a study using MRI imaging, Tebartz van Elste and colleagues (2000) noted that patients with epilepsy and severe aggression (referred to as intermittent explosive disorder) had a significantly higher incidence of encephalitic brain disease and left-handedness, more bilateral EEG abnormality and less frequent hippocampal sclerosis than controls. In the aggressive patients a subgroup showed severe amygdala atrophy. In a further analysis, voxel-based morphometry revealed reductions of grey-matter density over large areas of the left extratemporal neocortex, maximal in the left frontal neocortex (Woermann *et al.*, 2000).

A related condition is the episodic dyscontrol syndrome (Fenwick, 1986; Monroe, 1970), a synonym for episodic dyscontrol. This presents as sudden episodes of spontaneously released violence, often in the setting of minimal provocation, which tend to be short-lived. They may be provoked by small amounts of alcohol, and after the events, patients may feel remorse. Generally, the condition is associated with nonspecific abnormalities that are also seen in epilepsy, for example evidence of brain damage, low socioeconomic status and a disturbed upbringing. Evidence of minimal neurological damage, with soft neurological signs and abnormal EEGs, is often found, although there is no evidence that these episodes have the same pathophysiology as epileptic seizures.

Affective Disorders

Many people with epilepsy are miserable and unhappy, but this does not equate to a depressive illness. Further, many patients suffer from a chronic dysphoria, often provoked or exacerbated by the long-term administration of anticonvulsant drugs. However, interictal depressive states are frequent in epileptic patients, and postical affective states are becoming increasingly recognized. Several authors have commented on the frequency of suicide in epileptic patients (Blumer, 2004), the risk being approximately five times that expected, highest for those with temporal-lobe epilepsy. In patients assessed for self-poisoning, epileptic patients are overrepresented (Mackay, 1979), and frequent use of barbiturates for this purpose is noted. Anticonvulsant medications that act at the GABA receptor complex are highly implicated (Trimble, 1997).

Epidemiology

Assessing the frequency of epilepsy and depression from selected clinic samples gives a bias towards the more severely affected patients and also those on the most medication. In community studies, Edeh and Toone (1987) reported that 22% of unselected patients with epilepsy were rated as having a depressive disorder. A Canadian community health survey examined 253 people with epilepsy using a rating scale to identify a history of depression, noted a lifetime prevalence of depression at 22%; this was compared with 12% in the general population (Tellez-Zenteno *et al.*, 2005).

More recently, Ettinger *et al.* (2004) assessed depression in 775 people with epilepsy, and compared the incidence with patients with asthma, and also with healthy controls. In this study, a rating-scale assessment was again used (Centers of Epidemiological Studies – Depression Instrument). Symptoms of depression were significantly more frequent in the epilepsy group (36.5%) than in those with asthma (27.8%) and the controls.

Several studies have noted a correlation with seizure frequency. In an epidemiological study, Jacoby *et al.* (1996) noted that depression occurred in 4% of seizure-free patients, in 10% of patients with less than one seizure a month, and in 21% patients with higher seizure frequency. O'Donoghue *et al.* (1999) noted that patients with epilepsy with continuing seizures were significantly more likely to suffer from depression than those in remission (33% vs 6%).

There are a number of studies from selected patient groups, for example tertiary centres, and from those awaiting surgery for epilepsy, which note in these populations an even higher frequency of depression (Jones *et al.*, 2005; Victoroff *et al.*, 1994). Another finding, which has been verified, is the association between depressive symptomatology and quality of life in people with epilepsy. Depressive symptoms tend to be the most important predictor of quality of life, and were a more powerful predictor than the actual seizure frequency (Gilliam *et al.*, 1997).

Some studies have shown patients with temporal-lobe epilepsy to be more prone to depression than other groups, but other investigations have failed to confirm this. Quiske *et al.* (2000) found that patients with temporal-lobe epilepsy who had mesial temporal sclerosis were more likely to report depression. In general terms, there is greater agreement that patients with complex partial seizures are more likely to have a depressive disorder (Robertson, 1998).

There are also studies linking frontal-lobe dysfunction to the depression of epilepsy. These have emerged from investigations using brain imaging (PET or SPECT) and neuropsychological batteries. Hermann *et al.* (1991) noted that patients with temporal-lobe epilepsy and depression were more likely to perform poorly on frontal-lobe neuropsychological tasks, especially with a left-sided seizure focus. Schmitz *et al.* (1997) noted similar frontal changes and localizations using SPECT, and Bromfield *et al.* (1990), using PET, reported that patients with temporal-lobe epilepsy and associated depression revealed bilateral reductions of frontal-lobe metabolism. Theodore *et al.* (2007) have reported decreased 5-HT$_{1A}$ binding in the ipsilateral hippocampus of depressed epilepsy patients, unrelated to the presence of medial temporal sclerosis or laterality of focus. These data relate well to the findings in non-epileptic bipolar patients (Chapter 8).

Although these studies, of necessity, were on a limited number of patients, the concordance between the findings does support an anatomical association between temporal-lobe epilepsy, depression and frontal-lobe dysfunction.

With regard to the temporal-lobe association with depression, it is of interest that there are a number of studies outside the field of epilepsy which suggest that hippocampal volume loss is associated with affective disorders (see Chapter 8). Although further research in this area is needed, neuroimaging studies are revealing an underlying neurocircuitry of depression in psychiatric patients without a neurological disorder. This neurocircuitry includes the hippocampus, in keeping with the findings in subgroups of patients with epilepsy.

Recent data have suggested a bidirectional relationship between epilepsy and several co-morbid conditions. In other words there is an increased risk of patients with anxiety, depression or schizophrenia developing epilepsy after the psychiatric disorder (Hesdorffer *et al.* 2006). This has led to a renewed interest in these biological links.

The Relationship of Antiepileptic Drugs to Depression

There is an older literature which links barbiturate-related drugs to depression, but more recent data suggest that it is possible to distinguish between AEDs with the potential to have positive effects on mood, such as carbamazepine, lamotrigine and valproic acid, and these older compounds. The AEDs most

associated with this effect seem to be those which act at the benzodiazepine–GABA receptor complex, and include tiagabine, gabapentin topiramate and vigabatrin. Since in psychiatric practice it is known that benzodiazepines and other GABA agonists are associated clinically with depression, and that abnormalities of CSF GABA have been reported in patients with depression (Trimble, 1996), the link between sudden cessation of seizures (Forced Normalization), GABAergic agents and the onset of depression seems reasonably secure. Further, these studies have revealed that patients with epilepsy and a prior history of an affective disorder are the more likely to develop depression in these circumstances.

Bipolar Disorder and Epilepsy

It used to be confidently stated that bipolar disorder was rare in patients with epilepsy (Wolf, 1982). Such statements were made prior to the use of standardized diagnostic manuals such as the DSM IV, and were also based upon clinical impression rather than assessment on rating scales. It was accepted however that in the context of the postictal state, patients could develop a postictal psychosis, the features of which were often manic or hypomanic, although more generally the presentation was one of a mixed affective state, often with psychotic features. Kanner *et al.* (2004) noted postictal hypomanic symptoms in 22% of patients, often with associated psychotic phenomenology. In the study of Ettinger *et al.* (2005), bipolar symptoms were revealed in 12.2% of the epilepsy patients, which was twice as much as in patients with asthma, and seven times as much as in the healthy comparison group. Of those who in the screening process were rated as potential patients with bipolar symptoms, nearly 50% were rated by a physician as having a bipolar disorder.

These data raise some doubts about the previous suggestions that bipolar disorder is rare in people with epilepsy, and about our knowledge of the association between these two disorders. However, the older discussions related more to classical manic–depressive disorder, as opposed to the more recently developed concepts of the bipolar spectrum, which is currently the focus of psychiatric interest.

Interictal Dysphoric Disorder (IDD)

The issue of phenomenology of depression in epilepsy is very much a matter of debate. In general terms, it is reasonable to hypothesize that patients with epilepsy can experience forms of mood disorder identical to those of patients without epilepsy and classifiable with standardized diagnostic manuals. However, it is equally reasonable to assume that the underlying brain pathology can influence the expression of mood-disorder symptoms, making less evident some aspects and emphasizing others.

Comorbid anxiety symptoms have been identified in 73% of patients with epilepsy and depression (Robertson *et al.*, 1987). This is very important clinically, since they may worsen the quality of life of depressed patients and significantly increase the risk of suicide (Kanner, 2006).

Mendez *et al.* (1986) investigated the clinical semeiology of depression in 175 patients with epilepsy, and reported that 22% could be classified as having atypical features. In particular, classic endogenous-type depressive symptoms, such as feelings of guilt, '*Gefühl der Gefühllosigkeit*' and a circadian pattern of symptom severity were rarely reported. Kanner *et al.* (2000) showed that 71% of patients with refractory epilepsy and depressive episodes severe enough to need a psychopharmacological treatment failed to meet criteria for any DSM IV axis 1 diagnosis. A study of 199 consecutive patients with epilepsy revealed that 64% failed to meet any DSM IV criteria using two structured clinical interviews, namely the Structured Clinical Interview for DSM IV Axis I (SCID-I) and the Mini International Neuropsychiatric Interview (MINI) (Kanner *et al.*, 2004).

The peri-ictal cluster of symptoms may to some degree account for the atypical features of affective disorders in epilepsy, but the possibility that in some cases the mood disorder of epilepsy has unique characteristics has plausibility. Kraepelin (1923) and then Bleuler (1949)

Table 10.7 Main symptom clusters of the interictal dysphoric disorder

Labile depressive symptoms	*Labile affective symptoms*	*Specific symptoms*
Depressed mood	Fear	Euphoric moods
Anergia	Anxiety	Paroxysmal irritability
Pain		
Insomnia		

were the first authors to describe a pleomorphic pattern of symptoms in epilepsy, including affective symptoms with prominent irritability intermixed with euphoric mood, fear and anxiety, as well as anergia, pain and insomnia. Blumer (2000) coined the term 'interictal dysphoric disorder' (IDD) to refer to this type of depressive disorder in epilepsy. It is characterized by eight key symptoms grouped in three major categories (Table 10.7): labile depressive symptoms (depressive mood, anergia, pain, insomnia), labile affective symptoms (fear, anxiety) and supposedly 'specific' symptoms (paroxysmal irritability, euphoric moods). Blumer used the term 'dysphoria' to stress the periodicity of mood changes and the presence of irritability and outbursts of aggressive behaviour as key symptoms. The dysphoric episodes are described as occurring without external triggers and without clouding of consciousness. They begin and end rapidly and recur fairly regularly in a uniform manner, occurring every few days to every few months and lasting a few hours up to two days.

The theoretical framework suggested by Blumer goes beyond a narrow IDD profile, and he speculated that affective symptoms in epilepsy exist along a continuum, from a dysphoric disorder with fleeting symptoms to a more severe disorder with transient psychotic features, to an even more debilitating disorder with prolonged psychotic states. It seems possible that IDD patients have several features in common with a specific subset of non-epileptic cyclothymic subjects, where depressive periods and labile–angry–irritable moods dominate the clinical picture. In a recent study investigating the prevalence and psychopathological features of IDD in patients with epilepsy compared with a group of patients with migraine (Mula *et al.*, 2008) it was diagnosed in 20% of patients, making it one of the most common mood disorders in epilepsy.

Seizures and Laterality

In his classic study, Flor-Henry (1969, 1983) examined 50 patients with temporal-lobe epilepsy awaiting temporal lobectomy who at one time had been psychotic, and compared them with 50 nonpsychotic cases with the same form of epilepsy. Where the lateralization could be determined, he noted that 18% were lateralized to the right hemisphere, and the majority of those had manic–depressive psychoses. He suggested that affective disorders were more likely to reflect nondominant-hemisphere pathology. While generalized tonic–clonic seizures were more often the only ictal manifestations in the affective-disorder group, the occurrence of psychomotor seizures was lowest. Flor-Henry suggested this implied that infrequently-released seizures were somehow related to the expression of the psychopathology. This is in keeping with the observations of decreased seizure frequency prior to the onset of a depressive illness (Betts, 1974), a finding noted in 43% of patients in the study of Robertson (1986).

The suggested link of affective disorder with the nondominant hemisphere in Flor-Henry's studies has been criticized not only on the grounds that the patients selected were all awaiting temporal-lobe surgery, but also because of the small numbers. It has received partial support from some studies (for example Taylor, 1975), but was not confirmed by others (Altschuler *et al.*, 1990; Robertson, 1986). If anything, the studies tend to suggest an association to a left-sided focus. Part of the confusion relates to diagnostic issues: Flor-Henry was referring to bipolar patients, others to depressive illness. Further, surface-electrode EEG is quite an unreliable method of establishing laterality. The instructive case study of Hurwitz *et al.* (1985) supports this. He described a case study of a patient with bilaterally independent

foci. During right temporal discharges she reported euphoria, but with left-sided changes depression was noted. The association between mania and euphoria and right-sided cerebral lesions is discussed further in Chapter 8.

Other Findings

Low serum, red cell and CSF folate levels have been reported in a high proportion of patients with epilepsy (Reynolds, 1976), associated with the taking of anticonvulsant drugs, in particular phenobarbitone, phenytoin and primidone. While the deficiency rarely leads to a megaloblastic anaemia, there are several studies which show a high incidence of low folate levels in epileptic patients with mental symptoms (Reynolds, 1976). Psychoses and dementia are often reported, but several studies note the link with depression (Edeh and Toone, 1985; Robertson, 1986; Rodin and Schmaltz, 1983; Trimble *et al.*, 1980). Reynolds (1986) has pointed out that folate deficiency and depression have also been reported in non-epileptic patients, not wholly explained by poor diet, and that *S*-adenosylmethionine (SAM), a methyl donor involved in folate metabolism, has anti-depressant properties.

Interictal Psychosis

A difficulty with the literature on psychosis and epilepsy is that few authors specify their precise diagnostic criteria for psychosis, and recognized research criteria are rarely quoted. Many continental authors refer to 'organic brain syndromes' in the context of epileptic psychosis, whereas British authors tend to use this phrase to refer to a psychosis in the setting of unclear consciousness. Generally authors distinguish between schizophrenia-like presentations and manic–depressive presentations. Further, a clear dissociation between ictal and interictal psychoses is not always clear, and issues such as Forced Normalization must be accommodated in any overall concept of understanding the psychoses of epilepsy.

Perez and Trimble (1980) used the present-state examination (PSE) of Wing to document the phenomenology of 24 epileptic patients prospectively referred with a psychosis in clear consciousness. Of the sample, 50% were categorized as having a schizophrenic psychosis, 92% having a profile of nuclear schizophrenia (NS), the diagnosis being based on the first-rank symptoms of Schneider. The syndrome profile of patients with schizophrenia-like symptoms and epilepsy, when compared to those with schizophrenia and no epilepsy, shows few significant differences, emphasizing the similarity of the clinical presentation of these two disorders. Similar findings have been reported in a retrospective study by Toone *et al*. (1982b).

Some differences between process schizophrenia and the schizophrenia-like psychoses of epilepsy were emphasized by Slater and Beard (1963), who noted the retention of affective warmth in the latter, patients showing less personality deterioration. They reported on 69 patients with a schizophrenia-like illness and epilepsy, and suggested, on statistical grounds, that the association was more than just coincidence. They noted an absence of premorbid schizoid personality traits and an absence of family history of psychiatric disturbance that might suggest a predisposition to schizophrenia. Forty-six had a psychosis that was highly typical of paranoid schizophrenia, and 12 had a hebephrenic presentation. Eleven of their series had a chronic psychosis that had been preceded by recurrent short-lived confusional states. The mean onset of the psychosis was 29.8 years, which occurred after the epilepsy had been present for a mean of 14.1 years. In 25% of the cases, the psychotic symptoms appeared as the frequency of generalized seizures was falling, and there was a preponderance of temporal-lobe abnormalities on neurological investigations.

Epidemiology

Stefansson *et al*. (1998), in a case-control study, compared the prevalence of nonorganic psychiatric disorders in patients with epilepsy to those with other somatic diseases, the groups being taken from a disability register in Iceland. Although the difference in psychiatric diagnoses overall was not significant, there was a higher rate of psychoses, particularly schizophrenia and paranoid states, among males with epilepsy.

Qin *et al*. (2005), in a study from Denmark, have confirmed the increased risk of schizophrenia and schizophrenia-like psychoses in epilepsy; in this study a family history of psychoses and a family history of epilepsy were significant risk factors for psychosis. Bredkjaer *et al*. (1998) in a record-linkage study looked for associations between epilepsy from the national patient register of Denmark and the equivalent psychiatric register. The incidence of nonorganic, nonaffective psychoses, which included schizophrenia and schizophrenia-spectrum disorders, was significantly increased in epilepsy, even when patients with learning disability or substance misuse were excluded.

Higher prevalence rates for psychoses were found in studies of much more select populations such as hospital case series. Thus, Gureje (1991), in patients attending a neurological clinic, quoted that 37% were psychiatric cases, and that 29% of these were psychotic. Mendez *et al*. (1993), in a retrospective investigation, reported that interictal psychotic disorders were found in over 9% of a large cohort of patients with epilepsy, in contrast to just over 1% in patients with migraine.

Risk Factors

Risk factors for interictal psychosis are shown in Table 10.8. The pathogenesis of psychosis in epilepsy is likely to be heterogeneous and the literature on risk factors is highly controversial. Studies are difficult to compare because of varying definitions of the epilepsy, the psychiatric disorder and the investigated risk factors.

There is some evidence for a genetic predisposition for the psychoses of epilepsy. The interval between age at onset of epilepsy and age at first manifestation of psychosis has been reported as similar in several studies – around 11–15 years. This interval has been used to postulate the etiologic significance of the seizure disorder and suggest a kindling-like mechanism.

There is a clear excess of temporal-lobe epilepsy in most case series of patients with epilepsy and psychosis, and focal seizure

Table 10.8   Risk factors for interictal psychosis

Age of onset	Early adolescence
Interval	Onset of seizures – psychosis Around 14 years
Seizure type	Complex partial, automatisms, visceral auras
Seizure frequency	Declining, but poor control over the years
Seizure focus	Temporal/limbic
Neurology	Sinistrality Gangliogliomas
EEG	Forced Normalization in a subgroup Temporal mediobasal focus (sphenoidal)

symptoms that indicate ictal mesial temporal or limbic involvement are overrepresented in patients with psychosis. There are several studies showing that psychoses in generalized epilepsies differ from psychoses in temporal-lobe epilepsy (Trimble, 1991). The former are more likely to be of short duration and confusional. There is also a general consensus that psychoses are less common in patients with neocortical extratemporal epilepsies.

Stevens and Hermann (1981) suggested the following important variables: age of onset, an abnormal neurological examination, automatisms and visceral auras, sphenoidal spike activity on EEG, and the presence of multifocal spikes. While some of these may reflect merely more cerebral disturbance, the automatisms with specific auras and the high incidence of sphenoidal spike activity would suggest the involvement of medial temporal structures in the psychosis. In particular, the study of patients with auras of fear by Hermann *et al.* (1982) showed that patients with temporal-lobe epilepsy and such auras displayed markedly raised elevations of some MMPI scales, especially for schizophrenia.

In support of these findings, in a study specifically looking at hippocampal and amygdala volumes, Tebartz van Elst *et al.* (2002) examined 26 patients with epileptic psychoses, 24 with temporal-lobe epilepsy and no psychosis, and 20 healthy controls. The psychotic patients had significantly increased amygdala sizes in comparison with the other two groups, which were bilateral, and not related to the laterality of the focus, or the length of epilepsy history. No hippocampal differences were noted in this study. In a complementary study on the same groups, Rüsch *et al.* (2004) was unable to find any neocortical–cortical volumetric differences.

Schmitz and Trimble (2007) identified the following risk factors for developing psychosis in epilepsy: complex partial and absence seizures, multiple seizure types, poor seizure control and a history of generalized status epilepticus. Age of onset of epilepsy in late childhood and early adolescence emerges from several studies (see Toone, 1981), while other data suggest that the relationship is not between temporal-lobe epilepsy and partial seizures, but between temporal-lobe pathology and complex partial seizures that lead to secondary generalized attacks.

In a follow-up study of 249 patients with temporal-lobe epilepsy who had earlier had a temporal lobectomy, Roberts *et al.* (1990) reported on 25 that had a schizophrenia-like psychosis before or after surgery. They noted associations of the psychosis with pathological lesions affecting the medial temporal lobe, which were developmental and present foetally or perinatally, and led to an early onset of epilepsy. Gangliogliomas seemed to be overrepresented pathologically.

In the only other pathological study of epileptic psychosis, Bruton *et al.* (1994) reported that psychosis was associated with larger cerebral ventricles, excessive periventricular gliosis and more focal cerebral damage than nonpsychotic controls, and that brains from patients with schizophrenia-like psychosis had more white-matter softenings. However, most of their small number of patients did not have the schizophrenia-like psychosis defined by Slater.

Laterality

Flor-Henry (1969) suggested that a left-sided temporal-lobe focus was more likely to be associated with a schizophrenia-like psychosis, contrasting this with the right-sided abnormality linking with an affective disorder. The evidence for the former is more substantial than the latter, although there are negative studies (Schmitz and Wolf, 1991).

Studies supporting the laterality hypothesis of epilepsy-related psychosis have been made using surface EEG, depth-electrode recordings, computed tomography, neuropathology, neuropsychology, positron-emission tomography (PET) and more recently MRI. Trimble (1991) summarized the earlier literature; of 14 studies with 341 patients, 43% had left, 23% right, and 34% bilateral abnormalities. This is a striking bias toward left lateralization. However, lateralization of epileptogenic foci was not confirmed in all controlled studies. Again, it may be that certain symptoms rather than any syndrome are associated with a specific side of focus. Trimble (1991) pointed out that a specific group of hallucinations and delusions, defined by Schneider, and referred to as first-rank symptoms, which usually (but by no means exclusively) signify schizophrenia, may be relevant. He suggested that these may be signifiers of temporal-lobe dysfunction, representing as they do disturbances of language and symbolic representation. In this sense he equated them to a Babinski sign for a neurologist, pointing to a location and lateralization of an abnormality in the CNS. These laterality findings have received support from brain-imaging studies. Using PET and oxygen-15, Trimble and colleagues (Trimble, 1986a) have reported data on patients with complex partial seizures, comparing a psychotic with a nonpsychotic subgroup. Generally, psychotic patients showed lower values for oxygen metabolism, but maximal differences were seen in the left hemisphere, across the entire temporal cortex. The majority of this sample had schizophrenia-like psychoses with Schneiderian symptoms.

Mellers (1998), using a verbal fluency activation paradigm and HMPAO SPECT, compared patients with schizophrenia-like psychoses of epilepsy with schizophrenia, epilepsy and no psychoses. The psychotic epilepsy patients showed lower blood flow in the superior temporal gyrus during activation than the other two groups. Using MR spectroscopy, Maier *et al.* (2000) were able to compare hippocampal–amygdala volumes and hippocampal N-acetyl aspartate (NAA) levels in patients with temporal-lobe epilepsy and schizophrenia-like psychoses of epilepsy, temporal-lobe epilepsy and no psychoses, schizophrenia and no epilepsy, and matched normal controls. The psychotic patients showed significant left-sided reduction of NAA; this was more pronounced in the psychotic epilepsy group. Regional volume reductions were noted bilaterally in this group, and in the left hippocampus–amygdala in the schizophrenic group.

Flügel *et al.* (2006) examined 20 psychotic and 20 nonpsychotic cases with temporal-lobe epilepsy using magnetization transfer imaging. They reported significant reductions of the magnetization transfer ratio (an index of signal loss) in the left superior and middle temporal gyri in the psychotic patients; this was unrelated to volume changes, and best revealed in a subgroup with no focal MRI lesions.

Summarizing these data, it appears that several authors, using independent samples and differing techniques, show a link between dominant-hemisphere pathology in patients with temporal-lobe epilepsy and a schizophrenia-like psychosis. It should be noted that the emphasis is on Schneiderian symptoms, presentation being with positive symptoms, and lack of deterioration and negative features.

Antagonism and the Concept of Forced Normalization

An earlier idea that schizophrenia and epilepsy had an inverse relationship has caused confusion. Essentially, this antagonism, observations of which led von Meduna to introduce convulsive seizures as a therapy for schizophrenia, was between seizures and the symptoms of psychosis, rather than between epilepsy and schizophrenia (Wolf and Trimble, 1985).

Landolt (1958) recorded changes in the EEG during preseizure dysphoric episodes and limited periods of frank psychosis lasting days or weeks in epileptic patients. He noted improvement in EEG activity during such episodes and referred to this as 'Forced Normalization'. He defined Forced Normalization thus: 'the phenomenon characterized by the fact that, with the recurrence of psychotic states, the EEG becomes more normal, or entirely normal, as compared with previous and subsequent EEG findings.' Forced Normalization was thus essentially an EEG phenomenon. He suggested that similar changes could be provoked by anticonvulsant drugs, and noted that, at the end of a psychotic episode, the EEG returned to being abnormal. Although initially he discussed this in relation to temporal-lobe epilepsy, he later drew attention to its occurrence with generalized epilepsies, in particular the precipitation of psychosis in patients with generalized absence seizures by ethosuximide. Although Forced Normalization is generally associated with psychosis, variant forms include prepsychotic dysphorias, depressive, manic, hypochondriacal and twilight states (Wolf and Trimble, 1985). A preferred term is perhaps 'paradoxical normalization'. Thus, as a general rule in epilepsy, if the behaviour deteriorates, so does the EEG. However, in the case of Forced Normalization, the EEG improves but paradoxically the behaviour becomes worse.

The clinical counterpart of forced normalization is referred to as alternative psychosis, in which less attention is paid to EEG phenomena and more to the presence or absence of seizures in association with the psychosis. Clinically, such states can be very problematic, since control of seizures leads to an even more disturbing and often difficult-to-control problem, namely the development of a psychosis. This sometimes has a schizophrenia-like presentation, but more often it appears as a paranoid or even manic psychosis. In lesser forms, the problem may merely present as an exacerbation or precipitation of behavioural problems as seizures remit. The disturbed behaviour may last days or weeks. It is often terminated by a seizure, and the EEG abnormalities then return.

Mechanisms

There appears to be some association between the development of an epileptic focus in one or other temporal lobe, expressed around early adolescence, and the development of a later psychiatric illness. The evidence implicates the dominant hemisphere in patients who develop a schizophrenia-like psychosis with positive symptoms, and suggests that in some patients there is an inverse relationship between the expression of the seizures and the expression of the psychosis. The latter is not only noted with Forced Normalization, but is also seen in patients with chronic psychosis, some of whom develop the psychosis as their seizure frequency declines. This holds for affective disorder (Flor-Henry, 1969) and for the schizophrenia-like conditions (Slater and Beard, 1963).

Most authors have used EEG or functional imaging to assess the side and site of the epileptic focus associated with psychopathology, which implies some disturbance of CNS function. This is supported by the inverse relationship to seizures and by the early observations of authors such as Heath (1962) and Kendrick and Gibbs (1957) of abnormal EEG discharges from deep limbic sites in patients who have psychosis, whether or not epilepsy is present. Heath, in work which is now barely quoted, but is important as it is unlikely ever to be repeated, emphasized the involvement of the septal region (the area we would now call the accumbens) in the development of psychosis, and showed that, while during interictal periods epileptic patients show paroxysms of abnormal activity, particularly in the hippocampus and amygdala, as psychosis becomes apparent these spread to involve the septal region. Schizophrenic patients also show spiking and slow-wave activity, primarily in this area, but to a lesser extent in the hippocampus and amygdala. The spiking is relatively infrequent in schizophrenic patients, but in epileptic psychosis there are dramatic high-amplitude spikes frequently associated with pronounced slow-wave activity. Thus, although differences were noted in the electrical patterns, the same anatomical regions are involved in psychosis whether or not the patient has epilepsy.

There are two main contrasting hypotheses to explain the development of the psychoses of epilepsy. The first, supported by the above, suggests that they are truly epileptic in origin and should be referred to as 'epileptic psychoses'.

The second says that they are a manifestation of organic neurological damage, and not specifically of epilepsy. The former view has been most strongly expressed by Flor-Henry (1969), supported by the observations of the link between seizure frequency and psychosis and the depth-electrode data. Slater and Beard (1963) advocated the second hypothesis, noting a significant proportion of psychotic patients had a defined organic basis for their epilepsy; a similar view was taken by Kristensen and Sindrup (1978) and Bruton *et al.* (1994).

CT and MRI studies do not add further information. Thus, patients with epilepsy tend to show a high frequency of abnormalities, with or without psychosis. Toone *et al.* (1982a) and Conlon *et al.* (1990) reported a tendency towards the reporting of more left-sided structural abnormalities in patients with schizophreniform psychosis of epilepsy, and hallucinations were exclusively reported in those with left-sided CT lesions. The studies with SPECT, PET and MRS quoted above lend further support to the concept that the psychoses are associated with disturbed function as opposed to structure. In general, patients with localization-related epilepsies, in particular temporal-lobe epilepsy, show hypometabolic areas at the site of the seizure focus, as demonstrated on the EEG. However, the extent of the underlying pathology, assessed during temporal lobectomy, tends to be much smaller than the zone of hypometabolism. This suggests a widespread functional disturbance in the associated brain regions of such patients. Further, these hypometabolic areas become hypermetabolic during an ictus. They do not appear to be dependent on seizure frequency, duration or clinical expression. In epileptic psychosis, these functional disturbances tend to be greater, and with schizophrenia-like presentations they involve the left side more than the right.

Neuropathological data (Stevens, 1986) do not clarify the situation much further. Thus, a common finding in epilepsy is mesial temporal sclerosis, with pyramidal cell loss in the CA1 area of the hippocampus. Although most common in patients with temporal-lobe epilepsy, this is also seen following status epilepticus. It is suspected to be aetiological for partial seizures with a temporal-lobe origin, but may also occur as a secondary consequence of recurrent seizures. Mesial temporal sclerosis has been reported occasionally in brains from schizophrenic patients who have never had seizures, and in epilepsy is associated with pathology elsewhere, such as Purkinje cell loss in the cerebellum.

Patients with epilepsy and psychosis are reported to have gliosis and degenerative changes in such areas as the pallidum, the brainstem, the tegmentum and the periaqueductal and periventricular regions of the basal forebrain, similar to the changes observed in patients with schizophrenia (Bruton *et al.*, 1994) (see Chapter 7).

Thus, mesial temporal sclerosis alone is insufficient for the development of psychosis, and other areas, in particular periventricular and forebrain sites which receive projections from the amygdala and hippocampus, would seem important. Further evidence for this stems from clinical observations that patients who have had temporal lobectomy sometimes develop psychosis postoperatively, which clearly implicates other areas of the brain than the medial temporal structures in the overall pathogenesis of the psychoses (Trimble, 1991).

Symonds (1962) pointed to the 'epileptic disorder of function'. It was, he suggested, not the loss of neurones in the temporal lobe that was responsible for the psychosis, but the disorderly activity of those that remained. One possibility is that chronic temporal-lobe ictal lesions lead to kindling of activity in other regions of the brain, especially forebrain limbic areas – changes which lead to the gradual development of the psychosis. Such a hypothesis fits with the intracerebral recording studies of Heath (1962), as well as observations that it is difficult to kindle epileptic seizures in certain parts of the limbic system, particularly those that are catecholaminergic such as the dopamine-rich areas of the limbic forebrain. In such sites, kindled behaviour changes rather than seizures are seen (Stevens and Livermore, 1978). The data of Ring *et al.* (1993) with IBZM binding (a D_2 ligand) to basal ganglia structures in psychotic epileptic patients compared with controls are in support of this hypothesis. These data are important for understanding the pathogenesis of schizophrenia since the temporal-lobe-epilepsy model of schizophrenia-like psychosis is one for the 'positive symptoms' of psychosis, and draws attention to the medial temporal lobes and forebrain limbic system in the development of some schizophrenic symptomatology.

COGNITIVE DETERIORATION AND EPILEPSY

It has long been recognized that some patients with epilepsy undergo dilapidation of their intellect, in particular showing disturbances of memory, which later may progress to intellectual deterioration and dementia. In some cases this may be related to a progressive encephalopathy. It may reflect an underlying neuropathology, such as a lipid storage disorder, which leads to both seizures and intellectual deterioration. Examples of epileptic syndromes such as West's syndrome have been noted already. Alternatively, recurrent head injuries, bouts of anoxia and intracranial bleeds may over time lead to deterioration. Some dementias, such as Alzheimer's disease, are associated with seizures, and links between Down's syndrome, early dementia and seizures are noted (Brown, 2004). Autism and autistic-spectrum disorders such as Asperger's syndrome are associated with a later development of seizures in about 25% of cases, comorbidity depending upon the age and type of disorder. Major risk factors for seizure occurrence are learning disability and additional neurological disorders. Autism with regression has been reported in one-third of children with previously normal or nearly-normal development. Epilepsy may be present, resulting in so-called autistic epileptiform regression (Canitano, 2007).

Attention has been drawn to anticonvulsant-induced encephalopathies, sometimes seen with phenytoin and sodium valproate, in the latter being associated with hyperammonemia. Diagnosing an anticonvulsant-induced encephalopathy can be difficult, since it may produce a typical picture of dementia, sometimes associated with focal neurological signs and dyskinesias, in association with a raised CSF protein. Since this represents one possible reversible cause of dementia, it should always be considered in patients with epilepsy who, for unclear reasons, are becoming cognitively impaired.

Most studies of non-institutionalized epileptic patients show a near-normal distribution of the IQ, with skewing at the lower end of the scale. On formal testing, people with epilepsy often show memory disturbances, particularly for more recent events, and there is some evidence of a laterality effect, patients with left-sided foci having memory deficits for verbal material and right-sided lesions for nonverbal material. Other selective deficits include impairment of attention, poor perceptuomotor scores, deficient arithmetical and reading ability, and a generalized slowing of cognitive processes. References to the latter have long been noted, and have been described as viscosity and stickiness of thought, referring to the prolonged speed of cerebration noted in some patients with epilepsy (Trimble and Thompson, 1985).

Factors influencing cognitive performance in epilepsy include length of seizure history, presence of hippocampal sclerosis, an early age of onset of seizures, an increasing frequency of seizures and associated neuropsychiatric handicaps such as depressive illness (Jokeit and Ebner, 2004). With regard to seizure types, generalized absence seizures seem less damaging than generalized tonic–clonic seizures, and patients with partial seizures seem more likely to show impairments of memory function. Patients with frontal epilepsies reveal deficits on testing frontal executive functions (Helmstaedter, 2004).

The more subtle adverse effects of anticonvulsant drugs on neuropsychological abilities have become appreciated (Trimble and Reynolds, 1984). Phenobarbitone, phenytoin and more recently topiramate have been most implicated, and carbamazepine the least. Topiramate seems to produce in around 7% of patients a reversible aphasia-like syndrome, associated with left-sided onset of seizures (Mula *et al.*, 2003). Polytherapy itself, particularly with older anticonvulsants, would appear detrimental, and significant improvements in both cognitive performance and affective symptoms can be brought about in patients by rationalizing polytherapy, or by substituting patients on polytherapy with more sedative compounds such as carbamazepine as monotherapy (Thompson and Trimble, 1982a).

SOME OUTSTANDING ISSUES

The last 30 years have seen a sea change with regards to the acceptance that epilepsy and psychopathology can be closely biologically linked. This has been due in part to a shift in neurological thinking, many neurologists now accepting that there is a neuroanatomy of emotion, and that the limbic circuitry is involved in many neurological disorders. Temporal-lobe epilepsy remains a paradigm. Further, as special epilepsy centres and clinics have developed, the behavioural syndromes of epilepsy have not only become more apparent to treating physicians, but have been the subject of much more scientifically-based research. The neuroanatomy outlined in Chapters 2 and 3 has also opened up the underlying mechanisms whereby such behavioural changes arise; the circuitry is clear, especially with regards to limbic-based syndromes.

Better definitions of some of the epilepsy-related behavioural syndromes are required. The characteristics, frequency and comorbidities of the IDD are unclear, as is its relationship to atypical depressions and bipolar disorder. This has very important implications. Thus, it is known that many patients with bipolar disorder in the absence of epilepsy respond to antiepileptic medications (see Chapter 12), although this is not a class effect, and is limited mainly to carbamazepine, sodium valproate and lamotrigine. In fact, antiepileptic drugs that are GABA agonists are likely to provoke or maintain depressive symptoms and not be mood-stabilizing. One possibility is that the non-epilepsy mood-disordered patients respond because they have atypical bipolar disorders – for which

there is some evidence – and that the effect of the antiepileptic drugs has to do with their influence at limbic structures. Carbamazepine, sodium valproate and lamotrigine all have an effect on the amygdala, are central in regulating mood and are involved in the neurobiology of many epilepsy syndromes.

The relationship between the interictal psychoses of epilepsy and schizophrenia have been partially sorted out, but more work is needed to examine neurobiological similarities and differences in greater detail. The underlying pathology is different, an absence of gliosis in the hippocampus and related structures characterizing schizophrenia. Thus, the site of the pathology, the timing of the lesions developmentally, and the consequent functional changes in the brain may all be crucial to the later development of any behaviour changes in both epilepsy and schizophrenia.

The recent evidence then, especially from brain-imaging studies, suggests that Slater's original hypothesis regarding the structural basis for the syndromes was part right but part wrong. The interictal psychoses seem different from schizophrenia, especially with regards to the admixture with affective symptoms and the long-term social prognosis, which is better. While hippocampal changes may relate to both disorders, the increased amygdala size – bilateral and around 17–20% – and the lesser volumetric changes in the hippocampus in the epileptic psychoses suggest the two psychopathological states are biologically quite different. While the laterality findings with regards to the functioning of the left hemisphere seem to hold up, the data point away from fundamentally cortical abnormalities in these psychoses, and show the amygdala and related structures to be central in pathogenesis.

This raises questions as to the relationship of the schizophrenia-like syndromes of epilepsy to disturbances of affect, and the way the concept of the IDD fits into this scheme, since Blumer considers a spectrum of IDD which includes psychotic presentations. However, these clinical and pathological differences perhaps reflect on the prognosis of the various disorders, and should be telling us something about the role of the amygdala vis-à-vis the hippocampus in psychotic states.

The phenomenon of Forced Normalization is still held in doubt by a number of physicians, in spite of considerable evidence for its occurrence clinically and a neurobiological explanation, namely switching off the cortical expression of the EEG and diverting electrochemical forces through limbic–limbic forebrain structures. It is certainly found less often than made out by Landolt, and specific studies are few and far between. It is difficult to document cases precisely, EEG recordings being difficult to obtain at the right times. However, studies which systematically analyse the aetiology in consecutive case series identify Forced Normalization or alternative psychoses as accounting for about 10% of psychotic cases (Schmitz *et al.*, 1999). The importance of the condition cannot be overemphasized, either clinically or theoretically. The concept brings psychiatry uncomfortably close to neurology for some people, revealing a close biological link between seizures and psychosis. It also affects treatment. Thus, if, in some patients, suppression of seizures provokes psychopathology, it reinforces the fact, often ignored or misunderstood, that seizures and epilepsy are not synonymous, and that an understanding of the epileptic process and its treatment goes far beyond the control of seizures. In clinical practice, to ignore the fact that some patients manifest these problems as their seizures come under control can lead to the continuation of severe behaviour disturbances, with all of the social disruption that then emerges, and a failure to manage the epilepsy appropriately.

The term 'dementia of epilepsy' is also controversial. It is clear that some syndromes (such as ESES) reveal a direct relationship between seizures and a dementia syndrome, perhaps reversible. But the controversy was over whether or not a slow cognitive decline occurred due to the direct effect of seizures damaging neurones. This seems accepted, with the understanding of the toxic effects of calcium influx with excess neuronal excitability, and clinical evidence of cognitive decline over the long term in some patients.

Finally, the Gastaut–Geschwind syndrome has been much debated. However, the concept that an organic brain syndrome secondary to a temporal-lobe/limbic disorder of function could manifest has to be seen alongside the ready acceptance of the Klüver–Bucy syndrome and a raft of frontal-lobe behavioural syndromes. The presence of such features as hyperreligiosity and hypergraphia, deep feelings of personal destiny and epiphanic experiences leads the interested to the borderlands of brain–behaviour relationships, and touches on fundamental neuroscience issues that are coming to the forefront of research, namely neuroaesthetics, neurotheology and the neurology of human consciousness (Trimble, 2007b).

11
The Dementias

INTRODUCTION

Progress in our understanding of the neuro-pathological and neurochemical bases of the dementias has been substantial in the last two decades. New forms of dementia have been discovered, and the fundamental molecular biology, especially with regards to tau and amyloid protein, has been valuable in directing potential diagnostic methods and interventions.

DEFINITION

Dementia refers to a syndrome. Over the years, many authors have attempted definitions, and most agree on the following characteristics: it is acquired and chronic, thus distinguishing it from learning disability and acute organic brain syndromes, and in most cases it is irreversible, being secondary to structural changes in the brain. Further, it is distinguished by a decline in intellectual capabilities, in addition to changes in other areas of behaviour, notably emotional and motor. The emphasis is on social decline and failure to cope with an independent life.

Lishman (1987) defined dementia as 'an acquired global impairment of intellect, memory and personality but without impairment of consciousness' (p. 6).

Cummings and Benson (1992) refer to 'an acquired persistent impairment of intellectual function with compromise in at least three of the following spheres of mental activity; language,

memory, visuospatial skills, emotion or personality, and cognition (abstraction, calculation, judgement, etc.)' (p. 1).

ICD 10 refers to dementia as a syndrome 'due to disease of the brain, usually of a chronic or progressive nature, in which there is disturbance of multiple higher cortical functions, including memory, thinking, orientation, comprehension, calculation, learning capacity, language and judgement. Consciousness is not clouded' (p. 45). ICD and DSM IV-TR both subclassify according to type (dementia in Alzheimer's disease, etc.).

DSM IV-TR notes the essential feature of dementia to be the development of multiple cognitive deficits, which include memory impairment and at least one of aphasia, apraxia, agnosia or a disturbance in executive functioning. These deficits must be severe enough to impair occupational or social functioning. But Cummings and Benson (1992) consider this too restrictive: it excludes patients in early phases of dementia who still function well, it fails to include dementias such as Pick's disease where memory disturbances appear late and it does not include the dementias associated with psychiatric illness.

One feature of the various definitions is their descriptive nature, the concept being, initially at any rate, clinical. Another is the global nature of the impairments; this distinguishes dementia from persistent focal brain syndromes such as aphasias or amnesias. Although several of the dementias present with signs of focal brain damage, their resulting incapacity is clearly much more extensive than purely focal dysfunction would allow.

PREVALENCE

Most agree that dementia is posing one of the most rapidly increasing medical problems in the Western world. This is on account of the rising age of the population, the tendency towards a nuclear family structure, leaving many elderly people without the support of the extended family, and an increased awareness of diagnosis.

Prevalence rates rise with age, some 6% of the population over 65 being affected (Kay *et al.*, 1970), essentially doubling with every five-year increase of age over 65. Over 75 the prevalence increases rapidly, to around 40% by the age of 95. In geriatric units, over one-third of patients show evidence of mental impairment, and many in retirement communities and residential homes are affected. The prevalence is higher in women than in men, except in those with younger onset, when this is reversed. The incidence rate is variously estimated at around 0.5–7.0% per annum, again dependent on age.

Although the majority of cases, between 22 and 60%, are diagnosed as Alzheimer's disease (Cummings and Benson, 1992), these estimates are invariably made on selected referral patients, the diagnosis being clinical and rarely supported by post-mortem confirmation. The second most common diagnosis is multi-infarct dementia (MID), accounting for around 10% of cases. However, the growing recognition and importance clinically of dementia syndromes such as fronto-temporal dementia and dementia with Lewy bodies, along with increased clinical acumen, is altering these earlier estimates.

DIAGNOSIS AND CLASSIFICATION

Not all dementias show the same presentation, and one of the advances in recent years has been in the identification of different subtypes, based on clinical presentation, which appears to conform to underlying pathological processes.

In the classical picture, memory disorder is the initial complaint, especially for new events. This emerges gradually, although the family may report a dramatic behavioural event early on in the condition which signalled to them that something was wrong with their relative. Over time, other features of intellectual impairment become apparent, including a lack of spontaneity, concrete thinking and an impairment of abstract reasoning. Disorientation is a frequent early cognitive sign, patients easily losing their way, often in familiar surroundings.

As the disorder progresses, thought disorder may emerge, with delusions, often of persecution, and illusions or hallucinations, usually of a fleeting nature. Ultimately patients may become floridly psychotic.

Affective symptoms are present early in many cases, with lability of affect, tearfulness, withdrawal and frank depressive symptoms. In some presentations, distinction from major affective disorder may be difficult (see below). Hypochondriacal complaints, often with bizarre presentations, may arise.

Focal symptoms such as aphasia or apraxia are common, and as the disorder progresses abnormal neurological signs may appear. Motor signs, in particular Parkinsonism, can lead to a poverty of facial expression and postural disorders, and add to the slowness of movement and impaired ability to act. The development of Parkinsonism (suggestive of either Parkinson's disease with dementia or Lewy-body dementia), or of lateralizing signs (suggestive of cerebrovascular or fronto-temporal dementia), assumes clinical importance. Premorbid personality traits are exaggerated, irritability and aggression common, but the focal deficits may give rise to a more clearly defined change of personality, for example frontal-lobe pathology leading to disinhibition and perseveration. As time progresses, apathy, personal neglect and vacuousness come to dominate the clinical picture.

Identification of dementia in its early stages can be difficult. Often the patient is well supported by a relative, who, while noting the failing powers of their companion, will cover up for any deficits. The loss of such support, for example with the death of a spouse, may lead to a crisis, but by this time the disorder is well advanced.

It is clear that in the diagnosis of dementia, especially in the early stages, the witness account of a third party, especially one who knows the patient well, is essential. A full mental status and neurological evaluation are then followed by a series of special investigations. These include specialized neuropsychometry, with assessment of both the premorbid and the current level of functioning, skull and chest X-ray, and now MRI scanning, EEG investigations and, where necessary, more specialized techniques such as SPECT, PET or angiography. Laboratory investigations include haematology and electrolytes, B_{12} and folate levels, serology, thyroid-, liver- and renal-function tests, and an ESR. CSF is becoming of value, usually showing elevation of proteins, but also biological markers. Examination of the CSF will help exclude an inflammatory process.

The above introduction is a starting point, from the clinical point of view, for detecting the development of a dementia. Unlike in the other chapters of this book, diagnostic entities will here be discussed separately, as it has become clear that clinical, pathological and in some cases molecular biological differences can be made. Soon it may be possible to classify the dementias within a genetic, molecular and neuroanatomical biological framework, which will override clinical considerations.

ALZHEIMER'S DISEASE

This is the most commonly diagnosed of the dementias. Described in 1907 by Alzheimer, it is now used by many to refer to a dementia which is not confined to any particular age group but increases in incidence with age. It is often referred to as dementia of the Alzheimer type (DAT). In life, the diagnosis is still made by exclusion, there being as yet no confirmatory test, although with brain imaging and biological markers case identification is more certain (see below).

Familial cases have been described suggesting an autosomal dominant inheritance, and there are several reports of identical twins with the disorder, confirmed histologically (Kilpatrick *et al.*, 1983). In such reports the cases usually present in the presenile period (under 65). There tends to be an increase in cases among relatives of probands, especially with a presenile onset, and, further, relatives have an excess of Down's syndrome, lymphoma and immune-system disorders (for example rheumatoid arthritis, lupus erythematosus) compared to that expected from a control group (Heston *et al.*, 1981). The link with Down's syndrome is the more interesting in that it is now established that, if patients with the trisomy 21 survive long enough, they will almost certainly develop a dementia, the pathological features of which are typical for Alzheimer's disease. Mosaicism for trisomy 21 can present with no or minimal manifestations of Down's syndrome, and it may be an underdiagnosed cause of early-onset Alzheimer's disease.

Studies of the molecular genetics of Alzheimer's disease have, to date, revealed several candidate genes linked with the rarer early-onset familial disorder. These are those for the amyloid-beta precursor protein (APP), presenilin-1 (chromosome 14) and presenilin-2. The latter two form the catalytic core in gamma-secretase complexes, and mutations lead to abnormal formation of APP and to an accumulation of the beta-amyloid in the brain (see Figure 11.1). However, these account for less than 5% of all Alzheimer's disease cases. Susceptibility genes associated with the sporadic forms of the disease include apolipoprotein E (Apo E) alleles, which are associated with late-onset and familial Alzheimer's disease. The genes for Apo E are localized to chromosome 19, and Apo E is found in plaques, tangles and amyloid deposits. Intracellularly it is thought to stabilize tau protein, which binds perihelical filaments, and hence stabilizes minitubules (see below). There are three alleles: Apo E 2, 3 and 4. The latter is present in about 15–20% of the population, but the E4–E4 genotype occurs in about 1%, and in 40% of patients with Alzheimer's disease. Thus, homozygosity for Apo E E4 leads to an eightfold risk for the disease, and most homozygotes will develop Alzheimer's disease before the age

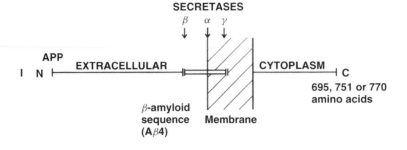

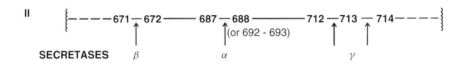

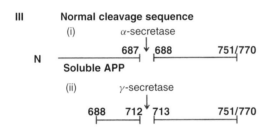

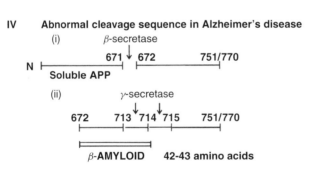

Figure 11.1   Schematic representation of possible cleavage sites of APP by secretases leading to the production of beta-amyloid protein. Section I shows APP molecules in aminoacid chain lengths (695, 751 or 770); much is extracellular. Section II is an enlargement of the beta-amyloid sequence. Section III shows the cleavage, normally of APP, by alpha-secretase releasing extracellular APP. The remaining molecule is broken down by gamma-secretase, yielding two short proteins that are broken down. In Section IV beta- rather than alpha-secretase splits off the extracellular APP to leave insoluble beta-amyloid (Webster *et al.*, 2002, p. 390)

of 80. Several other genetic associations have been reported but not confirmed.

   Although it may present in the fourth decade, the disease typically comes on later, and is more common in women. It progresses slowly over 5 to 10 years, with early signs of amnesia and lack of spontaneity. The course is steady, with the emergence of additional intellectual deficits, and finally extrapyramidal signs, seizures and advanced dementia. Focal neuropsychological disorders are prominent, and the presentation with aphasia or disorientation is seen. Depressive symptoms, irritability and aggression may be early signs, and slight infections or centrally active medications may provoke an acute organic brain syndrome.

The memory disturbance in Alzheimer's disease has been studied in detail by Kopelman (1985). He compared this condition to Korsakoff's psychosis and normal controls on a battery of memory tasks, and provided evidence that in the dementia, primary (short-term) memory was impaired, and there was also an increase in the rate of forgetting. Secondary (long-term) memory was also impaired, Alzheimer's patients showing a higher rate of false-positive errors. However, like Korsakoff's patients, those with the dementia, if allowed, could acquire memory by prolonged exposure to the stimulus material. Thus the Alzheimer's-disease patients showed defects in both memory systems: notably primary memory capacity and retention, and secondary memory acquisition. Tests of working memory (such as digit span) are retained, at least early on. One interpretation given by Kopelman was that these data support the clinical impression that the forgetfulness of these patients is due to a failure to take in information. Delayed memory recall is the most sensitive measure of the disorder, but with progression, semantic memory declines. Further, the existence of these multiple memory deficits may explain the failure of cholinergic replacement therapy, which primarily acts on secondary memory systems. The retrograde amnesia with loss of memory for faces and events from the distant past that patients develop remains unaccounted for.

Language disturbances are almost universal. Anomia is the commonest impairment, followed by comprehension difficulties. Speech is characterized by being fluent but irrelevant, with a high incidence of semantic jargon (Appell *et al.*, 1982). A consistent relationship has been reported between the impairment of language and the severity of the dementia, but not to duration of symptoms (Cummings *et al.*, 1985). The pattern of the aphasia resembles transcortical sensory aphasia, albeit usually

with a diminished output, being fluent and paraphasic, and with the ability to repeat remaining intact. In the later stages of the illness, echolalia, palilalia and verbigeration may occur, and finally mutism.

The personality in Alzheimer's disease remains relatively preserved in the early phases of the illness, and patients may retain social graces, in spite of severe impairments. This may be quite deceptive, the patient making good cognitive deficits by employing polite replies to questions and avoiding further interrogation. Sim (1979) outlined some of the early behavioural patterns seen in Alzheimer's disease in response to questions. These were: (a) perseverative movements, such as snapping of the fingers, indicating the answer to a question is on the tip of the patient's tongue; (b) the offering of entirely irrelevant answers; (c) simply smiling in response to a question in the hope that an alternative, less demanding one will be asked; (d) a display of anger, or a reply such as 'I'm not a child to be asked these silly questions'; (e) tearfulness; (f) a full catastrophic reaction, patients acting violently, with anger or tearfulness.

Wells (1979) noted such features as over-expression of satisfaction with trivial achievements, the increased reference to diaries and calendars for everyday events, and the abandonment of interest in hobbies and other topics, patients noting that this is so that others, for example the younger generation, can keep up with them. Gradually changes become obvious, and in the later stages features of frontal- or temporal-lobe disease appear. Fragments of the Klüver–Bucy syndrome may be recognized.

The EEG is invariably abnormal, with reduction of alpha rhythm, and later rhythmical theta and delta discharges – particularly over frontal and temporal regions – or diffuse slowing being recorded. There is some correlation between the degree of the dementia and the degree of slowing of the background rhythms. Of importance is the observation that, except in some conditions such as fronto-temporal dementia, the EEG tends to deteriorate over time in most forms of dementia. The investigation is thus essential for assessing difficult cases with regards to clarifying diagnosis over time, and may give an impression of the rate of the progression of the disease (Gordon, 1968). There are several reports that the P300 of the evoked potential shows increased latency and diminished amplitude, greater than that seen in aging (St Clair *et al.*, 1985), although to date no diagnostically specific findings have been noted.

The CT or MRI scan usually, but not always, reveals enlarged ventricles and enlarged cortical sulci. Nonetheless, like the EEG, the CT or MRI scan is an essential technique in investigating the disorder. First, it will reliably rule out many other causes of dementia (see below), some of which are potentially reversible. Second, it is of help in assessing the course of the condition in difficult-to-diagnose or established cases. Third, a normal scan in the presence of severe dementia should alert the physician to the possibility that the problem is a pseudodementia (apparently a dementia but actually a severe depression), still one of the commonest causes of a misdiagnosis of dementia.

Generally, brain atrophy as shown on the CT or MRI scan tends to correlate with the degree of dementia, although using planimetric measurements considerable overlap is seen when comparing patients with Alzheimer's disease and age-matched controls (Jacoby and Levy, 1980a), and correlations to cognitive tasks vary. Dementia associated with more severe atrophy has a poorer prognosis (Fox *et al.*, 1975), especially with marked parietal atrophy (Jacoby and Levy, 1980a). The latter is in keeping with the clinical data, implying a shorter survival in those with low scores on parietal tests (McDonald, 1969) and lower attenuation densities in the right parietal region (Naguib and Levy, 1982).

MRI studies have shown smaller cortical volumes and larger ventricular size. Hippocampal loss of volume on MRI is particularly important (although not specific, being seen also in Lewy-body dementia and some cases of frontotemporal dementia), and the finding of mesial temporal atrophy predicts those high-risk people with mild cognitive impairment (see below) who convert to Alzheimer's disease (Figure 11.2) (Korf *et al.*, 2004; Scher *et al.*, 2007). More recent MRI methods segment grey matter, white matter

and CSF, allowing for quantification of brain atrophy, calculating the boundary shift in brain structures on repeated scanning.

CBF and PET have also yielded interesting data. Mean-hemisphere CBF is decreased with increasing cognitive deterioration, especially grey-matter flow. Further, some correlations to cognitive tasks have been detected, with decreased temporal CBF with impaired memory scores, and a reduction in occipito-parietotemporal areas with verbal and symbolic language defects. In addition, a positive correlation between rCBF reduction in the postcentral areas and increasing EEG abnormalities has been shown in patients with post-mortem histological confirmation of their diagnosis (Johannesson *et al.*, 1977). In Alzheimer's disease, SPECT abnormalities are maximal in the postcentral region, predominantly in the area of the parietal lobes.

The PET studies confirm the decreased CBF, but also note low oxygen and glucose uptake. In general they confirm that the extent of the abnormalities reflects the degree of the dementia (Frackowiak *et al.*, 1981), and in Alzheimer's disease reveal early abnormalities in the parieto-temporal regions and later frontal-lobe involvement, with relative preservation of metabolic activity in the primary motor and sensory areas. Some groups are even using FDG PET as a disease marker, comparing an individual's scan against a gender- and age-matched healthy database (a jack-knife or individual-to-group comparison), looking for individual reductions greater than one standard deviation compared to the group, especially in the parietal cortex (Small *et al.*, 2000).

Recently it has become possible to visualize amyloid with PET using tracers such as F-18 FDDNP and C11PIB – called the Pittsburgh compound. It is possible to look at amyloid-beta deposition in the brain, although F-18 FDDNP visualizes both beta-amyloid plaques and neurofibrillary tangles (see below). Correlations have been shown between the binding of the latter tracer and the degree of dementia (Kepe *et al.*, 2006; Shoghi-Jadid *et al.*, 2005).

Much interest has been generated by the neuropathological findings of Alzheimer's

Alzheimer's Disease   FrontoTemporal Dementia   Huntington's Disease

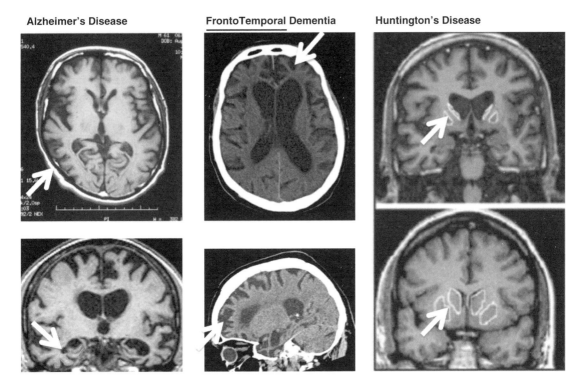

Figure 11.2 Hallmark pathological changes seen in several of the dementias. On the top-left a transverse T_1-weighted MRI scan shows the characteristic atrophy of the parietal cortex in a patient with Alzheimer's disease (arrow). Below that, a coronal MRI scan shows the hippocampal atrophy (arrow and outlined). In the centre panel, in contrast, are images from a patient with fronto-temporal dementia showing the prominent frontal atrophy (arrows on the transverse (top) and sagittal images (below)). The images on the right depict the characteristic atrophy of the caudate nucleus, with relative preservation of the rest of the brain in Huntington's chorea. The top-right image shows the caudate atrophy (arrow), with the bottom-right image showing the caudate of a healthy control (fronto-temporal dementia courtesy of Dr Donna Roberts, MUSC; Alzheimer's disease from www.medscape.com; Huntington's chorea from Ruocco *et al.*, 2006)

disease. Macroscopically there may be atrophy, especially in the temporoparietal region, and histologically there is loss of neurones, proliferation of astrocytes and the presence of senile plaques and neurofibrillary tangles. Granulovacuolar degeneration, in particular in the hippocampal pyramidal cells, is also seen. Tangles appear as coils of parallel bundles which stain intensively with silver; on electron microscopy they are seen to be made up of paired helical filaments. The tangle is composed of hyperphosphorylated tau protein, which derives from microtubules. The latter normally are both a transport system and provide structural support for the neurone, but in Alzheimer's

disease the tau protein is abnormally phosphorylated and less soluble. It becomes unable to bind to microtubules, presumably altering microtubule structure. Alzheimer's disease is thus one of the tauopathies, others being shown in Table 11.1.

The plaques are degenerating nerve terminals, astrocytes and microglia with an amyloid centre. Amyloid is seen as playing a central role in the pathology of Alzheimer's disease. Beta-amyloid is a protein of 39–43 amino acids, and is a fragment of the larger precursor protein APP. The latter is cleaved by beta and gamma secretases, but is also actually prevented from this by alpha secretase. It is an insoluble 40/42 amino

Table 11.1 The tauopathies

1. Alzheimer's disease	
2. Sporadic	Progressive supranuclear palsy
	Corticobasal degeneration
	Pick's disease
	Neurofibrillary form of senile dementia
3. Familial	

acid, and accumulates in plaques and cerebral blood vessels (amyloid angiopathy).

Tau protein is involved in the polymerization on neurotubules and tau accumulates in the neurones in several disorders, referred to collectively as the tau-opathies. Abnormal tau is found in neurofibrillary tangles, in Pick bodies, and can also be identified in astrocytes in some conditions. Microtubules are stabilized by tau–tubulin interactions. In Alzheimer's disease, tau pathology is most likely secondary; the proximate cause is unknown. However, amyloid-beta protein precursor is somehow involved.

There is some relationship between the site of pathology and clinical presentation. Forstl *et al.* (1994) reported that misidentifications (e.g. Capgras phenomena) were associated with lower neurone counts in the CA1 region of the hippocampus, but delusions and hallucinations were found in those patients with less cell loss in the parahippocampal gyrus and more in the raphe nucleus.

The tangles are in the cell body, usually close to the axon hillock, and the plaques are often located near to blood vessels. This situation of the tangles may lead them to block the normal movement of the macromolecules from the neurones to the terminal.

These changes are maximal in the cortex, especially in the temporo-parieto-ocipital region and in limbic-related cortex, hippocampus and amygdala, but also occur in some brainstem nuclei such as the locus coeruleus. Most tangles are seen in the entorhinal cortex, and the amygdala is also affected (lateral but not centro-medial nuclei), but primary sensory cortices are least affected. The earliest site of tangle

formation is in the entorhinal cortex and CA1 hippocampus, and a staging system of the progression of the disorder has been developed by Braak and Braak (Braak and Braak, 1997; Braak *et al.*, 1994a, 1994b). Plaques in noncortical structures are most numerous in the mammillary bodies

Although plaques and tangles are an essential feature of the pathology of Alzheimer's disease, they are not exclusive to that condition. Tangles are found, albeit in smaller numbers, in association with normal aging, and with such pathologies as dementia pugilistica, postencephalitic Parkinson's disease, progressive supranuclear palsy (the Steele–Richardson syndrome), subacute sclerosing panencephalitis and Down's syndrome. This raises the question as to whether or not they represent some nonspecific response to a variety of insults. Plaques, too, have been seen in Down's syndrome, Creutzfeldt–Jakob disease and with lead encephalopathy (Cummings and Benson, 1992).

What is unclear at present is the relationship between the findings that relate to Apo E E4, tau protein and the development of amyloid abnormalities, tangles and plaques. The E4 allele is a normal polymorphism in the population which confers increased risk of Alzheimer's disease, but it is possible that the Apo E2 allele confers protection. The relationship may involve enhanced aggregation or decreased clearance of amyloid-beta peptides, since Apo E enhances the proteolytic clearance of soluble beta-amyloid from the brain, and this ability is dependent upon the Apo E isoform.

The other line of pathological research has been the discovery of the neurochemical defects in Alzheimer's disease. The first to be defined was an abnormality of cholinergic mechanisms. Thus, it is now known that in Alzheimer's disease there is a widespread loss of presynaptic cholinergic activity, notably in the hippocampus, amygdala and neocortex (Bowen and Davison, 1986). The principal abnormality detected is a deficit of the synthesizing enzyme choline acetyl transferase, and a significant relationship exists between the decline in activity and an increasing number of plaques (Perry and Perry, 1980). This contrasts with the presence of normal muscarinic cholinergic (M1)-receptor activity. It is thought that the loss reflects degeneration of cholinergic neurones from the nucleus basalis, the projections of which are widespread. These cortical cholinergic deficits are not found in some other dementias, for example multi-infarct dementia or Huntington's chorea, but do occur in Creutzfeldt–Jakob disease and alcoholic dementia (Bowen and Davison, 1986).

Although some have suggested that Alzheimer's disease is a disorder of cholinergic innervation (Coyle *et al.*, 1983), several other neurotransmitter deficits have now been described (see Table 11.2). These include diminished noradrenergic and serotonergic innervation to the cortex, with associated neuropathological findings in the locus coeruleus and raphe nuclei (Adolfsson *et al.*, 1979; Mann *et al.*, 1980). Low levels of GABA, dopamine (Adolfsson *et al.*, 1979), dopamine beta hydrolase (Cross *et al.*, 1981), somatostatin (Francis and Bowen, 1985) and neurotensin with an increase in substance P (Perry and Perry, 1982) have all been reported. A low uptake of 5-HT by neocortical biopsy tissue has also been noted (Benton *et al.*, 1982), as has decreased 5-HT$_4$ receptor binding to frontal and temporal cortices (Cross *et al.*, 1984). All these changes may have relevance for the symptomatology of the disease, and are relevant in terms of defining therapies. Not all neurotransmitters are reduced, however, and some peptides such as cholecystokinin and VIP seem normal (Rossor *et al.*, 1980). NMDA binding is variable but often normal.

Decreased glutamate terminals in cortical and hippocampal areas from Alzheimer's-disease

brains have been reported, suggesting dysfunction of excitatory amino-acid-release pathways from neocortical neurones (Bowen and Davison, 1986; Hardy *et al.*, 1987). Such data implicate the cortex as a possible site of the primary pathology, loss of descending projections leading to secondary changes in subcortical structures.

Bowen and colleagues argue that since cognitive decline can be related to reduced synthesis of acetylcholine and other monoamine abnormalities have not been so clearly related to the cognitive changes, these latter changes are not the primary neuropathological events in the disease (Francis *et al.*, 1985).

CSF studies in general have led to conflicting results with regard to monoamine findings. However, the search for biomarkers has seen a renewed interest in CSF data (see below). On the basis of genetic clinical and biochemical findings, several forms of Alzheimer's disease are being defined. Rossor *et al.* (1984) examined brains of Alzheimer's-disease patients and controls, and noted various changes in the former, including decreased choline acetyl transferase, GABA, noradrenaline and somatostatin levels. However, older patients, dying in their ninth and tenth decades, had a relatively pure cholinergic deficit with additional decreases in somatostatin, reductions being confined to the temporal cortex. There was no cholinergic loss in the frontal cortex. The younger patients had more widespread changes with regard to acetylcholine and the other neurotransmitters. Rossor *et al.* suggested that Alzheimer's disease in those under 80 may be a distinct form. Bondareff *et al.* (1981) also provided data showing that neuronal dropout in the locus coeruleus characterizes a subgroup with a younger age, more severe disease and earlier death. Mahendra (1984) has developed the concept further. He suggests that one type of Alzheimer's dementia is characterized by earlier onset, signs and symptoms of parietal lobe and language disorders, and cortical and subcortical pathology. In the other, of later onset, the pathology is restricted to subcortical sites, and the presence of the parietal-lobe signs is minimal. The genetic studies seem to provide some support for these ideas. Some of the differences are shown in Table 11.3.

Table 11.2 Summary of some neurotransmitter and receptor changes in Alzheimer's disease

	Transmitter	Receptor
Acetylcholine	↓	N
Noradrenaline	↓	N
Dopamine	↓	N
5-HT	↓	N
Glutamate	↓	↑
Somatostatin	↓	↓
GABA	↓	?

Table 11.3   Summary of some changes in Alzheimer's disease and normal aging

	Old age	Alzheimer's early onset	Alzheimer's late onset
Plaques in cortex	+	+++	++
Tangles in cortex	−	+++	++
CAT decrease	±	+++	++ (temporal)
↓ cells in locus coeruleus		+++	+
↓ cells in nucleus basalis	−	+++	−
Noradrenaline ↓	−	++	+
GABA ↓	+	+++	+
5-HT ↓	+	+++	+
Somatostatin ↓	−	++	+ (temporal only)
Cholecystokinin	−	−	−
VIP	−	−	−
Genetics	−	14,21	19 (chromosome number)
Apo E E4	−	?	+

−, no change; + through +++, significant change; CAT = choline acetyl transferase.

In spite of this growing knowledge of the pathology and chemistry of Alzheimer's disease, the aetiology remains obscure. The suggestion that it represents premature aging is not compatible with the evidence from clinical, radiological and pathological comparisons of elderly people and patients with dementia. The presence of plaques and tangles, and possible biochemical links between them, may suggest a common genetic defect that leads to their formation, the consequent disruption of neuronal activity then leading to the clinical picture. Others suggest that the plaques are due to degeneration from their cells of origin in the nucleus basalis, the latter being the crucial site of pathology. Rossor (1981) has proposed that the disease should be conceptualized as a 'disorder of the isodendritic core'. The 'isodendritic core' refers to the fact that cells of the locus coeruleus, substantia nigra, substantia innominata and septal nuclei all share a generalized pattern of dendritic spread, intermingling with other neuronal elements, thus forming a continuous isodendritic core from the spinal cord to the basal forebrain. This idea links Alzheimer's disease and Parkinson's disease, each of which represents a different region of loss of the core, and may explain the frequent presence of extrapyramidal motor symptoms in Alzheimer's disease and the high frequency of cognitive impairment in Parkinson's disease. While tangles are not a regular feature of the latter, profound losses of neurones in the nucleus basalis are seen.

At one time, the cortical/subcortical location of the pathology of the dementias led to the suggestion that there were two types of dementia, one primarily cortical, presenting with focal cortical signs such as aphasia and apraxia, and the other subcortical, with dilapidation of cognition, memory problems and slowing. This placed Alzheimer's disease firmly with the cortical dementias. However, the pathological studies have emphasized the subcortical basis for much of the neurochemical change in Alzheimer's disease, and the dichotomy is no longer held to be valid.

Pathogenic agents discussed have included aluminium intoxication, immunological abnormalities and slow viruses, although no convincing data have supported such ideas. Certainly to date there are no substantial reports of transmission of a similar disease from Alzheimer's-disease brain tissue to animals, and the immunological abnormalities reported may well be secondary (Cummings and Benson, 1992).

Biomarkers

In the context of this section, 'biomarkers' refers to possible clinically-useful biological markers of Alzheimer's disease, as opposed to, for example, genetic linkages. The latter confer risk factors but not state markers. The idea is to better identify the disorder, especially with treatment in mind, and possibly to monitor progress. There are several candidates, and they relate to amyloid and tau. CSF beta-amyloid is low and total tau protein is high, the combination having high sensitivity and specificity for Alzheimer's disease. Either alone is less useful since although CSF amyloid-beta$_{1-42}$ differentiates Alzheimer's disease from healthy controls, it is much less discriminating against some other types of dementia (Schipper, 2007, 2009). There may be some association of the combination to Apo E E4 status.

DEMENTIA OF FRONTAL-LOBE TYPE

Pick described a form of dementia in 1892 associated with a circumscribed atrophy of the frontal and temporal lobes. Neary and colleagues (1988) suggested that this was one form of a wider spectrum of dementing illness in which the primary pathology was frontal. These patients present a clinical picture suggestive of progressive frontal damage, an absence of Alzheimer's pathology and decreased frontal-lobe CBF with brain imaging. They have few neurological signs. As a group, patients with dementia of frontal-lobe type are younger than patients with Alzheimer's disease, and a family history of dementia is reported in 46%. In the familial variant with autosomal dominant inheritance, around 20% have mutations in the MAPT gene which encodes tau protein,

This is a clinical designation, not a pathological diagnosis. Clinical features are shown in Table 11.4. Pick's disease itself is much less common than Alzheimer's disease. It is more common in females. Inheritance is said to be through a single autosomal dominant gene, although most cases are sporadic.

There are distinguishing features that reflect the underlying pathology and separate fronto-temporal dementia from Alzheimer's disease (see Table 11.5). Thus abnormalities of behaviour, emotional changes and aphasia are frequently the presenting features, as opposed to memory impairments. Some have noted elements of Klüver–Bucy syndrome at one stage or another of the disease (Cummings

Table 11.4 Clinical diagnostic features of fronto-temporal dementias (adapted from Brun *et al.*, 1994)

Behaviour disorder
Affective symptoms
Speech disorder
Spatial orientation and praxis preserved
    Physical signs:
        Early: incontinence, primitive reflexes
        Late: akinesia, rigidity
Investigations:
    EEG: normal
    Imaging: predominantly fronto-temporal change
    Neuropsychology: failure on frontal tests
Supportive features:
    Onset before 65 in 80%
    Positive family history 20% autosomal
        dominant inheritance
    Bulbar palsy

and Benson, 1992). Interpersonal relationships deteriorate, insight is lost, and the jocularity of frontal-lobe damage may even suggest a manic picture. The aphasia is reflected in word-finding difficulties, empty, flat, nonfluent speech and paraphasias. With progression the cognitive changes become apparent, including memory deterioration, but several higher cortical functions are intact – for example, a patient may continue to play bridge or even to work at a technical job. Cases are described of an output of creativity, such as painting or poetry, and obsessions, hoarding, compulsive eating and unusual rituals may be seen (Mendez and Shapira, 2008, 2009). Ultimately, extrapyramidal signs, incontinence and widespread cognitive decline are seen.

The EEG tends to remain normal in fronto-temporal dementias, even when the behaviour changes are advanced, and the CT or MRI may provide confirmatory evidence of lobar atrophy (see Figure 11.2). Likewise, the PET picture shows diminished metabolism in the frontal and temporal areas. Neuropsychological testing will reveal appropriate abnormalities on frontal-executive tasks.

Pathologically, the brunt of the change in frontotemporal dementias is borne by the frontal and temporal lobes, and mainly takes the form of neurone loss with gliosis and spongiform changes. In some cases there is predominant

Table 11.5   The differential diagnosis of dementia (from Trimble, 1981, p. 118)

	Alzheimer's disease	Dementia of frontal type	Creutzfeldt–Jakob' disease	Arteriosclerotic	Hydrocephalic
Early signs	Memory	Behaviour change, aphasia, incontinence	Neurological signs and symptoms	Acute focal deficit	Memory, psychomotor showing, ataxia, incontinence
Focal deficits	++	+	+	++	– –
Orientation difficulties	Early	Late	–	–	–
Personality change	Late	Early	Early	Late	Early
Extrapyramidal signs	+	–	+	+	±
CBF	Posterior hemisphere	Anterior hemisphere	Multiple areas of hypoperfusion	Multiple areas of hypoperfusion	
EEG	Abnormal	Often normal	Always abnormal	Abnormal	Abnormal
Other features	'Mirror sign'	Hyperalgesia	Myoclonus	Pseudobulbar signs	Ventricular enlargement

–, no change; + through +++, significant change.

tau pathology, in others ubiquitin changes are in evidence, and in a third group there is no distinguishing pathology. Mutation of the tau gene has been identified in most familial cases with tau pathology, although this is only the minority of cases with familial fronto-temporal dementia. Cases with tau-gene mutation can be distinguished from typical Pick pathology with the characteristic 'balloon' cell, which contains disorganized neurofilaments and neurotubules, and also the Pick bodies, which are silver-staining and are also composed of neurofilaments, tau protein and tubules. The latter are particularly prominent in the mediotemporal and limbic frontal areas. Plaques and tangles are not a feature of this disease, and the aetiology is unknown.

FOCAL CORTICAL ATROPHIES

Pick's disease is one of a number of focal atrophies that lead to a dementia syndrome. The clinical picture is related to the site and speed of the developing pathology. Semantic dementia is a subtype of fronto-temporal dementia which presents with predominant language impairments, with the same demographic features and MRI evidence of atrophy of the left anterior temporal lobe. There is an anomia but a fluent aphasia, and often a reading difficulty with an inability to read words with irregular spellings (such as yaught). Progressive nonfluent aphasia is associated with left perisylvian atrophy. There is a variant associated with motor-neurone disease, with bulbar palsy, weakness, wasting and muscular fasciculations. Corticobasal degeneration has cortical and basal-ganglia pathology, with an associated extrapyramidal syndrome; in some cases the cortical presentation may be mainly parietal. The pathology resembles Pick's disease. Other variants are with a posterior atrophy, but with Alzheimer-like pathological changes.

Progressive subcortical gliosis is a disorder with a primarily frontal presentation and gliosis of frontal and subcortical structures.

DEMENTIA WITH LEWY BODIES

This is a syndrome of dementia with extrapyramidal rigidity, associated with Lewy bodies as a pathological finding. Lewy bodies occur with or without associated plaques or tangles. They are identified with alpha-synuclein antibodies and are typically found in the substantia nigra in Parkinson's disease, but in dementia with Lewy bodies they are scattered throughout the cortex, especially in the parahippocampal gyrus and temporal, frontal and insular cortices. They are round hyaline bodies with a pale peripheral halo, found in the cell cytoplasm. The presentation of the dementia is often with hallucinations or delusions, and it may be much more common than as yet diagnosed. The distinction between Parkinson's disease with dementia and dementia with Lewy bodies can be difficult, but the latter has a far shorter history of Parkinsonism before the onset of the dementia. Other suggestive signs of dementia with Lewy bodies include the presence of REM-sleep behaviour disorder, early autonomic dysfunction and sensitivity to neuroleptic drugs.

In comparison with Alzheimer's disease, basal-ganglia imaging with ligands for the dopamine transporter (FP-CIT) will often be abnormal, while imaging of medial temporal structures is normal.

VASCULAR DEMENTIAS

The concept of vascular dementia has undergone significant changes in recent years, most notably with the recognition that chronic ischaemic changes in the brain are rarely, if ever, responsible for dementia. It is now thought that multiple cerebral infarctions are a common cause of dementia, and that separation of this type of deterioration from Alzheimer's disease is possible on clinical grounds and has therapeutic and prognostic relevance. However, ischaemic changes are frequently found in association with Alzheimer's disease or Lewy-body dementia, and may contribute to the clinical picture.

The vascular dementias comprise three main groups: first, multi-infarct dementia (MID) associated predominantly with multiple cortical infarcts; second, MID with mainly subcortical infarcts; and third, that type which affects white matter diffusely, Binswagner's disease. In reality the first two types are frequently combined.

The pattern of the presentation relates to the occurrence of multiple infarcts, their site of extracranial origin and their location in the CNS. The most common cause is emboli from the extracranial arteries and the heart, and typically the progression is of a stepwise dementia, often with a history of hypertension and evidence of recurrent strokes. On examination there may be evidence of focal deficits in neurological function, and increased muscular tone, hyperreflexia and Babinski responses may be found. A pseudobulbar state may be apparent, and emotional lability present. Unlike Alzheimer's disease, there is an equal sex preponderance.

The Hachinski score is now an accepted method for helping establish a diagnosis, and is used widely in research (Hachinski *et al.*, 1975). Application of this scale, the features of which are shown in Table 11.6, leads to a score: the ischaemia score. If over seven, the diagnosis is more likely to be MID, while a score of under four suggests parenchymatous dementia. There are criticisms of the method and the scale, especially with regard to identification of early cases. Follow-up studies have been carried out which suggest that four features, namely abrupt onset, stepwise deterioration, focal neurological symptoms and a history of hypertension, are the best discriminators for MID.

In the cortical presentations of MID, the signs and symptoms depend on the site of the lesions. The middle cerebral-artery territory is most involved, leading to aphasias, apraxias,

Table 11.6 The Hachinski scale (from Hachinski *et al.*, 1975)

Abrupt onset	2
Stepwise deterioration	1
Fluctuation	2
Nocturnal confusion	1
Relative preservation of personality	1
Depression	1
Somatic complaints	1
Emotional lability	1
Hypertension	1
History of stroke	2
Focal symptoms	2
Focal signs	2
Other arteriosclerotic signs	1

visuospatial problems and other signs and symptoms of cortical pathology. In contrast, the subcortical variant affects the basal ganglia, thalamus and internal capsule. It is usually the consequence of infarction of tissue supplied by the lenticulostriate arteries of the middle cerebral artery and other small perforating vessels from the posterior communicating and posterior cerebral arteries.

The pattern of the disorder is progressive, with acute deterioration in the mental and cognitive state of the patient, followed by recovery. The latter is rarely to the state prior to the infarct, so a continuous but interrupted decline occurs. Patients often retain insight to their difficulties, and personality is quite preserved initially. Affective changes are common, and these must be distinguished from the lability of pseudobulbar palsy. Psychotic episodes with paranoid delusions may be seen, and may be the only or initial sign of an infarct. Hypochondriacal complaints may be an early sign. The cognitive state is one of memory impairment, psychomotor slowing and general dilapidation of performance. As the condition advances, motor symptoms are clear, including a Parkinsonian syndrome.

The pathology in MID reveals areas of softening and cavitation, and when these are multiple in the basal ganglia the condition is referred to as a lacunar state.

The EEG usually shows severe changes, and focal slow activity is not uncommon. The CT and MRI scan reveal multiple infarcts, bilaterally distributed, some of which may be seen in the basal ganglia.

With PET, clearer differences between vascular and nonvascular cases have been noted (Frackowiak *et al.*, 1981). In contrast to the fronto-parietal distribution of Alzheimer's disease, MID showed more scattered areas of focal infarction, although in mild dementia the parietal areas were involved in both groups. In general, a low frontal pattern was characteristic of the Alzheimer's-disease group. Of importance were the findings that changes in oxygen uptake in the MID patients were coupled to the CBF, the ratio of extracted oxygen (OER) remaining in the normal range. This demonstrates that the pathology is not related to ischaemia where the OER increases, and raises doubts about the feasibility of using agents that increase blood flow in treatment. One possible consequence of this finding is that episodes of hypotension may cause ischaemia in zones of decreased perfusion.

'Binswagner's encephalopathy' refers to a form of dementia of vascular aetiology with predominantly white-matter changes. The cerebral cortex appears well preserved, and patients have a past history of hypertension. The presentation is of a slowly-developing dementia, often in the presenium, with a history compatible with multiple small strokes. Neurological signs, pseudobulbar lability and psychopathology are seen. The latter includes affective changes, paranoid delusions and hallucinations.

Pathologically there is loss of myelin and gliosis, and accompanying blood vessels are arteriosclerotic (Janota, 1981). The EEG is usually abnormal, with generalized slowing or focal changes, and the CT scan may reveal decreased white-matter attenuation. MRI shows increased T_2 signal from periventricular areas and associated white-matter hemisphere lesions The white-matter changes are reflected by low oxygen uptake with a PET scan (Frackowiak *et al.*, 1981).

'Leucoaraiosis' refers to small areas of white-matter change that can be seen on CT, or better with MRI, and are commonly visualized in the elderly. These may represent either increased water content of myelin without alteration of function, or myelin loss, and thus their presence has a poor correlation with cognition. It is associated with hypertension, but may result from hypoperfusion, and there is a genetic link in some cases. Cerebral autosomal dominant arteriopathy with subcortical infarcts and leucoencephalopathy (CADASIL) is related to a mutation on chromosome 19 (notch-3 gene) which affects the smooth muscle of the walls of affected cerebral blood vessels. It has a young age of onset, with recurrent ischaemic attacts, and there is often a history of migraine. However, there may be a history of psychiatric disorder, especially depression, preceding the obvious vascular lesions by a number of years.

The causes of the vascular occlusions responsible for the vascular dementias are legion (Cummings and Benson, 1992). Included are haematological conditions, inflammatory disorders and infections, and cardiac disease, all of which may lead to emboli, and the prominent role of hypertension has been noted above. This is of utmost relevance for evaluation and treatment. Thus, since vascular dementia is a secondary form of dementia, elicitation of any underlying pathology is of prime importance, especially if the condition is treatable in its own right. This underlines the importance of a full and proper evaluation and investigation of patients with dementia. Ruling out cardiovascular disease, and especially hypertension, may require specialized investigations and repeated estimations of blood pressure. Rarer causes such as systemic lupus erythematosus, giant cell arteritis, atrial myxomas and sarcoid should be thought of, as well as the commoner diabetes, and emboli from silent myocardial infarctions and atrial fibrillation. While survival may relate to the underlying condition, it seems that it is longer in Alzheimer's disease (5–10 years) than in MID.

OTHER FORMS OF DEMENTIA

The primary dementias of Alzheimer and Pick can be distinguished from dementia associated with other CNS conditions such as Huntington's chorea and Parkinson's disease, and from the secondary dementias such as those due to vascular (for example MID), infective (for example syphilis, AIDS), traumatic, metabolic, neoplastic and metabolic causes. In addition, one form of dementia, potentially reversible, is now clinically identifiable secondary to hydrocephalus. Some of these conditions are described here (see Table 11.7).

Huntington's Chorea

The main features of this disease are dementia, chorea and a family history of a similar disorder. There is a high frequency of associated psychopathology, notably depression, personality

Table 11.7 Some treatable causes of dementia (from Trimble, 1981, p. 125)

Traumatic	Head injury, hydrocephalus after head injury, subdural
Infective	Neurosyphilis, chronic meningitis, parasitic and fungal infections, AIDS – secondary infections
Deficiencies	Vitamin B_{12}, folic acid
Neoplasia	Primary or metastatic
Intoxications	Barbiturates, anticonvulsants, alcohol
Metabolic	Hormonal (thyroid, parathyroid, adrenal)
	Wilson's disease
	Renal failure
	Hepatic failure
	Pulmonary or cardiac failure
Dynamic	Hydrocephalus
Other	Embolic: Sarcoid: SLE
	Whipple's disease
	Lyme disease
	Behçet's disease
	Giant cell arteritis
	Systemic vasculitides

disorder and a schizophrenia-like or paranoid disorder (Trimble, 1981a). The condition has an age of onset typically in the fourth or fifth decade, although juvenile forms are seen. Psychiatric states are the earliest manifestations of the disease in about one-third of patients, and memory disturbance occurs early, though it is qualitatively different from that of Alzheimer's disease. In Huntington's chorea there are both encoding and retrieval deficits.

Huntington's chorea is a genetic disorder, with an autosomal dominant pattern of inheritance, and a gene abnormality on the short arm of chromosome 4. It is known that CAG repeats are expanded, and the abnormal protein is referred to as huntingtin. In normal chromosomes, there are 9–39 CAG repeats, but in Huntington's chorea there are usually over 40. The number is related to the age of onset of the disease, larger numbers relating to earlier onset.

Gradual atrophy of the neostriatum is the hallmark of the condition, and medium spiny projection neurones (containing GABA and substance P) degenerate first and most severely. The small spiny cells are inhibitory GABA neurones, with a high density of NMDA receptors. Nuclear inclusions that label for ubiquitin and huntingtin are seen. The latter is a widely-distributed protein, and is involved in intracellular transcription and transport. It also has anti-apoptotic properties. There are decreased concentrations of GABA and glutamic acid decarboxylase, with a relative increase of dopamine function. CSF GABA is also decreased. Some neurotransmitters are increased in levels, including 5-HT and peptide Y (Beal *et al.*, 1988). Receptor studies reveal reduced binding in the basal ganglia for NMDA, dopamine, GABA and acetylcholine (Young *et al.*, 1988). One hypothesis is that NMDA excitotoxicity is involved in pathogenesis, although how this relates to the genetic findings is unknown.

CT and MRI will reveal loss of bulk in the head of the caudate, and PET studies show decreased metabolism in the caudate, even before structural changes are visible (Figure 11.2). Presymptomatic patients often show subtle motor impairments, subtle clumsiness, brief choreiform movements and ocular motor impairment, and on imaging it may be possible to show a decrease in size of the corpus striatum. Genetic testing for CAG repeats is definitive, and it is now possible to estimate the years to clinical diagnosis from the current age of the patient and the CAG-repeat length.

CNS Syphilis

Although rare, this condition is still encountered as a cause of dementia in the Western world, and it is advisable to test serology appropriately in all cases. In its florid form, GPI presents as a progressive deterioration with associated psychopathology. The latter may resemble manic illness, schizophrenia or a depressive illness. The disorder starts insidiously, some 10–15 years after the primary infection, but soon loss of judgement and delusions, sometimes with the well-known grandiosity, appear. It may resemble the euphoria of the frontal-lobe syndrome, but the grandiosity is quite distinctive from the mood-congruent behaviour of mania. On examination, apart from the abnormal mental state, tremor of the lips, tongue and outstretched hands may occur. Dysarthria is common. The typical Argyll–Robertson pupil is seen in about 50% of cases. If associated with tabes dorsalis, neurological features of this, such as loss of vibration and position sense in the limbs, will be found. Convulsions may occur.

Pathologically there is marked atrophy with neuronal loss and gliosis, and iron pigment in the microglia and perivascular spaces is specific for the disease (Catterall, 1977). Treponema pallidum can be seen in the cortex in about 50% of cases.

In the CSF there is elevation of total protein and lymphocyte count, a paretic (first-zone) rise in the Lange colloidal gold curve and positive serology. An oligoclonal antibody pattern is also seen. Blood screening with WR or the VDRL is essential, but these give both false-positive and negative results. The treponema pallidum immobilization test (TPI) and the fluorescent antibody test (FTA) are much more reliable. After treatment, the VDRL and the WR usually become normal, but this may take several years. The FTA, however, may remain positive, but prior to relapse the clinical manifestations are normally preceded by further CSF changes, notably a rise in cells and protein, and increasing antibody titres.

Another spirochete that is associated with dementia is borrelia burgdorferi, which causes Lyme disease. As with treponema pallidum, this organism can invade many organs, including the brain, leading to inflammatory changes.

HIV Encephalopathy

This condition, also referred to as the AIDS–dementia complex, is caused by the virus HTLV-111 (HIV, human immunodeficiency virus), which invades T-helper lymphocytes and damages them. Briefly, the T-helper cells promote immunological responses to infection. They have a surface glycoprotein which binds to the envelope glycoprotein of HIV. The HIV is a retrovirus, one which destroys cells it invades by transcribing its own RNA into the DNA of the host cell using the enzyme reverse transcriptase. The depletion of T-helper (T_4) lymphocytes leads to loss of the infected person's immunological competence; neurotoxins are secreted and secondary 'opportunistic' infections develop, many of which affect the brain, for example toxoplasmosis or cryptococcal meningitis. An alternative expression is the development of certain tumours, for example CNS lymphoma. The pathological hallmarks of HIV dementia are microglial nodules and multinucleated giant cells which are HIV-infected macrophages.

It is known that the virus itself is neurotropic and can be isolated from the brains and CSF of patients. It may lead to an acute encephalopathy, associated with malaise, mood changes and seizures. However, an insidious dementia may occur with initial features of psychopathology such as lethargy, loss of libido, affective changes and cognitive blunting. Eventually, neurological signs become clear, the EEG changes often showing bilateral slowing, and MRI may reveal evidence of atrophy and periventricular white-matter lesions. The CSF may show a rise of the white-cell count and protein. In the final stages, mutism, dementia, incontinence and paraplegia may result. Highly-active antiretroviral therapy (HART), introduced in the mid-1990s, has led to a remarkable decline in the incidence of HIV-associated dementia.

The virus is a blood-borne pathogen, and high-risk patients are intravenous drug abusers, homosexuals and haemophiliacs. It is identified by testing for HIV antibodies, the viral load and an abnormal ratio of T_4 to T_8 lymphocytes. Less than 400 T_4 cells per cu mm is considered abnormal.

Creutzfeldt–Jakob Disease and Prions

The original descriptions of this condition were of a dementia with pyramidal and extrapyramidal manifestations. It is a rare cause of dementia, males being affected more than females. Rarely, familial cases are described, and autosomal dominant inheritance is suggested (Masters *et al.*, 1979).

Although sudden onset is seen, usually, in the initial phase, there may be only vague somatic complaints followed by mood and personality changes. The progression of the disorder may be fairly rapid, many patients dying within six months of the diagnosis. Soon the dementia is apparent, and localized cortical deficits such as aphasia or apraxia may occur. The accompanying signs are those of extrapyramidal and pyramidal dysfunction, but cerebellar abnormalities and frontal-lobe features may also be seen. Muscle wasting, convulsions (particularly myoclonic jerking), delusions and hallucinations form part of the clinical picture. A startle response to sudden loud noises is an interesting sign that may help provide a clue to diagnosis.

Several different forms of the dementia have been described. These include a cerebellar form, an amyotrophic form with marked lower motor-neurone signs, and the amaurotic variant of Heidenhain. However, some prefer not to split the disorder in this way, regarding the disease as a single entity with various presentations.

The CSF is usually unremarkable, although 14-3-3 protein may be elevated. The EEG is always abnormal, with increased slow-wave activity and diminution of the alpha rhythm. A pattern of slow sharp-wave discharges is seen, which may be locked to the myoclonic jerks. Although these may be seen in other conditions such as metabolic encephalopathies, SSPE and some viral encephalitides, their presence with the above clinical picture confirms the diagnosis of Creutzfeldt–Jakob disease. The CT and MRI scans may be normal, although they mostly show atrophy and ventricular dilatation, while on PET there are multifocal areas of hypometabolism (Cummings and Benson, 1992). Biopsies of the tonsils can identify prion protein, and a brain biopsy will confirm the diagnosis.

Of interest has been the transmission of the condition from human brain material to primates. The first degenerative condition of the human CNS to be transmitted to primates was Kuru. This disorder, found among aborigines in New Guinea, causes a pathological state similar to the human disease in the primate brains. In Creutzfeldt–Jakob disease this consists of neuronal loss and gliosis, and status spongiosus – the microscopic appearance of vacuoles leading to a spongiform picture. Abnormal proteinaceous particles representing prions can be detected. This disorder has now been transmitted to several species, and there are reports of man-to-man inoculation during neurosurgical procedures (Bernoulli *et al.*, 1977) and from human growth hormone extracts. The pathological agent responsible is a prion (small proteinaceous infectious agent). The human prion diseases include Creutzfeldt–Jakob disease (sporadic and familial forms), Kuru and the Gerstmann–Straussler–Scheinker syndrome, and are referred to as transmissible cerebral amyloidoses. The latter is an autosomal dominant disorder which presents in the third or fourth decade with cerebellar symptoms, with later onset of extrapyramidal features and dementia (Collinge *et al.*, 1990). Familial fatal insomnia, with progressive insomnia, autonomic dysfunction and dementia is another prion disorder with pathological changes largely in the thalamus.

Variant Creutzfeldt–Jakob disorder appeared in the UK, and is thought to be related to ingestion of beef from cows with bovine spongiform encephalopathy. It differs from other forms of Creutzfeldt–Jakob disease by an earlier age of onset (mean 28 years) and presentation initially with behavioural problems. It produces a characteristic MRI picture with high signal bilaterally in the posterior thalamus (the pulvinar sign). Homozygosity at codon 129 has been noted in most cases, the gene being on chromosome 20.

Prions are resistant to heat, ultraviolet and ionizing radiation and formaldehyde treatment, but are inactivated by agents that hydrolyse proteins. There is no associated nucleic acid, and they do not evoke an inflammatory reaction. They are thought to be glycoproteins, essentially isoforms of normal host-membrane glycoproteins (prion proteins), which are broken down by proteases. PrP 27–30 has been identified as the infective agent (Prusiner, 1987). The cDNA has been found, and has been shown to be a single gene on the short arm of chromosome 20 that codes for the normal membrane protein. In the prion disorders, the protease-resistant insoluable isoform of the protein accumulates (PrP^{sc}/PrP^{res}/PrP^{P}), a process which is autocatalytic; in other words, the abnormal protein acts as a template for its further production.

Although clearly genetic, with mutations leading to autosomal dominant disease, prion diseases can also be transmitted by inoculation of exogenous prion protein.

It is now recognized that multiple mutations of the gene that encodes the prion protein (PrP or PRNP) can occur, and over 50 different mutations have been reported in the familial cases. The commonest mutation is reported at codon 200. Since prion diseases can have very variable presentations, the extent to which other dementias may be prion-related has yet to be determined.

Hydrocephalic Dementias

Although not exactly understood, the dynamics of CSF flow are as follows. The majority is produced by the choroid plexi of the ventricular system, and flow is from the lateral and third ventricles, through the Sylvian aqueduct to the fourth ventricle, and then out from the interstices of the brain to the subarachnoid space. It then goes either upwards, over the surface of the brain to be absorbed into the saggital sinus, or downwards over the spinal cord. Interference with this flow pattern can lead to hydrocephalus, with accumulation of excess CSF within the ventricular system. Two main varieties of hydrocephalus are recognized: obstructive and non-obstructive (see Table 11.8).

The non-obstructive conditions refer to those traumatic, destructive or degenerative states that lead to ventricular enlargement. The obstructive varieties are of two main types. In noncommunicating hydrocephalus, the CSF flow is impeded within the ventricular system, leading to increased pressure in the ventricles and secondary enlargement. Such states have long been recognized in childhood, but it is now clear that a variety of processes may lead to similar pathology in adulthood, and dementia is

Table 11.8 Hydrocephalic dementias (after Benson, 1975)

Non-obstructive	Degenerative, e.g. Alzheimer's disease
	Destructive, e.g. arteriosclerotic
Obstructive	Noncommunicating with ventricular obstruction
	Communicating – normal-pressure hydrocephalus

one result. Pathologies include tumours, intracranial haemorrhage, colloid cysts of the third ventricle, ectatic basilar artery and periventricular inflammation. The link between stenosis of the aqueduct, a very vulnerable site, and a schizophreniform illness has been noted (see Chapter 8). In communicating hydrocephalus there is no obstruction of the flow within the ventricular system or its exits, but a failure of absorption of the CSF back into the saggital sinus through blockage occurs. Either the fluid is unable to reach the convexity of the brain or absorption through the arachnoid villi is abnormal. There are several causes of this, including cerebral trauma, previous meningitis, neoplasia or, most commonly, subarachnoid haemorrhage. Normal-pressure hydrocephalus was described by Adams *et al.* (1965), and referred to a dementia seen several years after a head injury or subarachnoid haemorrhage with characteristic clinical features. These include gait disturbance and incontinence, and a normal CSF pressure. The dementia was often of recent onset, and was more related to a psychomotor slowing than to memory and higher cognitive deficits. Patients lost initiative, became apathetic, and in some cases their behaviour resembled a state of depression.

It is now recognized that the clinical picture can be varied. Spasticity, especially of the lower limbs (feet glued to the floor), difficulty in initiating movement, frontal-lobe signs, and incontinence and ataxia in the presence of dementia should alert to the possibility of this diagnosis, even in the absence of the above associated events in the patient's history, idiopathic cases being well recognized.

The EEG is usually abnormal, showing diffuse slowing, and a CT or MRI scan reveals large ventricles, often maximally blown in the frontal and temporal regions, in the presence of normal or small cortical sulci. Isotope cisternography will reveal the abnormal pattern of flow, and monitoring intracranial CSF pressure may help identify patients who will benefit from shunting.

The possibility of shunting the CSF to either the atrium of the heart or the peritoneal cavity has been tested, but with variable success.

FURTHER CAUSES OF DEMENTIA

The causes of dementia are legion, and some of the more common ones have already been defined. Every physician is looking to exclude a treatable cause, some of which are shown in Table 11.7. Tumours, especially meningiomas, must always be ruled out. Both folic acid and vitamin B_{12} deficiencies can lead to neuropsychiatric change and dementia, and this can occur in the absence of an anaemia. Nicotinic acid deficiency can lead to a pellagra-like state with dermatological changes, gastroenterological symptoms and dementia. Anticonvulsant drugs, notably phenytoin, in epileptic patients have been implicated with an encephalopathy (Trimble and Reynolds, 1976) and the dementia of chronic alcoholism is recognized (Ron *et al.*, 1979). Intoxication with psychotropic drugs can lead to cognitive dulling, for example with lithium, and rarely major tranquillizers can provoke or exacerbate a dementia-like syndrome. Creutzfeldt–Jakob-like symptoms are described with tricyclic antidepressant intoxication and lithium.

Hormone disturbances can lead to dementia, especially hypothyroidism, which is usually accompanied by other signs of myxoedema. Thyroid function tests will be abnormal, serum cholesterol raised and thyroid antibodies may be present in the serum.

More pervasive causes of dementia include those secondary to such cerebral insults as trauma and anoxia, and the dementia of demyelinating conditions such as multiple sclerosis.

SOME OUTSTANDING ISSUES

Differential Diagnosis

It used to be suggested that to try and diagnose the cause of dementia in life is a futile exercise. It was asserted that the post-mortem diagnosis is the only valid one, and that clinical diagnosis is often at variance with this. It was further implied that dementia is irreversible and that treatments are ineffective, and hence the diagnosis is purely an academic exercise.

There are several reasons why such views are no longer tenable. Thus, the dementias do differ in their clinical presentation. While the broader issue of cortical and subcortical dementia is discussed below, it seems that there are some forms of dementia that primarily present with cortical destruction, with apraxias and aphasias, while in others there is gradual cognitive slowing, difficulties with planning a future event and impairment of the grasp of complex issues – often initially with minimal memory impairment. Alzheimer's and fronto-temporal dementia can be distinguished in many cases, the latter showing behavioural complications in the presence of a relatively well-preserved memory and absence of the parietal signs. EEG and MRI data aid this distinction. An important sequel to this is to allow for and expect more florid behavioural problems with frontal dementias, which has consequences not only for management, but also medicolegally.

Both of these forms of dementias must be distinguished from a cortical aphasia syndrome, which may be very difficult in the so-called angular gyrus syndrome, or following an infarct in the dominant hemisphere of a left-handed patient, in whom the clinical picture of the aphasia can be misleading. The angular gyrus syndrome is caused by a lesion of the left hemisphere in the region of that gyrus. Patients have combinations of fluent aphasias, apraxias, alexia and parts of Gerstmann's syndrome, comprising acalculia, right–left disorientation, finger agnosia and agraphia. Such focal syndromes are most likely, particularly if they are due to a vascular cause, to be nonprogressive, and thus carry a very different prognosis to the dementias.

Distinguishing primary parenchymatous dementias from secondary dementias is of utmost importance, especially in view of the number of reversible causes that exist. The separation of the different types of vascular dementia has prognostic and treatment implications. The number of toxic, metabolic and hormonal causes should be remembered, and patients with dementia should be offered the same medical facilities for investigation as other patients, irrespective of their age. The distinction of an acute organic brain syndrome (delirium) from dementia can sometimes be difficult, but the possibility that an established dementia may be exacerbated by such a state must always be borne in mind, and significant improvements of the mental state can be seen with resolution of the offending causes (infections, drug treatments, etc.).

The relevance of careful clinical investigation is apparent with follow-up studies. The commonest missed condition is depression and the best discriminator of this diagnosis is a previous history of depressive illness, and affective features on admission. Psychometric tests, with marked verbal/performance discrepancy (but not memory tasks), radiological evidence of cerebral (particularly cortical) atrophy and EEG abnormalities are of maximum value in discriminating between those with and without reversible dementia.

For some conditions, specific treatments are needed. For example, cerebrosyphilis requires antibiotics, usually large doses of penicillin, although steroids are often given in addition to prevent the Herxheimer reaction. This is an acute febrile state with intensification of symptoms that comes on soon after treatment. A patient with hydrocephalus should be referred to an interested surgeon for consideration of shunting, and tumours will require similar referral. Attempts should be made to correct any endocrine or metabolic causes discovered, and intoxicants, especially any unnecessary drugs, should be removed. It should be remembered that the aging brain, especially one affected by a dementing process, is easily decompensated by such factors, and an acute organic brain syndrome thus complicates the underlying deficits. Respiratory and urinary-tract infections are notorious offenders, although in patients that have ceased to care for themselves and have no one to look after them, nutritional deficiencies may be paramount.

Subtle head injuries may occur, either causing a dementia syndrome, for example with the development of subdural haematomas, or exacerbating an existing condition. Alcohol dependency or misuse should never be overlooked; many elderly early demented patients take an excess, with poor food intake, worsening confusion and potentiating falls and head injuries. Diagnosis of MID should lead to a search for the site of origin of any emboli, and any hypertension requires cautious treatment. Stopping smoking is important. Treating cardiac arrythmias and using lipid-lowering agents and aspirin helps prevent further strokes, and may even protect against dementia (Erkinjuntti and Gauthier, 2009; Gouw *et al.*, 2008). Some advocate even more aggressive anticoagulant treatment – an area of considerable unresolved controversy. In a few selected cases, where the problem relates to carotid artery stenosis, carotid endarterectomy has been tried, although the evidence that this brings lasting benefit in many cases is not clear.

Reversible/Irreversible

In older definitions of dementia, the criterion that it shall be an irreversible syndrome is often noted. One distinguishing feature between a delirium and a dementia was thus thought to be the acute reversible nature of the former and the chronic irreversibility of the latter. However, the feature of irreversibility can no longer be accepted. This arises from the structural impairment, and if the pathogenesis is functional (altered neuronal function) then the possibility of reversibility can be entertained. There are many examples of reversible dementia noted above, and early treatment may prevent significant morbidity, or prevent secondary structural changes from developing.

Dementia/Pseudodementia

The presentation of a major affective disorder with a picture resembling dementia has already been discussed (Chapter 8). It has also been noted that follow-up studies indicate that patients diagnosed with dementia who do not deteriorate tend to have an affective disorder in retrospect. Although the term 'pseudodementia' refers to this condition, it is arguably incorrect. Thus, if it has the hallmarks of dementia, it should be so diagnosed, recognizing that dementia is the beginning not the end of the diagnostic process. Depression, in addition to several other conditions, is a cause of reversible dementia. Others include mania, the depressive 'pseudodementia' of Ganser's syndrome,

hysteria, simulation and anxiety disorders. The acknowledgement that these conditions must be considered in the differential diagnosis of dementia will hopefully lead to their presence being sought and the correct diagnosis of a potentially treatable condition being made.

Cortical/Subcortical

In this chapter, reference has been made to subcortical dementia. It has been suggested that damage to subcortical nuclei (basal ganglia, thalamus) and deep white matter may lead to a dementia syndrome, the presentation of which differs from those disorders that mainly influence cortex. Albert *et al.* (1974) described the features of subcortical dementia as emotional and personality changes, memory disorder, a defective ability to manipulate acquired knowledge and a slowness in the rate of information processing. In contrast to the cortical dementias, aphasias, apraxias and similar symptoms are not seen. This clinical picture may be seen in progressive supranuclear palsy (Steele–Richardson syndrome), Parkinson's disease, Huntington's chorea, Wilson's disease, some vascular dementias and the AIDS–dementia complex. The dementia of depression also has similar features. Albert *et al.* supported this concept by quoting evidence that surgical lesions of the basal ganglia impair performance and problem-solving tasks, and that stimulation of subcortical structures impairs cognitive performance. They also noted the similarity of the symptom complex of subcortical dementia to the behavioural syndrome seen in patients with frontal-lobe damage. Pointing to the unique reciprocal connections between the frontal cortex and the limbic system, they also referred to this as frontolimbic dementia.

The concept of the subcortical dementias is most strongly advocated by Cummings and Benson (1992). They give as prominent clinical features 'mental slowness, inertia and lack of initiative, forgetfulness, dilapidation of cognition, and mood disturbance' (p. 95). The memory changes are more of forgetfulness and difficulty of spontaneous recall, and the cognitive state may demonstrate a difficulty with processing of complex problems, 'failing to synthesize the elements properly to achieve the correct answer. . .' (p. 10). They also include as causes hydrocephalus and toxic/metabolic disorders that disrupt basal ganglia function, and note that many conditions may lead to a combined picture of both cortical and subcortical deficits.

The concept of subcortical dementias has not gained universal acceptance. This stems in part from a traditional reluctance to view some subcortical structures, such as the basal ganglia, as anything but motor in function, and the long-held view that 'higher' cognitive function is the prerogative only of the cortex. Further, the pathological studies viewed above have led to a questioning of the value of the term 'subcortical' in the context of pathology of most syndromes. Anatomically the close links between the basal-ganglia structures and cortex are well established (Chapter 2) and disruption of cerebral circuits in pathology involves cortical and subcortical structures. However, the concept does emphasize that disruption of cognition can be the result of damage to the deeper nuclear structures of the brain and that dementia has presentations other than the classical one seen in association with Alzheimer's disease.

Senile/Presenile

The term 'senile dementia' referred arbitrarily to patients developing dementia over the age of 65. If no other underlying condition was found, it was labelled parenchymatous senile dementia, and was thought to present in a similar fashion to the presenile dementia of Alzheimer, but in a milder form. Those who wish to uphold differences between the latter and parenchymatous senile dementia note the genetic difference, and comment clinically on the relative absence of focal cortical signs, extrapyramidal disorder and seizures in the senile group. Others have argued there were neuropathological differences, noting the higher density of plaques and tangles in the temporal neocortex, amygdala and hippocampus from brains of Alzheimer's disease patients. The alternative view, that the senile dementia and Alzheimer's disease were the same condition,

emerged from the early neurochemical studies, in which cholinergic deficits were seen irrespective of age (Bowen *et al.*, 1979).

The concept of presenile/senile based on arbitrary age limits was poorly conceived, and the unravelling of different pathologies – for example of fronto-temporal dementia, with different age of onset from classical Alzheimer's disease – plus potential classifications that are moving towards a pathological (tauopathies) or even a genetic basis render it redundant.

Dementia, Aging and Mild Cognitive Impairment

A related issue is the extent to which disorders such as Alzheimer's disease merely represent accelerated aging. This view is almost certainly incorrect. It is true that elderly people develop cognitive impairments, notable slowing and memory difficulty, but cognition is often intact in advanced old age, and the other disturbances found in Alzheimer's disease are not seen.

The concept of mild cognitive impairment (earlier called 'benign senescent forgetfulness') refers to a transitional state between the cognitive changes of normal aging and early dementia. Thus, on history taking, those who later get a diagnosis of Alzheimer's disease reveal cognitive problems before the diagnosis is made, but not all aging people with memory complaints will go on to develop dementia. The concept of mild cognitive impairment is thus defining a high-risk group. On cognitive testing members of this group perform below age–education norms on at least one cognitive test (>1.5 standard deviations), but they have no impairments of activities of daily living, and function independently. The prevalence increases with age, but the conversion to dementia is given at between 2.7 and 15% per year, perhaps revealing the difficulty of defining mild cognitive impairment in practice. Further, some distinguish different forms, for example an amnestic variety. Prognostic studies suggest poor verbal memory, cerebral or regional brain atrophy on MRI (especially in hippocampus and entorhinal cortex), and progression of the latter over time, as well as decreased glucose uptake in posterior cingulate/temporoparietal areas, are significant. The Apo E allele status is also relevant.

A confounding factor is that depression is also comorbid with mild cognitive impairment, and with the considerable publicity given to Alzheimer's disease, concern, worry and hypochondriacal issues can cloud the picture.

Neuropathological data reveal that plaques and tangles are common in the brains of elderly nondemented people, and even Lewy bodies are reported, but plaques are usually in smaller numbers and tangles are only rarely found in the cortex. There seems to be a common mechanism underlying several degenerative disorders, with aggregation and deposition of misfolded insoluble proteins, which lead to amyloid deposition. These changes seem to accumulate slowly over the years, but how the misfolded proteins lead to neurodegeneration remains to be discovered. Cell loss is seen, but, compared to Alzheimer's disease, it is less extensive, and where there is a reduction of dentritic arborization an increase in synaptic contact is noted (Tomlinson, 1982). Pathological follow-up studies suggest that those with amnestic mild cognitive impairment are most likely to progress to Alzheimer's disease, but some develop other disorders such as Lewy-body dementia (Jicha *et al.*, 2008; Josephs *et al.*, 2009; Whitwell *et al.*, 2007).

Some decline in muscarinic binding sites occurs with aging, but choline acetyltransferase activity is not characteristically diminished, and nor is the ability to synthetize acetylcholine. The losses of noradrenaline and somatostatin seen in Alzheimer's disease are not a feature of aging (Rossor *et al.*, 1984) (see Table 11.3). The CSF changes shown in Alzheimer's disease are not as yet defined in mild cognitive impairment and are not found in normal aging. One interpretation of this is that in spite of some neuronal loss and diminution of biochemical activity with aging, the remaining neurones can cope with the demands on them by increasing their activity, while the neurones in mild cognitive impairment in those who progress to Alzheimer's disease do not possess this reserve capacity.

The introduction of mild cognitive impairment in many ways simply shifts the problem of when the process of dementia begins, and the borders between it, healthy aging and early Alzheimer's disease remain unclear. Further, we do not know what the first step in any pathology is, or where it begins. Amyloid precursor protein is a normal synaptic constituent, and the first problems may therefore be synaptic.

Mixed Types and Thresholds

In spite of attempts to clearly distinguish various types of dementia, mixed types are frequently seen. Thus Pick's and Alzheimer's pathology have been seen in the same brain (Smith and Lantos, 1983), and the existence of low attenuation areas on CT scans or areas of increased T_2 signed intensity on MRI in patients with presumed Alzheimer's disease are common (Coffey and Figiel, 1991; Jacoby and Levy, 1980a). The acute onset of Alzheimer's disease following head injury or illness is reported (Hollander and Strich, 1970), and several pathogenic influences seem to be linked to the formation of both plaques and tangles. The presence of plaques in normal aging and their correlation broadly with the cognitive performance has led to the suggestion that there are thresholds beyond which dementia occurs. Thus, aging processes provide the nidus upon which other insults operate to increase the changes and eventually throw the brain into 'brain failure', analogous to the development of cardiac failure. The insults could be many, including a vascular episode, minor head injury or anoxia. In spite of the attractiveness of these ideas to explain some of the clinical phenomena, they are not supported by the biochemical evidence accumulated to date.

Incidence Rates

Finally, since the population is getting older, and the incidence rates rise with age, will everyone who reaches the age of 120 be demented? One study of an elderly community living in Cache county, Utah noted a peak in incidence in the 90–92 age group, with a decline thereafter (Onyike *et al.*, 2007; Tschanz *et al.*, 2006).

12
Biological Treatments

INTRODUCTION

Most of the treatment modalities used in biological psychiatry attempt to modify brain circuitry and behaviour. They can be grouped into one of several types. By and large they generally approach the allocortex.

There are treatments that directly interact with the brain and cause direct physical changes. Included in this class are the old and new brain-stimulation techniques: electroconvulsive therapy (ECT), vagus-nerve stimulation (VNS), deep-brain stimulation (DBS) and transcranial magnetic stimulation (TMS).

In contrast, there are treatments where there is an indirect physical intervention. This class includes the talking therapies (psychoanalysis, cognitive behavioural therapy), various forms of biofeedback, and even techniques like aromatherapy. We also include in this indirect physical class the indirect medications used as treatments.

Psychopharmacology, or allopathy, has been a cornerstone of biological psychiatry and will continue to be so for the next decade at least. We will discuss psychopharmacology first, and deal with the newer direct physical treatments at the end of the chapter.

PHARMACOLOGY: PHARMACOKINETICS AND PHARMACODYNAMICS

Of the several ways that drugs are administered to patients, the oral route is the most common. Following absorption from the gastrointestinal tract, the drug passes to the liver via the portal system, where metabolism may occur, usually by oxidation, reduction, hydrolysis or conjugation. This metabolism is referred to as 'first-pass metabolism', and drugs which are given intramuscularly, intravenously or with a skin patch avoid this 'first-pass' effect. For oral compounds, the rate of absorption of a drug from the stomach depends upon a number of factors, including the concentration of the active compound, the carrying medium with which the compounds are given (including whether or not they are taken with food), the pH of the gastrointestinal tract, associated disease of the gut and other active medications which may compete with uptake across the gastrointestinal cell membranes.

Ionization is an important factor determining uptake, since only non-ionized drug crosses cell membranes freely, and, unless specific transport mechanisms exist, the rate of movement is proportional to the concentration of the drug across cell membranes. The proportion of ionized to non-ionized drug is dependent on both pH and its dissociation constant. It is immediately apparent how oral ingestion may lead to a wide variation in the amount of drug finally absorbed from the gut, and thus how oral dose does not necessarily relate to serum levels and can change over time even within the same individual.

Some drugs increase the activity of enzymes responsible for their metabolism or for the

Biological Psychiatry 3e   Michael R. Trimble and Mark S. George
© 2010 John Wiley & Sons, Ltd

metabolism of other drugs within the liver. Barbiturates, phenytoin, carbamazepine and steroids are particularly implicated; carbamazepine is known to induce its own metabolism.

Cytochrome P450 plays a major role in oxidative metabolism, and at least 19 forms exist in the human liver. Individual isoenzymes may metabolize different drugs, and inhibition of the metabolism of one drug by another using the same isoenzymes may result in high serum levels of the inhibited drug, and toxicity. Induction of the enzymes that metabolize one drug by another will lead to lower serum levels of the first. Although some 75% of drug metabolism is through the CYP system, much is not polymorphically expressed (e.g. CYP3A4/5) and the main polymorphisms of relevance, in other words those genetic variables that influence drug metabolism in humans, and may determine alterations of speed of metabolism, are CYP 2D6, 2C19 and 2C9.

From the bloodstream, drugs become widely distributed throughout the body. The distribution is initially determined by the relative blood flow of the various organs and the presence of the blood–brain barrier, which protects the brain from the effects of many neurotoxic compounds. Further, many drugs are bound to plasma proteins, especially albumin; the presence of the drug in plasma thus occurs in both bound and unbound (free) forms.

Many psychotropic drugs are secondary or tertiary amines and weak bases, and are absorbed better from the duodenum than the stomach. Since lipid solubility is important for passing through the blood–brain barrier, these drugs are highly lipid-soluble, but are also often highly protein-bound. P-glycoproteins are transporter proteins within the brain which effectively prevent drugs getting into it, and form part of the blood–brain barrier. They are encoded by selective genes (ABCB1) and studies are underway to see which genotypes may relate to response to psychotropic medications. P-glycoprotein status may be one cause of treatment nonresponsiveness.

Excretion of drugs is usually via the kidney, although the liver and other organs such as the lung may also be involved.

The half-life of a drug refers to the time it takes for its concentration to decrease in the plasma by 50%. The quicker the metabolism and elimination, the shorter the half-life. 'Zero-order' kinetics refers to a situation in which there is an exponential relationship between the dose of a drug and its serum levels (see Figure 12.1), while in 'first-order' kinetics the relationship is one of equivalence.

Zero-order kinetics occurs because the enzymes responsible for drug metabolism and excretion become saturated at levels required for the therapeutic effects. Phenytoin is one drug that follows such kinetics, whereas the majority of psychotropic medications show first-order kinetics. Knowledge of the half-life of a drug is useful, since it is recommended that the dose interval be equivalent to the half-life. The steady state, namely that in which the serum level of the drug reaches a steady plateau, excretion being in balance with intake, is approximately equivalent to four or five half-lives.

Since factors which influence drug metabolism include genetics, age, diet, coexistent medications and coexistent disease, careful consideration of pharmacokinetic principles is required, particularly in certain patients. These include those with diseases of the liver, kidney and heart, as well as the young and the elderly. In children, absorption from the stomach is faster than in adults, which may lead to higher peak drug concentrations and thus an increased risk of adverse effects. Plasma–protein binding is reduced because of lower albumin and globulin contents of the blood, values comparable to those of adults being reached between the ages of 10 and 15. The enzyme systems responsible for drug degradation are faster than those of adults in early childhood, and decrease slowly with age, such that adult clearance values develop around puberty. The increased metabolism of drugs in childhood means dosing requirements need careful adjustment.

In elderly patients, the body composition has altered, with a generally leaner body mass and an increase in adipose tissue. This means that lipid-soluble drugs are more extensively distributed, particularly in elderly women, as the fraction of the total body weight composed of

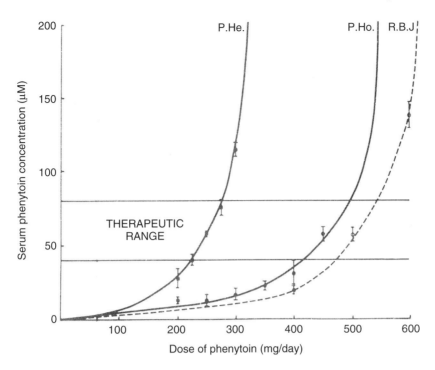

Figure 12.1 An example of zero-order kinetics. Dose/serum-level relationship for phenytoin in three patients in whom steady-state concentrations were measured at several doses of the drug. Each point represents the mean ±SD of three to seven separate estimations. The curves were fitted by computer using the Michaelis–Menten equation. The therapeutic range suggested by Buchthal *et al.* (1960) has been drawn in to illustrate the steepness of the relationship within this range. Note: 4 mM = 1 mg/ml (*Biol Psych*, 2 Ed, p. 326)

adipose tissue increases more in women than in men. Alteration of gastrointestinal-tract activity, with reduction of gastroparietal cell function and impaired acid secretion with an elevated pH, leads to impaired absorption of certain drugs. Hepatic and renal activity may also be altered. In particular, the hepatic microsomal enzymes responsible for oxidative metabolism, principally hydroxylation and n-dealkylation, may be diminished in this age group, leading to reduced clearance and higher steady-state plasma concentrations with multiple drug dosage. Further, reduced hepatic blood flow occurs, on account of reduced cardiac output, with a further decline of clearance. Elderly patients may have diminished plasma albumin with reduced total protein binding, and elimination of drugs by renal clearance is increased since there is a fall of glomerular filtration rate and decreased tubular secretion and absorption

capacity of the renal tubules. All of these factors mean alterations in the volume of the drug distribution (the hypothetical volume relating the amount of drug in the body to the plasma concentration at all times after the attainment of distribution equilibrium) and reduced clearance, with considerable danger of drug toxicity if dosages employed for younger patients are not modified.

'Pharmacodynamics' is a term that refers to the biochemical, physiological and behavioural effects of drugs, which in many cases bear no direct relation to pharmacokinetics. 'Behavioural toxicity' refers to specific side effects of drugs, leading to impaired performance. These problems, frequently encountered in clinical practice, include a whole spectrum from minor mood changes, impairment of psychomotor performance, fatigue and drowsiness, through to severe agitation and psychoses.

ANTIDEPRESSANTS

These are divided into two major categories: the monoamine oxidase inhibitors (MAOI) and non-MAOI drugs. The non-MAOI medications are traditionally further divided into tricyclic and nontricyclic, while the MAOIs may be subdivided either by chemical structure into hydrazines and nonhydrazines, in reference to their enzyme selectivity as MAOA or MAOB inhibitors, or in relation to their reversibility of enzyme inhibition.

MAOI Antidepressants

These compounds, the first of which was isoniazid, were introduced for the treatment of tuberculosis, but were soon recognized to be energizing in their effects. The early forerunners were all hydrazines, and were notable because of their hepatotoxicity and the 'cheese reaction'. The mechanism of the latter is as follows. Monoamine oxidase is widely distributed throughout the body, and together with catechol-*O*-methyl transferase (COMT) is responsible for the detoxification of absorbed primary amines. Some sympathomimetic amines, in particular tyramine, exert a hypertensive effect by releasing noradrenaline from tissue. Although the main problem is tyramine, other amines and amine precursors such as tyrosine, histamine and dopamine may also be involved, and such products may derive from protein-containing foods that have undergone degradation, or from other drugs.

MAOIs will minimize the degradation of these amines in the gut wall, and thus one explanation for the 'cheese effect' relates to an increased presence of these amines in the circulation. Alternatively, inhibition of MAO in adrenergic nerve endings delays the metabolism of tyramine and noradrenaline, and thus increases their effects.

It is now known that MAO exists in both A and B forms. The substrates for MAOA include noradrenaline and 5-HT, while phenylethylamine is a substrate for MAOB. Tyramine and dopamine are substrates for both forms, but it has been suggested that selective inhibition of only one form of MAO may minimize the chances of a hypertensive reaction. The symptoms of this reaction include headache, sweating, nausea, vomiting and a rise in blood pressure that can lead to cerebral bleeding. The foods most often involved contain tyramine, although fatalities have almost always been associated with cheese.

Currently-marketed hydrazine derivatives include isocarboxide, nialamide and phenelzine; the nonhydrazine groups include tranylcypramine and pargyline. The selective compounds include deprenyl for MAOB and clorgyline, cimoxatone and moclobemide for MAOA. The place of MAO drugs in the treatment of depression has been evaluated in several reviews (Tyrer, 1976; Pare, 1985). Generally they are recommended for patients with 'atypical depressions', although the exact features that respond are often less than clearly defined. Tyrer (1976) suggested that the clinical profile most commonly associated with a good response includes hypochondriasis, somatic anxiety, irritability, agoraphobia, social phobias and anergia. A poor result is associated with guilt, depressed mood, ideas of reference and nihilistic delusions. Most clinicians agree that a patient with typical major affective disorder and endogenous features is the least appropriate for this class of drugs, while additional anxiety or phobic symptoms, or mixed anxiety–depressive states, may respond. The presence of somatic symptoms, of the phobic anxiety–depersonalization syndrome and of panic attacks suggests a good response. Following administration there is often a delay before improvement, sometimes of days or even weeks, although this is less with the nonhydrazine drugs. These compounds suppress REM sleep, and the onset of the clinical improvement often coincides with the change in sleep pattern. Dosage is particularly important, and some negative results of earlier trials stemmed from inadequate prescriptions. It is usual to start with doses in the medium range and then increase after one or two weeks, depending on the patient's response. However, doses of up to 90 mg of phenelzine, 20–40 mg of tranylcypromine and 50 mg of isocarboxazid may be necessary. Once treatment has been started it may continue for several years if necessary, and apart from the limitations of interactions with foodstuffs and other drugs, long-term side effects appear to be rare.

The drugs are metabolized by acetylation, and the speed (fast and slow) at which this is carried out is a polygenetically inherited trait. In the United Kingdom, some 40% of the population comprises fast acetylators, but the clinical relevance of this is unclear.

MAOI drugs may be combined with tricyclic or other antidepressants in certain clinical situations. Although this may lead to unwanted effects, especially hypotension, used carefully such combinations can be useful, particularly with resistant depressions. In general, a patient on a tricyclic antidepressant may be started on an MAOI, but more caution needs to be exercised when patients are already on the latter and need to be given additional tricyclic therapy. Both drugs may be started simultaneously, but it is wise to start each drug at a lower dose than would be used when given alone. It has been suggested that clomipramine, ecstasy (MDMA 3,4 methylenedioxymethamphetamine), meperidine, tramadol, dextromethorphan and St John's wort should not be combined with an MAOA inhibitor. Selective 5-HT reuptake inhibitors (SSRIs) should be used with caution, and after a washout period.

Apart from the hyper- and hypotensive reactions, other side effects noted include tremor, weakness, dizziness, hyperreflexia, irritability, ataxia, impotence, hypotension, micturition problems, sweating, hyperpyrexia, rashes and, rarely, convulsions. The drugs are contraindicated in liver disease, congestive heart failure and following cerebrovascular accidents. The hypertensive complications respond to alpha adrenergic blocking drugs, such as phentolamine or chlorpromazine.

The newer generation of MAOI drugs currently being investigated shows selectivity for one or other of the enzymes. Most work has been carried out with selegeline, which appears to possess antidepressant properties (Mendlewicz and Youdim, 1983), which can be shown to inhibit platelet MAOB, an effect that may be related to the clinical response. The selectivity for MAOB is probably related to lack of the hypertensive effect with tyramine and lack

of postural hypotension as a side effect. The main use of selegeline is in Parkinson's disease; a transdermal delivery product is available, which is also approved for depression. A similar agent is rasagiline.

Reversible inhibitors of monoamine oxidase (RIMAs) are selective MAOA inhibitors that are themselves inhibited in action by the presence of high levels of natural substrate. Thus, high released or ingested endogenous amines would continue to be peripherally metabolized, and not provoke a hypertensive reaction. MAO in the brain would continue to be inhibited, exerting the therapeutic effect. Several of these compounds have been tested (toloxatone, brofaromine). The only one clinically available is moclobemide.

There is no dietary restriction with moclobemide: an average meal contains 25 mg of tyramine, and doses of up to 100 mg of the latter have been given with moclobemide safely. However, caution is advised with clomipramine or deprenyl, and a serotoninergic syndrome has been reported in combination with SSRIs. The starting dose is 300 mg, with target doses of 450–600 mg, and single daily dosing is possible. Moclobemide has a half-life of 1–4 hours, and is generally nonsedative. It is unclear whether these compounds are effective for the atypical presentations that are responsive to the earlier generation of MAOIs, their use at present being for depression and social phobias.

Non-MAOI Antidepressants

The first of these to be synthesized and used was imipramine, followed shortly by amitriptyline. These two drugs are probably still the most widely used of the non-SSRI antidepressants. The early members of this group were all variations of the tricyclic nucleus, but more recently drugs have been developed with nontricyclic structures.

Tricyclic Drugs

Traditionally, the tricyclic drugs were thought to act by inhibition of monamine uptake into the presynaptic neurone, thus enhancing the availability of monoamines within the synaptic

Table 12.1 Properties of some antidepressant drugs

	Inhibition of uptake			Affinities for receptor	
	5-HT	NA	DA	Muscarinic anticholinergic	Anti-histaminic
Amitriptyline	++	+++	±	+++	+++
Clomipramine	+++	+	−	++	±
Imipramine	++	+	±	+	+
Maprotiline	−	+++	±	±	+
Desipramine	+	+++	−	+	−
Nortriptyline	+	+++	±	+	+
Bupropion	−	−	++	−	−
L-tryptophan	−	−	−	−	−
Mianserin	−	+	+	−	++
Viloxazine	−	+	+	−	−
Paroxetine	+++	−	−	±	−
Fluvoxamine	+++	−	−	−	−
Sertraline	+++	−	−	−	−
Citalopram	+++	−	−	−	+
Escitalopram	+++	−	−	−	−
Fluoxetine	+++	−	−	−	−
Trazadone	+	−	−	−	±
Iprindole	−	−	±	−	−
Dothiepin	+	+	±	±	+++
Protriptyline	+	+++	±	+++	±
Lofepramine	−	++	−	+	?
Venlafaxine	++	++	±	−	−
Nefadozone	++	++	−	−	−
Mirtazepine	+	−	−	±	+

cleft. Further, it was taught that drugs which are tertiary amines have more of an effect on 5-HT uptake, while the secondary amines are more potent with regards to catecholamine uptake. The spectrum of action of this group and of some other antidepressants in relationship to biochemical effects is shown in Table 12.1.

Lofepramine is a tricyclic antidepressant which is metabolized *in vivo* into desipramine; hence its pharmacological and clinical profile is similar to the other tricyclic drugs, but it has an apparently excellent safety profile, including in overdose.

Anticholinergic effects are noted, particularly with amitriptyline, clomipramine and protriptyline. These relate not only to their side effects, but also to their clinical efficacy if patients find them difficult to take. Antihistaminic effects also vary as shown.

Nontricyclic Drugs

In view of the problematic side effects of the tricyclic drugs, many alternative antidepressants have been marketed. Most investigated are the SSRIs, developed largely on the basis of the 5-HT hypothesis of depression (see Chapter 8).

Trazadone

This is a triazolopyridine with an added phenylpiprazine group. It has no anticholinergic properties and is free from cardiovascular side effects, but is a 5-HT$_2$ antagonist, a 5-HT uptake inhibitor and an alpha-2 adrenoceptor antagonist. It is thus serotoninergic. It is rapidly and completely absorbed following oral administration and its metabolites are inactive. The half-life is about four hours, and its clinical dosage is approximately twice that of tricyclic drugs, up to a maximum of 600 mg per day. It has similar efficacy to tricyclic antidepressants, but is sedative, and relatively safe when taken in overdose. It is reported to provoke priapism in males (Scher *et al.*, 1983) and may increase libido in females (Gartrell, 1986). Nefazodone is chemically related to trazadone. In addition to its effects inhibiting the uptake of 5-HT and noradrenaline, it blocks 5-HT$_2$ receptors.

Amoxapine

This is a demethylated metabolite of the antipsychotic drug loxapine, a tricyclic drug of the dibenzoxazepine class. It is rapidly absorbed following oral administration, and has a half-life of eight hours. It has minimal anticholinergic properties, but does block dopamine receptors, which contributes to its side-effect profile. This includes extrapyramidal reactions and hyperprolactinaemia, but in addition seizures may be a problem.

L-tryptophan

Some of the literature that relates to the antidepressant properties of tryptophan is discussed in Chapter 8. It is an essential amino acid, and its antidepressant effects, potentiated in particular by MOAI drugs, form part of the evidence for implication of 5-HT mechanisms in depression. It possesses no anticholinergic, antiadrenergic or dopaminergic properties, with a half-life of around four hours. It may, in addition, be usefully combined with tricyclic drugs, in particular amityriptyline and clomipramine. It has few side effects other than drowsiness, although it has been linked to the development of an eosinophilic myalgia syndrome, which has limited its availability, although it is readily available as a nonprescription product.

Venlafaxine

This selectively blocks the reuptake of 5-HT and noradrenaline. It has no muscarinic or histaminic effects. It has a half-life of between one and six hours, and an active metabolite. It is given twice daily, with a dose range of 75–300 mg. Nausea, anorexia and insomnia are the main side effects.

While it does not affect cardiac conduction, there are reports of increased blood pressure with the drug, especially with higher doses. A once-daily preparation of the major metabolite des-venlafaxine has a half-life of 11 hours and the recommended dose range is 50–400 mg daily.

Selective Serotonin Reuptake Inhibitors (SSRIs)

The main SSRIs in clinical practice are citalopram, escitalopram, fluoxetine, fluvoxamine, paroxetine and sertraline (see Table 12.2). As noted below, they block the 5-HT transporter, but this effect occurs in a matter of hours, the activity of the 5-HT neurones slowly recovering over the next 14 days (Montigny and Blier, 1985).

Fluoxetine is a bicyclic drug with high selectivity for inhibition of 5-HT uptake and virtually no effect on catecholamine neurones. It is the least potent of the SSRIs for the inhibition of 5-HT uptake. It is highly protein-bound (95–99%) and has an active metabolite, norfluoxetine giving a long half-life of 6–14 days. It reduces REM sleep and increases REM latency. There is a 90 mg extended-release formulation of this compound to be given once per week.

Fluvoxamine is a single-ringed compound with no anticholinergic properties which is rapidly absorbed after oral administration and has a half-life of approximately 15 hours. It is extensively metabolized and its metabolites also have no effect on the catecholamine uptake

Table 12.2 Some properties of SSRI antidepressants

Drug	5-HT*	5-HT/NA**	Half-life	Active metabolite	Protein binding
Citalopram	2.6	1500	36 hours	None	50%
Escitalopram	1.2	2000	30 hours	None	60%
Fluoxetine	25	20	1–3 days	7–15 days	94%
Fluvoxamine	6.2	180	15 hours	none	77%
Paroxetine	1.1	320	20 hours	none	95%
Sertraline	7.3	190	25 hours	66 hours	99%

*Impramine = 100: inhibition of uptake.
**Ratio of 5-HT to noradrenaline uptake inhibition.

process. Gastrointestinal side effects appear to be a particular problem, although it has minimal effect on the EEG profile (Saletu *et al.*, 1983). It has a half-life of approximately 15 hours, and can therefore be given on a once-daily basis.

Paroxetine is one of the more highly selective of the group for 5-HT, and has no active metabolites. It does however inhibit its own clearance; its half-life therefore increases with higher dose. Agitation as a side effect is not reported.

Sertraline has long-acting metabolites, and sexual side effects have been more prominent. It too is highly protein-bound (98.5%) and has a half-life of 13–45 hours.

Citalopram is sold as a racemic mixture, consisting of 50% R-(−)-citalopram and 50% S-(+)-citalopram. Only the S-(+) enantiomer has the desired antidepressant effect, so it has been marketed by itself as escitalopram.

The main advantage of the SSRIs is the lack of cardiac effects, weight gain or sedation. The main side effects that limit their use are nausea, diarrhoea, agitation or increased anxiety, and delayed orgasm and reduced sexual drive. Others are mainly CNS-related, including insomnia, dizziness, tremor and extrapyramidal reactions (see below). The SSRIs do show an effect on dopamine uptake, this being strongest for sertraline and weakest for fluvoxamine and citalopram.

The metabolites of citalopram, fluvoxamine, paroxetine and sertraline are inactive, and the potential for interactions with other drugs is therefore less than with fluoxetine. It is recommended that at least a four-week interval is allowed when switching from fluoxetine to an MAOI.

The dose prescribed depends on the product, but, unlike the tricyclics, there is often little to be gained when treating depression by increasing the dose if a response is not obtained with the recommended prescription. Markedly higher doses of the SSRIs do have clinical benefits in patients with OCD. Some of the SSRIs are now being introduced as extended-release preparations.

Clinically the SSRIs have also been used to treat OCD, social phobia, migraine, bulimia and panic disorder, the indications varying in different countries.

Some Other Novel or More Recently Introduced Antidepressants

Viloxazine has minimal anticholinergic properties. It is rapidly absorbed after oral administration, with maximal blood levels between 1 and 4 hours and a half-life of 2–5 hours. In animal models it is a stimulant, and is a weak inhibitor of noradrenergic uptake. It has limited antihistaminic and anticholinergic properties, but is mildly sympathomimetic. Its main disadvantages are nausea and vomiting, but, of the antidepressants, it has minimal convulsant potential (Trimble, 1978). However, its use in epilepsy is inhibited because of its adverse pharmacokinetic interaction with carbamazepine (Pisani *et al.*, 1984).

Mianserin is a tetracyclic compound whose main mode of action appears to be as an antagonist at the presynaptic alpha-adrenoceptor. It has antihistaminic but only minimal anticholinergic and serotonergic activity. Its biochemistry confers certain advantages, for example minimal anticholinergic side effects and thus cardiotoxicity, although it is epileptogenic.

It is rapidly absorbed following oral administration, peak plasma concentrations occurring in 2–3 hours. Its half-life is 10–17 hours, and it is highly protein-bound. It possesses antidepressant activity at doses between 30 and 120 mg daily, and it is customary to prescribe it as a single night-time dose.

Blood dyscrasias have been noted, including agranulocytosis, which are usually reversible but are an indication for blood monitoring.

Maprotiline is a tetracyclic drug which has selectivity for blocking noradrenergic reuptake. It is low in anticholinergic effects, and may even have cardiac antiarrhythmic properties. It is well absorbed after oral administration, peak plasma levels being reached between 6 and 19 hours, with a half-life around 30 hours. This makes it ideal for single daily administration. It has antidepressant effects equivalent to tricyclic drugs, but seizures are a specific problem, particularly at higher doses (Trimble, 1980).

Iprindole is a weak inhibitor of both noradrenaline and 5-HT uptake, with relatively weak antidepressant action. Like mianserin, its lack of effect on traditional monoamine systems is one piece of evidence which has led to questioning of the classical neurotransmitter hypothesis of affective disorder.

Bupropion has a single-ring novel structure that has no effect on 5-HT or noradrenaline uptake, and does not inhibit monoamine oxidase. It may block dopamine reuptake and has a chemical structure which resembles amphetamine. It is not associated with weight gain or sexual dysfunction but at higher doses it provokes seizures. It has comparable efficacy in depression to the SSRIs and is also used for nicotine craving. It is available as a slow-release preparation.

Mirtazapine has a tetracyclic chemical structure. It is a noradrenergic, being an antagonist at alpha-2 receptors, and is a specific serotonergic agent acting as an antagonist of 5-HT2 and 5-HT3 receptors (NaSSA). It has minimal anticholinergic, 5-HT-related or adrenergic side effects, but antihistaminic effects (drowsiness and weight gain) are prominent. The alpha-2 receptors, located in the locus coeruleus, control the firing rate of serotonergic neurones; the drug thus increases hippocampal 5-HT release.

Novel drugs with antidepressant action include the 5-HT$_{1A}$ agonist *buspirone*, the tricyclic *tianeptine*, the phosphodiesterase-inhibitor *rolipram* and the 5-HT–noradrenaline-reuptake inhibitor (SNRI) *duloxetine*. Tianeptine is described as a selective 5-HT-reuptake enhancer (SSRE) since, unlike conventional tricyclic antidepressants or SSRIs, tianeptine enhances the reuptake of 5-HT instead of inhibiting it. It does not bind to adrenergic or dopaminergic receptors or transporters but may influence glutaminergic transmission, and its effects on the stress-induced neuronal changes in the hippocampus in particular have been a focus of interest.

The Mode of Action of Antidepressant Drugs

The mode of action of tricyclic drugs has traditionally been related to their ability to inhibit monoamine uptake within neurones of the CNS, or to influence the uptake and distribution of other neurotransmitters. This is shown by example in Figure 12.2, which shows various compounds that influence the glutamate system and Figure 1.14 for the 5-HT system. Certainly this is a common biological activity that most of them share. However, it occurs acutely, while their therapeutic effect may take several weeks to become apparent. In addition, compounds such as mianserin and iprindole minimally inhibit amine uptake *in vivo*. Attention has been paid to the chronic effects of these and other antidepressant treatments on the sensitivity of catecholamine receptors, in particular downregulation of β-receptor activity. This leads to a decrease in glycogenolysis in the postsynaptic cell, small changes at the receptor being magnified through the coupler, effector and amplifier system of the postsynaptic cell membrane into larger dynamic changes. It is known that an intact 5-HT system is required for the beta-receptor changes to occur. These data have led to hypotheses that relate depressive illness to a supersensitivity at these receptor sites, itself related to decreased intrasynaptic levels of neurotransmitters, such as 5-HT. The mechanism of the downregulation and subsensitivity of noradrenergic receptors by antidepressants is unclear, but it could be related to a change of affinity, a reduction of density or interference with cyclic AMP coupling or activity.

However, several antidepressants, such as mianserin, paroxetine, citalopram and fluoxetine, fail to downregulate beta receptors, implying that these changes alone are not sufficient. Another theory relates to the alpha-2 adrenergic receptor, since long-term but not short-term antidepressant treatment reduced the sensitivity of the alpha-2 autoreceptor. The functional effect of this is to increase noradrenergic impulse flow and turnover with behavioural activation (Charney *et al.* 1983). Although some antidepressants, for example amitryptiline, desipramine and imipramine, have been shown to reduce alpha-2 autoreceptor sensitivity, at present information on other drugs, particularly in patient studies, is limited. Nonetheless, these findings are in keeping with a hypothesis that

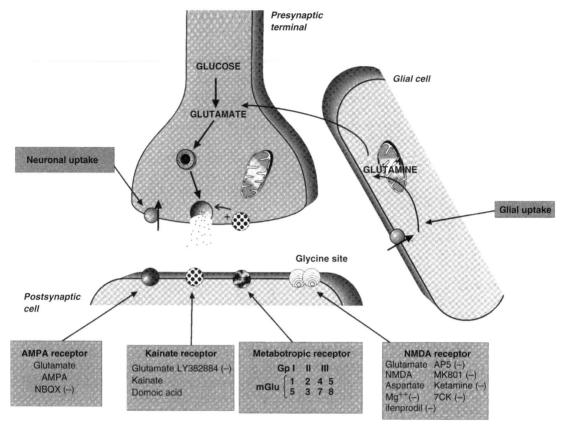

Figure 12.2   Synaptic cleft, showing the influence of some drugs on the glutamate system (reproduced with permission from Webster, 2002)

hypersensitivity of the presynaptic receptors in depression is associated with decreased release of neurotransmitters and upregulation of the postsynaptic beta receptor. Antidepressants thus regulate the presynaptic receptor and normalize the postsynaptic receptor. The association of these findings to the decreased post-synaptic alpha-2 activity in depressed patients (Siever and Uhde, 1984) is unclear. It is of interest that mianserin is an alpha-2 presynaptic receptor antagonist, an action which may be relevant to its antidepressant action.

There has been much interest in serotonergic mechanisms since the introduction of the SSRIs. It is not known how these drugs work, but some findings are secure. All types of antidepressant therapy, including ECT, MAOI and lithium, increase 5-HT neurotransmission. The effects of antidepressant action can be reversed

by reducing brain 5-HT through the technique of tryptophan depletion (Delgado *et al.*, 1990). Following administration of an SSRI there is considerable acute release of 5-HT into the synaptic cleft, and this is followed by a dramatic decrease of related neuronal activity. Gradually the functions of the neurones resume, and the 5-HT$_2$ receptors are normalized (see Figure 12.3).

There is considerable debate over where these effects take place, and what is primary. It has been speculated (see Chapter 8) that in depression, with reduced 5-HT turnover, there is decreased transmission at the pre- and postsynaptic 5-HT$_{1A}$ receptors and the 5-HT$_2$ receptor is upregulated. With SSRIs, the biological effect is seen mainly at the raphe nuclei, which have a high density of 5-HT$_{1A}$ autoreceptors. One speculation is that SSRIs block the transporter at the raphe, increasing the release of 5-HT around the

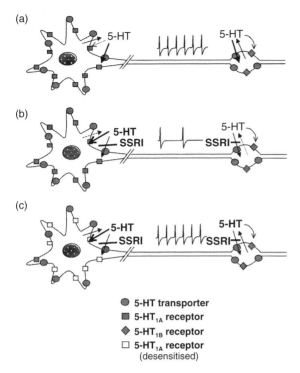

5-HT transporter

5-HT$_{1A}$ receptor

5-HT$_{1B}$ receptor

5-HT$_{1A}$ receptor
(desensitised)

Figure 12.3 Schematic representation of the effects of SSRI drugs on 5-HT neurones. (a) 5-HT is released from neurones within the raphe nuclei and taken up by the 5-HT transporter. (b) Blockade of the transporter increases the concentration of 5-HT and activates the 5-HT$_{1A}$ autoreceptors, which hyperpolarises the neurone, reducing 5-HT release from forebrain terminals. (c) The increased extracellular 5-HT concentration with continuous treatment desensitises the raphe 5-HT$_{1A}$ autoreceptors, allowing the 5-HT neurones to recover cell-firing and the terminal release of 5-HT (reproduced with permission from Webster, 2002, p. 445)

raphe, probably from the local dendrites, which then acts as an agonist, activating the autoreceptor, and decreasing cell firing and the release of 5-HT. With continued treatment there is desensitization of the autoreceptor (leading to increased 5-HT synaptic transmission) and resumption of normal firing. Further, postsynaptic 5-HT$_{1A}$ receptors in the hippocampus and 5-HT$_2$ receptors are also normalized (see Figure 12.3).

The 5-HT$_{1A}$ receptor is the main 5-HT inhibitory receptor, and is found in high concentrations in the raphe but also in the pregenual cingulum, temporal cortex, anterior cingulum, orbitofrontal cortex and olfactory cortex. It can be quite reliably imaged with ligands such as 11C-WAY and 18-F MPPF and is reduced in depression, panic disorder and social-anxiety disorder, all of which are conditions that respond to SSRIs. As noted, the effect of the SSRIs at the 5-HT$_{1A}$ raphe receptors is partly responsible for their action, somehow leading to a resetting of the neuronal system with eventual increased release of 5-HT into the synaptic space (Neumeister *et al.*, 2006). 5-HT$_{1A}$ partial agonists (gepirone, vilazedone) are thus being examined as potential antidepressants when combined with SSRIs, to see if the effect of the latter can be advanced or enhanced.

The importance of the 5-HT$_{1A}$ receptor for therapeutics goes beyond the antidepressants however, since some of the atypical antipsychotics (ziprazidone, quetiapine, clozapine) also possess 5-HT$_{1A}$ partial agonist activity, although others (sertindole, risperidone) have low affinity, as do the first-generation antipsychotics. Since some of the atypical antipsychotics have an effect on mood stabilization (see below), the 5-HT$_{1A}$ receptor activity may be relevant to their therapeutic effect.

The role of the 5-HT transporter (5-HTTLRP) in clinical antidepressant response is being investigated. Thus, those with the 5-HTTLRP ss allele have a threefold decrease in transporters and 5-HT uptake (Hariri *et al.*, 2002). On imaging, these depressed subjects with the short allele have been shown to have more responsive amygdala to angry and fearful faces than do the long-allele ll carriers, and show enhanced startle responses. At present, investigations into drug-responsiveness and phenotypic status are ongoing.

Tricyclic drugs may not act in the same way; one suggestion is that their response is more via the hippocampal postsynaptic 5-HT$_{1A}$ receptors. In any case, enhanced responsivity of forebrain 5-HT neurones seems to be a common response to long-term treatment with both the SSRIs and tricyclic drugs.

Most antidepressants decrease the receptor density of 5-HT$_2$ receptors in the frontal cortex, an effect which distinguishes them from ECT, which increases 5-HT$_2$ receptors. As a generalization, therefore, antidepressants and ECT downregulate alpha-2, beta and 5-HT$_1$ receptors, but their action on the 5-HT$_2$ receptor differs.

One major difficulty for the discovery of new antidepressant treatments has been to find an animal model for depression that closely resembles the human condition. The most widely used are the forced swim test, in which animals are placed in water and the length of time they struggle before giving up is measured, and the learned helplessness model, a state provoked by enforced foot shock. Further, for two generations drugs which act on monoamine systems have been targeted for investigation, but the trend has been to develop drugs with more than one monoamine target, with minimal effect at other receptors, which may relate to side effects. However, antidepressants have an effect on glutamate receptors, tricyclics, ECT, MAOIs and some SSRIs, decreasing NMDA receptor function (Kilts, 1994). Sigma receptors modulate several central neurotransmitters, including glutaminergic and monoaminergic systems, and they have been considered possibly relevant for the action of some antidepressants. Fluvoxamine is the most potent sigma-receptor agonist; sertraline has low affinity or may even be an antagonist; and venlafaxine has no effect.

The CRF system has been a longstanding focus of interest, although disappointing in terms of new medications that act within it. Essentially, stress leads some people to depression, and the hypothalamic–pituitary–adrenal (HPA) axis is involved in this relationship. In animals, CRF increases locomotor activity and enhances stress-induced freezing. Increased activity of the HPA axis leads to increased cortisol release, decreasing central glucocorticoid receptors and potentially doing harm to some cerebral structures, notably the hippocampus. Chronic increased CRF secretion may underlie these HPA axis changes noted in depression. However, CRF-receptor antagonists to date have been ineffective in depression and anxiety clinical trials.

Observations that structural changes in the brain may accompany depression, in part related to the altered HPA-axis activity, notably in the amygdala, hippocampus and prefrontal cortex (see Chapter 8), have coincided with findings from animal models that several psychotropic agents, especially antidepressants, may induce synaptogenesis or neurogenesis. Neuroplasticity has become an exciting area of research, and may be one mechanism of antidepressant action.

Attention is also now focussing on transcription factors that mediate between receptor activity and cellular genetic expression. CREB, the translocation of glucocorticoid receptors to the cell nucleus and alteration of m-RNA expression after antidepressant administration in animal models are all current areas of research.

There are several genetic candidates which may link outcome of treatment with antidepressants, including genes related to the 5-HT transporter, polymorphisms of 5-HT-receptor genes and the val/met polymorphism of the BDNF gene (Lee *et al.*, 2009; Kim *et al.*, 2008).

Some General Principles of Treatment

Although many of the newer drugs seem to have equivalent clinical efficacy with the established tricyclic drugs, their main benefit may lie in having less side effects, particularly those related to anticholinergic activity. Many of them, for example mianserin and the SSRIs, are much safer in overdose. Some 15% of all fatal poisonings are due to tricyclic drugs, and 3.3% of tricyclic overdoses have a fatal outcome. Amitriptyline and related tricyclics are responsible for approximately 1.66 deaths by suicide per 10 000 patients prescribed the drug, whereas the comparable figure for mianserin is around 0.13; historically before the widespread use of SSRIs 82% of deaths from antidepressant overdose were due to two drugs, amitryptiline and dothiepin (Henry *et al.*, 1995). There are also major differences between the drugs in regard to their sedative properties, some of which are related to their antihistaminic action. The more sedative compounds include amitriptyline, trimipramine, dothiepin, clomipramine, mianserin and mirtazepine, while less sedative are protriptyline and some of the newer selective 5-HT uptake inhibitors and their successors. The clinical implications of this are that patients with depression that require sedation, either because of anxiety, agitation or insomnia, may do better on the more sedative compounds, whereas those with psychomotor retardation require less sedation. If insomnia is prominent then the whole of the prescribed dose should be given at night-time, so that maximum sedation is obtained without the need for additional hypnotic drugs. Some patients, especially the elderly or those with heart or urinary problems, will be unable to tolerate the anticholinergic properties of some of the drugs, and those with minimal anticholinergic activity will be required.

Choice of antidepressant needs therefore to take into account the clinical pattern of the depression, the age of the patient and additional medical diagnoses. It is helpful to take a drug history from the patient and to find out if any close relative has had a depressive illness and, if so, to which drug they have responded. If a patient has been reliably treated before on a particular compound and has suffered few side effects from it, it is logical to start on the same preparation, unless there are contraindications. Potential suicide risk may be one of these, and drugs which are safe in overdose such as the SSRIs have obvious advantages. Venlafaxine is more associated with seizures, and citalopram leads to a prolonged QT interval following overdose, related to its metabolite didesmethylcitalopram.

It is wise, especially if the patient has previously experienced side effects or has some associated medical problem such as a seizure disorder, to start on low doses and build up the prescription over the ensuing one or two weeks. Polypharmacy should be avoided, however, and no patients should require an additional hypnotic to an antidepressant if a sedative antidepressant can be given as a single night-time dose. Useful combinations, apart from those with MAOI drugs, include L-tryptophan (if available) and clomipramine, or clomipramine and lithium in intractable cases. Some preparations are still available which combine antidepressants and phenothiazines, for example motival, which is fluphenazine and nortriptyline. If possible, these should be avoided. In non-responding patients, higher than usual doses may be prescribed, the increments being given until side effects occur or a clinical response is obtained. Once started, an antidepressant should be continued, if successful, for 6–12 months.

Pharmacology

Serum-level monitoring of antidepressant drugs can be undertaken. It is usually carried out using gas–liquid chromatography, although radio-immunoassay and mass spectrometry are also used. With regards to the tricyclic drugs, following absorption they are metabolized by methylation and hydroxylation in the liver, before passing into the circulation, where they are strongly protein-bound. Tertiary tricyclics, for example imipramine and amitriptyline, are demethylated to secondary amines, which themselves possess antidepressant properties. They are absorbed well and rapidly, peak plasma concentration occurring in 2–6 hours, although marked variation between patients is noted in terms of the serum levels for identical doses of medication. The half-lives are variable, from 8 hours for imipramine to over 80 hours for protriptyline. They are highly bound to plasma protein, with about 10% circulating as free drug.

Most of the studies that have examined the relationship between clinical response and serum levels have measured total rather than free levels. Further, since the presence of metabolites has to be taken into account, it is hardly surprising that the results obtained are difficult to interpret. Some authors have claimed that a therapeutic window exists, such that levels below or above this lead to poor results. This has mainly been noted with nortriptyline (Sørensen *et al.*, 1978). In contrast, for imipramine, the relationship is linear, levels below 150 ng ml^{-1} (540 nmol l^{-1}) being less effective (Glassman *et al.*, 1977). In general it may be said that high levels of drugs are more likely to lead to side effects, while patients with low levels respond poorly.

Table 12.3 CYP enzymes inhibited by different psychotropic drugs

CYP isoenzyme	Antidepressants	Antipsychotics
CYP1A2	Fluvoxamine	
CYP2C9/10/19	Fluoxetine	Thioridazine
	Sertraline	Clozapine
	Fluvoxamine	
	Moclobemide	
CYP2D6	Fluoxetine	Thioridazine
	Paroxetine	Haloperidol
	Sertraline	Clozapine
		Olanzapine
		Risperidone
CYP3A4	Fluoxetine	Chlorpromazine
	Sertraline	Thioridazine
	Nefazodone	Haloperidol
		Risperidone
		Thioridazine

In practice, measurement of serum levels is helpful in patients not responding as expected on good clinical doses of the drug, or in patients apparently experiencing side effects on small doses. It may also be useful in monitoring compliance where this is suspect. Interactions between tricyclic drugs and others show that barbiturates and some other anticonvulsants lower, while major tranquillizers raise, the serum levels of antidepressants, these effects mainly occurring by alteration of activity of metabolizing enzymes in the liver.

The SSRIs tend to have nonlinear pharmacokinetics, but this has little clinical relevance, and to date no relationships have been shown between serum levels and either clinical response or side effects.

The cytochrome 450 isoenzymes 1A2, 2C, 2D6 and 3A4 are important in the metabolism of psychotropic drugs, especially 2D6. Fluoxetine, paroxetine and sertraline have similar inhibitory effects on the 2D6 enzyme, and increased levels of some concomitantly prescribed drugs, for example tricyclic drugs or some antipsychotics, may be expected. Sertraline and fluoxetine inhibit 3A4, which mediates the metabolism of carbamazepine, and thus may increase levels of the latter if both classes are coprescribed. A list of enzymes is shown in Tables 12.3 and 12.4.

A general list of side effects with antidepressants is shown in Table 12.5. Some of these occur

Table 12.4 CYPs enzymes involved in psychotropic drug metabolism

CYP1A2	CYP2C9/10	CYP2C19	CYP2D6	CYP3A4
Antidepressants	*Anticonvulsants*	*Antidepressants*	*Antidepressants*	*Antidepressants*
Amitriptyline	Phenytoin	Amitriptyline	Fluoxetine	Amitriptyline
Clomipramine	*Antipsychotics*	Citalopram	Paroxetine	Clomipramine
Imipramine	Thioridazine	Clomipramine	Mianserin	Desipramine
Trazodone	Olanzapine	Imipramine	Venlafaxine	Imipramine
Fluvoxamine		Moclobemide	Trazodone	Norclomipramine
Antipsychotics		*Anticonvulsants*	Nefazodone	Nortriptyline
Chlorpromazine		Mephenytoin	Amitriptyline	Trimipramine
Haloperidol		Esobarbital	Clomipramine	Nefazodone
Clozapine		Mephobarbital	Desipramine	Fluoxetine
Olanzapine			Imipramine	Sertraline
Ziprasidone			Norclomipramine	Venlafaxine
			Nortryptiline	*Antipsychotics*
			Trimipramine	Haloperidol
			Maprotiline	Clozapine
			Sertraline	Risperidone
			Antipsychotics	Ziprasidone
			Chlorpromazine	Iloperidone
			Thioridazine	Quetiapine
			Haloperidol	*Anticonvulsants*
			Olanzapine	Carbamazepine
			Risperidone	
			Iloperidone	
			Quetiapine	

Table 12.5 Some side effects of non-MAOI antidepressant drugs

Sedation	Dyskinesia
Dry mouth	Myopathy, neuropathy
Palpitations and tachycardia, changes on the ECG	Convulsions
Visual difficulties	Ataxia
Postural difficulties	Delirium
Postural hypotension	Agitation
Nausea, vomiting, heartburn, G. I. bleeding	Transient hypomania
Constipation	Depersonalization
Glaucoma	Aggression
Urinary retention, impotence, delayed ejaculation	Jaundice (cholestatic)
Paralytic ileus	Weight gain
Galactorrhoea	Impairment of cognitive function
Sweating	Rashes
Fever	Extrapyramidal reactions
Tremor	Psychosis

frequently but may be tolerable, for example dry mouth, while others are rarer and can be very discomforting, such as dyskinesias or seizures. Some may be used therapeutically, for example the hypnotic effect. As noted, generally the SSRIs have less side effects than tricyclic antidepressants.

Much attention in the past has been paid to some specific side effects, in particular cardiac and neurological problems. Tricyclic drugs increase the atrioventricular conduction time (Burrows *et al.*, 1976) and can convert a partial to a complete heart block. In overdose they provoke a variety of arrhythmias, these being the commonest cause of death from overdose. The antidepressants with minimal anticholinergic effects, including the newer selective-uptake inhibitors, are safer in this regard. In one study, a comparison between fluoxetine and amitriptyline, an increased heart rate and prolongation of the P–R interval and QRS complex were noted with the tricyclic drug but not with fluoxetine (Fisch, 1985). Venlafaxine has been associated with a mildly increased blood pressure, especially in doses above 300 mg per day,

Nearly all the non-MAOI antidepressants lower the seizure threshold and may precipitate

seizures, with the possible exception of viloxazine and nomifensine (Trimble, 1978). The mechanism of this side effect is not understood, although it may be related to interference with monoamine or GABA activity. Thus patients with organic neurological disease, who may have a lowered seizure threshold, should be prescribed tricyclic drugs with caution. The management of epileptic patients is discussed below.

Impairment of cognitive function and performance on psychological tests probably occurs with most of the non-MAOI drugs, although this has not been well evaluated. Most studies are single-dose or short-term in volunteers, and while patient data tend to show improvement of cognitive function on antidepressant therapy, this may well be due to the relief of the cognitive effects of the depression rather than the antidepressant per se. Evidence from healthy volunteers suggests differences between drugs, for example imipramine, amitriptyline and mianserin give the most detrimental effects, while nomifensine and viloxazine are associated with the least problems (Thompson and Trimble, 1982b). The SSRIs are also more beneficial in this regard and there are reports of alerting effects with some of them (sertraline, fluoxetine, paroxetine).

Flu-like reactions have been described with several compounds, including zimelidine and nomifensine, with headaches, joint pains and elevation of liver enzymes. The 5-HT syndrome is a potentially life-threatening adverse effect that may occur following therapeutic use of SSRIs, notably with inadvertent interactions with other agents such as the MAOIs or with overdoses. It is related to excess 5-HT activity in the CNS and peripheral nervous system. The main symptoms, which can be mild and come on quite quickly, are flu-like, but include tachycardia, mydriasis, myoclonic jerks and increased superficial reflexes on neurological examination. When more severe, there is hypertension and fever, and behavioural agitation. Severe cases may lead to rhabdomyolysis, seizures, renal failure and rarely disseminated intravascular coagulation. There are similarities in the presentation of this syndrome and the neuroleptic malignant syndrome (see below), although CPK changes are usually not raised in the 5-HT syndrome.

Weight gain is a particularly difficult problem for patients, and this is not solely attributable to an increase in appetite. With the SSRIs weight may initially be lost, then regained later in treatment, in some cases leading to weight gain. A withdrawal syndrome on stopping antidepressants after long-term treatment has been reported. Symptoms include anxiety, panic, abdominal cramping, vertigo, dysasthesias, vomiting and diarrhoea. In addition, insomnia with nightmares, some restlessness, and occasionally hypomanic, manic or even psychotic pictures have been described. These flu-like withdrawal syndromes generally tend to occur in patients who have been on higher doses for long periods of time and who stop their drugs suddenly. They can be avoided by careful reduction of dosage and by warning the patient at the time of initial prescription not to suddenly stop taking their medication. With the SSRIs they are reported most with paroxetine, and are also noted with venlafaxine.

It has been known for many years that paradoxical excitation and increased motor activity can be seen with the prescription of antidepressants, and that this may lead the immobile depressed but suicidal patient to become active and act on their suicidal ideation. Similar activation has been reported with some of the SSRIs, and there is a continuing controversy as to whether they may induce suicide in some patients. There are analyses which suggest that the odds ratio of suicide attempts is increased with the SSRIs compared with placebo, but not against tricyclic agents (Fergusson *et al.*, 2005), and some epidemiological data note that the suicide rate has fallen with increasing use of SSRI prescriptions (Gibbons *et al.*, 2005). The FDA inserted a black-box warning concerning these in children and adolescents, and prescriptions fell. These data imply a need to closely observe patients as they are started on antidepressants for signs of increasing suicidal ideation.

ANTIPSYCHOTIC DRUGS

The term 'antipsychotic' for this group of drugs implies that their most important action is to lyse psychotic symptoms. Other terms that have been used for this class include 'major tranquilizer' (to be contrasted with 'minor tranquilizer') and 'neuroleptic' (a compound that tranquilizes but does not sedate).

These drugs naturally fall into four groups: phenothiazines, butyrophenones, thioxanthines and others. The phenothiazines have a tricyclic nucleus in which different configurations of the side chain lead to alteration of their properties. Three subgroups are recognized, one with an aliphatic side chain, such as chlorpromazine, one with a piperidine side chain, such as thioridazine, and one with piperazine side chains, such as trifluoperazine. The thioxanthines have a structure similar to the phenothiazines and include clopenthixol, flupenthixol, thiothixine and related drugs.

The butyrophenones, such as haloperidol, and related diphenylbutylpiperidines, such as pimozide, fluspiriline and penfluridol, have a different chemical structure, and some drugs, for example fluspiriline and penfluridol, are long-acting oral preparations. Other antipsychotics include molindone, reserpine, tetrabenazine, oxypertine, loxapine and the so-called atypicals, which include clozapine and the substituted benzamides, such as sulpiride.

The distinguishing property of all the standard antipsychotic drugs is their ability to block dopamine receptors. In addition they may evoke extrapyramidal symptoms of various types. They all inhibit apomorphine-induced stereotypy and agitation in animal models; provoke an acute increase in dopamine turnover with raised HVA levels in areas such as the corpus striatum, nucleus accumbens, olfactory tubercle and frontal cortex; block the stimulation of dopamine-sensitive adenylate cyclase; and displace receptor binding with H_3 dopamine or H_3 spiroperidol at postsynaptic dopamine receptor sites. The relative receptor binding profiles for some of these drugs are shown in Table 12.6.

The most potent dopamine-receptor antagonist used clinically is benperidol, while pimozide is the most specific. With few exceptions, the ability of these drugs to block the receptor correlates with their clinical antipsychotic action. Since the majority readily provoke extrapyramidal effects, it has been

Table 12.6 Receptor-binding properties of neuroleptics

	DA	5-HT	Alpha adrenergic	Histamine	ACh
Benperidol	+++++	±	±	−	−
Droperidol	+++++	+	+	−	−
Haloperidol	+++++	−	±	−	−
Pimozide	+++++	−	−	−	−
Bromperidol	+++++	−	±	−	−
Fluspiriline	+++++	+	−	−	−
Thiothixine	++++	+	±	+	−
Trifluoperazine	++++	±	±	±	−
Perphenazine	++++	+	−	+	−
Flupenthixol	++++	+	+	±	−
Fluphenazine	+++	+	+	+	−
Penfluridol	+++	−	−	−	−
Chlorprothixine	+++	++	++	++	++
Clozapine	+++	++	++	+++	+++
Risperidone	+++	+++	++	++	−
Thioridazine	++	+	++	+	++
Chlorpromazine	++	++	+++	+++	++
Sulpiride	+	−	−	−	−
Promazine	±	+	+++	+++	+++
Quetiapine	+	+	+	+	+
Ziprasidone	+	++	++	+	−
Olanzapine	+++	++	+	+	+
Aripiprazole	+	+	+	+	−

suggested that the antipsychotic potential is due to antagonism of dopamine receptors in the mesolimbic or mesocortical areas of the brain, while the motor effects relate to the nigrostriatal system. There are a few drugs that appear to possess minimal potential to evoke extrapyramidal effects, especially thioridazine and clozapine. One explanation for this has been the anticholinergic potential of these drugs, which may counteract the tendency to provoke extrapyramidal symptoms. Alternatively, it has been suggested that some, especially the atypicals, preferentially act on dopamine receptors in mesolimbic areas, rather than at the striatum. Although studies examining dopamine metabolites do not confirm a preferential increase in levels when comparing mesolimbic to striatal structures for various neuroleptics, those examining the disappearance or release of dopamine from selective sites do support a suggestion of a more preferential action in mesolimbic areas for these compounds (Leysen and Niemegeers, 1985; Scatton and Zivkovic, 1984). Since for example sulpiride does not have anticholinergic properties, it would seem that

the most likely explanation for these differing clinical effects of some of the antipsychotics relates to differential blockade of dopamine receptors in limbic as opposed to striatal areas.

These biochemical differences have given rise to the concept of atypical neuroleptics. These drugs weakly antagonize dopamine-induced stereotypies, but do not induce catalepsy. They do not lead to an upregulation of D_2 receptors in striatal structures or to the development of tolerance of increased dopamine turnover with chronic treatment. Clozapine is the paradigm.

When typical neuroleptics are given chronically, it is shown in animal models that tolerance occurs, and in patients initially elevated HVA levels in the CSF tend to decrease after a few weeks of drug administration (Post and Goodwin, 1975). However, it seems that this tolerance is observed in the striatum but not in mesolimbic and mesocortical dopaminergic systems (Scatton and Zivkovic, 1984), possibly explaining the clinically effective antipsychotic action of these drugs, which persists over time.

It should be noted that of the various subclasses of dopamine receptors described,

Table 12.7 D_1 and D_2 receptor-site antagonism

	D_1	D_2
Pimozide	+	+ + + +
Butaclamol	+ + + +	+ + + +
Chlorpromazine	+ +	+ + +
Thioridazine	+ +	+ + +
Flupenthixol	+ + + +	+ + +
Haloperidol	+ +	+ + + +
Sulpiride	−	+ + +
Clozapine	+ +	+ +
Fluphenazine	+ + +	+ + +
Risperidone	±	+ + +
Quetiapine	+	+
Aripiprazole	+	+
Ziprasidone	+ +	+ +
Olanzapine	+ +	+ +

antagonism of the D_2 receptor is related to many behavioural effects. Table 12.7 shows a comparison of the antagonism at D_1 and D_2 receptors for some neuroleptic drugs. However, clozapine shows equal occupancy at the D_1 and D_2 receptors, and has a potent effect at D_4 receptors (Seeman, 1992). Risperidone has high affinity for D_2, D_4, 5-HT$_2$ and alpha-adrenergic receptors, but acts only weakly at the D_1 site. Quetiapine is antagonistic at the D_1 and D_2 dopamine receptor, the alpha-1 and alpha-2 adrenergic receptor, the histamine H_1 receptor and the 5-HT$_{1A}$ and 5-HT$_2$ 5-HT receptor subtypes. PET data have shown that the D_2 receptor occupancy of quetiapine rapidly dissociates, which theoretically may minimize the risk of extrapyramidal and prolactin-related side effects. Ziprasidone has a high affinity for D_1 and D_2, 5-HT$_{2A}$ and alpha-adrenergic receptors and a medium affinity for histaminic receptors. Amisulpiride is quite specific for D_2 and D_3 receptors, but like other benzamides activates the endogenous GABA receptor. Olanzapine is structurally similar to clozapine, and has a higher affinity for 5-HT$_2$ receptors than D_2 receptors, with lower affinity for histamine, cholinergic muscarinic and alpha-adrenergic receptors. Aripiprazole is a partial D_2 and 5-HT$_{1A}$ agonist, and a 5-HT$_{2A}$ antagonist with moderate affinity for histamine and alpha-adrenergic receptors, and no appreciable affinity for cholinergic muscarinic receptors. Zotepine and sertindole are other

atypicals with both D_2 and 5-HT$_2$ antagonist effects, which are marketed in some countries.

In general, the rank order of the potency of the drugs for interaction with the D_1 receptor is unrelated to any of the behavioural tests of measuring dopaminergic activity, and as yet the relationship of this receptor to CNS function is undetermined. However, the D_2-receptor binding does correlate with effects on behavioural tests of dopaminergic function, and probably relates to their antipsychotic function. Following treatment with these drugs, it has been shown in animal models that the number of D_2-receptor binding sites increases, and on drug withdrawal slowly revert to pretreatment values (Leysen and Niemegeers, 1985). Other effects mediated by the D_2 receptor are dopamine-activated locomotion, prolactin release, dopamine-induced vomiting and impaired learning, noted following administration of dopamine antagonists. The alpha-1 adrenergic blockade is related to cardiovascular problems including hypotension, tachycardia and sedative effects; the latter may be enhanced by any antihistaminic effect.

Although the effects of clozapine at the D_4 receptor have stimulated considerable interest as a significant potential interaction site to explain its properties, it also antagonizes 5-HT$_2$ receptors. This, and the fact that other atypicals also antagonize the 5-HT$_2$ system, has led to a renewed interest in the role of 5-HT in schizophrenia.

SPECT and PET data have shown that clinical response to neuroleptics in schizophrenia is not directly related to the amount of D_2 blockade (Pilowsky et al., 1992), although low occupancy ($<50\%$) is more likely in nonresponders and the occurrence of extrapyramidal side effects is more likely with high occupancy (Nordstrom et al., 1993).

Following oral administration, chlorpromazine is easily absorbed and metabolized by the liver, with peak plasma level occurring in 1–3 hours. Its half-life is 17 hours. Some metabolites, such as the sulfoxide, have little pharmacological activity, while others, for example the hydroxy derivatives, are more potent. It is strongly protein-bound, and preferentially accumulates in the brain with a brain:plasma ratio of about 5:1. After termination of treatment, excretion of the drug or one of its metabolites may continue for several months.

Haloperidol is less rapidly absorbed, maximal concentrations occurring around 5 hours, with a half-life of 13–20 hours. It is 90% protein-bound, and does not induce its own metabolism. Pimozide has a half-life of over 50 hours, and it is possible to give the drug on less than a daily basis. Once-weekly treatment has been tried successfully in maintenance therapy for psychotic patients.

Clozapine is well absorbed, with peak plasma levels at 1–4 hours. It is 95% protein-bound, and metabolized through the liver with a half-life of about 14 hours. It is started at low doses (25 mg once or twice daily) and increased as necessary up to 300–600 mg a day. Because of the problem of agranulocytosis, it is essential to monitor blood counts, and the risk of seizures is increased with larger doses (5–10% over 600 mg). Other drugs which may be associated with agranulocytosis such as carbamazepine should be avoided. The incidence of extrapyramidal reactions, especially tardive kinesia, is low, although there are reports of the neuroleptic malignant syndrome associated with this drug, and akathisia is common. Patients often nonresponsive to other antipsychotics have been reported to respond to clozapine; in particular, patients with negative symptoms have done well. There may be a relationship between a low ratio of CSF HVA to 5-HIAA and better response (Pickar *et al.*, 1992).

Risperidone is also rapidly absorbed, with a half-life of about 24 hours. It has an active metabolite, 9-hydroxyrisperidone. It seems to have maximal antipsychotic efficiency at doses of 6–10 mg daily, but with increasing doses it provokes Parkinsonism, and dystonias and akathisia are reported. Ziprasidone has a short half-life of 2–4 hours, quetiapine 6 hours, olanzapine 20–50 hours and aripiprazole 6 days. The latter also has an active metabolite, dehydro-aripiprazole. The incidence of side effects with these drugs varies, but generally the extrapyramidal ones are less than with the older compounds. Quetiapine is available as a sustained-release preparation, while paliperidone is an extended-release preparation, being the main active metabolite of risperidone.

The dose of antipsychotic prescribed needs to be titrated for individual patients against their symptoms, but in some cases large doses are necessary. With drugs that are alpha-adrenergic blockers, for example chlorpromazine, clozapine and risperidone, such doses may lower blood pressure and monitoring of the latter may be necessary. It is usual in clinical practice to start patients on oral medications, and often once-daily prescription is possible. Following control of psychotic symptoms with oral therapy, especially if the patient has schizophrenia, a change to intramuscular preparations may be preferred.

Esterified drugs, mostly dissolved in oil, are given intramuscularly, and released over a varying period of time, up to about four weeks. They include the older decanoate preparations of haloperidol, fluphenazine, flupenthixol, and clopenthixol and fluspiriline. These drugs provoke the same incidence of extrapyramidal problems as do oral preparations, although the onset may be more rapid (Ayd, 1974). It may have been expected that the use of intramuscular preparations would have increased compliance and thus response. However, early trials comparing patients on injectable preparations to oral pimozide suggest little difference in relapse rate (McCreadie *et al.*, 1980), and the growth in the use of intramuscular therapies waned with the introduction of the atypicals. Recently however, a number of the latter have become available as intramuscular preparations (risperidone, olanzapine, ziprazadone) and some have been developed with different delivery systems, such as oral olanzapine, which dissolves on the tongue. In schizophrenia, once treatment has been started, it probably needs to be continued indefinitely. Discontinuation of therapy leads to relapse in approximately 20% of patients in six months and 45% of patients at one year (Curson *et al.*, 1985). It is estimated that some 60–65% of patients will relapse over a 24-month period if not taking drugs, comparable data for those in maintenance therapy being 35%. Poor response to treatment relates to younger age of onset of illness, prominent initial negative symptoms, impairment of cognitive performance and an enlarged ventricular:brain ratio on the CT or MRI scan.

A relationship between clinical response to serum levels of antipsychotics or plasma prolactin has not been demonstrated in schizophrenia (Kolakowska *et al.*, 1985). Maintenance with low dose may reduce the long-term incidence of side effects. Low doses of these drugs have been used in other conditions, for example depressive illness, borderline personalities and anxiety disorders, although the use of those with a high potential for extrapyramidal or metabolic side effects should be discouraged. The preferential response of monosymptomatic psychoses to pimozide has been reported (Riding and Munroe, 1975), and for aggression, in particular in patients with brain damage, clopenthixol may have special value.

Antipsychotics are also used in the management of acute or chronic organic brain syndromes, and may be used in alcohol withdrawal states, although their potential to lower seizure threshold is a problem in this setting. Their use in the management of personality disorders remains controversial, and their use in the elderly is discouraged unless the indications for use are very clear. An increased risk of cerebrovascular disease, stroke and bone fractures has been reported with the atypicals in the geriatric population. They should be used sparingly and with caution in elderly patients.

There has been an accepted tendency to use atypical antipsychotic medications in the management of bipolar-spectrum disorders. In the past, on account of the high prevalence of extrapyramidal side effects of the first generation drugs, this was not considered good practice, except in the rapid resolution of acute manic behaviours. The atypicals also have good acute antimanic efficacy, and all are acceptable for use in acute states, with the exception of clozapine. The more difficult question relates to their chronic use to prevent manic relapses. The licences for use vary across countries, but the profile of effects is similar in clinical trials, even for side effects; again the exception is clozapine. Quetiapine seems to have the lowest potential to provoke extrapyamidal reactions. In clinical practice, an atypical antipsychotic or valproic acid is added to lithium, but no study has tested the hypothesis that two drugs are better than one in this situation. Several of the atypical antipsychotics have been shown to have antidepressant effects in bipolar depression, and they are thus now used widely for bipolar patients who struggle with depression.

In some cases it is necessary to tranquillize patients rapidly, and intramuscular or intravenous doses may be given. In these situations, changeover to oral therapy should be carried out as soon as possible. Side effects, such as acute dystonias, seem to be rare.

Side Effects

The side effects of the antipsychotics are similar to those listed for antidepressants (Table 12.5). Of particular interest, however, are the extrapyramidal syndromes, which include dystonias, akinesia, akathisia, Parkinsonism and tardive syndromes.

In general, these disorders fall into two groups, as shown in Table 12.8. In practice, some admixture of symptoms is seen, and the division may not be so clear. The acute disorders include acute dystonias, akathisia, akinesia and Parkinsonism. The chronic ones are mainly tardive dystonia and tardive dyskinesia. Acute dystonia is one of the earliest extrapyramidal side effects and usually occurs within the first two or three days of treatment. Typically, the movements are uncoordinated and spasmodic, and may involve the body, the limbs, the head and the neck. The jaws may be tightly clenched together, the tongue may be forcibly protruded and facial

Table 12.8 Extrapyramidal effects of psychotropic drugs

Acute	*Chronic*
Dystonia	Tardive dyskinesia
Akathisia	Tardive dystonia
Akinesia	
Parkinsonism	
Rabbit syndrome	

grimaces occur. Retrocollis, torticollis, antecollis, oculogyric crises or opisthotonos may all be seen. Males are preferentially affected and some suggest that up to 50% of patients may develop some form of reaction following treatment with high-potency neuroleptics (Winslow *et al.*, 1986). There are repeated spasms of muscles with hypertonicity between attacks, and the condition can be distressing and painful. Dystonia is usually treated by intramuscular or intravenous administration of an anticholinergic drug such as benztropine or orphenadrine, although benzodiazepines are also effective; it is thought to be caused by increased dopamine turnover that occurs following acute administration of dopamine antagonists, stimulating dopamine receptors not blocked by the action of the drugs and thus provoking the movement disorder.

Much more common is akinesia, which is usually seen within 24 hours of starting the drugs. Patients have diminished spontaneous movements, reduced facial expression and may complain of fatigue. Muscle tone is not increased, and the clinical picture may be mistaken for an increasing apathy of depression or schizophrenia. It is usually helped by lowering the dose of the antipsychotic or adding an anticholinergic drug.

Akathisia is sometimes less acute, but occurs very frequently, affecting over 50% of patients. It is characterized by a subjective sense of restlessness and presents as motor hyperactivity, with shifting posture and inability to sit or stay still for more than a few moments. It thus resembles agitation, and may lead to a mistaken diagnosis of agitated depression, or a deterioration of the psychosis if unrecognized. Some patients have added orofacial dyskinesia; thus both disorders can occur in the same patient. Akathisia usually responds to a reduction of dose or to the administration of anticholinergic or benzodiazepine drugs. Since similar clinical pictures have been reported in patients following L-dopa therapy in Parkinson's disease, it is thought that it somehow relates to abnormalities of dopamine transmission in the basal ganglia.

The classical picture of Parkinsonism, with increased muscle tone, rigidity, increased salivation, and gait and posture disturbances, may

be seen in patients prescribed antipsychotic drugs, and over 60% of patients may have mild symptoms. In contrast to idiopathic Parkinson's disease, tremor tends to occur late in the picture and is less common than rigidity and akinesia. Akathisia may also be associated with the Parkinsonian picture. The Parkinsonism tends to come on gradually, and may be preceded by complaints of weakness or limb pains. Females are more affected than males. A variant is the so-called 'rabbit syndrome', in which rapid chewing-like movements of the lips occur, which resemble a rabbit eating. This is to be distinguished from tardive dyskinesia.

It has been suggested that the incidence of Parkinsonism, and indeed some of the other extrapyramidal syndromes, may be diminished by the administration of routine prophylactic anticholinergic drugs. However, it may be argued that since anticholinergic drugs may exacerbate some motor disorders (for example tardive dyskinesia), provoke a toxic psychosis, delay gastric emptying and, by neurochemical antagonism of the dopamine blocking potential of the antipsychotic drugs, diminish their therapeutic potential, such routine prescription should be avoided. It is clinically accepted that the atypical antipsychotic drugs provoke less in the way of Parkinsonism and other extrapyramidal side effects than the older compounds

Other conditions seen after varying time intervals following introduction of neuroleptic drugs include the blepharospasm–oromandibular–dystonia syndrome (Meige's or Bruegel's syndrome), catatonic reactions and the neuroleptic malignant syndrome. The blepharospasm–oromandibular–dystonia syndrome is characterized by prolonged spasms of the jaw and mouth, usually in association with blepharospasm, which is seen both as an idiopathic form and following neuroleptic treatment. Females are more affected than males, and the onset is usually in the sixth decade. The dystonia can be extremely painful, the teeth being forced together and sometimes damaged, or alternatively tongue biting can occur. The mouth may be forced into an open position for varying periods, which if severe may lead to difficulties with speaking and eating, and sometimes jaw dislocation. Tongue protrusion, lip pouting and occasionally dystonic posturing in other parts of the body may also be noted. The pathogenesis is unknown, but again it is thought to be related to abnormalities of dopamine activity within the basal ganglia. It is one of a group of tardive dystonias, which include other forms of dystonic posturing, spasmodic dysphonia and abnormal vocalizations, which sometimes are in association with tics, a tardive form of Gilles de la Tourette's syndrome.

Catatonic reactions involve posturing, waxy flexibility, withdrawal, mutism and associated Parkinsonism, which may be severe and life-threatening, and can be misinterpreted as an exacerbation of the underlying psychosis.

The neuroleptic malignant syndrome is one of the most serious of the extrapyramidal complications, presenting as hyperpyrexia and rigidity. It may emerge from a catatonic reaction and be associated with a variety of other abnormal involuntary movements. Autonomic disturbances including cardiovascular and respiratory difficulties, perspiration, salivation and incontinence may be seen, and death may occur from respiratory, cardiac, hepatic or renal failure. It can develop quite suddenly and has been described following a single injection of an antipsychotic. Its appearance may be facilitated by the combined administration of lithium. Its pathogenesis is not understood, but presumably relates to dopamine-receptor blockade in the basal ganglia and hypothalamus. In view of its high mortality (5–30%), attention to the patient's medical state is extremely important. Leucocytosis and elevated creatine kinase levels in the presence of abnormal liver-function tests are often found. Treatment with bromocryptine, dantrolene, amantadine and ECT have all been tried.

Tardive Dyskinesia

This condition is a chronic disorder secondary to the administration of antipsychotics, although idiopathic forms with an identical clinical picture are noted. In addition, it has been associated with the taking of antihistamines, anticholinergic drugs, anticonvulsants, particularly phenytoin, and the tricyclic antidepressants. It usually comes on after about three months of therapy, and its appearance is gradual. In some patients, the first movements are noted following reduction of drug dosage. This withdrawal dyskinesia is frequently seen in patients who have been on neuroleptic medication for a long period of time.

The characteristic features of tardive dyskinesia are persistent abnormal muscular movements, predominantly affecting the tongue and perioral region, but, in addition, choreiform and athetoid movements in the limbs, and occasionally the trunk. There is smacking of the lips with masticatory jaw movements and protrusion of the tongue, often in combination. Sometimes the only clinical manifestation is increasing writhing movements of the lips. In other patients, blepharospasm, blinking, tics, abdominal movement and laryngeal spasms may also be noted. More rarely, particularly in younger patients, a to-and-fro clonic-type movement of the spine is seen. Although it is sometimes stated that the condition does not cause much stress, and it is true that patients often lightly dismiss the dyskinesia, putting their problems down to 'denture difficulties', it is nevertheless very uncomfortable in some patients and may be socially quite disabling.

Tardive dyskinesia is found more frequently in patients receiving antipsychotics than in control populations, is commoner in females and is found with increasing frequency with age. Younger patients tend to have involvement of the extremities and trunk, occasionally with bizarre postures and ballistic movements with gait abnormalities and rocking, while in the elderly a perioral distribution with associated limb movements is the more frequent picture. In some cases the dyskinesia is persistent, although a withdrawal dyskinesia will tend to disappear over weeks to months, following cessation of the neuroleptic. Present estimates suggest that about 50% of patients with tardive dyskinesia will remain unchanged at follow-up. No convincing association between duration, dose and type of antipsychotic drug treatment has emerged, but these pictures are seen less frequently with the atypicals. There is a suggestion that patients who develop tardive dyskinesia are more likely to show impairments on psychological testing (Struve and Willner, 1983; Wegner *et al.*, 1985) and an increased incidence of CT-scan changes, including ventricular dilatation (Owens *et al.*, 1985).

The pathogenesis of tardive dyskinesia has yet to be clarified. The facts that it is commonly related to drugs whose principal action is dopamine antagonism and that it is a tardive disorder have led to the suggestion that it is related to the development of postsynaptic dopamine-receptor supersensitivity. This is supported by observations that similar movements may be seen following L-dopa therapy for Parkinson's disease and that L-dopa itself may exacerbate the movements of tardive dyskinesia. However, there are serious shortcomings to the concept that the condition is simply related to some form of receptor-disuse supersensitivity. These include the discrepancies between the development of the clinical syndrome and the time of the increase in dopamine receptors following the beginning of treatment, which can be shown to occur rapidly in animal models. Further, all animals given neuroleptics develop supersensitivity, whereas only some 20% of patients develop the persisting dyskinesia. In addition, in animal models where increased receptor sensitivity is shown, no equivalent of tardive dyskinesia has been seen. The receptor changes tend to revert to normal after withdrawal, but again, in patients, persistence of the syndrome can continue for many years. Finally, in patient post-mortem studies, no difference in binding has been shown with respect to either D_1 or D_2 receptors in the brain when patients with schizophrenia with or without movement disorders are compared (Waddington *et al.*, 1985).

An alternative hypothesis relates to an alteration of GABA, since significant reductions in GAD activity have been shown in the globus pallidus, subthalamus and substantia nigra of primates receiving long-term neuroleptic therapy (Gunne *et al.*, 1984). This deficit appeared related to abnormal orofacial movements in the animals. The hypothesis receives some support from early suggestions that GABA agonists may improve some of the symptoms of tardive

dyskinesia in patients (Casey *et al.*, 1980). These data have recently been replicated using vigabatrin in studies in which dyskinetic schizophrenic patients were reported to show lower CSF GABA levels than those without dyskinesias (Thaker *et al.*, 1987). Although no consistent abnormalities or neuropathological changes at post mortem have been described, there are several reports of microscopic changes in some basal-ganglia areas, including the substantia nigra in patients receiving long-term neuroleptics (Christensen *et al.*, 1970), perhaps suggesting that the clinical picture arises from the combination of some form of intrinsic neuronal damage in these crucial regions of the brain and long-term dopamine-receptor blockade.

A large number of drugs have been tried in the treatment of tardive dyskinesia, but success has been limited. Most of the studies have been continued for a few weeks only, and the majority are not double blind. Antipsychotic drugs, especially an atypical, are the most effective method of suppressing the symptoms, although in the long term it seems hardly logical to use them. Anticholinergic drugs exacerbate the symptoms, and withdrawal should be undertaken if they are concurrently prescribed in a patient with the syndrome (Burnett *et al.*, 1980).

Other Side Effects

Agranulocytosis, due to a direct toxic effect of phenothiazines on the bone marrow, may occur, and depression of the white-cell count is often encountered. The estimated incidence of this with clozapine is 1–2% of patients. This mainly occurs within four months of treatment, and is reversible in most cases on stopping the drug. Photosensitivity may be a problem with chlorpromazine, and may lead to a pattern of contact dermatitis or skin eruptions on exposure to sunlight. Retinal pigmentation has been described with thioridazine. Combinations of lithium and haloperidol may lead to an organic psycho-syndrome.

Cardiac arrhythmias are noted with pimozide, necessitating an EEG examination prior to commencing therapy. The finding of a prolonged QT interval, or prescription of other drugs that may increase the QT interval, which includes other antipsychotics, are contraindications to its use. The concern over cardiac conduction problems has lead to the failure of some antipsychotics reaching clinical practice. Ziprasidone leads to a prolongation of the QT interval and should not be given to patients with a QT interval >500 ms or with other drugs which have an action on this ECG period (such as methadone, some tricyclic drugs, lithium). Torsade de points is a ventricular tachycardia associated with a long QT interval, which may lead to loss of consciousness, and rarely to death. Sudden death in patients on antipsychotic drugs has been reported, and this may be due to cardiac problems. Findings at post mortem are usually negative.

A withdrawal syndrome has been seen after long-term treatment with the antipsychotics, with insomnia, anxiety, restlessness and the already-mentioned movement disorders. A depressive illness has been reported to occur in some patients treated with antipsychotics, although the exact relationship between the medication and the depression is unclear, since postpsychotic depression is a well-recognized clinical entity. One suggestion is that suppression of the psychotic symptoms permits the expression of pre-existent affective symptoms.

One problem that has emerged with the atypical antipsychotics relates to metabolic abnormalities. These include weight gain, hyperlipidaemia, glucose intolerance, increased insulin levels and type-2 diabetes mellitus. The latter has been reported to lead to episodes of ketoacidosis, a medical emergency which can lead to death. Weight gain is reported less with risperidone, aripiprazole and ziprasidone, and more for clozapine and olanzapine, the latter two having the higher risk for diabetes (Jin *et al.*, 2006). In prospective studies the risk for diabetes with typical agents is also shown to be increased, but not in all studies, and less so than with the atypical antipsychotics.

What is unclear is whether schizophrenia itself raises the risk for diabetes, and its relationship to weight gain. The metabolic syndrome, which represents a clinical picture of abdominal obesity, raised triglyceride and lowered HDL-cholesterol levels, hypertension and raised fasting glucose, puts patients at high risk for cardiovascular disease and diabetes mellitus, and is overrepresented in psychiatric patients, including those diagnosed with schizophrenia. In many cases the diabetes develops before weight gain, and it may emerge soon after the onset of therapy. It is unclear at present to what extent patients beginning to take atypical antipsychotics should be screened for the metabolic syndrome, but attention to family history, weight, fasting blood sugar, the lipid profile and blood pressure would seem sensible, and the vulnerable should be notified of the risk and appropriately monitored.

Antipsychotic Drugs in Development

Asenpaine is a novel atypical drug which has higher affinity for several 5-HT and D3 and D4 receptors. The trend has been to develop D_2 antagonists or partial agonists with high-affinity antagonism for other receptors such as 5-HT (5-HT$_{1A}$, 5-HT$_{2a}$ 5—HT$_{2c}$, 5-HT$_3$, etc.) or for noradrenaline, or selective agonists at D_1 or D_4, nicotinic and GABA$_a$ receptors. However, other potential treatments include COMT inhibitors such as tolcapone, and drugs that act on the glutaminergic system such as glycine, D-serine, D-cycloserine and ampakine. Of these, only the co-agonists glycine and D-serine show any promise; these seem effective on negative as opposed to positive symptoms (Tuominen *et al.*, 2006).

Another strategy is to target symptoms, especially those derived from endophenotypic research (such as cognition), or negative symptoms, moving away from using DSM IV-TR approaches to patient selection. Genetic research may in the future allow molecular libraries of potential targets for pharmaceuticals to be established, with genetic profiling of patients most likely to respond.

ANXIOLYTICS AND HYPNOTICS

Three main groups are included: barbiturates, benzodiazepines and others. They are the most widely used drugs in psychiatry, and possess sedative and anticonvulsant properties in addition to being anxiolytic. The main differences between the barbiturates and the benzodiazepines reside in the lack of suicide potential with the latter and the greater tendency to addiction with the former.

Barbiturates include phenobarbitone, butobarbitone and amylobarbitone. They are rapidly absorbed from the GI tract and are powerful hepatic enzyme inducers. Their duration of action is around eight hours, but their generalized effect on the brain leads to respiratory depression, which may cause death in overdose. Since the introduction of the benzodiazepines they have been used far less frequently, although occasional patients still benefit from the prescription of a hypnotic barbiturate in very selected circumstances. Although phenobarbitone at one time was an important drug in the management of epilepsy, its use these days is not encouraged.

The benzodiazepines have a common structure, but differ with respect to their metabolites (see Figure 12.4). Ultimately, they are conjugated with glucuronic acid, and a number of the metabolic products themselves are active compounds. However, some of the benzodiazepines (particularly the short-acting ones) tend not to have active intermediaries. Many of the longeracting ones have desmethyldiazepam as their active metabolite, which has a half-life of some 50 hours. However, benzodiazepines differ both with regards to their half-life and with their potential for anxiolytic, anticonvulsant, musclerelaxant, sedative and amnesic effects. Some

Table 12.9 Half-life of different benzodiazepines

	Hours
Temazepam	8
Oxazepam	8
Lorazepam	12
Medazepam	6–20
Flurazepam	10–20
Chlordiazepoxide	24
Diazepam	30
Chlorazepate	30–60
Nitrazepam	48
Triazolam	2
Clonazepam	53
Clobazam	18

of these differences are shown in Tables 12.9 and 12.10.

On the basis of their half-lives, they may be divided into long, intermediate and short duration of action. Some of these pharmacokinetic differences are shown in Table 12.11. In general, those with a long duration of action tend to be prescribed as anxiolytics, while those in the short-acting class are hypnotics. The clearance of many of these drugs is increased with age, although oxazepam, lorazepam and temazepam show only minor differences in their kinetics with advancing years. The metabolism of lorazepam and oxazepam is little influenced by liver disease.

The discovery of the benzodiazepine receptor led to a clearer understanding of their mode of action (Braestrup and Nielsen, 1982). The benzodiazepine binding site, thought to represent part of the GABA–receptor chloride ionophor complex, is in some way related to the behavioural actions of these drugs,

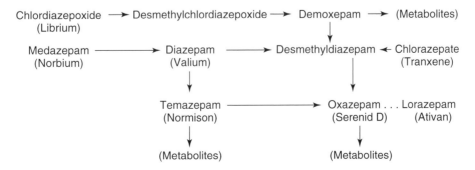

Figure 12.4 The pathway of benzodiazepine metabolism (*Biol Psych*, 2 Ed, p. 358)

Table 12.10 Differential effects of different benzodiazepines

Drug	Anxiolytic	Anti-convulsant	Muscle relaxing	Sedative	Amnesic
Lorazepam	++	+++	+	+	+++
Diazepam	++	+	+++	++	+
Temazepam	+	±	+	+++	±
Clonazepam	±	+++	++	+	±
Nitrazepam	+	++	+	+++	±
Clobazam	++	+++	+	±	±

Table 12.11 Pharmacokinetic differences among benzodiazepines

Long	Intermediate	Short
Chlordiazepoxide	Alprazolam	Brotizolam
Clorazepate	Bromazepam	Midazolam
Clobazam	Flunitrazepam	Triazolam
Diazepam	Lorazepam	
Flurazepam	Lormetazepam	
Ketazolam	Nitrazepam	
Medazepam	Oxazepam	
Prazepam	Temazepam	

although it does not explain all of their effects. For example, meprobamate and alcohol, both effective anxiolytics, do not bind to the receptor. This is one element of the argument which has led Gray (1982) to suggest that at least the anxiolytic effect of the benzodiazepines is related to enhancement of the GABA transmission, probably at selective sites within the CNS, but that interaction with other neurotransmitter systems, in particular the ascending monoamines, is also involved (Iversen, 1983). Benzodiazepine antagonists counteract some of the effects of benzodiazepines, and provoke anxiety in humans (Dorrow *et al.*, 1983). Respiratory depression does not appear to be a complication of benzodiazepine therapy, and after overdose, if taken alone, benzodiazepines rarely result in death.

The existence of multiple potential configurations of the benzodiazepine–GABA receptor has allowed further understanding of the spectrum of benzodiazepine effects. These range from full agonism to partial agonism, to antagonism and inverse agonism, as illustrated in Figure 12.5. This has allowed partial agonists to be developed, such as abecarnil and bretazenil, although as yet none have found clinical approval. The differing profile of benzodiazepines is reflected in two compounds, namely clobazam and alprazolam. Clobazam is a 1,5-benzodiazepine, in which the nitrogen on the heterocyclic ring is moved from the 4 to the 5 position. This appears to confer a better therapeutic potential of the drug with regards to its anticonvulsant effect, the drug possessing minimal sedative, myorelaxant and cognitive side effects

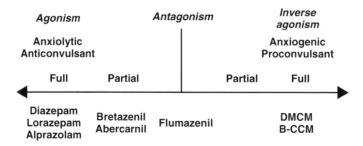

The spectrum of benzodiazepine activity

Figure 12.5 The spectrum of benzodiazepine effects (reproduced from Cummings and Trimble, 1995; *Biol Psych*, 2 Ed, p. 361)

(Trimble, 1986b). Alprazolam is a triazolobenzodiazepine, which in addition to its anxiolytic properties is reported to be effective in the control of panic disorder and may possess antidepressant properties (Judd *et al.*, 1986). It appears that most benzodiazepines are ineffective for panic attacks, while tricyclic antidepressants, SSRIs, MAOI drugs and alprazolam are therapeutically useful. Alprazolam is antidepressant for patients with reactive or neurotic depression (Imlah, 1985) and mania has been reported as a side effect (Arana *et al.*, 1985).

Concern has been expressed about benzodiazepine dependence. This has been reported after as short a time as six weeks of treatment, although it tends to occur in patients who have been on high doses for prolonged periods. Withdrawal symptoms may occur, particularly if the dose of the drug is withdrawn at an inappropriate rate. The withdrawal syndrome in many cases actually represents a return of earlier anxiety, although some authors have suggested that perceptual distortions and feelings of depersonalization are characteristic (Ashton, 1984). Withdrawal seizures are certainly one manifestation, although again, in the clinical setting, they probably reflect too rapid a decrease in dose. The presence of the withdrawal syndrome suggests how effective these compounds are biologically, and thus how they should be used judiciously in clinical practice. It has been reported that premorbid personality characteristics may be important in predicting those patients who will show withdrawal reactions, those with passive and dependent personality traits being more susceptible than those showing premorbid conscientiousness, rigidity or even premorbid anxiety proneness (Tyrer *et al.*, 1983).

Other side effects include oversedation, problems with concentration and memory, and in the elderly, ataxia and confusion, particularly with the longer-acting and more sedative compounds. The shortest-acting benzodiazapines, such as midazolam, are powerful amnestic agents and are commonly used in brief surgeries and procedures. Longer-term confusional states have been reported in the elderly, even after brief exposure to the shortest-acting

agents. Depression has been reported, but it is also seen following long-term benzodiazepine withdrawal (Olajide and Lader, 1984). Release of aggression has also been noted in both animals and humans.

Other anxiolytics include meprobamate, which is absorbed rapidly, induces its own metabolism and has a half-life of about 12 hours. It is approximately halfway between the barbiturates and the benzodiazepines in terms of producing tolerance, sedation and cortical depression. Other hypnotics include chloral hydrate, dichloralphenazone, glutethamide, paraldehyde and chlormethiazole. The latter may be particularly useful in the management of alcohol withdrawal syndromes.

The azapirones are nonbenzodiazepine anxiolytics which include gepirone, ipsapirone, binospirone and buspirone. They act as agonists at the 5-HT$_{1A}$ receptor, and seem also to possess antidepressant properties (see above). The role of the 5-HT receptors in anxiety is actively under investigation at present, and some 5-HT$_2$ antagonists such as mianserin and ritanserin may diminish anxiety. It is thought that the downregulation of 5-HT$_2$ receptors by antidepressants may be related to the anxiolytic effects of these drugs. 5-HT$_3$ antagonists such as ondansetron may be effective in some anxiety states, although the clinical use of the later is as an antiemetic.

Buspirone is well absorbed and widely distributed throughout the body. It has a half-life of approximately 2–3 hours, and although a weak dopamine antagonist, does not appear to be antipsychotic, and lacks sedative, muscle-relaxant and anticonvulsant effects.

Zopiclone is a cyclopyrrolone that acts at subunits of the benzodiazepine A receptor, with sedative and anticonvulsant properties. It is one of a group of drugs, including zaleplon and zolpidem, which were thought to have less addictive potential than the benzodiazepines, but cases of dependence are reported. These drugs have short half-lives (3–6 hours) and are used as hypnotics. Dysgeusia is a particular problem with zopiclone, and a tentative association with carcinoma has been suggested. A related drug, alpidem, is not hypnotic but has anxiolytic properties.

When using anxiolytics, doses of drugs have to be based on clinical judgement, and for tranquillization once-daily or twice-daily regimes can be used. Although some patients develop tolerance to these drugs, requiring increasing doses over time, this is not usual and many patients continue to get clinical benefit on small doses. However, it is important that they should not be given for longer than is necessary, and that when withdrawal is undertaken it should be done slowly and with care.

Recently, increased knowledge of the heterogeneity and complexity of the GABA receptor, especially regarding extrasynaptic receptors, has led to a resurgence of interest in GABA agonists as psychotropic agents, but beyond anxiolysis, with even potential antipsychotic effects. More subtype-selective benzodiazepines are being explored.

With regard to hypnotics, there has been a growing interest in cerebral rhythms, especially circadian ones controlled by the suprachiasmatic nucleus of the hypothalamus. This nucleus receives light stimuli via the eye, and regulates a number of bodily rhythms including temperature and sleep–wake cycles. Melatonin receptors (M_1 and M_2) are found in the supachiasmatic nucleus, and act through adenylate cyclase to regulate oscillations of neuronal activity. Melatonin levels are high at night-time and low in the daytime.

Melatonin itself can induce sleep, and is used by many people as a hypnotic. Ramelteon selectively binds to M_1 and M_2 receptors. Agomelatine is an M_1 and M_2 agonist with high affinity for the 5-HT_{2c} receptor, and no affinity for 5-HT or dopamine transporters, or histaminic and muscarinic receptors. The 5-HT_{2c} receptor effect is thought to release noradrenaline and dopamine in frontal cortex, contributing to an antidepressant effect. This compound increases slow-wave sleep and is nonsedative.

BETA-ADRENERGIC BLOCKERS

Beta-adrenergic blockers, such as propranolol, are widely used in the management of cardiovascular disorders, and clinically decrease the heart rate, lower the blood pressure and may cause bronchial constriction. Their use in the management of anxiety disorders has been advocated, one suggestion being that they influence the somatic symptoms such as palpitations, sweating and diarrhoea, as opposed to psychic symptoms (Tyrer and Lader, 1974). However, improvement of psychic symptoms has also been reported (Kathol *et al.*, 1980), and the suggestion that their effect is primarily on peripheral receptors may need revision. Some beta-blockers such as practolol, with little ability to cross the blood–brain barrier, also appear to be effective anxiolytics. They are of little value in agoraphobia and panic attacks and do not influence lactate-induced panic (Gorman *et al.*, 1983). There has been interest in their use in schizophrenia, but the results of various trials are contradictory. They are contraindicated in patients with respiratory and cardiac disorders, where beta blockade may lead to deterioration of the clinical state, and are poorly tolerated by some people, who develop a severe malaise and lethargy, which, if unrecognized, may be taken for further symptoms of the underlying psychiatric disturbance. A withdrawal syndrome has been described with abrupt termination of treatment. Their use as single doses (40 mg of oxprenolol) to quell stage fright and other brief-lived episodes of stress-induced anxiety may be helpful, but generally in the management of patients with anxiety, benzodiazepines are preferred, particularly by patients (Tyrer and Lader, 1974).

LITHIUM

Lithium carbonate was first introduced for the treatment of manic–depressive illness in 1949 and is the drug of choice for prophylactic management of manic–depressive psychosis. Following ingestion, it is absorbed rapidly, peak concentrations occurring in 1–2 hours, with a half-life of approximately 24 hours. It is mainly excreted in the urine, and thus patients with renal disease readily become intoxicated. Since it is reabsorbed with sodium into the proximal renal tubules, any drug that leads to a negative sodium balance, such as a diuretic, will lead to increased retention of lithium. This also occurs with alteration of the diet, heavy sweating and diseases that reduce sodium intake. For a hypertensive patient, a beta-blocker or clonidine is preferred, and thiazide diuretics should be avoided.

Its mode of action is still unknown in spite of its widespread use, but it does reduce the sodium content of the brain, increase central 5-HT synthesis and noradrenaline turnover, increase platelet 5-HT uptake (Coppen *et al.*, 1980), and reduce urinary noradrenaline, MHPG, VMA and whole-body noradrenaline turnover (Linnoila *et al.*, 1983a). Lithium also affects the PI intracellular transduction system, perhaps interfering with neurotransmitter-stimulated PI metabolism. This may thus downregulate, for example, an overactive dopamine system. Since dopamine-induced stimulation of PI can also be inhibited by dopamine antagonists, one explanation for the effects of both neuroleptics and lithium in mania is through this common mechanism. Rangel-Guerra *et al.* (1983) reported using MRI, that T_1 proton relaxation time was reduced from elevated levels in 20 patients with bipolar affective disorder following lithium therapy of 900 mg per day for 10 days.

The main indication for lithium is in bipolar affective disorder, although it is now known to be useful in the management of recurrent unipolar affective disorder. It may also be used in the acute treatment of affective disorder, especially mania, when it is usually started in combination with an antipsychotic. Other uses of lithium include recurrent aggressive disorders, migraine, cluster headaches, cycloid psychoses and organic mental disorders with secondary affective symptoms. In one trial (Coppen *et al.*, 1978), lithium was found to be superior to mianserin in the long-term maintenance treatment of depressive illness.

Lithium has a number of toxic effects, which are shown in Table 12.12. Although these are minimized by regular monitoring of serum lithium levels, with a suggested nontoxic range of 0.6–1.5 mmol l^{-1}, severe toxicity has been described at lower levels, and coexistent medication such as phenytoin, carbamazepine and

Table 12.12 Toxic effects of lithium

Neuropsychiatric	Drowsiness
	Confusion
	Psychomotor retardation
	Restlessness
	Stupor
	Headache
	Weakness
	Tremor
	Ataxia
	Myasthenia gravis syndrome
	Peripheral neuropathy
	Choreoathetoid movements
	Cerebellar syndrome
	Dysarthria
	Dysgeusia
	Blurred vision
	Seizures
	Dizziness, vertigo
	Impaired short-term memory and concentration
Gastrointestinal	Anorexia, nausea, vomiting
	Diarrhoea
	Dry mouth, metallic taste
	Weight gain
Renal	Microtubular lesions
	Impairment of renal concentrating capacity
Cardiovascular	Low blood pressure
	ECG changes
Endocrine	Myxoedema
	Hyperthyroidism
	Hyperparathyroidism
Other	Polyuria and polydipsia
	Glycosuria
	Hypercalcinuria
	Rashes

haloperidol may be related to this. Ibuprofen, indomethacin, mefenamic acid, diclofenac and piroxicam inhibit lithium excretion, and diuretics cause lithium retention, which may increase serum levels. Patients with cardiac or renal disease, or in other situations that may interfere with the clearance of lithium, will obviously need regular monitoring, and prior to starting therapy it is customary to assess renal and hepatic function. Thyroid function is also checked since hypothyroidism, sometimes associated with goitre or even advanced myxoedema, has been observed. Lithium therapy may decrease thyroxine and T_3 and increase TSH levels, which may lead to abnormalities of thyroid-function tests even in the absence of clinical signs of hypothyroidism. If lithium-maintenance therapy is essential then supplementary thyroxine treatment will be required if the patient develops myxoedema.

Although a teratogenic effect of lithium in humans has not been demonstrated, there are reports of a high incidence of congenital malformations in babies born to mothers who take lithium, and it should probably be discontinued if possible during pregnancy.

One of the commonest side effects relates to altered renal function, with polyuria and polydipsia. Urinary-concentrating ability is impaired, which may be exacerbated by combination with neuroleptics. The polyuria may result in compensatory increases in antidiuretic hormone secretion, although occasionally a picture of nephrogenic diabetes insipidus is seen. In spite of these findings, long-term follow-up does not suggest that serious renal damage occurs with prolonged therapy.

Severe intoxication may lead to an organic brain syndrome with hyperactive reflexes, seizures and tremor. On occasion, unilateral neurological abnormalities have been reported, which may be interpreted as an alternative neurological diagnosis. If toxicity results in coma, dialysis should be considered, especially if clearance is in any way delayed. On stopping the drug, the serum concentration usually falls by about half each day, and after routine therapy withdrawal symptoms including irritability and emotional lability have been described (King and Hullin, 1983). For reasons that are not clear, lithium is the only medication that appears to have a distinct anti-suicide effect. This was noted by Baldessarini in a large meta-analysis (22 studies, 6000 patients) and has now been confirmed in several studies, one involving a large California health-maintenance organization (HMO) (21 000 patients). In the HMO study, bipolar patients on valproic acid had a suicide rate three times higher than those taking lithium.

ANTICONVULSANTS

These compounds are also referred to as antiepileptic drugs, although there is no evidence that they affect the underlying processes of epilepsy. They are antiseizure agents, but have a much broader clinical spectrum, and some are used widely in neuropsychiatry beyond epilepsy, particularly for mood stabilization in bipolar patients. Some of the anticonvulsant drugs presently in use are shown in Table 12.13. The older barbiturate-related compounds and phenytoin have been largely replaced by drugs such as carbamazepine and sodium valproate, and newer agents which include gabapentin, lamotrigine, levetiracetam, oxcarbazepine, pregabalin, tiagabine, topiramate, vigabatrin and zonisamide.

As a generalization, the four main modes of action are by blockade of voltage-dependent sodium channels, antagonism of excitatory aminoacid receptors, potentiation of GABA transmission and blockade of calcium channels (see Table 12.14). New findings with gabapentin and pregabalin are that these agents inhibit the action of the alpha-2-delta component of the calcium channel and that levetiracetam binds to a synaptic vesicle protein, SV2A. These new findings may lead to the development of different antiseizure agents.

Phenytoin is highly plasma-bound and cleared from the plasma by hepatic metabolism. Varying serum levels may be noted amongst different patients on the same dose, and small increments in prescription can lead to rapidly escalating serum levels on account of its zero-order pharmacokinetics (Figure 12.1). In spite of its long use, its mechanism of action is still unclear, although there are suggestions that it may interact with sodium or calcium channels in excitable neurones, thus limiting the potential for high-frequency neuronal discharges. It is a membrane stabilizer and also possesses some benzodiazepine binding, and thus has some influence at the GABA receptor, particularly at higher concentrations.

Primidone is partially converted to phenobarbitone, although the primidone component itself probably exerts independent anticonvulsant activity. Phenobarbitone also influences the transcellular transport of sodium, calcium and potassium ions and influences the neurotransmitter release of GABA, glutamate

Table 12.13 Some anticonvulsant drugs in current use

Name	Half-life (hours)	Recommended serum level (mmol l^{-1})	Indications
Carbamazepine	8–45	16–50[*]	Generalized seizures: simple or complex partial seizures; secondary generalized seizures
Clobazam	22	–	As for carbamazepine
Clonazepam	20–40	–	Myoclonic epilepsy
Ethosuximide	30–100	300–700	Generalized absence seizures
Phenobarbitone	36	6–180[*]	Generalized or simple partial seizures
Phenytoin	22	40–80[*]	Generalized seizures: simple or complex partial seizures
Primidone	3–12	–	Generalized: complex or simple partial seizures
Sodium valproate	10–15	–	Generalized absence seizures: myoclonic epilepsy; simple or complex partial seizures
Newer Agents			
Gabapentin	5–7	–	Intractable, partial and generalized seizures
Lamotrigine	22–36	–	Intractable, partial and generalized seizures
Levetiracetam	6–9	–	Intractable partial aand generalised seizures
Oxcarbazepine	8–15	–	Adjunctive therapy for partial seizures
Pregabalin	5–6	–	Intractible partial and generalised seizures
Tiagabin	4–13	–	Intractible partial and generalised seizures
Topiramate	20–30	–	Intractible partial and generalised seizures
Vigabatrin	5–7	–	Intractable, partial and generalized seizures
Zonisamide	50–70	–	Intractible partial and generalised seizures

[*]Conversion factor for μg/ml: carbamazepine 4.2, phenobarbitone 4.3, phenytoin 4.0.

Table 12.14 The principal modes of action of anticonvulsant drugs (adapted from Perucca, 2002)

	Blockade of voltage dependent sodium channels	Antagonism of excitatory aminoacid receptors	Potentiation of GABA transmission	Blockade of calcium channels (channel type)
Older AEDs				
Benzodiazepines	–	–	+	–
Carbamazepine	+	–	–	–(L)
Ethosuximide	–	–	–	+(T)
Phenobarbital	–	–	+	–
Phenytoin	+	–	–	?
Valproic acid	+	–	+	+(T)
Newer AEDs				
Felbamate	+	+	+	+
Gabapentin/Pregabalin	+(?)	–	+(gbp)	+
Lamotrigine	+	–	–	+(L,N,P)
Levetiracetam	–	–	–	+(N)
Oxcarbazepine	+	–	–	+(L)
Tiagabine	–	–	+	–
Topiramate	+	+	+	+(L)
Vigabatrin	–	–	+	–
Zonisamide	+	–	–	+

gbp = gabapentin.

and aspartate. Further, it enhances GABA postsynaptic inhibition, interacting at the benzodiazepine–GABA receptor.

Carbamazepine is structurally related to the tricyclic antidepressants, and has a mode of action different from phenytoin and phenobarbitone. This drug also acts at the sodium channel, but in addition its biochemical actions include partial agonism of adenosine receptors; it acutely increases the firing of the locus coeruleus and decreases CSF somatostatin and HVA accumulation after probenacid (Post and Uhde, 1986; Post et al., 1986). Further, in animal models, carbamazepine is shown to be relatively more effective than other anticonvulsants in inhibiting the seizures developed from amygdala kindling, suggesting some limbic-system selectivity for the drug (Albright and Burnham, 1980). Sodium valproate is a GABA agonist in some animal models, but clinically this is not thought important, and the mechanism of its antiseizure action is unknown at the present time. It also reduces sodium and potassium conductance, reducing the excitability of nerve membranes. The role of benzodiazepines in the management of epilepsy has been largely restricted to acute use in status epilepticus (e.g. midalozam). However, clonazepam, clobazam and nitrazepam have been used for oral therapy. Clonazepam finds more use in childhood, but is markedly sedative in contrast to clobazam, a nonsedative 1,5-benzodiazepine. Clobazam has effective antiepileptic properties in a subgroup of patients who are nonresponsive to other drugs, and is used as adjunctive therapy. Gabapentin probably acts at extrasynaptic GABA receptors.

Gabapentin and pregabalin have a novel mechanism of action, not influencing directly postsynaptic GABA receptors, and binding to the alpha-2-delta subunit of the calcium channel. This leads to a decrease in the release of monoamines and glutamate. Lamotrigine was originally developed as a folate antagonist, but is now thought to act by reducing the release of excitatory amino acids from presynaptic terminals. Oxcarbazepine is structurally related to carbamazepine; it is a 10-keto analogue, possessing an extra oxygen atom on the dibenzazepine ring. This reduces the liver-enzyme induction, and decreases the risk of some side effects, including the agranulocytosis that is occasionally associated with carbamazepine. Vigabatrin was the first important designer drug for epilepsy, being developed as a suicide inhibitor of GABA transaminase, the main enzyme that metabolizes GABA in neurones and glial cells. It reliably increases GABA in the CSF and CNS, an effect detected by MRS (Preece et al., 1994). It was later shown to lead to irreversible partial loss of vision (scotoma) in about 30% of patients, an effect of GABA on the retina, which has markedly restricted its use. Despite this concern, it is currently being investigated as an anti-craving drug for cocaine users. Drugs such as tiagabine, topiramate and zonisamide have several mechanisms of action that may be relevant to their antiseizure effects.

All of the newer drugs are advocated for use in intractable epilepsy, usually as add-on therapy, although several are licensed for use in monotherapy, their availability depending on the country of use.

The side effects of anticonvulsants are many; they are given often for many years and in combination with other anticonvulsants. Table 12.15 sets out the neuropsychiatric side effects, attributed to the older generation of drugs, although many are still in use in various countries. These include an encephalopathy and deterioration of intellectual function, as well as apathy, depression, dysphoria, irritability and occasionally hyperactivity, which are particularly seen in association with the barbituates and polytherapy. Chronic dyskinesias are occasionally seen, while an acute dystonic reaction has been noted with carbamazepine. Sodium valproate has been associated with liver failure in a small number of young patients, and also produces a reversible alopecia and weight gain. Carbamazepine may be associated with water intoxication and hyponatraemia, although the mechanism of this is not clear. This is in contrast to the polyuria provoked by lithium, and emphasizes the different pharmacological profiles of lithium and carbamazepine, even though both have mood-stabilizing effects.

The profile of the side effects with the newer drugs is given in Table 12.16. Some exacerbate or even initiate generalized (especially myoclonic)

Table 12.15   Chronic toxic effects of some anticonvulsant drugs (reproduced from Reynolds, 1975)

Nervous system	Cerebellar atrophy (?)
	Peripheral neuropathy
	Encephalopathy
	Other mental symptoms,
	depression, agitation,
	psychoses
Haemopoietic	Folic acid deficiency
system	Coagulation defects
	Agranulocytosis
	Aplastic anaemia
Skeletal system	Metabolic bone disease
	Vitamin D deficiency
Connective tissue	Gum hypertrophy
	Facial skin changes
	Wound healing
	Dupytren's contracture
Skin	Hirsutism
	Pigmentation
	Hair loss
	Acne
Liver	Enzyme induction; failure
Endocrine system	Pituitary–adrenal
	Thyroid–parathyroid
	Hyperglycaemia
	(diabetogenic)
Other metabolic	Vitamin B_6 deficiency(?)
disorders	
Immunological	Lymphotoxicity
disorders	Lymphadenopathy
	Systemic lupus
	erythematosus
	Antinuclear antibodies
	Immunoglobulin changes(?)
	Immunosuppression

seizures (vigabatrin, lamotrigine). Behavioural problems have limited the use of some, in particular the exacerbation or precipitation of aggression, depression and psychoses. Such adverse reactions may be linked with the phenomenon referred to as 'Forced Normalization' (see Chapter 10). They may occur with all of the drugs, but are particularly prominent with GABAergic agents such as vigabatrin, topiramate, gabapentin and tiagabine, and attempted or completed suicide has been reported. The link between anticonvulsant drugs and suicide has been of such concern that in the USA the FDA has instructed all companies marketing these drugs to include a warning about suicide in their data and information sheets. Of particular concern has been the use of some of these compounds 'off label' in patients with mood disorders.

Topiramate has been associated with cognitive blunting, and particularly with a reversible aphasia-like syndrome, presenting with word-finding difficulties.

Interactions between anticonvulsants and other drugs, or between different anticonvulsants, may present problems in management. Of particular importance are the drugs that elevate phenytoin levels and might lead to phenytoin toxicity (see Table 12.17), and interactions with psychotropic drugs (Tables 12.3 and 12.4). There is some evidence that patients on phenytoin, because of induced hepatic enzymes, will have lower serum levels of antidepressants, and that thus prescription of the usual dose may be subtherapeutic. Serum levels of neuroleptics may likewise be significantly lower in patients treated with anticonvulsants than in controls. Carbamazepine intoxication can also be caused by cimetidine, dextropopoxyphene, erythromycin and verapamil, and SSRIs. Of the new drugs, only lamotrigine has significant interactions. Its metabolism is inhibited by sodium valproate, so when it is given with that drug, the dose of lamotrigine that is needed is much lower. Some of the hepatic enzyme inducers, such as carbamazepine, oxcarbazepine and topiramate, will lower serum oestrogen levels, and contraceptive protection may be lost unless high-dose oestrogen pills are prescribed.

It is generally accepted that in epilepsy, newly diagnosed patients should be treated by the prescription of only one anticonvulsant drug if possible. Upwards of 80% of new patients with appropriate serum-level monitoring and adequate serum levels will be satisfactorily controlled on monotherapy. It is not clear that addition of a second drug will lead to better management of seizures in those who continue to have attacks, with exceptions. Recent research has suggested that patients who have further seizures are likely to do so within a year of presentation with the first attack, and it is thus to some extent predictable who is likely to suffer from chronic uncontrolled seizures. It is such patients who are liable to receive polytherapy, and, in the long term, to suffer neuropsychiatric

Table 12.16 Summary of the main side effects of the newer generation of anticonvulsant drugs (adapted from Perruca, 2002)

Felbamate	Gabapentin+	Lamotrigine	Levetiracetam	Oxcarbazepine	Tiagabine	Topiramate	Vigabatrin	Zonisamide
Nausea	Dizziness	Dizziness	Dizziness	Fatigue	Dizziness	Dizziness	Visual field constriction (30%)***	Fatigue
Vomiting	Fatigue	Blurred vision	Fatigue	Headache	Fatigue	Somnolence	Somnolence	Somnolence
Headache	Somnolence	Diplopia	Headache	Dizziness	Headache	Mental slowing	Weight gain	Dizziness
Dizziness	Behavioural disorders**	Insomnia	Somnolence	Ataxia	Tremor	Impaired concentration	Fatigue	Ataxia
Insomnia	Ataxia	Somnolence	Nervousness	Sedation	Nervousness	Somnolence	Dizziness	Anorexia
Behavioural disturbances	Tremor	Ataxia	Behavioural disturbances**	Nausea	Impaired concentration	Paresthesiae	Behavioural disturbances	Nausea
Weight loss	Weight gain	Headache		Hyponatraemia	Abdominal pain	Dysnomia/anomia	Depression	Mental slowing
Aplastic anaemia (1:5,000)		Fatigue		Mild skin rashes	Depression	Weight loss	Psychosis	Impaired concentration
Hepatotoxicity (1:26,000)		Nausea		*Serious hypersensitivity reactions*		Anorexia		Agitation
Other serious hypersensitivity reactions		Mild skin rashes				Nausea		Irritability
		*Stevens-Johnson syndrome (1:1,000)**				Ataxia		Confusion
		Other serious hypersensitivity reactions				Fatigue		Dysnomia/anomia
						Nephrolithiasis (1–2%)		Paresthesias
						Metabolic acidosis		Skin rashes
						Depression		Nephrolithiasis (1–2%)

*Higher incidence in children (1,100 to 1,300).

**Especially in patients with learning disability or a history of behavioural disorders.

***Incidence of symptomatic visual field constriction is about 1–3%.

+Similar for pregabalin.

N.B. Suicidality and self-harm have been linked with AED prescriptions (see text).

Table 12.17 Anticonvulsant interactions

(a) Clinically significant interactions with carbamazepine and phenytoin

Drugs which may cause elevation of anticonvulsant levels of carbamazepine or phenytoin	Allopurinol Carbamazepine*† Chloramphenicol Chlorpromazine Cimetidine Co-trimoxole Dextropropoxyphene Diltiazem Disulfiram Erythromycin Imipramine Metronidazole Miconazole Sulphonamides Thioridazine Topiramate Troleandomycin Verapamil Viloxazine
Drugs which have their effect reduced by phenytoin or carbamazepine	Amitriptyline Dexamethasone Diazepam Doxepin Haloperidol Hydrocortisone Oral contraceptives Pethidine Phenobarbitone Primidone Prednisolone Sodium valproate Theophylline Warfarin

(b) Other significant anticonvulsant interactions

Sodium valproate	Levels reduced by carbamazepine and phenytoin Increases free phenytoin levels Increases lamotrigine levels Increases phenobarbitone levels

*Phenytoin levels can be increased or decreased when carbamazepine is added.
†Carbamazepine induces its own metabolism.

complications and become candidates for either surgical resection or treatment with VNS.

A number of new anticonvulsant drugs are in development, which are either structural variables of existing compounds or novel chemicals. The structural variables include (with marketed product in brackets): breviracetam (levetiracetam), which in addition to binding at the SV2A protein interacts with voltage-gated sodium channels; eslicarbazepine, the l-isomer of oxcarbazepine; and fluorofelbamate (felbamate). The new compounds include: lacosamide, an amino acid which enhances the slow inactivation of sodium channels; retiagabine, which acts on voltage-gated K-channels, increasing the M-current and stabilizing resting and subthreshold membrane potentials; and ganaxolone, a neurosteroid.

The question of which anticonvulsant drug to use for which type of seizure is often a matter of clinical choice, but some guidelines are clear. In some instances, for example the use of steroids or ACTH for infantile spasms and the almost exclusive use of ethosuximide for generalized absence seizures, there is high specificity. However, for the majority of seizures, there is more overlap, as noted in Table 12.13. There is some evidence that carbamazepine has superiority over the other drugs for the management of complex partial seizures, but aside from this the choice of prescription relates to side effects and the patient's tolerability. Phenytoin is particularly unsuitable for a number of patients because of its side effects, including cognitive dulling, hirsutes, gum hypertrophy and acne, with coarsening of the facial features. Teratogenic effects also occur with anticonvulsant drugs, and several follow-up pregnancy registers have been set up to examine this. The rate of major malformations is higher in children born to women who were on polytherapy during the pregnancy, and sodium valproate in particular has been associated with major malformations, especially spina bifida. This restricts the use of this drug in women. Another gender-related problem is the polycystic ovary syndrome. Polycystic ovaries (PCO) are diagnosed when more than ten 2–8 mm ovarian cysts are found on abdominal examination. The syndrome is diagnosed when the cysts are associated with hyperandrogenism (hirsuitism, acne and male pattern baldness), along with raised serum androgen.

During pregnancy, serum levels of anticonvulsants may fall, and they thus need to be carefully monitored if control of the epilepsy proves difficult. The best clinical use and the full spectrum of side effects of the new drugs are still being evaluated.

Ever since carbamazepine's introduction for the management of epilepsy it has been reported to have psychotropic properties, and its use as a mood stabilizer in manic–depressive illness has been widely investigated and reviewed (Post and Uhde, 1986). It appears to be as effective as conventional neuroleptics in the acute management of mania, and to be equivalent to lithium in the long-term prophylaxis of bipolar affective disorder. Although some trials have been carried out on patients who are lithium-resistant, neither this nor the presence of EEG abnormalities is related to a beneficial clinical response. Rapid-cycling patients and those with secondary mania may respond well. Some patients respond to a combination of carbamazepine and lithium, but not to either drug alone. Carbamazepine is also used in schizoaffective disorders, in the management of aggression and episodic dyscontrol, and in some schizophrenic patients. Trials in the latter condition are sparse and the indications for its use are not clear.

Other anticonvulsants seem to possess mood-stabilizing properties. However, this is not a class effect, and it has been most revealed through studies in patients with affective disorders with sodium valproate and lamotrigine. The latter drug seems better for type-2 as opposed to type-1 bipolar disorder, especially treating the depressed phase, and because of the problem of rashes with rapid increases of serum levels it is not suitable for acute disorders. A summary of the data on anticonvulsant use in psychiatric conditions is given in Table 12.18.

Dosage of the drugs will vary with each individual, although generally it is wise to start with a small dose and increase gradually until satisfactory serum levels are achieved. Many anticonvulsants can be given on a once-daily or twice-daily regime; some are available as extended-release preparations and compliance may be enhanced by this prescription.

Table 12.18   A summary of the effects of anticonvulsant drugs in psychiatric disorders

	Depression	Mania	Bipolar prophylaxis	Anx'y
Carbamazapine	0	+	+	0
Oxcarbazapine	0	+	0	0
Valproate	0	+	?	0
Lamotrigine	0	0	+	0
Gabapentin	0	−	−	0
Topiramate	0	−	0	0
Tiagabine	0	−	0	0
Pregabalin	0	0	0	+

0 = no evidence of effect.
+ = effect shown.
− = no studies.

DRUGS FOR THE TREATMENT OF DEMENTIA

Many drug therapies have been used for failing brains, but most of those advocated in the past are symptomatic and of little value. Several drugs are reported to improve blood flow or metabolism, although the evidence that they help dementia is minimal. The futility of merely increasing blood flow in Alzheimer's disease or MID has been demonstrated by the PET studies. Cycladenate, isoxsuprine, co-dergocrine mesylate, pentifylline and naftidrofuryl are past examples. Hydergine, an ergot alkaloid, appears to possess mixed dopamine agonist–antagonist properties, and has been reported in several short-term trials (up to 8 mg daily) to improve behaviour, rather than cognition (MacDonald, 1982). Piracetam, thought to enhance acetylcholine release, is another compound for which claims have been made.

Among the most important drugs used in management are the psychotropics. Depression or a depressive component often responds to antidepressants, although choice of drug is difficult. Their anticholinergic properties may increase cognitive problems and lead to urinary retention. Imipramine, starting with as small a dose as 10 mg a day, has been popular; the SSRIs however are also of value. ECT is not contraindicated.

Of the antipsychotics, the atypicals are drugs of choice, but warnings over side effects (especially stroke with typical antipsychotics and olanzapine and risperidone), maximized in the elderly, must be heeded. Benzodiazepines should be used with caution, and certainly no patient should be on more than two at the same time. For nocturnal sedation, the shorter-acting drugs are preferred, while in the daytime, drugs whose pharmacokinetics are minimally influenced by aging and which have minimal effect on cognition are needed. Oxazepam and clobazam are examples. Chlormethiazole can provide a useful alternative to the benzodiazepines, but barbiturates should be avoided.

The demonstration of the significant reduction in the density of muscarinic and nicotinic receptors in the brain of Alzheimer's-disease patients led to the development of receptor agonists. However, since other transmitter systems are involved in the pathology, the acetylcholine abnormalities, while they may link to memory changes, do not necessarily reflect on the other behavioural changes so characteristic of dementia. Further, as Kopelman (1985) has shown, even the memory deficits are more pervasive than those provoked by artificial disruption of acetylcholine activity.

Treatments have either been with choline precursors such as choline, deanol or lecithin, or with anticholinesterases. The main drugs available are tacrine, donazepil, rivastigmine and galantamine. Rivastigmine and galantamine (extended release) are given once daily, but there is no evidence that either is more potent than the other. Both are available as a transdermal preparations. It is inadvisable to use more than one of these drugs at a time. Side effects include nausea and vomiting, anorexia, tremor, weight loss and fatigue. The gastrointestinal effects can be minimized by taking the prescription with food.

Memantine is a partial NMDA antagonist. It may be better tolerated than the anticholinesterases, and can be combined with them. Other therapeutic strategies sometimes employed include giving L-dopa and a decarboxylase inhibitor (sinemet, madopar) to help motor impairments.

Problems inhibiting trials of such treatments were until recently lack of any *in vivo* diagnostic technique for the vast majority of people with dementia, and the inclusion into trials of such

heterogenous pathological subtypes. Further complicating the area is the lack of a reliable biomarker that predicts disease progression. Also, the assessment techniques are variable, but a standard assessment scale in clinical trials is the ADAS-Cog (0–70, a higher score implying greater impairment). None of the drugs recommended in Alzheimer's disease are licensed for the other dementias, although they may bring benefit, and trials are underway. Anticholinesterase inhibitors may however make the symptoms of fronto-temporal dementia worse.

Future strategies are concentrating more on amyloid-related changes, and ways to deal with either its accumulation or its resorption. Therapies in development include those evolved from a better understanding of the cascade of molecular events underlying amyloid deposition, and concepts derived from the developing genetics of the disorder. Strategies include inhibition of beta- and gamma-secretases, amyloid-lowering agents (tarenflurbil) and decreasing the production or deposition of β amyloid. Immune therapies are being investigated; these target β amyloid, and include immunization with synthetic β amyloid or monoclonal antibody infusion. Targeting tau is another potential strategy. Varenicline is an antismoking drug which targets nicotinic anticholinergic receptors, and is one of a group of new nicotinic receptor compounds which are being tried in the dementias.

MEDICATIONS FOR THE ADDICTIONS

Researchers have made good progress over the past decade in developing several medications useful in the treatment and management of the addictions. These can be divided into medications useful in detoxification, and those designed to block craving and prevent relapse.

Each of the substances of abuse has its own characteristic withdrawal pattern, and the drugs used in managing withdrawal are substance-dependent. For example, opiate withdrawal is typically managed by replacing the short-acting opiate with slower-acting agents such as methadone. More recently, clinicians have used buprenorphine. For many years alcohol withdrawal was accomplished by administering benzodiazapines, particularly to block alcohol-withdrawal seizures. However, some worried that it made little clinical sense to replace an addictive compound (alcohol) with a medication that might itself be addictive. More recent studies have now shown that alcohol withdrawal can be treated with nonbenzodiazapine GABAergic compounds such as carbamazepine, valproic acid and other nonaddicting medications such as beta-blockers. Cocaine withdrawal is managed with amantadine, bromocriptine or clonidine.

Classically, alcohol-relapse prevention has been accomplished with self-help groups combined with disulfiram, which interacts with alcohol to create nausea and flushing. There is now intense interest in developing specific anticraving medications for alcoholism. These include acamprosate, naltrexone, buproprion and verenacline. These agents may also be of value for various other addictions. Pharmacological agents such as GABA agents (topiramate, tiagabine, baclofen and vigabatrin) and agonist-replacement agents (modafinil, disulfiram, methylphenidate) seem to be the most promising in treatment of cocaine dependence. Trials of antipsychotics are largely negative. Preliminary results of human studies with an anticocaine vaccine, N-acetylcysteine, and ondansetron are promising, as are several compounds in pre-clinical development. While opioid dependence has more treatment agents available than other abused drugs, none are curative. They can, however, markedly diminish withdrawal symptoms and craving, and block opioid effects due to lapses. The most effective withdrawal method is substituting and then tapering methadone or buprenorphine. Alpha-2 adrenergic agents such as clonidine can ameliorate untreated symptoms or substitute for agonists if not available. Shortening withdrawal by precipitating it with narcotic antagonists has been studied, but the methods are plagued by safety issues and persisting symptoms. Neither the withdrawal agents nor the other methods are associated with better long-term outcome, which appears mostly related to post-detoxification treatment. Excluding those with short-term habits, the best outcome occurs with long-term maintenance on

methadone or buprenorphine accompanied by appropriate psychosocial interventions. Those with strong external motivation may do well on the antagonist naltrexone. Currently, optimum duration of maintenance on either is unclear.

BRAIN-STIMULATION THERAPIES

The device-based treatments involving brain stimulation have certain advantages over classical oral medications. Because the devices deliver focal electricity to specific brain regions, there are less or no systemic side effects, and there is less worry about drug–drug interactions.

Convulsive Therapy

Although the original observations of von Meduna led to the introduction of convulsive therapy with camphor, electroconvulsive therapy (ECT) was introduced by Cerletti and Bini for the treatment of schizophrenia. However, it was clear that it gave better results in depressive illness, the main indication of its use today. Although it was eclipsed by the successful introduction of antidepressants in the 1960s, more recently there has been an upsurge of interest. This has stemmed partly from the realization that antidepressant drugs may be ineffective in severe affective disorder, and further from the troublesome side effects of psychotropic drugs that can be seen with long-term treatment – sometimes required in psychotic patients – for example the extrapyramidal complications of neuroleptic drugs. Its current place in therapy has been extensively reviewed (Fink, 1986; Malitz and Sackheim, 1986; Coffey, 1993). The conclusions of an NIH consensus-development conference stated: 'ECT is demonstrably effective for a narrow range of severe psychiatric disorders in a limited number of diagnostic categories; delusional and severe endogenous depression and manic and certain schizophrenic syndromes' (Consensus Development Conference Statement, 1986).

Fink (1986) refers to the changes in behaviour that occur consequent on ECT, dividing them into those which are seizure-dependent and those which are subject-dependent.

The seizure-dependent effects are a direct result of the seizure or the seizure-induction method and include neurophysiological and hormonal consequences, the majority of which are usually transient, returning to pretreatment levels within days or a few weeks of the seizures. The subject-dependent effects are related to the state of the patient at the time of administration of the seizure, one of the most persistently observed consequences being elevation of mood in severely depressed patients, an effect particularly noted in patients who are suicidal or psychotic.

Stimulus parameters have received considerable attention, as has the issue of unilateral or bilateral electrode placement. Waveforms, either sine waves or brief pulse stimuli (short current bursts with lower energy content), have been compared, as have different stimulus intensities. At present there is no evidence of a difference in therapeutic outcome between high- and low-energy stimuli, although the latter provoke less acute cognitive and electrophysiological abnormalities (Weiner, 1986). Caffeine is proconvulsant, and increases seizure duration.

The issue of whether unilateral ECT is as effective as bilateral ECT has been the subject of considerable investigation. Memory disruption is considerably greater with bilateral electrode placement, as are other side effects such as postseizure confusion and headache. Unilateral nondominant-hemisphere seizure discharge seems to be associated with less intracerebral current and less postictal suppression of the contralateral hemisphere, and with treatment about six times higher than seizure threshold is roughly equivalent to bilateral ECT.

Although its use has been established for many years, several double-blind controlled trials of ECT have been carried out (see Crow and Johnstone, 1986). The majority of these have been in affective disorder, and demonstrate a significant benefit for ECT. A consistent predictor of response has been the presence of delusions, although clinically 'endogenicity' has been a valuable guide.

Generally, while the prognosis seems unrelated to the pretreatment DST status, normalization of an abnormal DST suggests a good clinical outcome and failure to normalize should be cause for concern. Prolactin has been shown to rise following the seizure (Trimble, 1978), elevations being greater for bilateral as opposed to unilateral electrode placement. Abrahams and Schwartz (1985) have reported an inverse relationship between the prolactin release at 15 minutes of the first four treatments and clinical outcome. Those with good response showed lower peak prolactin elevations than poor responders.

Trials against simulated ECT have also been reported for schizophrenia (Taylor and Fleminger, 1980), demonstrating the benefit of the seizure, and successful use of nondominant-hemisphere unilateral ECT in manic episodes has been shown (Small *et al.*, 1986). Other situations where ECT has occasionally been helpful have been in the management of Parkinson's disease, organic mental disorders (particularly associated with severe affective disorder), delirium and epilepsia partialis continua (where it is used in order to bring the seizure to an end).

The mechanism of action of ECT is not known. Changes of brain function evolve over time, reflected in the usual clinical practice of administering therapy two or three times a week. The antidepressant effect was initially thought to be directly related to the seizure activity (Ottosson, 1960), cumulative seizure duration being an important variable. Maletsky (1978) estimated that if total seizure time was less than 201 seconds, no response was noted; most patients respond after 1000 seconds, with little additional improvement beyond this being noted. However, seizures for ECT, while necessary, are not sufficient. For example, Sackeim and colleagues have shown in several studies that generalized seizures triggered by electrodes over the parietal lobe are ineffective, as are some inadequate doses of prefrontal treatment. Clearly the therapeutic effects of ECT must involve an interplay between local charge density in certain prefrontal regions and the results of the actual seizure. This line of reasoning then directly intersects with the other brain-stimulation techniques that are influencing brain activity in these same regions.

ECT has an anticonvulsant effect, greater with bilateral as opposed to unilateral treatment. With the former, this averages 87% during a course of treatment, but it does not seem to be persistent over long periods of time after the end of ECT (Nobler and Sackheim, 1993).

In animal models a consistent effect is down-regulation of presynaptic 5-HT$_{1A}$, alpha-2 and beta-adrenergic receptor sites, and enhanced behavioural responses to 5-HT, possibly related to increased numbers of 5-HT$_2$ receptors, have been noted. Dopamine-related behaviours are also shown to be enhanced by repeated seizures (Green, 1986). Other reported changes include increased release of GABA and increased GABA$_b$ binding, increased opioid binding and increased limbic neuropeptide-Y and TRH levels (Mikkelsen *et al.*, 1994; Nutt and Glue, 1993). Both the GABA and the opiate changes may explain the inherent anticonvulsant properties of ECT. While some of the effects, especially on the adrenergic receptors, which may reflect on increased synaptic noradrenergic activity, are similar to the effects of other antidepressants, the effects of ECT at the 5-HT$_2$ receptor are the opposite.

In man, Slade and Checkley (1980) examined growth-hormone responses to clonidine and methylamphetamine in patients with affective disorder before and after a course of ECT. No significant changes were noted. The effects of ECT on neuroendocrine responses to apomorphine have also been reported but are variable.

ECT increases CSF 5-HIAA and HVA (Rudorfer *et al.*, 1988), and enhances the prolactin response to fenfluramine, suggesting increased 5-HT activity (Shapira *et al.*, 1992).

The effects of ECT on CBF using SPECT and PET show consistent increases immediately, with postictal hypoperfusion. The latter is not evenly distributed over the cortex, and is related to the site of electrode placement. Further, it persists after a full course of treatment, and the degree of acute reduction, especially in frontal cortex, predicts response, nonresponders showing no CBF decline (Rubin *et al.*, 1994).

Contraindications to the use of ECT are few, but include the presence of intracranial tumours and a recent cerebrovascular accident. Since an increase in CSF pressure occurs during the seizure discharge, ECT is best avoided in conditions where raised intracranial pressure is suspected. It carries with it minimal risk of mortality, and the morbidity is more related to complications of the accompanying anaesthetic than to the therapy itself.

Two recent developments with ECT deserve note. Sackeim and colleagues have begun using ultrabrief pulse ECT, where the pulse width approaches the minimum necessary to cause depolarization. Importantly, right unilateral ultrabrief ECT appears as effective as bilateral regular-pulse ECT, without any of the associated cognitive side effects (Sackeim *et al.*, 2008).

The other trend with ECT has been in studying the relapse rates following a course of treatment and which maintenance medications work best. Most studies find a 50% relapse rate at six months, even with aggressive maintenance-medication treatment (Petrides *et al.*, 2001).

Transcranial Magnetic Stimulation (TMS)

This is perhaps the most interesting of the new brain-stimulation techniques, because the skull does not need to be opened in order to stimulate the brain, and to date there appear to be only limited side effects (George, 2002; George and Belmaker, 2000; George *et al.*, 2002). TMS involves creating a powerful electrical current near the scalp. The electricity flowing in an electromagnetic coil resting on the scalp creates an extremely potent (near 1.5 Tesla) but brief (microseconds) magnetic field. Although skin and bone act as resistors to impede electrical currents, magnetic fields pass unimpeded through the skull and soft tissue. The importance of this is that the TMS magnetic field enters the surface of the brain without interference. There it encounters nerve cells with resting potentials, and induces electrical currents to flow. Thus, electrical energy is converted to magnetic fields, which are then converted back into electrical currents in the brain (Bohning, 2000). TMS is thus sometimes called 'electrodeless electrical stimulation'.

The magnetic field acts to bridge the skull. Although magnetic fields do have biological effects on tissue, the vast majority of TMS effects likely derive not from the magnetic fields but rather from the induced electrical currents generated in the brain. TMS, with powerful but extremely brief magnetic fields, differs from wearing (or sleeping on) constant low-field magnets. TMS directly electrically stimulates the brain, while constant weak magnets do not induce currents.

The idea of using TMS, or something akin to it, to alter neural function goes back to at least the early 1900s. Pollacsek and Beer, psychiatrists working in Vienna at the same time as Freud, filed a patent to treat depression and neuroses with an electromagnetic device that looks surprisingly like modern TMS (Beer, 1902). The modern TMS era began in 1985 when Barker and colleagues, working in Sheffield, UK, created a focal electromagnetic device with sufficient power to induce currents in the spine (Barker *et al.*, 1985, 1987). They quickly realized that their device could also directly and non-invasively stimulate the human brain. It could only stimulate the surface of the brain, however, as the magnetic field falls off sharply with distance from the coil. Several researchers are working on more powerful TMS devices that might stimulate deeper.

A single pulse of TMS, applied over the motor cortex, produces a jerk-like movement in the hand, arm, face or leg, depending on where the coil is positioned. A single pulse applied over the back of the brain can produce a phosphene. However, that is about the extent of the immediate positive effect that single-pulse TMS can produce. TMS pulses applied in rhythmic succession are referred to as repetitive TMS or rTMS. rTMS can create behaviours not seen with single pulses, including the potential risk of causing an unintended seizure. Twenty seizures have occurred in the history of its use, twelve unintended, out of an unclear total amount of use. All seizures have occurred during stimulation, rather than later, and have been self-limited, with no sequelae. rTMS seizures are more likely to occur with certain combinations of TMS intensity, frequency, duration and interstimulus interval (Wassermann, 1997; Wassermann *et al.*, 1996).

Much research is underway to determine exactly which neurone TMS effects, and the cascade of neurobiological events that follows stimulation. Different factors such as gyral anatomy (how the brain is shaped), the distance from the skull to the brain (brain atrophy) and the orientation of nerve fibres relative to coil are all important.

One of the more interesting rTMS effects is that for brief periods of time, during stimulation, rTMS can block or inhibit a brain function. That is, rTMS over the motor area that controls speech can temporarily render the subject speechless (motor aphasia), only while the device is firing. Cognitive neuroscientists have used this knockout aspect or 'temporary lesioning' ability of rTMS to re-explore and test the large body of information gleaned from years of studying stroke patients. Additionally, two pulses of TMS in quick succession can provide information about the underlying excitability of a region of cortex. This diagnostic technique, called paired-pulse TMS, can demonstrate the behaviour of local interneurons in the motor cortex and serve as an indirect measure of GABA or glutamate activity.

Single nerve cells form themselves into functioning circuits over time through repeated discharges. Externally stimulating a single nerve cell with low-frequency electrical stimulation can cause long-term depression, where the efficiency of links between cells diminishes. High-frequency stimulation over time can cause the opposite effect, called long-term potentiation. These behaviours are thought to be involved in learning, memory and dynamic brain changes associated with networks. A very exciting aspect of TMS research, and of the other brain-stimulation techniques, is the examination of whether or not one can use external brain stimulation to change brain circuits over time in a manner analogous to long-term depression or long-term potentiation. Although this is still controversial and not fully resolved, there are a number of rTMS studies showing inhibition or excitation lasting for up to several hours beyond the time of stimulation. The clinical implications here are profound: one could begin to use TMS or other techniques to change learning and memory, or resculpt brain circuits. Some basic physiological studies indicate that one can best change a circuit while the behaviour is ongoing, and the cells involved in the various neural pathways are acting as a circuit (Barnes *et al.*, 1994; Bartsch and van Hemmen, 2001; Stanton and Sejnowsky, 1989). It is an important question whether rTMS should be delivered while patients are thinking about important topics or abreacting (Amat *et al.*, 2008). Thus, in the near future one might combine rTMS with modified forms of talking or cognitive behavioural therapy.

Animal and cellular studies with TMS reinforce that it is a powerful technique able to alter neuronal function. One stumbling block in using TMS in animals is that it is hard to make TMS coils that are the same size relative to humans. Small coils simply explode. Thus, most animal TMS studies have not really used focal TMS as in humans, especially small-animal studies. Nevertheless, studies have shown that rTMS enhances apomorphine-induced stereotypy and reduces immobility in the Porsolt swim test (Fleischmann *et al.*, 1996), and induces electroconvulsive shock (ECS)-like changes in rodent-brain monoamines, beta-adrenergic receptor binding and immediate early gene induction (Ben-Sachar *et al.*, 1997). Most recently, researchers have found that rTMS can induce neurogenesis (Jennum and Klitgaard, 1996).

A critically important area that will ultimately guide clinical parameters is to combine TMS with functional imaging to directly monitor TMS effects on the brain, and to thus understand the varying effects of different TMS use parameters on brain function. Since it appears that rTMS at different frequencies has divergent effects on brain activity, combining TMS with functional brain imaging will better delineate not only the behavioural neuropsychology of various psychiatric syndromes, but also some of the pathophysiologic circuits in the brain. In contrast to imaging studies with ECT, which have found that ECT decreased global and regional activity (Nobler *et al.*, 2001), most studies using serial scans in depressed patients undergoing rTMS have found increased activity in the cingulate and other limbic regions (Shajahan *et al.*,

2002; Teneback *et al.*, 1999). However, two studies have now found divergent effects of rTMS on regional activity in depressed patients, determined both by the frequency of stimulation and the baseline state of the patient (Mitchel, 2002; Speer *et al.*, 2000). That is, in patients with global or focal hypometabolism, high-frequency prefrontal stimulation increases brain activity over time. Patients with focal hyperactivity have been shown to have reduced activity over time following chronic daily low-frequency stimulation. Although these two small sample studies have numerous flaws, they simultaneously show the potential, and the complexity, surrounding the issue of how to use rTMS to change activity in defined circuits. They also point out an obvious difference with ECT, where the net effect of the ECT seizure is to decrease prefrontal and global activity (Nobler *et al.*, 2001).

Therapeutic Uses of rTMS

Although there is controversy, and much more work is needed, certain brain regions have consistently been implicated in the pathogenesis of depression and mood regulation (see Chapter 8). These include the medial and dorsolateral prefrontal cortex, the cingulate gyrus, and other regions commonly referred to as limbic (amygdala, hippocampus, parahippocampus, septum, hypothalamus, limbic thalamus, insula) and related cortex (anterior temporal pole, orbitofrontal cortex). A widely-held theory over the last decade has been that depression results from a dysregulation of these prefrontal cortical and limbic regions (see Chapter 8) (George *et al.*, 1994a, 1995a; Mayberg *et al.*, 1999). The very first uses of rTMS as an antidepressant were not influenced by this regional neuroanatomic literature, and stimulation was applied over the vertex (Beer) (Kolbinger *et al.*, 1995; Grisaru *et al.*, 1994). However, working within the prefrontal cortical limbic dysregulation theory outlined above, and realizing that theories of ECT action emphasize the role of prefrontal cortex effects (Nobler *et al.*, 2000), in 1995 George and Post performed the first open trial of prefrontal rTMS as an antidepressant, followed immediately by a crossover double-blind study.

Their reasoning was that chronic, frequent, sub-convulsive stimulation of the prefrontal cortex over several weeks might initiate a therapeutic cascade of events both in the prefrontal cortex and in connected limbic regions, thereby causing the dysregulated circuits to rebalance and normalize, alleviating depression symptoms (George and Wassermann, 1994). The imaging evidence previously discussed now shows that this hypothesis was largely correct: prefrontal rTMS sends direct neural information to important mood-regulating cerebral regions such as the cingulate gyrus, orbitofrontal cortex, insula and hippocampus. Thus, beginning with these prefrontal studies, modern TMS was specifically designed as a focal, nonconvulsive, circuit-based approach to therapy.

Since the initial studies, there has been continued high interest in rTMS as an antidepressant treatment. There are now over 30 published randomized controlled clinical trials (RCTs) in depression, and 5 independent meta-analyses of the published or public rTMS antidepressant literature, each differing in the publications included and the statistics used (Burt *et al.*, 2002; Holtzheimer *et al.*, 2001; Kozel and George, 2002; Martin *et al.*, 2002; McNamara *et al.*, 2001). These largely conclude that daily prefrontal TMS delivered over several weeks has antidepressant effects greater than sham treatment. Several studies have compared rTMS to ECT, without finding differences in efficacy in small sample studies. rTMS was clearly better tolerated than ECT, with no cognitive side effects and no need for repeated general anaesthesia. In a similar but slightly modified design, Pridmore (2000) reported a study comparing the antidepressant effects of standard ECT (three times a week) versus one ECT a week followed by rTMS on the other four weekdays. At three weeks he found that both regimens produced similar antidepressant effects. An Israeli group recently published that relapse rates in the six months following ECT versus rTMS were similar (Dannon *et al.*, 2002). In sum, these studies suggest that rTMS clinical antidepressant effects are in the range of other antidepressants, and persist as long as the clinical effects following ECT.

A multisite industry-sponsored RCT of 301 patients with major depression, medication-free, has recently been published (O'Reardon *et al.*, 2007). rTMS was delivered five times per week at 10 Hz frequency and 120% of motor threshold, for a period of 4–6 weeks. Active rTMS was significantly superior to sham TMS. rTMS was well tolerated, with a low dropout rate for adverse events (4.5%). The adverse events observed were mild, and limited to transient scalp discomfort or pain. There were no seizures. These data resulted in FDA approval in October 2008 of rTMS as a treatment for depression.

Although the literature suggests that prefrontal rTMS has an antidepressant effect greater than sham, and that the magnitude of this effect is in the range of other antidepressants, many issues are not resolved. Work done to date has shown clear evidence that prefrontal rTMS produces immediate (George *et al.*, 1999; Li *et al.*, 2002; Nahas *et al.*, 2001; Paus *et al.*, 2001; Strafella *et al.*, 2001) and longer-term (Teneback *et al.*, 1999) changes in mood-regulating circuits. Thus, the original hypothesis about its antidepressant mechanism of action is still the most likely explanation. What remains unclear is which specific prefrontal or other brain locations might be best targeted for treating depression, and whether this can be determined with a group algorithm or needs individual imaging guidance. For the most part, the coil has been positioned using the rule-based algorithm to find the prefrontal cortex that was used in the early studies (George *et al.*, 1995b). However, this method was shown to be imprecise in the particular prefrontal regions stimulated directly underneath the coil, depending largely on the subject's head size (Herwig *et al.*, 2001). Additionally, most studies have stimulated with the intensity needed to cause movement in the thumb (called the motor threshold). There is now increasing recognition that higher intensities of stimulation are needed to reach the prefrontal cortex, especially in elderly patients, where prefrontal atrophy may outpace that of motor cortex, the site at which the motor threshold is measured (Kozel *et al.*, 2000; McConnell *et al.*, 2001; Mosimann *et al.*, 2002; Padberg *et al.*, 2002). There is only limited data on using rTMS as a maintenance treatment in depression.

rTMS as a Treatment for Other Psychiatric Conditions

rTMS has also been investigated as a possible treatment for a variety of neuropsychiatric disorders. In general, the published literature in these conditions is much less extensive than for rTMS as an antidepressant, and therefore conclusions about the clinical significance of effects must remain tentative until large-sample studies are conducted. Hoffman and colleagues have used repeated daily session of low-frequency rTMS over the temporal lobes to treat hallucinations in patients with schizophrenia (Hoffman et al., 1998). Some but not all groups have replicated these effects (d'Alfonso et al., 2002; Fitzgerald et al., 2006; Hoffman et al., 1998, 2000; Jin et al., 2006; Rollnik et al., 2000).

Several studies have shown promise in using rTMS to treat OCD. In the initial study in the field, Greenberg et al. (1997) found that a single session of right-prefrontal rTMS decreased compulsive urges for eight hours. Mood was also transiently improved, but there was no effect on anxiety or obsessions. Two other studies have examined possible therapeutic effects of rTMS in OCD. A double-blind study using right-prefrontal slow (1 Hz) rTMS and a less-focal coil failed to find statistically significant effects greater than sham (Alonso et al., 2001). In contrast, a recent open study in a group of 12 OCD patients, refractory to standard treatments, who were randomly assigned to right- or left-prefrontal fast rTMS, found that clinically-significant and sustained improvement was observed in one-third of patients (Sachdev et al., 2001). Finally a recent group stimulated the supplemental motor area (SMA) and found clinical improvements in OCD and Gilles de la Tourette's syndrome (Mantovani et al., 2006).

Mood-regulating circuits in the brain highly overlap with the neural pathways involved in pain regulation, especially the regions involved in determining the subjective discomfort of the pain. Thus, some researchers have begun exploring whether rTMS might have a therapeutic

role in treating acute or chronic pain. There are reports that rTMS over either prefrontal cortex or motor cortex can acutely decrease pain in healthy adults or patients with chronic pain (Lefaucheur et al., 2001; Pridmore and Oberoi, 2000). A recent RCT found that a single 20-minute session of left-prefrontal rTMS given to patients in the recovery room following surgery reduced self-administered morphine use by 40% (Borckardt et al., 2006).

Overall, rTMS is a promising new therapy, as well as research tool. The bulk of clinical work to date has been in depression, where it is now FDA-approved, but research shows that it has potential applications in several other psychiatric disorders.

Vagus-nerve Stimulation (VNS)

TMS is non-invasive, focal and largely limited to different cortical sites, and is given intermittently. VNS is in some sense the opposite of this as it is invasive, requiring surgical implantation of a device in the chest wall and a wire in the neck. The brain region stimulated is always the same initial route: the vagus nerve in the neck. It is also a permanent implant in that it cannot easily be implanted and then removed without surgery. VNS has been approved for almost 15 years as a treatment for epilepsy (Ben-Menachem et al., 1994; George et al., 1994b; Salinsky et al., 1996; Uthman et al., 1993; Vagus Nerve Stimulation Study Group, 1995) and is also approved for the chronic treatment of recurrent treatment-resistant depression.

The vagus nerve helps regulate the body's autonomic functions, which are important in a variety of emotional tasks. For reasons that are unclear, most people are more familiar with the vagus nerve's efferent functions, where it serves as the messenger for signals from the brain to the viscera. Traditionally, the vagus nerve has been considered a parasympathetic efferent nerve (controlling and regulating autonomic functions such as heart rate and gastric tone). The afferent role of the vagus has been underemphasized in the traditional literature. The vagus is actually a mixed nerve, composed of about 80% afferent sensory fibres carrying information to the brain from the head, neck, thorax and abdomen (Foley and Dubois, 1937).

Over the past 100 years several different researchers have convincingly demonstrated the extensive projections of the vagus nerve via its sensory afferent connections in the nucleus tractus solitarius (NTS) to diverse brain regions (Ammons and Blair, 1983; Bailey and Bremer, 1938; Otterson, 1981; Rutecki, 1990; Zardetto-Smith and Gray, 1990). Reasoning in part from this body of literature, Zabara demonstrated an anticonvulsant action of VNS on experimental seizures in dogs (Zabara, 1992). Zabara hypothesized that VNS could prevent or control the motor and autonomic components of epilepsy. Penry and others ushered in the modern clinical application of VNS in 1988, using an implanted device to treat epilepsy (Penry and Dean, 1990; Uthman et al., 1993).

Although the route of entry into the brain is constrained, VNS offers the potential for modulating and modifying function in many brain regions, through trans-synaptic connections (Henry, 2002; George et al., 2000; Nemeroff et al., 2006). Briefly, incoming sensory (afferent) connections of the vagus nerve provide direct projections to many of the brain regions implicated in neuropsychiatric disorders. These connections provide a basis for understanding how VNS might be a portal to the brainstem and connected limbic and cortical regions. These pathways likely account for the neuropsychiatric effects of VNS, and they invite additional theoretical considerations for potential research and clinical applications. Functional imaging studies in patients with implanted VNS stimulators have largely confirmed this important neuroanatomy of the vagus (Bohning et al., 2001; Chae et al., 2003; Conway et al., 2006; Henry et al., 1998, 1999; Lomarev et al., 2002; Mu et al., 2004).

VNS Methods

VNS has been commercially available for the treatment of resistant partial-onset seizures in Europe since 1994, and in the USA since 1997. The surgery for implanting the VNS generator in the chest is much like inserting a cardiac pacemaker. In both VNS and cardiac pacemakers, a subcutaneous generator sends an electrical signal to an organ through an implanted electrode. With VNS, the electrical stimulation is delivered through the generator, an implantable, multiprogrammable, bipolar pulse generator (about the size of a pocket watch) that is implanted in the left chest wall to deliver electrical signals to the left vagus nerve through a bipolar lead. The electrode is wrapped around the vagus nerve in the neck, and is connected to the generator subcutaneously. The VNS generator can be controlled by a personal computer or PDA connected to an infrared wand. As a safety feature, the generator is designed to shut off in the presence of a constant magnetic field. Each patient is thus given a magnet that, when held over the pulse generator, turns off stimulation. When the magnet is removed, normal programmed stimulation resumes. This allows patients to control and temporarily eliminate stimulation-related side effects during key behaviours like public speaking (voice tremor) or heavy exercising (mild shortness of breath).

Therapeutic Uses of VNS

VNS has been most extensively studied as a treatment for epilepsy. Two double-blind studies have been conducted in patients with epilepsy, with a total of 313 treatment-resistant completers (Ben-Menachem et al., 1994; Handforth et al., 1998). In this difficult-to-treat group, the average decline in seizure frequency was about 25–30% compared to baseline. Interestingly, the longer the treatment was applied, the better the clinical response rates.

Most epilepsy patients with VNS have not been able to reduce or withdraw antiepileptic medications. Thus VNS, as now delivered, has not been shown to be a substitute for anticonvulsant medications, although in some patients the dosage levels or numbers of anti-epileptic medications have been decreased with the addition of VNS. VNS is increasingly being used in children with epilepsy, in part because of its lack of negative cognitive effects, which are common to other anticonvulsants (Helmers et al., 2001).

There are several different programmable variables in determining how to deliver VNS.

These 'use parameters' include the pulse width of the electrical signal (130, 250, 500, 750, 1000 μs), the intensity (0.25–4 mA is clinically tolerated), the frequency of stimulation (1–145 Hz), the length of stimulation (7–270 seconds) and the length of time between trains of stimuli (0.2 seconds to 180 minutes). In general, the initial epilepsy studies used settings that derived from the animal studies where anticonvulsant effects were found. These studies compared efficacy in two groups, based on different use parameters. There was a high-stimulation group (30 Hz, 30 seconds on, 5 minutes off, 500 μs pulse width) and a low-stimulation group (1 Hz, 30 seconds on, 90–180 minutes off, 130 μs pulse width). The majority of the VNS epilepsy efficacy and safety data come from trials with use parameters similar to those used in the high-stimulation group. Similarly, most of the data from other neuropsychiatric disorders (depression, anxiety) involve VNS at use parameters similar to those used in the initial epilepsy studies. It is difficult to imagine that these use parameters are the maximally effective choices, or that the same parameters work equally well in all conditions and all patients. Epilepsy physicians commonly switch nonresponding patients to use-parameter settings that are different from their current settings. However, there has been no clear demonstration that changing settings improves efficacy. Further work toward understanding the translational neurobiology of these use-parameter choices, and how they relate to clinical symptoms, is the key area for future growth of the field.

There is a long history in biological psychiatry where anticonvulsant medications (e.g. carbamazepine) or devices (e.g. ECT), have been found to have mood-stabilizing or antidepressant effects. In early 1998, there were several lines of evidence to suggest that VNS might have antidepressant effects. Anecdotal reports of mood improvement in VNS-implanted epilepsy patients, knowledge of vagus function and neuroanatomy, brain-imaging studies, work in animals and CSF studies all supported an initial pilot clinical trial in treatment-resistant depression (George *et al.*, 2000).

In June 1998, the first depression patient was implanted at MUSC in Charleston, launching an open study of VNS for the treatment of chronic or recurrent treatment-resistant depression (called D-01). This study involved four sites (MUSC, Charleston; Columbia PI, NY; UTSW, Dallas; Baylor, Houston) and initially involved 30 subjects (Rush *et al.*, 2000), with a later extension of 30 more subjects to clarify the effect size and look for response predictors (Sackeim *et al.*, 2001b). The study design involved selecting patients with treatment-resistant, chronic or recurrent major depressive episodes (MDEs) (unipolar or nonrapid cycling bipolar) and then adding VNS to a stable regimen of antidepressant medications or no antidepressant medications. No stimulation was given for the first two weeks following implantation, creating a single-blind placebo phase and allowing for surgical recovery. All patients met eligibility criteria by failing at least two adequate treatment trials in the current episode.

Ten weeks of VNS therapy were provided, with medications held constant. Of 59 completers (1 patient improved during the recovery period), the response rates were 30.5% for the primary Hamilton Rating Scale for Depression (HRSD$_{28}$) measure, 34.0% for the Montgomery–Äsberg Depression Rating Scale (MADRAS) and 37.3% for the Clinical Global Impression-Improvement score (CGI-I of 1 or 2). VNS was well tolerated in this group, with side effects similar to those encountered by epilepsy patients. The most common side effect was voice alteration or hoarseness (60.0%, 36/60), which was generally mild and related to the intensity of the output current. There were no adverse cognitive effects (Sackeim *et al.*, 2001a).

The only response predictor was prior treatment-resistance. VNS as used in this open study was more effective in depressed patients who were less treatment-resistant.

These encouraging initial results served as the basis for a US multisite double-blind trial of VNS for chronic or recurrent, low-to-moderate treatment-resistant depression. In this trial, active VNS failed to show a statistically significant difference in acute response from the sham group (Rush *et al.*, 2005). The sham response rate was 10%, with the active response 15%.

The longer-term response rates for VNS-implanted depression patients are encouraging (Nahas *et al.*, 2005) and appear better than would be expected in this population (Rush *et al.*, 2006). A parallel but nonrandomized comparison found that patients with VNS implanted had better outcomes at one year than a group receiving treatment as usual (George *et al.*, 2005). These data served as the basis for FDA approval of VNS for the chronic (not acute) treatment of chronic recurrent depression. Thus, VNS is FDA approved, although there is no double-blind evidence for VNS as an antidepressant in patients with depression. There are however open (Harden *et al.*, 2000) and double-blind (Elger *et al.*, 2000) studies showing that VNS has antidepressant effects in epilepsy patients with comorbid depression.

In conclusion, VNS has an important role in the treatment of epilepsy. However, the only clinical effects that have been shown with double-blind studies are in epilepsy for seizure control and depression occurring in the setting of epilepsy. There are many areas where more information would facilitate its adoption. Compared to psychotherapy, medications and even ECT, VNS requires a different approach to treating depression. Whereas other treatments can be begun and sampled and then easily abandoned if not effective, VNS, with the installation of an implant, requires careful consideration prior to initiating therapy. Currently there is no non-invasive method of VNS that could be tried prior to a permanent implant. Thus, it is crucial to determine from available data who will likely respond (or not). Additionally, because of the relatively large initial capital cost of implanting a VNS generator, data are needed to convince payers that VNS is cost-effective. An initial implantation fee of around US$20 000 (device and surgery) is about equal to one week of hospitalization, or a course of outpatient ECT. VNS would thus be cost-effective in those recurrent chronically-ill patients where implantation results in clinical improvements that eliminate the need for hospitalization, ECT or

more frequent and aggressive outpatient medication management. Another radical difference between VNS and medication treatments is that VNS facilitates almost 100% adherence. The device, once implanted, cycles on and off without problems for several years. Many studies have shown that even the best patients skip and forget medications, with resultant problems in their clinical course. VNS is thus a most interesting new approach to treating depression, but more information is critically needed.

Resective or Ablative Brain Surgery (Psychosurgery)

The early experiments of Fulton and Jacobsen (1935) demonstrated that primates with destruction of the frontal lobes became more placid and less anxious. Moniz (1936) became the first to sever connections between the frontal lobes and other areas of the limbic system in psychiatric patients, which led Freeman and Watts (1947) to develop a standardized leucotomy technique.

The early operations were radical frontal leucotomies in which a large section of white matter was severed between the frontal lobes and the rest of the brain, but since that time the operation has been remarkably refined. Restricted frontal leucotomy was followed by orbital undercutting in which only the medially-situated frontothalamic fibres were destroyed. Other selective lesions include cingulectomy, in which the anterior 4 cm of the cingulum is removed, and subcaudate tractotomy, in which lesions are placed beneath the head of the caudate nucleus. Stereotactic techniques have been used to place lesions with greater accuracy, and during some surgical procedures stimulation is carried out. This provokes subjective experiences in patients, but is also used to evaluate autonomic changes such as alteration of heart rate, blood pressure and forearm blood flow in order to locate sites for surgical destruction. In one procedure, multifocal leucocoagulation, patients have lesions made through chronically-implanted electrodes after various intervals of time, and the change in symptoms is continuously observed. When clinical status improves, further lesions are withheld. In cingulotomy, lesions are placed bilaterally in the cingulum bundle, and capsulotomy targets the anterior limb of the internal capsule. A stereotactic gamma unit in which radioactive cobalt rays are directed at a selected target using the gamma knife, can be used for the latter operation, which avoids the necessity of a craniotomy (Mindus and Nyman, 1991).

The main frontolimbic connections that are severed pass from the lower medial quadrant of the frontal lobe to the septal and nucleus accumbens regions, thalamus and hypothalamus. Additional target areas are the frontocingular connections passing to the cingulate gyrus and hippocampus. The subcaudate pathway interrupts frontal and temporal connections, in addition to the ascending monamine projections from the ventral tegmental area to the frontal cortex.

In capsulotomy, fibres between the frontal cortex and the limbic system and basal ganglia are lesioned.

Although the very early techniques had a mortality of around 6% and a high morbidity, the modified and restricted operations can be carried out safely. Mitchell-Heggs *et al.* (1976) presented data on 66 patients who had a limbic leucotomy; 73% were improved at 6 weeks and 76% at 16 months. The best results were in obsessional neurosis, anxiety and depression, although six of seven schizophrenic patients also responded, particularly if the schizophrenic symptoms were accompanied by anxiety, depression or obsessional states. In this follow-up, no intellectual deterioration was noted, and adverse personality changes were reported as minimal. Clinical improvements occurred gradually, for up to a period of a year. Patients with good premorbid personalities did better than those with poor preoperative adjustment. Patients with obsessional illness seemed to do particularly well with stereotactic limbic leucotomy.

Bridges *et al.* (1994) have reported on the results of a large series of patients after subcaudate tractotomy, with 40–60% of patients going on to live normal or near-normal lives. There was a 1% postoperative suicide rate, compared with 15% in cases of affective-disorder controls. Similarly, the follow-up data with capsulotomy (Mindus and Nyman, 1991) reveal 70% symptom-free or 'much improved' at 1–7 years of follow-up.

Postoperatively, marked frontal-lobe oedema can be seen on the MRI scan and a characteristic frontal slow-wave activity is seen on the EEG. The amount of this shortly after the operation correlates with a beneficial clinical outcome one year later (Evans *et al.*, 1981).

The indications for brain surgery for psychaitric disorders have been clarified. Patients should have had a severe psychiatric illness, be potentially suicidal and have been ill for an average of 10 years. Further, they must have been shown to have failed to respond to all alternative forms of therapy, including a good trial with available psychotropic medications. The best responses are seen in patients suffering from depression and obsessional neurosis, with good premorbid personalities, and from a stable home environment. Some schizophrenic patients do well, showing a reduction in the number of their psychotic episodes and a reduced need for phenothiazine medication. Psychopathy is an absolute contraindication, and patients who are addicted to drugs or alcohol are not suitable. Complications include cerebral haemorrhage, postoperative suicide, postoperative seizures, personality changes, urinary and faecal incontinence, increased weight, sleep disturbance and diabetes insipidus.

Other neurosurgical procedures used to ameliorate psychopathology include unilateral or bilateral amygdalotomy in patients with aggression, especially lesions of the medial amygdala in the relief of aggressive behaviour disturbances associated with epilepsy (Narabayashi, 1971). Thalamotomy has been used for obsessional illness, while placing lesions in the hypothalamus and stria terminalis has been tried for aggression.

Deep-brain Stimulation (DBS)

Instead of permanently resecting or lesioning an area of the brain, one can stimulate the region electrically with an electrode and temporarily 'knock out' its function. Because of its more favourable safety profile compared to resective surgery, and the potential for withdrawing the stimulator if the effects are not satisfactory, DBS has replaced resective brain surgery for OCD or depression. Typically the DBS electrodes are small wires with exposed terminals at the very end of the wire. These contacts are placed neurosurgically with MRI and CT image guidance. Once the wires are in place the electrodes are connected to external generators implanted under the skin in the chest. For the treatment of Parkinson's disease and dystonia, the DBS electrodes are implanted in the suthalamic nucleus (STN) or the globus pallidus interna (Gpi). The electricity is delivered at high frequency (>100 Hz) constantly. The anti-tremor effects are immediate in PD, while the anti-dystonia effects take weeks or months to emerge, even with constant high-frequency stimulation.

DBS has been studied for both OCD and depression. The evidence base for DBS in OCD is slightly greater than that for depression, but for both conditions the number of published cases is less than 100. For OCD, researchers have followed the neurosurgical literature and have implanted the electrodes in the anterior limb of the internal capsule, which then approaches the nucleus accumbens. The FDA refers to this electrode placement as the ALICNA; depending on which of the four electrode positions one uses, the same electrode can interfere with different brain regions. ALICNA implantation of refractory OCD has been granted a humanitarian device exemption by the US FDA. In the early OCD studies of the ALICNA location, researchers were struck by the antidepressant effects, and some have used this electrode location for treatment-resistant depression. Another location for depression involves implanting in the white-matter fibres immediately lateral to the subgenual cingulate. Further research is needed for these invasive and risky procedures, which are not yet clinical treatments.

SLEEP-DEPRIVATION THERAPY

It has been observed for some time that if a patient with a depressive illness is kept awake for the whole night, elevation of mood occurs. This is often only transient, although there are anecdotal reports of some patients having a sustained benefit. The technique can be used to help with diagnosis, the alteration of mood confirming the presence of an affective disorder.

Wu *et al.* (1992) reported that over 50% of patients with an affective disorder will show a response to deprivation, and in bipolar patients transient hypomania can be seen in up to 30%. They postulated that in sleep, an endogenous substance is released that causes depression, in contrast to an alternative theory that an endogenous antidepressant substance is released in wakefulness. In other studies it has been shown using PET that increased cingulate activity before deprivation predicts the antidepressant response (Ebert *et al.*, 1994).

13

Epilogue: Progress toward a Neuroanatomically, Biological-psychiatrically Informed Classification Scheme in Psychiatry

It is over 20 years since the first edition of *Biological Psychiatry* was published in 1987. The second edition followed in 1996. In the decade that has passed since there have been substantial developments in the field, which the authors of this edition believe justified the present endeavour to update knowledge. It is however worth taking a glimpse back in time to see just what has happened since the first edition, and to make some comments on the prides and pitfalls that have come to pass.

One of the most important advances has been the development of brain-imaging technologies. These were still in relative infancy at the time of writing the first edition, but as outlined in Chapter 4, the power of PET and MRI in various formats has transformed research and theoretical approaches to biological psychiatry. The first two editions contained much information on monoaminergic and other transmitter function, revealed by chemical challenge tests and blood measurements of hormones, CSF studies and a deal of neuropathology, with an emphasis on the findings from neurochemistry. Many of these data have been omitted from this current text, summaries of the results being given,

and the fuller complement of references can be found in earlier editions. This is not to criticize these research endeavours. Psychiatrists with an interest in biological psychiatry used the best techniques available to test their hypotheses, and the quite diverse methods nevertheless allow certain outcomes to form a continuing basis on which to build further hypotheses. In addition, they led to a refinement of therapies, especially in neuropsychopharmacology.

The field of genetics had progressed by the second edition, but was yielding few results not predicted from the earlier edition. This third edition finds much more space devoted to genetics and brain imaging, and the section on neuroanatomy has re-emphasized the importance of understanding advances in those fields to the overall enterprise of uniting brain and behaviour, in sickness and in health. The preface to the first edition noted 'one challenge for biological psychiatry is to unite information we now have regarding functional changes in the brain in psychopathology with that which we now know about brain–behaviour relationships and brain structure' (p. xi). It seems that the challenge can now be met, and the

Biological Psychiatry 3e   Michael R. Trimble and Mark S. George
© 2010 John Wiley & Sons, Ltd

following conclusions are put forward, not only to stimulate discussion and debate, but in a sincere attempt to raise important issues, some of which open up vistas of opportunity for future progress.

The first edition was bound into DSM III; by the second it was DSM IV; now we have DSM IV-TR. It may come as some surprise, but of the 176 diagnostic criteria sets that appear in both DSM IV and ICD 10, only one, namely transient tic disorder, has identical DSM IV and ICD 10 definitions. Throughout the text we have made some comments about the failure of such committee-driven manuals as the DSM or the ICD system to provide an adequate method with which to understand psychopathology, and we believe that it is now the time, with the imminent threat of DSM V and ICD 11, to move classification away from the sociological to the biological; from the phenotype to the endophenotype; from the epigenetic to the genetic; and underlying all of these, from the phenomenological to the anatomical. Hints at the possible structure of such a classification scheme have emerged throughout this book, and to a large extent have been made possible by the power of the new developments in neuroscience that have unveiled intimate knowledge of cerebral anatomy. As discussed in Chapter 2, a fuller understanding of the neuroanatomy of the limbic forebrain has exposed some of the difficulties of the older conceptions of the limbic system. This allows us, along with data culled from the new brain-imaging techniques discussed in Chapter 4, to progress towards a classification of psychopathology founded in neuroanatomy.

Attempts in this direction are not new. Yakovlev introduced his evolutionary view of the brain, citing three layers or levels of anatomical distinction, an inner core surrounding the central CSF space, an intermediate level and an outer layer. The latter essentially was neocortex, but of interest was his bringing together of the basal ganglia and the limbic structures of the brain within his middle layer. Based on these evolutionary anatomical principles, Cummings has developed clinical counterparts, namely autonomic disorders as a consequence of inner-layer abnormalities, while signature cortical syndromes such as aphasias and apraxias emerge from damage to the outer layer. However, alteration of structure and function of the middle layer results in paradigmatic neuro-psychiatric disorders from Parkinson's disease to schizophrenia, which involve the cortical–subcortical circuits outlined in Chapter 2 and clinically lead to a confluence of motor and psychological symptoms, disorders of motivation being central.

We believe that a similar but more precise anatomical framework can be given this classification. We start out by asking not what is happening in the brain, but *where* in the brain is it happening? An outline of the scheme is given in Table 13.1.

We begin with anatomy. The outline is not to suggest that the related phenotype involves only the anatomical structure in column one, but that this is the *fons et origo* of the disorder and most likely, even with progression of the disorder, to be the site of maximum neuroanatomical and neurophysiological change. It is becoming clear that the unfolding of the cerebral, neuronal and glial structures has a genetic basis, and in the future the second column may be replete with relevant genotypes which underpin the anatomical variants, but at present the cells are largely blank. The major psychopathological categories lend themselves to an influence from one or more of the main neurotransmitters, which drive behaviour and set our emotional tone. The identified ones at present are dopamine, GABA, glutamate, 5-HT, noradrenaline and acetylcholine. As other neuromodulators become identified, the list will probably fractionate, for example with different GABA, cholinergic or 5-HT subtypes, and even new potent chemopathologies, perhaps linked to intracellular dynamics. Again, we do not wish to naively suggest that the neurotransmitter is the cause of the phenotype, only that knowledge to date had pointed in certain directions; but ask not whether transmitter X is abnormal in the brain, we are urging to ask *where*!

We do not wish to imply that we support an old-fashioned modular view of brain function, a return to phrenology, with regards to cognition or disorders. Indeed throughout the

Table 13.1 A Proposed First Pass at a neuroanatomically, biological-psychiatrically informed classification scheme in psychiatry. Note that for all of the major psychiatric disorders, one can begin by understanding the relevant neuroanatomy, and how the disorder is an imbalance of the function or behaviour resulting from that region, falling along a spectrum often from hyperfunction to hypofunction of the behaviour. For example, both the addictions and apathy syndromes flow from a dysfunction of a medial frontal–cingulate–basal ganglia–nucleus accumbens circuit involved in appetitive drives. These behaviours prominently involve dopamine, without clear-cut genetic factors, can sometimes involve structural damage of the circuit, and may or may not be progressive or lateralized. We posit that a nosology that is neuroanatomically based, building out from known brain functions, would refocus our field back on brain systems and would aid in future understanding of the diseases within the field of biological psychiatry

Anatomy	*Genetics*	*Neurotransmitters*	*Structure*	*Progressiveness*	*Laterality*	*Behaviour*
Non-isocortical						
Amyg	5-HT	5-HT/GABA/BDZ	N	N	?	GAD/panic
HC	APO E	ACH	Y	Y	N	Alzheimer's
	N	N	Y	N	Bilat.	Amnestic disorder
HC/ParaHC	Y	DA	Y	Y	L	Psychosis
OF/BG	Y	DA/5-HT	N	N	N	Compulsive and obsessive
MedF/Cing/BG	N	DA	Y	Y or N	?	Hyper/hypomotivation +/− tics
MedF (B 25)	Y	5-HT	N	N	?	Depression
BG	Y	GABA	Y	Y	Bilat.	Huntington's
BG	Y	DA	Y	Y	Bilat.	Parkinson's
Isocortical						
FT	Y	?	Y	Y	R/L	FT dementias
Parietal	N	N	Y	Y/N	R/L	Signature syndromes (aphasia, etc.)

Y, yes; N, no; R, right; L, left; DA, dopamine; BG, basal ganglia; FT, front-temporal; OF, orbitofrontal; ?, uncertain; MedF, mediofrontal; Cing, cingulum; B, Brodmann; Amyg, amygdala; HC, hippocampus; ParaHC, parahippocampal gyrus

book we have espoused a view of circuitry and distributed function. However, we opine that at the outset of any disorder identification of any circuitry involved will likely be unclear, but this will become apparent as the disorder matures, as genetic unfolding of cortical anatomy continues (into late life?), and under environmental impressions.

Whether or not there are structural changes and whether or not they are progressive is vital to understanding prognosis. For years it was suggested that schizophrenia and epilepsy were not progressive disorders, and in some cases this is so. However, these two variables we believe should be part of a multiaxial classification, ending arguments over progression, but perhaps requiring new phenotypic designations.

Finally, in our list of variables we have included laterality. In spite of over 150 years of neuroscience progress since Broca first suggested laterality as being important for the development of psychological syndromes, and Flor-Henry's rejuvenation of the theme in the 1960s, no psychopathological classification scheme includes this, although some isocortical signature syndromes are clearly lateralized. Much imaging research fails to discuss laterality, even when findings are clearly lateralized, and we know that the two hemispheres of the human brain subserve widely divergent functions.

As a clear example, we take OCD. For quite unclear reasons this has been categorized under anxiety disorders, and yet as we show in Chapter 6, this is untenable. In comparison with generalized anxiety disorder and panic disorder, the sex ratio is different, the environmental triggers to symptoms are different, the genetics are different, the neurocognitive profile is different, the somatic/neurological associations are different, and the *anatomy* is different. In contrast to the underling amygdala and hippocampal associations with the other anxiety disorders, OCD primarily reflects frontal–basal ganglia dysfunction. It is a behavioural reflection of a different circuitry. There are obvious subdivisions of this designation, for example with associated tics (now referred to as Gilles de la Tourette's syndrome), or with body image distortions (dysmorphic syndromes).

With regards to current concepts of schizophrenia, it has been clear for decades that a simple phenomenologically-based classification is inadequate for both neuroscientific and clinical understanding. There is considerable evidence that the earliest *anatomical* changes in many people so classified by DSM IV are in the left medial temporal areas, affecting principally hippocampus and surrounding cortical structures. In a majority there is slow progression and then a defect state remains. Secondary changes involve distributed anatomical and functional brain changes, which may be genetically linked, and are contributed to by the neurotransmitter dopamine. The genetics of cerebral development combined with the focus of the initial pathology would explain the unfolding of the clinical syndrome through endophenotype deviance and tertiary cognitive embodiment. This hippocampal–temporal disorder is different from another, which at present is referred to as Alzheimer's dementia, where the pathology is different, the genetics are different, the spread of the anatomy with time is different, the neurocognitive changes are different, and the main neurotransmitter involved is acetylcholine. This pattern of unfolding of the clinical picture is again contrasted with those progressive or halting disorders that primarily involve frontal areas, or parietal cortex. There are syndromes which begin in basal ganglia and then spread to involve cortex, and so the classification can be developed.

We believe that such an approach to classification helps with the issue of spectrums. Thus it is now fashionable to discuss the schizophrenia spectrum or the bipolar spectrum, which embrace both DSM IV axis 1 and axis 2 categories. The spectrum however reflects on the biological variability, which our anatomically-based view provides, temperament to psychosis linking anatomy with progression, as a disorder unfolds in time and neurological space.

We offer this neuroanatomical approach to an understanding of psychopathology as a thoughtful challenge to the next committees who will revise existing manuals. We believe that the days of purely symptom-derived classifications in psychiatry are numbered, and go further to imply that, up to now, they have inhibited so much intelligent thought and research funding, and ossified our urge for an understanding of the brain in psychopathology in favour of the simple flexibility of check-list diagnoses. Like an emperor with no clothes, they have no substance (biological validity), but parading nakedly around the fringes of academic circles, seemingly unashamed, they have garnered the multitudes to worship them.

References

Abdulla, Y.H. and Hamadah, K. (1970) 3,5 cyclic adenosine monophosphate in depression and mania, *Lancet*, **i**, 378–81.

Abi-Dargham, A. and Guillin, O. (2007) Preface, *International Review of Neurobiology*, **78**, xiii–xvi.

Abrahams, R. and Schwartz, C.M. (1985) ECT and prolactin release: relation to treatment response in melancholia, *Convulsive Therapy*, **1**, 38–42.

Abrams, R. and Taylor, M.A. (1979) Differential EEG patterns in affective disorder and schizophrenia, *Archives of General Psychiatry*, **36**, 1355–8.

Adamec, R.E. (1989) Kindling, anxiety and personality. In T.E. Bolwig and M.R. Trimble (eds.), *The Clinical Relevance of Kindling*, Wiley, Chichester, pp. 117–35.

Adamec, R.E. and Stark-Adamec, C. (1983) Limbic kindling and animal behaviour, *Biological Psychiatry*, **18**, 269–93.

Adams, F. (1939) *The Genuine Works of Hippocrates*, Williams and Wilkins, Baltimore.

Adams, R.D., Fisher, C.M., Hakim, S. *et al.* (1965) Symptomatic occult hydrocephalus with normal CSF pressure. A treatable syndrome, *New England Journal of Medicine*, **243**, 117–26.

Addington, J., Cadenhead, K.S., Cannon, T.D. *et al.* (2007) North American prodrome longitudinal study: a collaborative multisite approach to prodromal schizophrenia research, *Schizophrenia Bulletin*, **33**, 665–72.

Adolfsson, R., Gottfries, C.-G., Oreland, L. *et al.* (1978) Monoamine oxidase activity and serotonergic turnover in human brain, *Progress in Neuropsychopharmacology*, **2**, 225–30.

Adolfsson, R., Gottfries, C.-G., Roos, B.E. *et al.* (1979) Changes in brain catecholamines in patients with dementia of the Alzheimer type, *British Journal of Psychiatry*, **135**, 216–23.

Akiskal, H.S. (2007) The emergence of the bipolar spectrum: validation along clinical-epidemiologic and familial-genetic lines, *Psychopharmacology Bulletin*, **40**, 99–115.

Akiskal, H.S. and Benazzi, F. (2006) The DSM-IV and ICD-10 categories of recurrent (major) depressive and bipolar II disorders: evidence that they lie on a dimensional spectrum, *Journal of Affective Disorders*, **92**, 45–54.

Albert, M.L., Feldman, R.G. and Willis, A.L. (1974) The 'subcortical dementia' of progressive nuclear palsy, *Journal of Neurology, Neurosurgery and Psychiatry*, **37**, 121–30.

Albright, P.S. and Burnham, W.I. (1980) Development of a new pharmacological seizure model: effects of anticonvulsants on cortical and amygdala-kindled seizures in the rat, *Epilepsia*, **21**, 681–9.

Aldencamp, A.P. (2004) Antiepileptic drug treatment and epileptic seizures: effects on cognitive function. In M.R. Trimble and B. Schmitz (eds.), *The Neuropsychiatry of Epilepsy*, Cambridge University Press, Cambridge, pp. 256–265.

Aleman, A., Swart, M. and Van Rijn, S. (2008) Brain imaging, genetics and emotion, *Biological Psychology*, **79**, 58–69.

Alexander, G.E., DeLong, M.R. and Strick, P.L. (1986) Parallel organisation of functionally segregated circuits linking basal ganglia and cortex, *Annual Review of Neuroscience*, **9**, 357–81.

Alexopoulos, G.S., Inturrisi, C.E., Lipman, R. *et al.* (1983) Plasma immunoreactive beta-endorphin levels in depression, *Archives of General Psychiatry*, **40**, 181–3.

Alheid, G.F. and Heimer, L. (1988) New perspectives in basal forebrain organisation of special relevance for neuropsychiatric disorders, *Neuroscience*, **27**, 1–39.

Allen, J.J., McKnight, K.M., Moreno, F.A. *et al.* (2009) Alteration of frontal EEG asymmetry during tryptophan depletion predicts future depression, *Journal of Affective Disorders*, **115**, 189–95.

Alonso, P., Pujol, J., Cardoner, N. *et al.* (2001) Right prefrontal TMS in OCD: a double-blind, placebo-controlled study, *American Journal of Psychiatry*, **158**, 1143–5.

Altemus, M., Piggott, T., Kalogeras, K.T. *et al.* (1992) Abnormalities in the regulation of vasopressin and corticotrophic releasing factor secretion in obsessive–compulsive disorder, *Archives of General Psychiatry*, **49**, 9–20.

Altschuler, L.L., Devinsky, O., Post, R.M. *et al.* (1990) Depression, anxiety and temporal lobe epilepsy, *Archives of Neurology*, **47**, 284–8.

Altschuler, L.L., Conrad, A., Hauser, P. *et al.* (1991) Reduction of temporal lobe volume in bipolar disorder, *Archives of General Psychiatry*, **48**, 482–3.

Altschuler, L.L., Bartzokis, G., Grieder, T. *et al.* (2000) An MRI study of temporal lobe structures in men with bipolar disorder or schizophrenia, *Biological Psychiatry*, **48**, 147–62.

Amaral, D.G., Price, J.L., Pitkanen, A. *et al.* (1992) Anatomical organisation of primate amygdaloid complex. In Aggleton (ed.), *The Amygdala*, Wiley Liss, New York, NY, pp. 1–66.

Amat, J., Paul, E., Watkins, L.R. *et al.* (2008) Activation of the ventral medial prefrontal cortex during an uncontrollable stressor reproduces both the immediate and long-term protective effects of behavioral control, *Neuroscience*, **154**, 1178–86.

Amen, D.G. and Carmichael, B.D. (1997) High-resolution brain spect imaging in ADHD, *Annals of Clinical Psychiatry*, **9**, 81–6.

American Psychiatric Association (1987) *Diagnostic and Statistical Manual of Mental Disorders*, 3rd edition revised, APA, Washington, DC.

American Psychiatric Association (1994) DSM-IV-TR: *Diagnostic and Statistical Manual of Mental Disorders*, APA, Washington, DC.

American Psychiatric Association (2000) DSM-IV-TR: *Diagnostic and Statistical Manual of Mental Disorders*, APA, Washington, DC.

Ammons, W.S. and Blair, R.W.F.R.D. (1983) Vagal afferent inhibition of primate thoracic spinothalamic neurons, *Journal of Neurophysiology*, **50**, 926–40.

Anand, A., Li, Y., Wang, Y. *et al.* (2005a) Activity and connectivity of brain mood regulating circuit in depression: a functional magnetic resonance study, *Biological Psychiatry*, **57**, 1079–88.

Anand, A., Li, Y., Wang, Y. *et al.* (2005b) Antidepressant effect on connectivity of the mood-regulating circuit: an fMRI study, *Neuropsychopharmacology*, **30**, 1334–44.

Anckarsater, H. (2006) Central nervous changes in social dysfunction: autism, aggression, and psychopathy, *Brain Research Bulletin*, **69**, 259–65.

Anden, N.E. (1975) Animal models of brain dopamine function. In W. Birkmayer and O. Hornykiewicz (eds.), *Advances in Parkinsonism*, Roche, Basle, pp. 169–77.

Andermann, E. (1980) Genetic aspects of epilepsy. In P. Robb (ed.), *Epilepsy Updated: Causes and Treatment*, Medical Year Book, Chicago, pp. 11–24.

Andreasen, N.C., Arndt, S., Swayze, V. *et al.* (1994) Thalamic abnormalities in schizophrenia visualized through magnetic resonance image averaging, *Science*, **266**(5183), 294–8.

Andreasson, S., Allebeck, P., Engstrom, A. *et al.* (1987) Cannabis and Schizophrenia: a longitudinal study of Swedish conscripts, *Lancet*, **ii**, 1483–6.

Andre-Obadia, N., Peyron, R., Mertens, P. *et al.* (2006) Transcranial magnetic stimulation for pain control: double-blind study of different frequencies against placebo, and correlation with motor cortex stimulation efficacy, *Clinical Neurophysiology*, **117**, 1536–44.

Angst, J., Felder, W. and Lohmeyer, B. (1979) Schizoaffective disorders: results of a genetic investigation, *Journal of Affective Disorders*, **1**, 139–53.

Annegers, J.F., Hauser, W.A., Coan, S.P. *et al.* (1998) A population based study of seizures after traumatic head injuries, *New England Journal of Medicine*, **338**, 20–24.

Anthony, M.M., Brown, T.A. and Barlow, D.H. (1997) Response to hyperventilation and 5.5% carbon-dioxide inhalation of subjects with types of specific phobia, panic disorder or no mental illness, *American Journal of Psychiatry*, **154**, 1089–95.

Appell, J., Kertesz, A. and Fishman, M. (1982) A study of language functioning in Alzheimer's patients, *Brain and Language*, **17**, 73–91.

Applebaum, J., Bersudsky, Y. and Klein, E. (2007) Rapid tryptophan depletion as a treatment for acute mania: a double-blind, pilot-controlled study, *Bipolar Disorders*, **9**, 884–7.

Arana, G.W. and Baldessarini, R.J. (1985) The dexamethasone suppression test for diagnosis and prognosis in psychiatry, *Archives of General Psychiatry*, **42**, 1193–204.

Arana, G.W., Pearlman, C. and Shader, R.I. (1985) Alprazolam induced mania, *American Journal of Psychiatry*, **142**, 368–3.

Arora, R.C. and Meltzer, H.W. (1989) Serotonergic measures in the brains of suicide victims, *American Journal of Psychiatry*, **146**, 730–6.

Åsberg, M., Träskman, L. and Thoren, P. (1976) 5-HIAA in the CSF: a biochemical suicide predictor, *Archives of General Psychiatry*, **33**, 1193–7.

Ashton, H. (1984) Benzodiazepine withdrawal: an unfinished story, *British Medical Journal*, **288**, 1135–40.

Ayd, F.J. (1974) Side effects of depot fluphenazines, *Comprehensive Psychiatry*, **15**, 277–84.

Aylward, E.H., Roberts-Twiddie, J.V., Barta, P. *et al.* (1994) Basal ganglia volumes and acute white matter hyperintensities in patients with bipolar disorders, *American Journal of Psychiatry*, **151**, 687–94.

Bach, Y., Rita, G., Lion, J.R. *et al.* (1971) Episodic dyscontrol: a study of 130 violent patients, *American Journal of Psychiatry*, **127**, 1473–8.

Bailey, P. and Bremer, F. (1938) A sensory cortical representation of the vagus nerve, *Journal of Neurophysiology*, **1**, 405–12.

Baker, L.A., Jacobson, K.C., Raine, A. *et al.* (2007) Genetic and environmental bases of childhood antisocial behavior: a multi-informant twin study, *Journal of Abnormal Psychology*, **116**, 219–35.

Baker, L.A., Raine, A., Liu, J. *et al.* (2008) Differential genetic and environmental influences on reactive and proactive aggression in children, *Journal of Abnormal Child Psychology*, **36**, 1265–78.

Ballenger, J.C., Goodwin, F.K., Major, L.F. *et al.* (1979) Alcohol and central serotonin metabolism in man, *Archives of General Psychiatry*, **36**, 224–7.

Banasr, M., Chowdhury, G.M., Terwilliger, R. *et al.* (2008) Glial pathology in an animal model of depression: reversal of stress-induced cellular, metabolic and behavioral deficits by the glutamate-modulating drug riluzole, *Molecular Psychiatry* (epub ahead of print, PMID: 18825147).

Bandler, R. and Keay, K.A. (1996) Columnar organization in the midbrain periaqueductal gray and the integration of emotional expression, Department of Anatomy and Histology, Institute for Biomedical Research, The University of Sydney, NSW, Australia, *Progress in Brain Research*, **107**, 285–300.

Banki, C.M., Vojnick, M. and Molnar, G. (1981) CSF biochemical examinations, *Biological Psychiatry*, **18**, 1033–44.

Bannon M.J., Reinhard, J.F., Bunney, E.B. *et al.* (1982) Unique response to antipsychotic drugs is due to absence of terminal autoreceptors in mesocortical dopamine neurones, *Nature*, **296**, 444–6.

Barch, D.M., Berman, M.G., Engle, R. *et al.* (2009a) CNTRICS final task selection: working memory, *Schizophrenia Bulletin*, **35**, 136–52.

Barch, D.M., Braver, T.S., Carter, C.S. *et al.* (2009b) CNTRICS final task selection: executive control, *Schizophrenia Bulletin*, **35**, 115–35.

Bares, M., Brunovsky, M., Kopecek, M. *et al.* (2007) Changes in qEEG prefrontal cordance as a predictor of response to antidepressants in patients with treatment resistant depressive disorder: a pilot study, *Journal of Psychiatric Research*, **41**, 319–25.

Barker, A.T., Freeston, I.L., Jalinous, R. *et al.* (1987) Magnetic stimulation of the human brain and peripheral nervous system: an introduction and the results of an initial clinical evaluation, *Neurosurgery*, **20**, 100–9.

Barker, A.T., Jalinous, R. and Freeston, I.L. (1985) Non-invasive magnetic stimulation of the human motor cortex, *Lancet*, **i**, 1106–7.

Barnes, C.A., Jung, M.W., McNaughton, B.L. *et al.* (1994) LTP saturation and spatial learning disruption: effects of task variables and saturation levels, *Journal of Neuroscience*, **14**, 5793–806.

Baron, M., Levitt, M. and Perlman, R. (1980) Low platelet MAO activity: a possible biochemical correlate of borderline schizophrenia, *Psychiatry Research*, **3**, 329–35.

Baron, M., Levitt, M., Greuen, R. *et al.* (1984) Platelet MAO activity and genetic vulnerability to schizophrenia, *American Journal of Psychiatry*, **141**, 836–42.

Bartsch, A.P. and van Hemmen, J.L. (2001) Combined Hebbian development of geniculocortical and lateral connectivity in a model of primary visual cortex, *Biological Cybernetics*, **84**, 41–55.

Bastini, B., Nash, F. and Meltzer, H.Y. (1990) Prolactin and cortisol responses to MK-212, a serotonin agonist, in obsessive–compulsive disorder, *Archives of General Psychiatry*, **47**, 833–9.

Battaglia, M., Przybeck, T.R., Bellodi, L. *et al.* (1996) Temperament dimensions explain the comorbidity of psychiatric disorders, *Comprehensive Psychiatry*, **37**, 292–8.

Baumgartner, A., Gräf, K.J. and Kurten, I. (1985) The dexamethasone suppression test in depression, in schizophrenia and during experimental stress, *Biological Psychiatry*, **20**, 675–9.

Baxter, L.R., Phelps, M.E., Mazziotta, J.C. *et al.* (1985) Cerebral metabolic rates for glucose in mood disorders, *Archives of General Psychiatry*, **42**, 441–7.

Baxter, L.R., Schwartz, J.M., Mazziotta, J.C. *et al.* (1988) Cerebral glucose metabolic rates in non-depressed patients with obsessive–compulsive disorder, *American Journal of Psychiatry*, **145**, 1560–3.

Baxter, L.R., Jeffrey, M.S., Phelps, M.E. *et al.* (1989) Reduction of prefrontal cortex glucose metabolism common to three types of depression, *Archives of General Psychiatry*, **46**, 243–50.

Baxter, L.R., Schwartz, J.M., Bergman, K.S. *et al.* (1992) Caudate glucose metabolic rate changes with both drug and behaviour therapy for obsessive–compulsive disorder, *Archives of General Psychiatry*, **49**, 681–96.

Beal, M.F., Mazurek, M.F., Ellison, D.W. *et al.* (1988) Somatostatin and its neuropeptide Y concentrations in pathologically graded cases of Huntington's disease, *Annals of Neurology*, **23**, 562–9.

Bear, D. (1986) Hemispheric asymmetries in emotional function: a reflection of lateral specialisation in cortical–limbic connections. In B.K. Doane and K.E. Livingstone (eds.), *The Limbic System: Functional Organization and Clinical Disorders*, Raven Press, New York, NY, pp. 29–42.

Bear, D. and Fedio, P. (1977) Quantitative analysis of interictal behaviour in temporal lobe epilepsy, *Archives of Neurology*, **34**, 454–67.

Beer, B. (1902) Über das Auftreten einer objectiven Lichtempfindung in magnetischen Felde, *Klinische Wochenzeitschrift*, **15**, 108–9.

Beghi, E., Carpio, A., Forsgren, L. *et al.* (2009) Recommendation for a definition of acute symptomatic seizure, *Epilepsia* (epub ahead of print), Mario Negri Institute, Milan, Italy.

Beghi E. and Sander, J.W. (2007) The natural history and prognosis of epilepsy. In J. Engel and T. Pedley (eds.), *Epilepsy: A Comprehensive Textbook*, 2nd edition, Lippincott Williams & Wilkins, New York, NY, pp. 65–70.

Bejjani, B.P., Damier, P., Arnulf, I. *et al.* (1999) Transient acute depression induced by high-frequency deep-brain stimulation [see comments], *New England Journal Of Medicine*, **340**, 1476–80.

Belanoff, J.K., Gross, K., Yager, A. *et al.* (2001) Corticosteroids and cognition, *J Psychiatr Res*, **35**, 127–45.

Ben-Ari, Y. (1981) Transmitters and modulators in the amygdaloid complex: a review. In Y. Ben-Ari (ed.), *The Amygdaloid Complex*, Elsevier, North Holland, pp. 163–74.

Benazzi, F. and Akiskal, H.S. (2008) How best to identify a bipolar-related subtype among major depressive patients without spontaneous hypomania: superiority of age at onset criterion over recurrence and polarity?, *Journal of Affective Disorders*, **107**, 77–88.

Benca, R.M., Obermeyer, W.H., Thisted, R.A. *et al.* (1992) Sleep and psychiatric disorders: a meta-analysis, *Archives of General Psychiatry*, **49**, 651–68.

Bench, C.J., Friston, K.J., Brown, R.G. *et al.* (1993) Regional cerebral blood flow in depression measured by positron emission tomography: the relationship with clinical dimensions, *Psychological Medicine*, **23**, 579–90.

Benedetti, F., Dallaspezia, S., Colombo, C. *et al.* (2008) A length polymorphism in the circadian clock gene Per3 influences age at onset of bipolar disorder, *Neuroscience Letters*, **445**, 184–7.

Benes, F.M. (2007) Searching for unique endophenotypes for schizophrenia and bipolar disorder within neural circuits and their molecular regulatory mechanisms, *Schizophrenia Bulletin*, **33**, 932–6.

Benjamin, J., Osher, Y., Kotler, M. *et al.* (2000) Association of tridimensional personality questionnaire (TPQ), and three functional polymorphisms: dopamine receptor D4 (DRD4), serotonin transporter promotor region (5-HTTLRP) and catechol *O*-methyltransferase (COMT), *Molecular Psychiatry*, **5**, 96–100.

Benkelfat, C., Nordahl, T.E., Semple, W. *et al.* (1990) Local cerebral glucose metabolic rates in OCD, *Archives of General Psychiatry*, **47**, 840–8.

Ben-Menachem, E., Manon-Espaillat, R., Ristanovic, R. *et al.* (1994) Vagus nerve stimulation for treatment of partial seizures: 1. a controlled study of effect on seizures, *Epilepsia*, **35**, 616–26.

Ben-Sachar, D., Belmaker, R.H., Grisaru, N. *et al.* (1997) Transcranial magnetic stimulation induces alterations in brain monoamines, *Journal of Neural Transmission*, **104**, 191–7.

Benson, D.F. (1975) The hydrocephalic dementias. In D.F. Benson and D. Blumer (eds.), *Psychiatric Aspects of Neurolgoic Disease*, Grune and Stratton, New York, NY, pp. 83–97.

Benson, D.F. (1979) *Aphasia, Alexia and Agraphia*, Churchill Livingstone, Edinburgh.

Benton, J.S., Bowen, D.M., Alien, S.J. *et al.* (1982) Alzheimer's disease as a disorder of isodendritic core, *Lancet*, **i**, 456.

Berman, K.F., Doran, A.R., Picker, D. *et al.* (1993) Is the mechanism of prefrontal hypofunction in depression the same as schizophrenia?, *British Journal of Psychiatry*, **162**, 183–92.

Berney, A., Sookman, D., Leyton, M. *et al.* (2006) Lack of effects on core obsessive–compulsive symptoms of tryptophan depletion during symptom provocation in remitted obsessive–compulsive disorder patients, *Biological Psychiatry*, **59**, 853–7.

Bernouilli, C., Siegfried, J., Baumgartner, G. *et al.* (1977) Danger of accidental person-to-person transmission of Creutzfeld–Jakob disease by surgery, *Lancet*, **i**, 478–9.

Berrettini, W.H., Numberger, J.I., Hare, T.A. *et al.* (1983) Reduced plasma and CSF GABA in affective illness: effect of lithium carbonate, *Biological Psychiatry*, **18**, 185–94.

Bertelsen, A., Harvald, B. and Hauge, M. (1977) A Danish twin study of manic depressive disorders, *British Journal of Psychiatry*, **130**, 330–51.

Betts, T.A. (1974) A follow-up study of a cohort of patients with epilepsy admitted to psychiatric care in an English city. In P. Harris and C. Mawdsley (eds.), *Epilepsy: Proceedings of the Hans Berger Centenary Symposium*, Churchill Livingstone, Edinburgh, pp. 326–38.

Bhatia, K.P., Bhatt, M.H. and Marsden, C.D. (1993) The causalgia-dystonia syndrome, *Brain*, **116**, 843–51.

Birkmeyer, W., Jellinger, K. and Riederer, P. (1977) Striatal and extrastriatal dopaminergic functions. In A.R. Cools *et al.* (eds.), *Psychobiology of the Striatum*, Elsevier, North Holland, pp. 141–52.

Biver, F., Goldman, S., Delvenne, V. *et al.* (1994) Frontal and parietal metabolic disturbances in unipolar depression, *Biological Psychiatry*, **36**, 381–8.

Bleuler, E. (1911) *Dementia Praecox or the Group of Schizophrenics* (Translated by J. Zenkin, 1950), New York International University Press.

Bleuler, E. (1924) *Textbook of Psychiatry* (Translated by A.A. Brill, 1924), Dover Publications.

Bleuler, E. (1949) *Lehrbuch der Psychiatrie*, 8th edition, Springer-Verlag, Berlin.

Blumer, D. (2000) Dysphoric disorders and paroxysmal affects: recognition and treatment of epilepsy-related psychiatric disorders, *Harvard Review Psychiatry*, **8**, 8–17.

Blumer, D. (2004) Suicide. In M.R. Trimble and B. Schmitz (eds.), *The Neuropsychiatry of Epilepsy*, Cambridge University Press, Cambridge, pp. 107–116.

Bodner, M., Shafi, M., Zhou, Y.D. *et al.* (2005) Patterned firing of parietal cells in a haptic working memory task, *European Journal of Neuroscience*, **21**, 2538–46.

Bohning, D.E. (2000) Introduction and overview of TMS physics. In M.S. George and R.H. Belmaker (eds.), *Transcranial Magnetic Stimulation in Neuropsychiatry*, American Psychiatric Press, Washington, DC.

Bohning, D.E., Lomarev, M.P., Denslow, S. *et al.* (2001) Feasibility of vagus nerve stimulation-synchronized blood oxygenation level-dependent functional MRI, *Investigative Radiology*, **36**, 470–9.

Bondareff, W., Mountjoy, C.Q. and Roth, M. (1981) Selective loss of neurones of origin of adrenergic projection to cerebral cortex in senile dementia, *Lancet*, **i**, 783–4.

Borckardt, J.J., Weinstein, M., Reeves, S.T. *et al.* (2006) Post-operative left prefrontal repetitive transcranial magnetic stimulation (RTMS) reduces patient-controlled analgesia use, *Anesthesiology*, **105**, 557–562.

Borgwardt, S.J., Dickey, C., Pol, H.H. *et al.* (2009) Workshop on defining the significance of progressive brain change in schizophrenia: December 12, 2008 American College of Neuropsychopharmacology (ACNP) All-Day Satellite, Scottsdale, Arizona, The Rapporteurs' Report, *Schizophrenia Research*.

Bottiglieri, T., Godfrey, P., Flynn, T. *et al.* (1990) CSF S-adenosylmethionine in depression, *Journal of Neurology, Neurosurgery and Psychiatry*, **53**, 1096–8.

Bowen, D.M. and Davison, A. (1986) Biochemical studies of nerve cells and energy metabolism in Alzheimer's disease, *British Medical Bulletin*, **42**, 75–80.

Bowen, D.M., Spillane, J.A., Curzon, G. *et al.* (1979) Accelerated ageing or selective neuronal loss as an important cause of dementia, *Lancet*, **i**, 11–13.

Boylan, L.S., Flint, L.A., Labovitz, D.L. *et al.* (2004) Depression but not seizure frequency predicts quality of life in treatment-resistant epilepsy, *Neurology*, **62**, 258–61.

Braak, H. and Braak, E. (1997) Frequency of stages of alzheimer-related lesions in different age categories, *Neurobiol Aging*, **18**, 351–7.

Braak, E., Braak, H. and Mandelkow, E.M. (1994a) A sequence of cytoskeleton changes related to the formation of neurofibrillary tangles and neuropil threads, *Acta Neuropathol*, **87**, 554–67.

Braak, H., Braak, E., Yilmazer, D. *et al.* (1994b) Amygdala pathology in Parkinson's disease, *Acta Neuropathol*, **88**, 493–500.

Braddock, L. (1986) The dexamethasone suppression test: fact and artefact, *British Journal of Psychiatry*, **148**, 363–74.

Braestrup, C. and Nielsen, M. (1982) Anxiety, *Lancet*, **ii**, 1030–4.

Brambilla, F., Smeraldi, F., Sacchetti, E. *et al.* (1978) Deranged anterior pituitary responsiveness to hypothalamic hormones in depressed patients, *Archives of General Psychiatry*, **35**, 1231–8.

Bredkjaer, S.R., Mortensen, P.B. and Parnas, J. (1998) Epilepsy and non-organic non-affective psychosis: national epidemiologic study, *British Journal of Psychiatry*, **172**, 235–8.

Breggin, P.B. (1964) The psychophysiology of anxiety, *Journal of Nervous and Mental Diseases*, **139**, 558–68.

Breiter, H.C., Weisskoff, R.M., Kennedy, D.N. *et al.* (1997) Acute effects of cocaine on human brain activity and emotion, *Neuron*, **19**, 591–611.

Bremner, J.D., Davis, M., Southwick, S. *et al.* (1993) Neurobiology of PTSD. In J.M. Oldham *et al.* (eds.), *Review of Psychiatry 12*, APA Press, Washington, DC, pp. 183–214.

Bremner, J.D., Randall, P., Scott, T.M. *et al.* (1995) MRI-based measurement of hippocampal volume in patients with combat-related PTSD, *American Journal of Psychiatry*, **152**, 973–81.

Bremner, J.D., Innis, R.B., Salomon, R.M. *et al.* (1997) PET measurement of cerebral metabolic correlates of depressive relapse, *Archives of General Psychiatry*, **54**, 364–74.

Bridges, P.K., Bartlett, J.R., Sepping, P. *et al.* (1976) Precursors and metabolites of 5-HT and dopamine in the ventricular CSF of psychiatric patients, *Psychological Medicine*, **6**, 399–405.

Bridges, P.K., Bartlett, J.R., Hale, A.S. *et al.* (1994) Psychosurgery: stereotactic subcaudate tractotomy, *British Journal of Psychiatry*, **165**, 599–611.

Briley, M.S., Langer, S.Z., Raisman, R. *et al.* (1980) Tritiated imipramine binding sites are decreased in platelets of untreated depressed patients, *Science*, **209**, 303–5.

Broadhurst, P.L. (1975) The Maudsley reactive and non-reactive strain of rats, *Behaviour and Genetics*, **5**, 299–319.

Bromfield, E., Altschuler, L. and Leiderman, D. (1990) Cerebral metabolism and depression in patients with complex partial seizures, *Epilepsia*, **31**, 625.

Brown, S.W. (2004) Dementia and epilepsy. In M.R. Trimble and B. Schmitz (eds.), *The Neuropsychiatry of Epilepsy*, Cambridge University Press, Cambridge, pp. 135–51.

Brown, W.A. and Laughren, T.P. (1981) Tolerance to the prolactin-elevating effect of neuroleptics, *Psychiatry Research*, **5**, 317–22.

Brown, G.L., Ballanger, J.C., Minichello, M.D. *et al.* (1979) Human aggression and its relationship to CSF 5HIAA, 3MHPG and HVA. In M. Sandler (ed.), *Psychopharmacology of Aggression*, Raven Press, New York, NY, pp. 131–48.

Brown, G.L., Ebert, M.H., Goyer, P.F. *et al.* (1982) Aggression, suicide and serotonin: relationship to CSF amine metabolism, *American Journal of Psychiatry*, **139**, 741–6.

Brown, R.G., Marsden, C.D., Quinn, N. *et al.* (1984) Alterations in cognitive performance and affect-arousal state during fluctuations in motor function in Parkinson's disease, *Journal of Neurology, Neurosurgery and Psychiatry*, **47**, 454–65.

Brun, A., Englund, B., Gustafson, L. *et al.* (1994) Clinical and neuropathological criteria for fronto-temporal dementia, *Journal of Neurology, Neurosurgery and Psychiatry*, **57**, 416–18.

Brunner, R., Henze, R., Parzer, P. *et al.* (2009) Reduced prefrontal and orbitofrontal gray matter in female adolescents with borderline personality disorder: is it disorder specific?, *Neuroimage*, **49**(1), 114–20.

Brusov, O.G., Fomenko, A.M. and Katasonov, A.B. (1985) Human plasma inhibitors of platelet serotonin uptake and imipramine receptor binding: extraction and heterogeneity, *Biological Psychiatry*, **20**, 235–44.

Bruton, C.J., Stevens, J.R. and Frith, C. (1994) Epilepsy, psychosis and schizophrenia, *Neurology*, **44**, 34–42.

Buchheim, A., Erk, S., George, C. *et al.* (2008) Neural correlates of attachment trauma in borderline personality disorder: a functional magnetic resonance imaging study, *Psychiatry Research*, **163**, 223–35.

Buchsbaum, M.S., Coursey, R.D. and Murphy, D.L. (1976) The biochemical high risk paradigm: behavioural and familial correlates of low platelet MAO activity, *Science*, **194**, 339–41.

Buchsbaum, M.S., Wu, J., Delisi, L.E. *et al.* (1986) Frontal cortex and basal ganglia metabolic rates assessed by PET with 18F-2-deoxyglucose in affective illness, *Journal of Affective Disorders*, **10**, 139–52.

Buchsbaum, M.S., Christian, B.T., Lehrer, D.S. *et al.* (2006) D2/D3 dopamine receptor binding with [F-18]fallypride in thalamus and cortex of patients with schizophrenia, *Schizophrenia Research*, **85**(1–3), 232–44.

Buckley, M.J., Booth, M.C., Rolls, E.T. *et al.* (2001) Selective perceptual impairments after perirhinal cortex ablation, *Journal of Neuroscience*, **21**, 9824–36.

Burnet, P.W., Sharp, T., Lecorre, S.M. *et al.* (1999) Expression of 5-HT receptors and the 5-HT transporter in rat brain after electroconvulsive shock, *Neuroscience Letter*, **277**, 79–82.

Burnett, G.B., Prange, A.B., Wilson, I.C. *et al.* (1980) Adverse effects of anticholinergic antiparkinsonian drugs in tardive dyskinesia, *Neuropsychobiology*, **6**, 109–20.

Burrows, G.D., Vohra, J., Hunt, D. *et al.* (1976) Cardiac effects of different tricyclic antidepressant drugs, *British Journal of Psychiatry*, **129**, 335–41.

Burt, T., Lisanby, S.H. and Sackeim, H.A. (2002) Neuropsychiatric applications of transcranial magnetic stimulation, *International Journal of Neuropsychopharmacology*, **5**, 73–103.

Bush, G., Luu, P. and Posner, M.I. (2000) Cognitive and emotional influences in anterior cingulate cortex, *Trends in Cognitive Sciences*, **4**, 215–222.

Bush, G., Whalen, P.J., Shin, L.M. *et al.* (2006) The counting Stroop: a cognitive interference task, *Nature Protocols*, **1**(1), 230–3.

Butler, P.W.P. and Besser, G.M. (1968) Pituitary–adrenal function in severe depressive illness, *Lancet*, **i**, 1234–6.

Buzsaki, G. (2006) *Rhythms of the Brain*, Oxford University Press, London.

Byne, W., Kidkardnee, S., Tatusov, A. *et al.* (2006) Schizophrenia-associated reduction of neuronal and oligodendrocyte numbers in the anterior principal thalamic nucleus, *Schizophrenia Research*, **85**(1–3), 245–53.

Byne, W., Hazlett, E.A., Buchsbaum, M.S. *et al.* (2009) The thalamus and schizophrenia: current status of research, *Acta Neuropathologica*, **117**, 347–68.

Caceda, R., Kinkead, B. and Nemeroff, C.B. (2006) Neurotensin: role in psychiatric and neurological diseases, *Peptides*, **27**, 2385–404.

Caceda, R., Kinkead, B. and Nemeroff, C.B. (2007) Involvement of neuropeptide systems in schizophrenia: human studies, *International Review of Neurobiology*, **78**, 327–76.

Caine, E. (1981) Pseudodementia: current concepts and future directions, *Archives of General Psychiatry*, **38**, 1359–64.

Callicott, J.H., Straub, R.E., Pezawas, L. *et al.* (2005) Variation in disc1 affects hippocampal structure and function and increases risk for schizophrenia, *Proceedings of the National Academy of Science U S A*, **102**, 8627–32.

Calloway, S.P., Dolan, R.J., Fonagy, P. *et al.* (1984) Endocrine changes and clinical profiles in depression: the TRH test, *Psychological Medicine*, **14**, 759–65.

Cameron, O.G., Smith, C.B., Hollingsworth, P.J. *et al.* (1984) Plasma alpha-2 adrenergic receptor binding and plasma catecholamines, *Archives of General Psychiatry*, **41**, 1144–8.

Cameron, N.M., Shahrokh, D., del Corpo, A. *et al.* (2008) Epigenetic programming of phenotypic variations in reproductive strategies in the rat through maternal care, *J Neuroendocrinol*, **20**, 795–801.

Canitano, R. (2007) Epilepsy in autism spectrum disorders, *European Child and Adolescent Psychiatry*, **16**, 61–6.

Cannon, W.B. (1927) The James–Lange theory of emotion: a critical examination and an alternative theory, *American Journal of Psychology*, **39**, 106–24.

Cannon, D.M., Ichise, M., Fromm, S.J. *et al.* (2006) Serotonin transporter binding in bipolar disorder assessed using [11c]DASb and positron emission tomography, *Biological Psychiatry*, **60**, 207–17.

Cannon, D.M., Ichise, M., Rollis, D. *et al.* (2007) Elevated serotonin transporter binding in major depressive disorder assessed using positron emission tomography and [11c]DASb: comparison with bipolar disorder, *Biological Psychiatry*, **62**, 870–7.

Capstick, N. and Seldrup, J. (1977) Obsessional states: a study in the relationship between abnormalities occurring at the time of birth and the subsequent development of obsessional symptoms, *Acta Psychiatrica Scandinavica*, **56**, 427–31.

Cardinal, R.N., Daw, N., Robbins, T.W. *et al.* (2002a) Local analysis of behaviour in the adjusting-delay task for assessing choice of delayed reinforcement, *Neural Networks*, **15**, 617–34.

Cardinal, R.N., Parkinson, J.A., Lachenal, G. *et al.* (2002b) Effects of selective excitotoxic lesions of the nucleus accumbens core, anterior cingulate cortex, and central nucleus of the amygdala on autoshaping performance in rats, *Behavioral Neuroscience*, **116**, 553–67.

Cardinal, R.N., Parkinson, J.A., Hall, J. *et al.* (2002c) Emotion and motivation: the role of the amygdala, ventral striatum, and prefrontal cortex, *Neuroscience & Biobehavioral Reviews*, 321–52.

Cardinal, R.N., Parkinson, J.A., Marbini, H.D. *et al.* (2003) Role of the anterior cingulate cortex in the control over behavior by Pavlovian conditioned stimuli in rats, *Behavioral Neuroscience*, **117**, 566–87.

Carey, G., Gottesman, I.I. and Robins, E. (1980) Prevalence rates for the neuroses: pitfalls in the evaluation of familiality, *Psychological Medicine*, **10**(3), 437–43.

Carroll, B.J., Greden, J.F., Haskett, R.F. *et al.* (1980) Neurotransmitter studies of neuroendocrine pathology in depression, *Acta Psychiatrica Scandinavica*, **61**, Suppl. 280, 183–200.

Carroll, B.J., Feinberg, M., Greden, J.F. *et al.* (1981) A specific laboratory test for the diagnosis of melancholia, *Archives of General Psychiatry*, **38**, 15–22.

Carroll, S.B., Prud'homme, B. and Gopel, N. (2008) Regulating evolution, *Scientific American*, 35–45.

Carter, C.S., Barch, D.M., Gur, R. *et al.* (2009) CNTRICS final task selection: social cognitive and affective neuroscience-based measures, *Schizophrenia Bulletin*, **35**, 153–62.

Casey, D., Gerlach, J., Magelund, G. *et al.* (1980) Gamma acetylenic GABA in tardive dyskinesia, *Archives of General Psychiatry*, **37**, 1376–9.

Caspari, D., Trabert, W., Heinz, G. *et al.* (1993) The pattern of regional cerebral blood flow during alcohol withdrawal: a single photon emission tomography study with 99TC-HMPAO, *Acta Psychiatrica Scandinavica*, **87**(6), 414–417.

Catterall, R.D. (1977) Neurosyphilis, *British Journal of Hospital Medicine*, **17**, 585–604.

Cavanna, A.E. and Trimble, M.R. (2006) The precuneus: a review of its functional anatomy and behavioural correlates, *Brain*, **129**, 564–83.

Cecconi, J.P., Lopes, A.C., Duran, F.L. *et al.* (2008) Gamma ventral capsulotomy for treatment of resistant obsessive–compulsive disorder: a structural MRI pilot prospective study, *Neuroscience Letter*, **447**, 138–42.

Cervenka, S., Backman, L., Cselenyi, Z. *et al.* (2008) Associations between dopamine D2-receptor binding and cognitive performance indicate functional compartmentalization of the human striatum, *Neuroimage*, **40**, 1287–95.

Chae, J.H., Nahas, Z., Lomarev, M. *et al.* (2003) A review of functional neuroimaging studies of vagus nerve stimulation (VNS), *Journal of Psychiatric Research*, **37**, 443–55.

Chalmers, R.J. and Bennie, E.H. (1978) The effect of fluphenazine on basal prolactin concentrations, *Psychological Medicine*, **8**, 483–6.

Champagne, D.L., Bagot, R.C., van Hasselt, F. *et al.* (2008) Maternal care and hippocampal plasticity: evidence for experience-dependent structural plasticity, altered synaptic functioning, and differential responsiveness to glucocorticoids and stress, *Journal of Neuroscience*, **28**, 6037–45.

Champagne, F.A. and Meaney, M.J. (2007) Transgenerational effects of social environment on variations in maternal care and behavioral response to novelty, *Behavioral Neuroscience*, **121**, 1353–63.

Chapman, A., Meldrum, B. and Mendes, E. (1983) Acute anticonvulsant activity of structural analogues of valproic acid and changes in brain GABA and aspartate content, *Life Sciences*, **32**, 2023–31.

Charney, D.S., Heninger, G.R., Sternberg, D.E. *et al.* (1981) Presynaptic adrenergic receptor sensitivity in depression, *Archives of General Psychiatry*, **38**, 1334–40.

Charney, D.S., Heninger, G.R. and Sternberg, D.E. (1983) Alpha-2 adrenergic receptor sensitivity and the mechanism of action of antidepressant therapy, *British Journal of Psychiatry*, **142**, 265–75.

Charney, D.S., Heninger, G.R. and Breier, A. (1984a) Noradrenergic function in panic anxiety, *Archives of General Psychiatry*, **41**, 751–63.

Charney, D.S., Heninger, G.R. and Sternberg, C.E. (1984b) The effect of mianserin on alpha-2 adrenergic receptor function in depressed patients, *British Journal of Psychiatry*, **144**, 407–16.

Checkley, S.A. (1979) Corticosteroid and growth hormone responses to methyl amphetamine in depressive illness, *Psychological Medicine*, **9**, 107–15.

Checkley, S.A. (1985) Biological markers in depression. In Granville–Grossman (ed.), *Recent Advances in Clinical Psychiatry*, Churchill Livingstone, Edinburgh, pp. 201–4.

Cheetham, S.C., Crompton, M.R., Katona, C.L.E. *et al.* (1988) Brain GABA-A benzodiazepine binding sites and glutamic acid decarboxylase activity in depressed suicide victims, *Brain Research*, **460**, 114–23.

Christensen, E., Møller, J.E. and Faurbye, A. (1970) A neuropathological investigation of 28 brains from patients with dyskinesia, *Acta Psychiatrica Scandinavica*, **46**, 14–23.

Christensen, N.J., Vestergaard, P., Sorensen, T. *et al.* (1980) CSF adrenaline and noradrenaline in depressed patients, *Acta Psychiatrica Scandinavica*, **61**, 178–82.

Christiansen, K.O. (1974) The genesis of aggressive criminality. In J. De Wit and W.W. Hastings (eds.), *Determinants and Origins of Aggressive Behaviour*, Moulton, The Hague, pp. 233–53.

Ciesielski, K.T., Beech, H.R. and Gordon, P.K. (1981) Some electrophysiological observations in obsessional states, *British Journal of Psychiatry*, **138**, 479–84.

Cloninger, C.R. (1987) A systematic method for clinical description and classification of personality variants, *Archives of General Psychiatry*, **44**, 573–88.

Cloninger, C.R. (2005) Antisocial personality disorder: a review. In M. Maj, H.S. Akiskal, J.E. Mezzich and A. Okasha (eds.), *Personality Disorders*, John Wiley and Sons, New York, NY, pp. 125–169.

Cloninger, C.R. (2008) The psychobiological theory of temperament and character: comment on Farmer and Goldberg (2008), *Psychological Assessment*, **20**, 292–9; Discussion 300–4.

Cloninger, C.R., Svrakic, D.M. and Przybeck, T.R. (1993) A psychobiological model of temperament and character, *Archives of General Psychiatry*, **50**, 975–90.

Cloninger, C.R., Przybeck, T.R., Svrakic, D.M. *et al.* (1994) *The Temperamental Character Inventory, A Guide to its Development and Use*. Washington University Center for Psychobiology of Personality, St Louis.

Cloninger, C.R., Adolfsson, R. and Svrakic, D.M. (1996a) Mapping genes for human personality, *Nature Genetics*, **12**, 3–4.

Cloninger, C.R., Przybeck, T.R. and Svrakic, D.M. (1996b) The tridimensional personality questionnaire: US normative data, *Psychological Reports*, **69**, 1047–57.

Coccaro, E.F., Silverman, J.M., Klar, H.M. *et al.* (1994) Familial correlates of reduced central serotonergic system function in patients with personality disorder, *Archives of General Psychiatry*, **51**, 318–24.

Coffey, C.E. (1993) *The Clinical Science of ECT*, American Physiological Society Press, Washington, DC.

Coffey, C.E. and Figiel, G.S. (1991) Neuropsychiatric significance of subcortical encephalomalacia. In B.J. Carroll and J.E. Barrett (eds.), *Psychopathology and the Brain*, Raven Press, New York, NY. pp. 243–63.

Coffey, C.E., Wilkinson, W.E., Weiner, R.D. *et al.* (1993) Quantitative cerebral anatomy in depression, *Archives of General Psychiatry*, **50**, 7–16.

Cohen, S.I. (1980) Cushing's syndrome: a psychiatric study of 29 patients, *British Journal of Psychiatry*, **136**, 120–4.

Collinge, J., Owen. F., Poulter, M. *et al.* (1990) Prion dementia without characteristic pathology, *Lancet*, **336**, 7–10.

Conlon, P., Trimble, M.R. and Rogers, D. (1990) A study of epileptic psychosis using MRI, *British Journal of Psychiatry*, **156**, 231–5.

Consensus Development Conference Statement (1986) *Electroconvulsive Therapy*, **5**(11), NIH.

Conway, C.R., Sheline, Y.I., Chibnall, J.T. *et al.* (2006) Cerebral blood flow changes during vagus nerve stimulation for depression, *Psychiatry Research*, **146**, 179–84.

Cook, I.A., Leuchter, A.F., Morgan, M.L. *et al.* (2005) Changes in prefrontal activity characterize clinical response in SSRI nonresponders: a pilot study, *Journal of Psychiatric Research*, **39**, 461–6.

Cooper, S.J., Kelly, J.G. and King, D.J. (1985) Adrenergic receptors in depression, *British Journal of Psychiatry*, **147**, 23–9.

Coppen, A.J. and Shaw, D.M. (1963) Mineral metabolism in melancholia, *British Medical Journal*, **ii**, 1439–44.

Coppen, A. and Wood, K. (1978) Tryptophan and depressive illness, *Psychological Medicine*, **8**, 49–57.

Coppen, A., Shaw, D.M. and Farrell, M.B. (1963) Potentiation of the antidepressive effect of a MAOI by tryptophan, *Lancet*, **ii**, 79–81.

Coppen, A.J., Malleson, A. and Shaw, D.M. (1965) Effects of lithium carbonate on electrolyte distribution in man, *Lancet*, **i**, 682–3.

Coppen, A., Prange, A.J., Whybrow, P.C. *et al.* (1972) Abnormalities of indoleamines in affective disorders, *Archives of General Psychiatry*, **26**, 474–8.

Coppen, A., Ghose, K., Rao, R. *et al.* (1978) Mianserin and lithium in the prophylaxis of depression, *British Journal of Psychiatry*, **133**, 206–10.

Coppen, A., Swade, S. and Wood, K. (1980) Lithium restores abnormal platelet 5-HT transport in patients with affective disorders, *British Journal of Psychiatry*, **136**, 235–8.

Coppen, A., Abou-Saleh, M., Milln, P. *et al.* (1983) DST in depression and other psychiatric illness, *British Journal of Psychiatry*, **142**, 498–504.

Coppen, A., Milln, P., Harwood, J. *et al.* (1985) Does the DST predict antidepressant treatment success?, *British Journal of Psychiatry*, **146**, 294–6.

Coursey, R.D., Buchsbaum, M.S. and Murphy, D.L. (1982) Two year follow up of subjects and their families defined as at risk for psychopathology on the bases of platelet MAO activities, *Neuropsychobiology*, **8**, 51–6.

Cowdry, R.W., Pickar, D. and Davies, R. (1986) Symptoms and EEG findings in the borderline syndrome, *International Journal of Psychiatry and Medicine*, **15**, 201–11.

Cowen, P. (1994) Antidepressant drugs and brain 5-HT function in humans, *Neuropsychopharmacology*, **10**, 45S.

Coyle, J., Prince, D.L. and DeLong, M.R. (1983) Alzheimer's disease: a disorder of cholinergic innervation, *Science*, **219**, 1184–90.

Crayton, J.W. and Meltzer, H.Y. (1976) Motor endplate alterations in schizophrenic patients, *Nature*, **264**, 658–9.

Cross, A.J., Crow, T.J., Perry, R.H. *et al.* (1981) Reduced dopamine beta hydrolase activity in Alzheimer's disease, *British Medical Journal*, **1**, 93–4.

Cross, A.J., Crow, T.J., Johnson, J.A. *et al.* (1984) Studies of neurotransmitter receptor systems in neocortex and hippocampus in senile dementia of the Alzheimer type, *Journal of the Neurological Sciences*, **64**, 109–17.

Crow, T.J. (1988) Sex chromosome for psychosis in the case of the pseudo-autosomal locus, *British Journal of Psychiatry*, **153**, 675–83.

Crow, T.J. (1991) The search of the psychosis gene, *British Journal of Psychiatry*, **158**, 611–14.

Crow, T.J. (2009) A theory of the origin of cerebral asymmetry: epigenetic variation superimposed on a fixed right-shift, *Laterality*, 1–15.

Crow, T.J. and Johnstone, E.C. (1986) Controlled trials of ECT. In S. Malitz and H.A. Sackeim (eds.), *ECT*, Annals of the New York Academy of Sciences, Vol. **462**, pp. 12–29.

Crow, T.J., Johnstone, E.C. and Owen, F. (1979a) Research on schizophrenia. In *Recent Advances in Clinical Psychiatry*, Churchill Livingstone, Edinburgh, pp. 1–36.

Crow, T.J., Baker, H.F., Cross, A.J. *et al.* (1979b) Monoamine mechanisms in chronic schizophrenia: post-mortem neurochemical findings, *British Journal of Psychiatry*, **134**, 249–56.

Crow, T.J., Delisi, L.E., Lofthouse, R. *et al.* (1994) An examination of linkage of schizophrenia and schizoaffective disorder to the pseudoautosomal region (Xp 22.3).

Crow, T.J., Paez, P. and Chance, S.A. (2007) Callosal misconnectivity and the sex difference in psychosis, *International Review Psychiatry*, **19**, 449–57.

Crow, T.J., Close, J.P., Dagnall, A.M. *et al.* (2009) Where and what is the right shift factor or cerebral dominance gene? A critique of Francks *et al.* (2007), *Laterality*, **14**, 3–10.

Cuesta, M.J., Peralta, V. and Caro, F. (1999) Premorbid personality in psychoses, *Schizophrenia Bulletin*, **25**, 801–11.

Cummings, J.L. (1985) *Clinical Neuropsychiatry*, Grune and Stratton, New York, NY.

Cummings, J.L. (1992) Depression and Parkinson's disease: a review, *American Journal of Psychiatry*, **149**, 443–54.

Cummings, J.L. and Benson, D.F. (1992) *Dementia: A Clinical Approach*, 2nd edition, Butterworths, London.

Cummings, J.L. and Trimble, M.T. (1995) *A Concise Guide to Neuropsychiatry and Behavioural Neurology*, APA Press, Washington, DC.

Cummings, J.L. and Trimble, M.R. (2002) *A Concise Guide to Neuropsychiatry and Behavioural Neurology*, 2nd edition, APA Press, Washington, DC.

Cummings, J.L., Benson, F., Hill, M.A. *et al.* (1985) Aphasia in dementia of the Alzheimer type, *Neurology*, **35**, 394–7.

Curson, D.A., Barnes, T.R.E., Bamber, R.W. *et al.* (1985) Long-term depot maintenance of chronic schizophrenic out patients, *British Journal of Psychiatry*, **146**, 464–80.

Curtis, D., Sherrington, R., Brett, P. *et al.* (1993) Genetic linkage analysis of manic depression in Iceland, *Journal of the Royal Society of Medicine*, **86**, 506–10.

Czeizel, A.E. (2009) The unitary nature of functional psychoses, *Lancet*, **373**, 809.

Dager, S.R., Marro, K.I., Richards, T.L. *et al.* (1994) Preliminary application of MRS to investigate lactate induced panic, *American Journal of Psychiatry*, **151**, 57–63.

Dahl, R.E., Kaufman, J., Ryan, N.D. *et al.* (1992) The dexamethasone test in children and adolescents, *Biological Psychiatry*, **32**, 109–26.

d'Alfonso, A.A., Aleman, A., Kessels, R.P. *et al.* (2002) Transcranial magnetic stimulation of left auditory cortex in patients with schizophrenia: effects on hallucinations and neurocognition, *Journal of Neuropsychiatry Clinical Neuroscience*, **14**, 77–9.

Damasio, H., Grabowski, T., Frank, R. *et al.* (1994) The return of Phineas Gage: clues about the brain from the skull of a famous patient, *Science*, **264**, 1102–5.

Dana-Haeri, J. and Trimble, M.R. (1984) Prolactin and gonadotrophin changes following partial seizures in epileptic patients with and without psychopathology, *Biologice Psychiatry*, **19**(3), 329–36.

Dannon, P.N., Dolberg, O.T., Schreiber, S. *et al.* (2002) Three and six-month outcome following courses of either ECT or rTMS in a population of severely depressed individuals: preliminary report, *Biological Psychiatry*, **51**, 687–90.

Davidson, R.J. (1995) Cerebral asymmetry, emotion, and affective style. In R.J. Davidson and K. Hugdahl (eds.), *Brain Asymmetry*, MIT Press, Cambridge, MA, pp. 361–88.

Davies, R.K. (1979) Incest: some neuropsychiatric findings, *International Journal of Psychiatric Medicine*, **9**, 117–21.

Davis, P. (1941) Electroencephalograms of manic-depressive patients, *American Journal of Psychiatry*, **98**, 430–3.

Deakin, J.F.W., Guimaraes, F.S., Wang, M. *et al.* (1991) Experimental tests of the 5-HT receptor imbalance theory of affective disturbances. In S.N. Sandler *et al.* (eds.), *5-HT in Psychiatry*, Oxford University Press, Oxford, pp. 143–57.

Debbane, M., van der Linden, M., Gex-Fabry, M. *et al.* (2009) Cognitive and emotional associations to positive schizotypy during adolescence, *Journal of Child Psychological Psychiatry*, **50**, 326–34.

Debruyn, A., Mendelbaum, K., Sandkuijl, L.A. *et al.* (1994) Nonlinkage of bipolar illness to tyrosine hydrolase, tyrosinease and D_2 and D_4 dopamine receptor genes on chromosome 11, *American Journal of Psychiatry*, **151**, 102–6.

de Geus, E.J., van 't Ent, D., Wolfensberger, S.P. *et al.* (2007a) Intrapair differences in hippocampal volume in monozygotic twins discordant for the risk for anxiety and depression, *Biological Psychiatry*, **61**, 1062–71.

de Geus, F., Denys, D.A., Sitskoorn, M.M. *et al.* (2007b) Attention and cognition in patients with obsessive–compulsive disorder, *Psychiatry Clinical Neuroscience*, **61**, 45–53.

Deicken, R.F., Calabrase, G., Merrin, E.L. *et al.* (1995) Basal ganglia phosphorous metabolism in chronic schizophrenia, *American Journal of Psychiatry*, **152**, 126–9.

de Kloet, C.S., Vermetten E., Geuze E., *et al.* (2008) Elevated plasma corticotrophin-releasing hormone levels in veterans with posttraumatic stress disorder, *Progress in Brain Research*, **167**, 287–91.

de la Fuente, J.M., Tugendhaft, P. and Mavroudakis, N. (1998) Electroencephalographic abnormalities in borderline personality disorder, *Psychiatry Research*, **77**, 131–8.

Delgado, J.M.R. (1966) Aggressive behaviour evoked by radio stimulation in monkey colonies, *American Zoologist*, **6**, 669–81.

Delgado, P.L. (2006) Monoamine depletion studies: implications for antidepressant discontinuation syndrome, *The Journal of Clinical Psychiatry*, **67**, Suppl. 4, 22–6.

Delgado, P.L., Charney, D.S., Price, L.H. *et al.* (1990) Serotonin function and the mechanism of antidepressant action, *Archives of General Psychiatry*, **47**, 411–18.

Delgado, P.L., Price, L.H., Miller, H.L. *et al.* (1991) Rapid serotonin depletion as a provocative challenge test for patients with major depression: relevance to antidepressant action and the neurobiology of depression, *Psychopharmacology Bulletin*, **27**, 321–30.

Delgado, P.L., Price, L.H., Miller, H.L. *et al.* (1994) Serotonin and the neurobiology of depression: effects of tryptophan depletion in drug-free depressed patients, *Archives of General Psychiatry*, **51**, 865–74.

Delgado-Escueta, A., Mattson, R.H., King, L. *et al.* (1981) The nature of aggression during epileptic seizures, *New England Journal of Medicine*, **305**, 711–16.

Delisi, L.E. (2008) The concept of progressive brain change in schizophrenia: implications for understanding schizophrenia, *Schizophrenia Bulletin*, **34**, 312–21.

Delisi, L., Wise, C.O., Bridge, T. *et al.* (1982) Monamine oxidase and schizophrenia. In E. Usdin and I. Hanin (eds.), *Biological Markers in Psychiatry and Neurology*, Pergamon Press, New York, NY, pp. 79–96.

Delisi, L.E., Sakuma, M., Maurizio, A.M. *et al.* (2004) Cerebral ventricular change over the first 10 years after the onset of schizophrenia, *Psychiatry Research*, **130**, 57–70.

Delisi, L.E., Szulc, K.U., Bertisch, H. *et al.* (2006a) Early detection of schizophrenia by diffusion weighted imaging, *Psychiatry Research*, **148**, 61–6.

Delisi, L.E., Szulc, K.U., Bertisch, H.C. *et al.* (2006b) Understanding structural brain changes in schizophrenia, *Dialogues in Clinical Neuroscience*, **8**, 71–8.

de Tiege, X., Bier, J.C., Massat, I. *et al.* (2003) Regional cerebral glucose metabolism in akinetic catatonia and after remission, *Journal of Neurology, Neurosurgery and Psychiatry*, **74**, 1003–4.

Devinsky, O., Cox, C., Witt, E. *et al.* (1991) Ictal fear in temporal lobe epilepsy, *Journal of Epilepsy*, **4**, 231–8.

Devinsky, O. and Luciano, D. (1993) The contributions of cingulate cortex to human behavior. In B.A. Vogt and M. Gabriel (eds.), *Neurobiology of Cingulate Cortex and Limbic Thalamus*, Birkhauser, Boston, MA.

Dinan, T.G. (1994) Glucocorticoids and the genesis of depressive illness, *British Journal of Psychiatry*, **164**, 365–71.

Doble, A. and Martin, I.L. (1992) Multiple benzodiazepine receptors, *TIPS*, **13**, 16–18.

Dolan, M. and Park, I. (2002) The neuropsychology of antisocial personality disorder, *Psychological Medicine*, **32**, 417–27.

Dolan, R.J., Galloway, S.P., Fonagy, P. *et al.* (1985a) Life events, depression and hypothalamic pituitary–adrenal axis function, *British Journal of Psychiatry*, **147**, 429–34.

Dolan, R.J., Calloway, S.P. and Mann, A.H. (1985b) Cerebral ventricular size in depressed subjects, *Psychological Medicine*, **15**, 873–8.

Dolan, R.J., Poynton, A.M., Bridges, P.K. *et al.* (1990) Altered magnetic resonance white matter T1 values in patients with affective disorder, *British Journal of Psychiatry*, **157**, 107–10.

Doran, A.R., Rubinow, D.R., Roy, A. *et al.* (1986) CSF somatostatin and abnormal response to dexamethasone administration in schizophrenic and depressed patients, *Archives of General Psychiatry*, **43**, 365–9.

Dorrow, R., Horowski, R., Paschelke, G. *et al.* (1983) Severe anxiety induced by FG 7142, *Lancet*, **ii**, 98–9.

Dorus, E. (1980) Variability in the Y chromosome and variability in human behaviour, *Archives of General Psychiatry*, **37**, 587–94.

Drevets, W.C., Videen, T.O., MacLeod, A.K. *et al.* (1992) PET images of blood flow changes during anxiety: correction, *Science*, **256**, 1696.

Drevets, W.C. (2003) Neuroimaging abnormalities in the amygdala in mood disorders, *Annals of the New York Academy of Sciences*, **985**, 420–44.

Drevets, W.C., Thase, M.E., Moses-Kolko, E.L. *et al.* (2007) Serotonin-1a receptor imaging in recurrent depression: replication and literature review, *Nuclear Medicine and Biology*, **34**, 865–77.

Drevets, W.C., Price, J.L. and Furey, M.L. (2008) Brain structural and functional abnormalities in mood disorders: implications for neurocircuitry models of depression, *Brain Structure & Function*, **213**, 93–118.

Driessen, M., Herrmann, J., Stahl, K. *et al.* (2000) Magnetic resonance imaging volumes of the hippocampus and the amygdala in women with borderline personality disorder and early traumatization, *Archives of General Psychiatry*, **57**, 1115–22.

Driessen, M., Wingenfeld, K., Rullkoetter, N. *et al.* (2008) One-year functional magnetic resonance imaging follow-up study of neural activation during the recall of unresolved negative life events in borderline personality disorder, *Psychological Medicine*, 1–10.

Drubach, D.A. and Kelly, M.P. (1989) Panic disorder associated with right paralimbic lesion, *Neuropsychiatry, Neuropsychology and Behavioural Neurology*, **4**, 282–9.

D'souza, D.C., Abi-Saab, W.M., Madonick, S. *et al.* (2005) Delta-9-tetrahydrocannabinol effects in schizophrenia: implications for cognition, psychosis, and addiction, *Biological Psychiatry*, **57**, 594–608.

Dubrovsky, B. (1993) Effects of adrenal cortex hormones on limbic structures: some experimental and clinical correlations related to depression, *J Psychiatry Neurosci*, **18**, 4–16.

Duman, R.S. (2005) Neurotrophic factors and regulation of mood: role of exercise, diet and metabolism, *Neurobiological Aging*, **26**, Suppl. 1, 88–93.

Dwivedi, Y., Rizavi, H.S., Conley, R.R. *et al.* (2003) Altered gene expression of brain-derived neurotrophic factor and receptor tyrosine kinase B in postmortem brain of suicide subjects, *Archives of General Psychiatry*, **60**, 804–15.

Dworkin, R.H. and Lenzenweger, M.F. (1984) Symptoms and the genetics of schizophrenia implications for diagnosis, *American Journal of Psychiatry*, **141**, 1541–6.

Ebert, D., Feistel, H., Kaschka, W. *et al.* (1994) SPECT assessment of cerebral dopamine D_2 receptor blockade in depression before and after sleep deprivation, *Biological Psychiatry*, **35**, 880–5.

Edeh, J. and Toone, B.K. (1985) Antiepileptic therapy, folate deficiency, and psychiatric morbidity: a general practice survey, *Epilepsia*, **26**, 434–40.

Edelman, G.M. (1989) *The Remembered Present*, Basic Books, New York, NY.

Eeg-Olofsson, O., Petersen, I. and Sellden, U. (1971) The development of the EEG in normal children from the age of 1 through 15 years, *Neuropaediatrie*, **2**, 375–404.

Egrise, D., Rubinstein, M., Schoutens, A. *et al.* (1986) Seasonal variation of platelet serotonin binding in normal and depressed subjects, *Biological Psychiatry*, **21**, 283–92.

Eichelmann, B. (1979) Role of biogenic amines in aggressive behaviour. In M. Sandler (ed.), *Psychopharmacology of Aggression*, Raven Press, New York, NY, pp. 61–93.

Elger, G., Hoppe, C., Falkai, P. *et al.* (2000) Vagus nerve stimulation is associated with mood improvements in epilepsy patients, *Epilepsy Research*, **42**, 203–10.

Eliez, S. (2007) Autism in children with 22q11.2 deletion syndrome, *Journal of the Amenice Academic of Child and Adolescent Psychiatry*, **46**, 433–4; Author Reply 434–4.

Ellis, P.M. and Salmond, C. (1994) Is platelet imipramine binding reduced in depression?, *Biological Psychiatry*, **36**, 292–300.

El-Mallakh, R.S. and Wyatt, R.J. (1995) The Na, K-ATPase hypothesis for bipolar illness, *Biological Psychiatry*, **37**, 235–44.

Emrich, H.M., Dose, M. and von Zerssen, D. (1984) Action of sodium valproate and of oxycarbazepine in patients with affective disorders. In H.M. Emrich *et al.* (eds.), *Anticonvulsants in Affective Disorders*, Excerpta Medica, Oxford, pp. 45–55.

Engel, J. (2006a) ILAE classification of epilepsy syndromes, *Epilepsy Research*, **70**, Suppl. 1, S5–S10.

Engel, J. (2006b) Report of the ILAE classification core group, *Epilepsia*, **47**, 1558–68.

Engel, J., Fejerman, N., Berg, A.T. *et al.* (2007) Classification of the epilepsies. In J. Engel and T. Pedley (eds.), *Epilepsy: A Comprehensive textbook*, 2nd edition, Lippincott Williams & Wilkins, New York, NY, pp. 767–72.

Engin, E., Treit, D. and Dickson, C.T. *et al.* in *Neuroscience*, **162**(4), 1438–9.

Erkinjuntti, T. and Gauthier, S. (2009) The concept of vascular cognitive impairment, *Frontiers of Neurology and Neuroscience*, **24**, 79–85.

Eser, D., Baghai, T.C., Schule, C. *et al.* (2008a) Neuroactive steroids as endogenous modulators of anxiety, *Current Pharmaceutical Design*, **14**, 3525–33.

Eser, D., Wenninger, S., Baghai, T. *et al.* (2008b) Impact of state and trait anxiety on the panic response to CCK-4, *Journal of Neurological Transmission*, **115**, 917–20.

Esler, M., Turbott, J., Schwartz, R. *et al.* (1982) The peripheral kinetics of norepinephrine in depressive illness, *Archives of General Psychiatry*, **39**, 295–300.

Esslinger, C., Walter, H., Kirsch, P. *et al.* (2009) Neural mechanisms of a genome-wide supported psychosis variant, *Science*, **324**, 605.

Ettinger, A., Reed, M., Cramer, J. and the Epilepsy Impact Project Group (2004) Depression and comorbidity in community-based patients with epilepsy or asthma, *Neurology*, **63**, 1008–14.

Ettinger, A.B., Reed, M.L., Goldberg, J.F. *et al.* (2005) Prevalence of bipolar symptoms in epilepsy vs other chronic health disorders, *Neurology*, **65**, 535–40.

Extein, I., Tallman, J., Smith, C.C. *et al.* (1979) Changes in lymphocyte beta adrenergic receptors in depression and mania, *Psychiatric Research*, **1**, 191–7.

Extein, I., Pottash, A.L.C. and Gold, M.S. (1981) Relation of TRH test and DST abnormalities in unipolar depression, *Psychiatry Research*, **4**, 49–53.

Extein, I., Pottash, A.L.C., Gold, M.S. *et al.* (1982) TSH response to TRH in unipolar depression before and after clinical improvement, *Psychiatry Research*, **6**, 161–9.

Fabricius, K., Wortwein, G. and Pakkenberg, B. (2008) The impact of maternal separation on adult mouse behaviour and on the total neuron number in the mouse hippocampus, *Brain Structure Function*, **212**, 403–16.

Farde, L., Wiesel, F.-A., Stone-Elander, S. *et al.* (1990) D2 dopamine receptors in neuroleptic-naive schizophrenic patients, *Archives of General Psychiatry*, **47**, 213–19.

Feighner, J.P., Robins, E., Guze, S.B. *et al.* (1972) Diagnostic criteria for use in psychiatric research, *Archives of General Psychiatry*, **26**, 57–63.

Fenton, G.W. (1972) Epilepsy and automatism, *British Journal of Hospital Medicine*, **7**, 57–64.

Fenwick, P. (1981) Precipitation and inhibition of seizures. In E.H. Reynolds and M.R. Trimble (eds.), *Epilepsy and Psychiatry*, Churchill Livingstone, Edinburgh, pp. 242–63.

Fenwick, P. (1986) Aggression and epilepsy. In M.R. Trimble and T. Bolwig (eds.), *Aspects of Epilepsy and Psychiatry*, John Wiley and Sons, Chichester, pp. 31–60.

Fergusson, D., Doucette, S., Glass, K.C. *et al.* (2005) Association between suicide attempts and selective serotonin reuptake inhibitors: systematic review of randomised controlled trials, *British Medical Journal*, **330**, 396.

Filbey, F.M., Toulopoulou, T., Morris, R.G. *et al.* (2008) Selective attention deficits reflect increased genetic vulnerability to schizophrenia, *Schizophrenia Research*, **101**, 169–75.

Fink, M. (1986) Convulsive therapy and epilepsy research. In M.R. Trimble and E.H. Reynolds (eds.), *What is Epilepsy?*, Churchill Livingstone, Edinburgh, pp. 217–28.

Finley, G.W. and Campbell, C.M. (1941) Electroencephalography in schizophrenia, *American Journal of Psychiatry*, **98**, 374–84.

Fisch, C. (1985) Effect of fluoxetine on the electrocardiogram, *Journal of Clinical Psychiatry*, **46**, 42–4.

Fitzgerald, P.B., Benitez, J., Daskalakis, J.Z. *et al.* (2006) The treatment of recurring auditory hallucinations in schizophrenia with rTMS, *World Journal of Biological Psychiatry*, **7**, 119–22.

Fleischmann, A., Sternheim, A., Etgen, A.M. *et al.* (1996) Transcranial magnetic stimulation down-regulates beta-adrenoreceptors in rat cortex, *Journal of Neural Transmission*, **103**, 1361–6.

Flor-Henry, P. (1969) Psychosis and temporal lobe epilepsy, *Epilepsia*, **10**, 363–95.

Flor-Henry, P. (1983) *Cerebral Basis of Psychopathology*, John Wright, Bristol.

Flügel, D., Cercignani, M., Symms, M.R. *et al.* (2006) Diffusion tensor imaging findings and their correlation with neuropsychological deficits in patients with temporal lobe epilepsy and interictal psychosis, *Epilepsia*, **47**, 941–4.

Foley, J.O. and Dubois, F. (1937) Quantitative studies of the vagus nerve in the cat: I. the ratio of sensory and motor studies. *Journal of Comparative Neurology*, **67**, 49–67.

Folstein, M.F., Maiberger, R. and McHugh, P.R. (1977) Mood disorder as a specific complication of stroke, *Journal of Neurology, Neurosurgery and Psychiatry*, **40**, 1018–20.

Fontaine, R., Breton, G., Dery, R. *et al.* (1990) Temporal lobe abnormalities in panic disorder: an MRI study, *Biological Psychiatry*, **27**, 304–10.

Forstl, H., Burns, A., Levy, R. *et al.* (1994) Neuropathological correlates of psychotic phenomena in confirmed Alzheimer's disease, *British Journal of Psychiatry*, **165**, 53–9.

Fountoulakis, K.N. and Akiskal, H.S. (2008) Focus on bipolar illness, *CNS Spectrums*, **13**, 762.

Fowler, C.J., von Knorring, L. and Oreland, L. (1980) Platelet MAO in sensation seekers, *Psychiatry Research*, 273–9.

Fox, J.H., Topel, J.L. and Huckman, M.S. (1975) Use of computerized axial tomography in senile dementia, *Journal of Neurology, Neurosurgery and Psychiatry*, **38**, 948–53.

Frackowiak, R.S.J., Lenzi, G.L., Jones, T. *et al.* (1980) Quantitative measurements of regional CBF and oxygen metabolism in man using 15 O and PET: theory, procedure and normal values, *Journal of Computer Assisted Tomography*, **4**, 727–36.

Frackowiak, R.S.J., Pozzilli, C., Legg, N.J. *et al.* (1981) Regional cerebral oxygen supply and utilisation in dementia, *Brain*, **104**, 753–8.

Francis, P.T. and Bowen, D.M. (1985) Relevance of reduced concentrations of somatostatin in Alzheimer's disease, *Biochemical Society Transactions*, **13**, 170–1.

Francis, P.T., Palmer, A.M., Sims, N.R. *et al.* (1985) Neurochemical study of early onset Alzheimer's disease, *New England Journal of Medicine*, **313**, 7–11.

Fredrikson, M., Wik, G., Greitz, T. *et al.* (1993) Regional cerebral blood flow during experimental phobic fear, *Psychophysiology*, **30**, 126–30.

Freeman, W. and Watts, J.W. (1947) Psychosurgery during 1936–46, *Archives of Neurology and Psychiatry*, **58**, 417–25.

Friedman, M.J., Stolk, J.M., Harris, P.Q. *et al.* (1984) Serum dopamine–beta-hydrolase activity in depression and anxiety, *Biological Psychiatry*, **19**, 557–70.

Friston, K.J., Frith, C.D., Liddle, P.F. *et al.* (1991) Comparing functional (PET) images: the assessment of significant change, *Journal of Cerebral Blood Flow and Metabolism*, **11**, 690–9.

Friston, K.J., Liddle, P.P., Firth, C.D. *et al.* (1992) The left median temporal region and schizophrenia, *Brain*, **115**, 367–82.

Friston, K.J., Holmes, A., Poline, J.B. *et al.* (1996) Detecting activations in PET and fMRI: levels of inference and power, *Neuroimage*, **4**, 223–35.

Frolich, E.D., Tarazi, R.C. and Dunstan, H.F. (1969) Hyperdynamic beta-adrenergic circulatory state, *Archives of Internal Medicine*, **123**, 1–7.

Fulton, J.F. and Jacobsen, C.G. (1935) The functions of the frontal lobes, a comparative study in monkeys, chimpanzees and men, *Advances in Modern Biology*, **4**, 113–23.

Fuster, J.M. (1980) *The Pre-frontal Cortex*, Raven Press, New York, NY.

Fuster, J.M. (1993) Frontal lobes, *Current Opinion in Neurobiology*, **3**, 160–5.

Fuster, J.M. (2004) Upper processing stages of the perception-action cycle, *Trends in Cognitive Sciences*, **8**, 143–5.

Gainotti, G. (1972) Emotional behaviour and hemispheric side of the lesion, *Cortex*, **8**, 41–55.

Garber, H.J., Anarth, J.V., Chiu, L.C *et al.* (1989) Nuclear magnetic resonance study of OCD, *American Journal of Psychiatry*, **146**, 1001–5.

Garcia-Sevilla, J.A., Athanasios, P.Z., Hollingsworth, P.J. *et al.* (1981) Platelet alpha 2 adrenergic receptors in major depressive disorder, *Archives of General Psychiatry*, **38**, 1327–33.

Garcia-Sevilla, J.A., Guimon, J., Garcia-Valleto, P. *et al.* (1986) Biochemical and functional evidence of supersensitive platelet alpha-2 adrenoceptors in major affective disorder, *Archives of General Psychiatry*, **43**, 51–7.

Gartrell, N. (1986) Increased libido in women receiving trazadone, *American Journal of Psychiatry*, **143**, 781–2.

Geisler, S. (2008) The lateral habenula: no long neglected, *CNS Spectrums*, **13**, 484–9.

Gentsch, C., Lichtsteiner, M. and Freer, H. (1981) 3-H diazepam binding sites in Roman high- and low-avoidance rats, *Experientia*, **37**, 1315–16.

George, M.S. (2002) Advances in brain stimulation: guest editorial, *The Journal of ECT*, **18**, 169.

George, M.S. and Belmaker, R.H. (2000) *Transcranial Magnetic Stimulation in Neuropsychiatry*, American Psychiatric Press, Washington, DC.

George, M.S. and Belmaker, R.H. (2006) *TMS in Clinical Psychiatry*, American Psychiatric Press, Washington, DC.

George, M.S. and Wassermann, E.M. (1994) Rapid-rate transcranial magnetic stimulation (rTMS) and ECT, *Convulsive Therapy*, **10**(4), 251–3.

George, M.S., Ring, H.A., Costa, D.C. *et al.* (1991) *Neuroactivation and Neuroimaging with SPET*, London, Springer-Verlag.

George, M.S., Ring, H.A., Costa, D.C. *et al.* (1992) Demonstration of human motor cortex activation using SPECT, *Journal of Neural Transmission*, **87**, 231–6.

George, M.S., Ketter, T.A., Gill, D.S. *et al.* (1993) Brain regions involved in recognizing facial emotion or identity: an oxygen-15 PET study, *Journal of Neuropsychiatry Clinical Neuroscience*, **5**, 384–94.

George, M.S., Ketter, T.A. and Post, R.M. (1994a) Prefrontal cortex dysfunction in clinical depression, *Depression*, **2**, 59–72.

George, M.S., Ketter, T.A. and Post, R.M. (1994c) Activation studies in mood disorders, *Psychiatric Annals*, **24**, 648–52.

George, M.S., Ketter, T.A. and Post, R.M. (1994d) Prefrontal cortex dysfunction in clinical depression, *Depression*, **2**, 59–72.

George, M.S., Post, R.M., Ketter, T.A. *et al.* (1995a) Neural mechanisms of mood disorders. In A.J. Rush (ed.), *Current Review of Mood Disorders*, Current Medicine, Philadelphia.

George, M.S., Wassermann, E.M., Williams, W.A. *et al.* (1995b) Daily repetitive transcranial magnetic stimulation (RTMS) improves mood in depression, *Neuroreport*, **6**, 1853–6.

George, M.S., Ketter, T.A., Parekh, P.I. *et al.* (1995c) Depressed subjects have abnormal right hemisphere activation during facial emotion recognition, *Journal of Neuropsychiatry Clinical Neuroscience*, **9**, 55–63.

George, M.S., Ketter, T.A. and Post, R.M. (1996) What functional imaging studies have revealed about the brain basis of mood and emotion. In J. Panksepp (ed.), *Advances in Biological Psychiatry*, Jai Press, Greenwich, CN, pp. 63– 113.

George, M.S., Huggins, T., McDermut, W. *et al.* (1998) Abnormal facial emotion recognition in depression: serial testing in an ultra-rapid-cycling patients, *Behavioral Modification*, **22**, 192–204.

George, M.S., Stallings, L.E., Speer, A.M. *et al.* (1999a) Prefrontal repetitive transcranial magnetic stimulation (rTMS) changes relative perfusion locally and remotely, *Human Psychopharmacology*, **14**, 161–70.

George, M.S., Teneback, C.C., Malcolm, R.J. *et al.* (1999b) Multiple previous alcohol detoxifications are associated with decreased medial temporal and paralimbic function in the postwithdrawal period, *Alcohol Clinical Experiment Research*, **23**, 1077–84.

George, M.S., Sackeim, H.A., Rush, A.J. *et al.* (2000) Vagus nerve stimulation: a new tool for brain research and therapy, *Biological Psychiatry*, **47**, 287–95.

George, M.S., Anton, R.F., Bloomer, C. *et al.* (2001) Activation of prefrontal cortex and anterior thalamus in alcoholic subjects on exposure to alcohol-specific cues, *Archives of General Psychiatry*, **58**, 345–52.

George, M.S., Myrick, H., Li, X. *et al.* (2002a) Assessing the brain sequelae of alcoholism using brain imaging. In B.A. Johnson, P. Ruiz and M. Galanter (eds.), *Alcoholism: A Practical Handbook*, Lippincott Williams & Wilkins, New York, NY, pp. 94–9.

George, M.S., Nahas, Z., Kozel, F.A. *et al.* (2002b) Mechanisms and state of the art of transcranial magnetic stimulation, *The Journal of ECT*, **18**, 170–81.

George, M.S., Rush, A.J., Marangell, L.B. *et al.* (2005) A one-year comparison of vagus nerve stimulation with treatment as usual for treatment-resistant depression, *Biological Psychiatry*, **58**, 364–73.

George, R., Salinsky, M., Kuzniecky, R. *et al.* (1994b) Vagus nerve stimulation for treatment of partial seizures: 2. long-term follow-up on first 67 patients exiting a controlled study, *Epilepsia*, **35**, 637–43.

Gerner, R.H., Fairbanks, L., Anderson, G.M. *et al.* (1984) CSF neurochemistry in depressed, manic and schizophrenic patients compared with that of normal controls, *American Journal of Psychiatry*, **141**, 1533–40.

Gershon, E. (1983) The genetics of affective disorders. In L. Grinspoon (ed.), *Psychiatry Update*, Vol. **2**, APA, Washington, DC, pp. 434–56.

Geschwind, N. (1979) Behavioural changes in TLE, *Psychological Medicine*, **9**, 217–19.

Ghose, K., Turner, P. and Coppen, A. (1975) Intravenous tyramine pressor response in depression, *Lancet*, **i**, 1317–18.

Gibbons, R.D., Hur, K., Bhaumik, D.K. *et al.* (2005) The relationship between antidepressant medication use and rate of suicide, *Archives of General Psychiatry*, 165–72.

Gilliam, F., Kuzniecky, R., Faught, E. *et al.* (1997) Patient validated content of epilepsy specific quality of life measurement, *Epilepsia*, **38**, 233–6.

Gilliam, F.G., Barry, J.J., Hermann, B.P. *et al.* (2006) Rapid detection of major depression in epilepsy: a multicentre study, *Lancet Neurology*, **5**, 399–405.

Gillin, J.C., Sitaram, N., Wehr, T. *et al.* (1985) Sleep and affective illness. In R.M. Post and J.C. Ballenger (eds.), *Neurobiology of Mood Disorders*, Williams and Wilkins, Baltimore, pp. 157–89.

Gilman, J.M. and Hommer, D.W. (2008) Modulation of brain response to emotional images by alcohol cues in alcohol-dependent patients, *Addiction Biology*, **13**, 423–34.

Gjerris, A. (1988) Baseline studies on transmitter substances in CSF in depression, *Acta Psychiatrica Scandinavica*, **73**, Suppl. 346.

Gjessing, R. (1947) Biological investigations in endogenous psychoses, *Acta Psychiatrica Neurologica Scandinavica*, Suppl. 47.

Glass, I.B., Checkley, S.A., Shur, E. *et al.* (1982) Effect of desipramine upon central adrenergic function in depressed patients, *British Journal of Psychiatry*, **141**, 372–6.

Glassman, A.H., Perel, J.M., Shostak, M. *et al.* (1977) Clinical implications of imipramine plasma levels for depressive illness, *Archives of General Psychiatry*, **34**, 197–204.

Glenn, A.L. and Raine, A. (2008) The neurobiology of psychopathy, *Psychiatric Clinics North America*, **31**, 463–75, vii.

Gloor, P., Olivier, A., Quesney, L.F. *et al.* (1982) The role of the limbic system in experiential phenomena of TLE, *Annals of Neurology*, **12**, 129–44.

Goldman-Rakic, P.S. (1994) Working memory dysfunction in schizophrenia, *Journal of Neuropsychiatry Clinical Neuroscience*, **6**, 348–57.

Gold, P., Kling, M.A., Demitrack, M.A. *et al.* (1988) Clinical studies with CRH. In D. Genten and D. Pfaff (eds.), *Current Trends in Neuroendocrinology*, Vol. **8**, Springer Verlag, Berlin, pp. 238–56.

Gomez, R.G., Fleming, S.H., Keller, J. *et al.* (2006) The neuropsychological profile of psychotic major depression and its relation to cortisol, *Biological Psychiatry*, **60**, 472–8.

Gonda, X., Fountoulakis, K.N., Rihmer, Z. *et al.* (2009) Towards a genetically validated new affective temperament scale: a delineation of the temperament phenotype of 5-HTTLPR using the Temps-A, *Journal Of Affective Disorders*, **112**, 19–29.

Gonul, A.S., Akdeniz, F., Taneli, F. *et al.* (2005) Effect of treatment on serum brain-derived neurotrophic factor levels in depressed patients, *European Archives of Psychiatry and Clinical Neuroscience*, **255**(6), 381–6.

Good, K., Lawrence, N.S., Thomas, C.J. *et al.* (2003) Dosage-sensitive X-linked locus influences the development of amygdala and orbitofrontal cortex and fear recognition in humans, *Brain*, **126**, 2431–46.

Goodwin, D.W. and Guze, S.B. (1984) *Psychiatric Diagnosis*, 3rd edition, Oxford University Press, Oxford.

Gordon, E.B. (1968) Serial EEG studies in presenile dementia, *British Journal of Psychiatry*, **114**, 779–80.

Gorman, J.M., Levy, G.F., Liebowitz, M.R. *et al.* (1983) Effect of acute beta adrenergic blockade on lactate-induced panic, *Archives of General Psychiatry*, **40**, 1079–82.

Gorman, J., Liebowitz, M.R., Fyer, A.J. *et al.* (1985) Platelet MAO activity in patients with panic disorder, *Biological Psychiatry*, **20**, 852–8.

Gorman, J.M., Liebowitz, M.R., Fyer, A.J. *et al.* (1989) A neuroanatomical hypothesis for panic disorder, *American Journal of Psychiatry*, **146**, 148–61.

Gottesman, I.I. (1962) Differential inheritance of the psychoneuroses, *Eugenics Quarterly*, **9**, 223–7.

Gottesman, I.I. and Bertelsen, A. (1989) Confirming unexpressed genotypes for schizophrenia, *Archives of General Psychiatry*, **46**, 867–72.

Gottesman, I.I. and Shields, J. (1972) *Schizophrenia and Genetics: A Twin Study Vantage Point*, Academic Press, London.

Gouw, A.A., van der Flier, W.M., Fazekas, F. *et al.* (2008) Progression of white matter hyperintensities and incidence of new lacunes over a 3-year period: the leukoaraiosis and disability study, *Stroke*, **39**, 1414–20.

Gray, J.A. (1982) *The Neuropsychology of Anxiety: An Enquiry into the Functions of the Septo-hippocampal System*, Oxford University Press, New York, NY.

Graybiel, A.M. (1990) Neurotransmitters and modulators in the basal ganglia, *TINS*, **13**, 244–54.

Greicius, M.D., Flores, B.H., Menon, V. *et al.* (2007) Resting-state functional connectivity in major depression: abnormally increased contributions from subgenual cingulate cortex and thalamus, *Biological Psychiatry*, **62**, 429–37.

Green, A.R. (1986) Changes in GABA biochemistry and the seizure threshold. In S. Malitz and H.A. Sackeim (eds.), *ECT*, Annals of the New York Academy of Sciences, Vol. **462**, pp. 105–18.

Green, T., Gothelf, D., Glaser, B. *et al.* (2009) Psychiatric disorders and intellectual functioning throughout development in velocardiofacial (22q11.2 deletion) syndrome, *Journal of American Academics of Child and Adolescence Psychiatry*, **48**(11), 1060–8.

Greenberg, D.B. and Brown, G.L. (1985) Mania resulting from brain stem tumour, *Journal of Nervous and Mental Diseases*, **173**, 434–6.

Greenberg, B.D., George, M.S., Dearing, J. *et al.* (1997) Effect of prefrontal repetitive transcranial magnetic stimulation (rTMS) in obsessive compulsive disorder: a preliminary study, *American Journal of Psychiatry*, **154**, 867–869.

Greenberg, B.D., Askland, K.D. and Carpenter, L.L. (2008) The evolution of deep brain stimulation for neuropsychiatric disorders, *Frontiers in Bioscience*, **13**, 4638–48.

Griesinger, W. (1867) *Mental Pathology and Therapeutics* (Translated by C. Lockhart Robertson and J. Rutherford), New Sydenham Society, London.

Grisaru, N., Yarovslavsky, U., Abarbanel, J. *et al.* (1994) Transcranial magnetic stimulation in depression and schizophrenia, *European Neuropsychopharmacology*, **4**, 287–288.

Groenewegen, H.J. (1997) Cortical-subcortical relationships and the limbic forebrain. In M.R. Trimble and J. Cummings, *Behavioural Neurology*, Butterworth-Heinemann, pp. 29–48.

Guay, J.P., Ruscio, J., Knight, R.A. *et al.* (2007) A taxometric analysis of the latent structure of psychopathy: evidence for dimensionality, *Journal of Abnormal Psychology*, **116**, 701–16.

Gunne, L.M., Haggstrom, J.E. and Sjoquist, B. (1984) Association with persistent neuroleptic-induced dyskinesia of regional changes in brain GABA synthesis, *Nature*, **304**, 347–9.

Gur, R.E., Calkins, M.E., Gur, R.C. *et al.* (2007) The consortium on the genetics of schizophrenia: neurocognitive endophenotypes, *Schizophrenia Bulletin*, **33**, 49–68.

Gureje, O. (1991) Interictal psychopathology in epilepsy: prevalence and pattern in a Nigerian clinic, *British Journal of Psychiatry*, **158**, 700–5.

Guy, J.D., Majorski, L.V., Wallaco, C.J. *et al.* (1983) The incidence of minor physical abnormalities in male schizophrenics, *Schizophrenia Bulletin*, **9**, 571–82.

Hachinski, V.C., Linnette, D., Zilhka, E. *et al.* (1975) Cerebral blood flow in dementia, *Archives of Neurology*, **32**(9), 632–7.

Haenschel, C., Bittner, R.A., Haertling, F. *et al.* (2007) Contribution of impaired early-stage visual processing to working memory dysfunction in adolescents with schizophrenia: a study with event-related potentials and functional magnetic resonance imaging, *Archives in General Psychiatry*, **64**, 1229–40.

Haenschel, C., Bittner, R.A., Waltz, J. *et al.* (2009) Cortical oscillatory activity is critical for working memory as revealed by deficits in early-onset schizophrenia, *Journal of Neuroscience*, **29**, 9481–9.

Hakola, H.P.A. and Iivanainen, M. (1978) Pneumoencephalographic and clinical findings of the XYY syndrome, *Acta Psychiatrica Scandinavica*, **58**, 360–6.

Hale, A.S., Hannah, P., Sandler, M. *et al.* (1989) Tyramine conjugation test for prediction of treatment response in depressed patients, *Lancet*, **i**, 234–6.

Hall, K.C.W. (1980) Depression. In R.C.W. Hall (ed.), *Psychiatric Presentations of Medical Illness*, MTP, Press, Lancaster, pp. 37–63.

Han, M., Deng, C., Burne, T.H. *et al.* (2008) Short- and long-term effects of antipsychotic drug treatment on weight gain and H1 receptor expression, *Psychoneuroendocrinology*, **33**, 569–80.

Handforth, A., Degiorgio, C.M., Schachter, S.C. *et al.* (1998) Vagus nerve stimulation therapy for partial-onset seizures: a randomized active-control trial, *Neurology*, **51**, 48–55.

Hanna, G.L., Yuwiler, A. and Cartwell, D.P. (1993) Whole-blood serotonin during clomipramine treatment of juvenile obsessive–compulsive disorder, *Journal of Child and Adolescent Psychopharmacology*, **3**, 223–9.

Harden, C.L., Pulver, M.C., Ravdin, L.D. *et al.* (2000) A pilot study of mood in epilepsy patients treated with vagus nerve stimulation, *Epilepsy and Behavior*, **1**, 93–9.

Hardy, J., Cowburn, R., Barton, A. *et al.* (1987) Glutamate deficits in Alzheimer's disease, *Journal of Neurology, Neurosurgery and Psychiatry*, **50**, 356–9.

Hare, R.D. (1999) Psychopathy as a risk factor for violence, *Psychiatric Quarterly*, **70**, 181–97.

Hariri, A.R., Mattay, V.S., Tessitore, A. *et al.* (2002) Genetic variation and the response of the human amygdale, *Science*, **297**, 400–3.

Harrison, W.M., Cooper, T.B., Stewart, J.W. *et al.* (1984) The tyramine challenge test as a marker for melancholia, *Archives of General Psychiatry*, **41**, 681–5.

Harro, J., Vasar, E. and Bradwejn, J. (1993) CCK in animal and human research on anxiety, *TIPS*, **14**, 244–9.

Hart, S.D. and Hare, R.D. (1997) Psychopathy: assessment and association with criminal conduct. In D.M. Stoff, J. Breiling and M.D. Maser (eds.), *Handbook of Antisocial Behavior*, John Wiley and Sons, New York, NY, pp. 22–35.

Harvey, I., Persand, R., Ron, M.A. *et al.* (1994) Volumetric MRI measurements in bipolars compared with schizophrenics and healthy controls, *Psychological Medicine*, **24**, 1–11.

Hauser, P., Altschuler, L.L., Berrettini, W. *et al.* (1989) Temporal lobe measurement in primary affective disorder by MRI, *Journal of Neuropsychiatry and Clinical Neuroscience*, **1**, 128–34.

Hauser, P., Matochik, J., Altshuler, L.L. *et al.* (2000) MRI-based measurements of temporal lobe and ventricular structures in patients with bipolar I and bipolar II disorders, *Journal of Affective Disorders*, **60**, 25–32.

Hauser, W.A. and Beghi, E. (2008) First seizure definitions and worldwide incidence and mortality, *Epilepsia*, **49**, Suppl. 1, 8–12.

Hayden, E.P. and Nurnberger, J.I., Jr (2006) Molecular genetics of bipolar disorder, *Genes, Brain, and Behavior*, **5**, 85–95.

Hazlett, E.A., Buchsbaum, M.S., Zhang, J. *et al.* (2008) Frontal-striatal-thalamic mediodorsal nucleus dysfunction in schizophrenia-spectrum patients during sensorimotor gating, *Neuroimage*, **42**, 1164–77.

Healy, D., Carney, P.A. and Leonard, B.E. (1983) Monoamine related markers of depression: changes following treatment, *Journal of Psychiatric Research*, **17**, 251–60.

Heath, R.G. (1962) Common characteristics of epilepsy and schizophrenia, *American Journal of Psychiatry*, **118**, 1013–26.

Heath, R.G. (1972) Pleasure and brain activity in man, *Journal of Nervous and Mental Diseases*, **154**, 3–18.

Heath, R.G. (1982) Psychosis and epilepsy: similarities and differences in the anatomic–physiologic substrate. In W.P. Koella and M.R. Trimble (eds.), *Temporal Lobe Epilepsy, Mania and Schizophrenia and the Limbic System*, Karger, Basle, pp. 106–16.

Heath, R.G., Dempesy, C.W., Fontana, C.J. *et al.* (1978) Cerebellar stimulation: effects on septal region, hippocampal and amygdala of cats and rats. *Biological Psychiatry*, **13**, 501–29.

Heimer, L. and Larsson, E. (1966) Impairment of mating behaviour in male rats following lesions in the pre-optic and anterior hypothalamic continuum, *Brain Research*, **3**, 248–63.

Heimer, L., van Hoesen, G.W., Trimble, M. *et al.* (2007) *Anatomy of Neuropsychiatry*, Academic Press, San Diego, CA.

Heinz, A., Braus, D.F., Smolka, M.N. *et al.* (2005) Amygdala pre-frontal coupling depends on a genetic variation of the serotonin transporter, *Nature Neuroscience*, **8**, 20–1.

Helmberg, G. and Gershon, S. (1961) Autonomic and psychic effects of yohimbine, *Psychopharmacologia*, **2**, 93–106.

Helmers, S.L., Wheless, J.W., Frost, M. *et al.* (2001) Vagus nerve stimulation therapy in pediatric patients with refractory epilepsy: retrospective study, *Journal of Child Neurology*, **16**, 843–8.

Helmstaedter, C. (2004) Behavioural and neuropsychological effects of frontal lobe epilepsy. In M.R. Trimble and B. Schmitz (eds.), *The Neuropsychiatry of Epilepsy*, Cambridge University Press, Cambridge, pp. 164–88.

Heninger, G.R., Charney, D.S. and Sternberg, D.E. (1984) Serotinergic function in depression, *Archives of General Psychiatry*, **41**, 398–402.

Henquet, C., di Forti, M., Morrison, P. *et al.* (2008) Gene–environment interplay between cannabis and psychosis, *Schizophrenia Bulletin*, **34**, 1111–21.

Henriksen, G.F. (1973) Status epilepticus partialis with fear as a clinical expression: report of a case and ictal EEG findings, *Epilepsia*, **14**, 39–46.

Henry, T.R. (2002) Therapeutic mechanisms of vagus nerve stimulation, *Neurology*, **59**, S15–S20.

Henry, J.A., Alexander, C.A. and Sener, E.K. (1995) Relative mortality from overdose of antidepressants, *British Medical Journal*, **310**, 221–4.

Henry, T.R., Bakay, R.A., Votaw, J.R. *et al.* (1998) Brain blood flow alterations induced by therapeutic vagus nerve stimulation in partial epilepsy: I. acute effects at high and low levels of stimulation, *Epilepsia*, **39**, 983–90.

Henry, T.R., Votaw, J.R., Pennell, P.B. *et al.* (1999) Acute blood flow changes and efficacy of vagus nerve stimulation in partial epilepsy, *Neurology*, **52**, 1166–73.

Herbert, J. (1984) Behaviour and the limbic system with particular reference to sexual and aggressive interactions. In M.R. Trimble and E. Zarifian (eds.), *Psychopharmacology of the Limbic System*, Oxford University Press, Oxford, pp. 51–67.

Herbert, J.D., Hope, D.A. and Bellack, A.S. (1992) Validity of the distinction between generalized social phobia and avoidant personality disorder, *Journal of Abnormal Psychology*, **101**, 332–9.

Hermann, B.P. and Riel, P. (1981) Interictal personality and behavioural traits in temporal lobe and generalized epilepsy, *Cortex*, **17**, 125–8.

Hermann, B.P. and Whitman, S. (1984) Behavioural and personality correlates of epilepsy: a review, methodological critique, and conceptual model, *Psychological Bulletin*, **95**, 451–92.

Hermann, B.P., Dickmen, S., Swartz, M.S. *et al.* (1982) Interictal psychopathology in patients with ictal fear: a quantitative investigation, *Neurology*, **32**, 7–11.

Hermann, B.P., Seidenberg, M., Haltiner, A. *et al.* (1991) Mood state in unilateral temporal lobe epilepsy, *Biological Psychiatry*, **30**, 1205–18.

Hermann, B.P., Wyler, A.R., Blumer, D. *et al.* (1992) Ictal fear, *Neuropsychiatry, Neuropsychology, Behavioural Neurology*, **5**, 205–10.

Herpertz, S.C., Dietrich, T.M., Wenning, B. *et al.* (2001) Evidence of abnormal amygdala functioning in borderline personality disorder: a functional MRI study, *Biological Psychiatry*, **50**, 292–8.

Herwig, U., Padberg, F., Unger, J. *et al.* (2001) Transcranial magnetic stimulation in therapy studies: examination of the reliability of 'standard' coil positioning by neuronavigation, *Biological Psychiatry*, **50**(1), 58–61.

Hesdorffer, D.C., Hauser, W.A., Ludvigsson, P. *et al.* (2006) Depression and attempted suicide as risk factors for incident unprovoked seizures and epilepsy, *Annals of Neurology*, **59**, 35–41.

Heston, L.L. (1966) Psychiatric disorders in foster home reared children of schizophrenic mothers, *British Journal of Psychiatry*, **112**, 819–25.

Heston, L.L., Mastri, A.R., Anderson, E. *et al.* (1981) Dementia of the Alzheimer type, *Archives of General Psychiatry*, **38**, 1085–90.

Hewitt, J.K., Silberg, J.L., Rutter, M. *et al.* (1997) Genetics and developmental psychopathology: 1. phenotypic assessment in the virginia twin study of adolescent behavioral development, *Journal of Child Psychology Psychiatry*, **38**, 943–63.

Higgins, E.S. and George, M.S. (2007) *The Neuroscience of Clinical Psychiatry: The Pathophysiology of Behavior and Mental Illness*, Lippincott, Baltimore, MD.

Higley, J.D., Mehlman, P.T., Taub, D.M. *et al.* (1992) CSF monoamine and adrenal correlates of aggression in free-ranging rhesus monkeys, *Archives of General Psychiatry*, **49**, 436–41.

Hill, D. (1950) Psychiatry. In D. Hill and G. Parr (eds.), *Electroencephalography*, MacDonald, London, pp. 319–63.

Hill, D. (1952) EEG in episodic psychotic and psychopathic behaviour, *Electroencephalography and Clinical Neurophysiology*, **4**, 419–42.

Hillbom, E. (1960) After-effects of brain injuries, *Acta Psychiatrica Neurologica Scandinavica*, **35**, Suppl. 142.

Hiller, W. and Fichter, M.M. (2004) High utilizers of medical care: a crucial subgroup among somatizing patients, *Journal of Psychosomatic Research*, **56**, 437–43.

Hoehn-Saric, R. (1982) Neurotransmitters in anxiety, *Archives of General Psychiatry*, **39**, 735–42.

Hoffart, A., Thornes, K. and Hedley, L.M. (1995) DSM IIR Axis I and II disorders in agoraphobic patients with and without panic disorder before and after psychosocial treatment, *Psychiatry Research*, **56**, 1–9.

Hoffman, R., Boutros, N., Berman, R. *et al.* (1998) Transcranial magnetic stimulation and hallucinated 'voices', *Biological Psychiatry*, **43**, 93–310.

Hoffman, R.E., Boutros, N.N., Hu, S. *et al.* (2000) Transcranial magnetic stimulation and auditory hallucinations in schizophrenia, *Lancet*, **355**, 1073–5.

Hokfelt, T., Johansson, O., Ljungdahl, A. *et al.* (1980) Peptidergic neurones, *Nature*, **284**, 515–21.

Hollander, D. and Strich, S.J. (1970) Atypical Alzheimer's disease with congophilic angiopathy, presenting with dementia of acute onset. In G.E.W. Wolstenholm and M. O'Connor (eds.), *Alzheimer's Disease and Related Conditions*, Ciba Symposium, Churchill, London, pp. 105–24.

Hollister, L.E., Davis, K.L. and Berger, P.A. (1980) Subtypes of depression based on excretion of MHPG and response to nortriptyline, *Archives of General Psychiatry*, **37**, 1107–10.

Holsboer, F., Gerkoen, A., Stall, G.K. *et al.* (1985) ACTH, cortisol and coricosterone output after ovine corticotropin-releasing factor challenge during depression and after recovery, *Biological Psychiatry*, **20**, 276–86.

Holtzheimer, P.E., Russo, J. and Avery, D. (2001) A meta-analysis of repetitive transcranial magnetic stimulation in the treatment of depression, *Psychopharmacology Bulletin*, **35**, 149–69.

Hommer, D., Momenan, R., Kaiser, E. *et al.* (2001) Evidence for a gender-related effect of alcoholism on brain volumes, *American Journal of Psychiatry*, **158**, 198–204.

Howard, R.C., Fenton, G.W. and Fenwick, P.B.C. (1984) The CNV, personality and antisocial behaviour, *British Journal of Psychiatry*, **144**, 463–74.

Howes, O.D. and Kapur, S. (2009) The dopamine hypothesis of schizophrenia: Version III The final common pathway, *Schizophrenia Bulletin*, **35**, 549–62.

Howes, O.D., Montgomery, A.J., Asselin, M.C. *et al.* (2009) Elevated striatal dopamine function linked to prodromal signs of schizophrenia, *Archives of General Psychiatry*, **66**, 13–20.

Hu, X.Z., Rush, A.J., Charney, D. *et al.* (2007) Association between a functional serotonin transporter promoter polymorphism and citalopram treatment in adult outpatients with major depression, *Archives of General Psychiatry*, **64**, 783–92.

Hughes, J.R. and Hermann, B.P. (1984) Evidence for psychopathology in patients with rhythmic mid-temporal discharges, *Biological Psychiatry*, **19**, 1623–34.

Hunter, A.M., Leuchter, A.F., Morgan, M.L. *et al.* (2006) Changes in brain function (quantitative EEG cordance) during placebo lead-in and treatment outcomes in clinical trials for major depression, *American Journal of Psychiatry*, **163**, 1426–32.

Hurwitz, T.A., Wada, J.A., Kosaka, B.D. *et al.* (1985) Cerebral localisation of affect suggested by temporal lobe seizures, *Neurology*, **35**, 1335–7.

Hutchings, B. and Mednick, S.A. (1975) Registered criminality in the adoptive and biological parents of registered male criminal adoptees. In R.R. Fieve, D. Rosenthal and H. Brill (eds.), *Genetic Research in Psychiatry*, Johns Hopkins Press, Baltimore, pp. 105–16.

Hyman, S.E. (2007) The neurobiology of addiction: implications for voluntary control of behavior, *American Journal of Bioethics*, **7**, 8–11.

Hyman, S.E., Malenka, R.C. and Nestler, E.J. (2006) Neural mechanisms of addiction: the role of reward-related learning and memory, *Annual Review of Neuroscience*, **29**, 565–98.

ILAE (1985) Proposal for classification of the epilepsies and epileptic syndromes, *Epilepsia*, **26**, 268–78.

Imbesi, M., Yildiz, S., Dirim Arslan, A. *et al.* (2009) Dopamine receptor-mediated regulation of neuronal 'clock' gene expression, *Neuroscience*, **158**, 537–44.

Imlah, N.W. (1985) An evaluation of alprazolam in the treatment of reactive or neurotic depression, *British Journal of Psychiatry*, **14**, 515–19.

Insel, T.T. (1992) Oxytocin, *Psychoneuroendocrinology*, **17**, 1–35.

Insel, T.R., Gillin, J.C., Moore, A. *et al.* (1982) The sleep of patients with obsessive–compulsive disorder, *Archives of General Psychiatry*, **39**, 1372–7.

Ishizuka, K., Paek, M., Kamiya, A. *et al.* (2006) A review of disrupted-in-schizophrenia-1 (disc1): neurodevelopment, cognition, and mental conditions, *Biological Psychiatry*, **59**, 1189–97.

Ito, Y., Teicher, M.H., Glod, C.A. *et al.* (1993) Increased prevalence of electroencephalographic abnormalities in children with psychological, physical and sexual abuse, *Journal of Neuropsychiatry and Clinical Neuroscience*, **5**, 401–8.

Ito, Y., Teicher, M.H., Glod, C.A. *et al.* (1998) Preliminary evidence for aberrant cortical development in abused children: a quantitative EEG study, *Journal of Neuropsychiatry and Clinical Neuroscience*, **10**, 298–307.

Iversen, S. (1983) Where in the brain do benzodiazepines act? In M.R. Trimble (ed.), *Benzodiazepines Divided*, John Wiley and Sons, Chichester, pp. 167–85.

Iversen, S.D. and Iversen, L. (1981) Substance P: a new CNS transmitter, *Hospital Update*, May, 497–506.

Jacoby, R. and Levy, R. (1980a) Computed tomography in the elderly: II. Senile dementia, *British Journal of Psychiatry*, **136**, 256–69.

Jacoby, R. and Levy, R. (1980b) Computed tomography in the elderly: III. Affective disorder, *British Journal of Psychiatry*, **136**, 270–5.

Jacoby, A., Baker, G.A., Steen, N. *et al.* (1996) The clinical course of epilepsy and its psychosocial correlates: findings from a UK community study, *Epilepsia*, **37**, 148–61.

Jalava, M. and Sillanpaa, M. (1996) Concurrent illnesses in adults with childhood-onset epilepsy: a population based 35 year follow-up study, *Epilepsia*, **37**, 1155–63.

Jang, K.L., Paris, J., Zweig-Frank, H. *et al.* (1998) Twin study of dissociative experience, *Journal of Nervous and Mental Disease*, **186**, 345–51.

Janota, I. (1981) Dementia, deep white matter damage and hypertension: Binswanger's disease, *Psychological Medicine*, **11**, 39–48.

Janowsky, D.S., Risch, S.C., Parker, D. *et al.* (1980) Increased vulnerability to cholinergic stimulation in affective disorder patients, *Psychopharmacology Bulletin*, **16**, 29–31.

Janz, D. (2002) The psychiatry of idiopathic generalized epilepsy. In M.R. Trimble and B. Schmitz (eds.), *The Neuropsychiatry of Epilepsy*, Cambridge University Press, Cambridge, pp. 41–61.

Jaspers, K. (1963) *General Psychopathology* (Translated by J. Hoenig and M.W. Hamilton), Manchester University Press, Manchester.

Jennett, B. (1975) *Epilepsy after Non-missile Head Injuries*, Heinemann, London.

Jennum, P. and Klitgaard, H. (1996) Effect of acute and chronic stimulations on pentylenetetrazole-induced clonic seizures, *Epilepsy Research*, **23**, 115–22.

Jicha, G.A., Parisi, J.E., Dickson, D.W. *et al.* (2008) Age and apoE associations with complex pathologic features in Alzheimer's disease, *Journal of Neurological Science*, **273**, 34–9.

Jimerson, D.C., Insel, T.R., Reus, V.I. *et al.* (1983) Increased plasma MHPG in dexamethasone resistant depressed patients, *Archives of General Psychiatry*, **40**, 173–6.

Jin, Y., Potkin, S.G., Kemp, A.S. *et al.* (2006) Therapeutic effects of individualized alpha frequency transcranial magnetic stimulation (rTMS) on the negative symptoms of schizophrenia, *Schizophrenia Bulletin*, **32**, 556–61.

Johannesson, G., Brun, A., Gustaffson, L. *et al.* (1977) EEG in presenile dementia related to cerebral blood flow and autopsy findings, *Acta Neurologica Scandinavica*, **56**, 89–103.

Johansen-Berg, H., Gutman, D.A., Behrens, T.E. *et al.* (2008) Anatomical connectivity of the subgenual cingulate region targeted with deep brain stimulation for treatment-resistant depression, *Cereb Cortex*, **18**, 1374–83.

Johannsson, O. and Hokfelt, T. (1981) Nucleus accumbens; transmitter neurochemistry with special references to peptide-containing neurones. In R.B. Chronister and J.F. de France (eds.), *The Neurobiology of the Nucleus Accumbens*, Haer Institute, Brunswick, NJ, pp. 147–72.

Johnson, S., Summers, J. and Pridmore, S. (2006) Changes to somatosensory detection and pain thresholds following high frequency repetitive TMS of the motor cortex in individuals suffering from chronic pain, *Pain*, **123**, 187–92.

Johnstone, E.C., Crow, T.J., Frith, C.D. *et al.* (1978) The dementia of dementia preacoc, *Acta Psychiatrica Scandanavica*, **57**, 305–24.

Jokeit, H. and Ebner, A. (2004) The risk of cognitive decline in patients with refractory temporal lobe epilepsy. In M.R. Trimble and B. Schmitz (eds.), *The Neuropsychiatry of Epilepsy*, Cambridge University Press, Cambridge, pp. 152–163.

Jones, E.G. and Powell, T.P.S. (1970) An anatomical study of converging sensory pathways within the cerebral cortex of the monkey, *Brain*, **93**, 793–820.

Jones, J.E., Hermann, B.P., Barry, J.J. *et al.* (2005) Clinical assessment of axis 1 psychiatric morbidity in chronic epilepsy: a multicentre investigation, *Journal of Neuropsychiatry of Clinical Neurosciences*, **17**, 172–9.

Jorge, R., Robinson, R., Arndt, S. *et al.* (1993) Comparison between acute and delayed-onset depression following traumatic brain injury, *Journal of Neuropsychiatry and Clinical Neurosciences*, **5**, 43–9.

Josephs, K.A., Ahlskog, J.E., Parisi, J.E. *et al.* (2009) Rapidly progressive neurodegenerative dementias, *Archives of Neurology*, **66**, 201–7.

Judd, L.L., Risch, C., Parker, D.C. *et al.* (1982) Blunted prolactin response, *Archives of General Psychiatry*, **39**, 1413–16.

Judd, F.K., Norman T.R. and Burrows, G.D. (1986) Pharmacological treatment of panic disorder, *International Clinical Psychopharmacology*, **1**, 3–16.

Juengling, F.D., Schmahl, C., Hesslinger, B. *et al.* (2003) Positron emission tomography in female patients with borderline personality disorder, *Journal of Psychiatric Research*, **37**, 109–15.

Kaabi, B., Gelernter, J., Woods, S.W. *et al.* (2006) Genome scan for loci predisposing to anxiety disorders using a novel multivariate approach: strong evidence for a chromosome 4 risk locus, *American Journal of Human Genetics*, **78**, 543–53.

Kalivas, P.W. and Volkow, N.D. (2005) The neural basis of addiction: a pathology of motivation and choice, *American Journal of Psychiatry*, **162**, 1403–13.

Kallmann, F. (1946) The genetic theory of schizophrenia, *American Journal of Psychiatry*, **103**, 309–22.

Kallmann, F. (1954) Genetic principles in manic–depressive psychosis. In J. Zubin and P. Hoch (eds.), *Depression: Proceedings of the American Psychopathological Association*, Grune and Stratton, New York, NY.

Kanemoto, K. (2002) Post-ictal psychoses revisited. In M.R. Trimble and B. Schmitz (eds.), *The Neuropsychiatry of Epilepsy*, Cambridge University Press, Cambridge, pp. 117–34.

Kanner, A.M. (2006) Depression and epilepsy: a new perspective on two closely related disorders, *Epilepsy Currents*, **6**, 141–6.

Kanner, A.M., Kozac, A.M. and Frey, M. (2000) The use of sertraline in patients with epilepsy: is it safe?, *Epilepsy Behavior*, **1**, 100–5.

Kanner, A.M., Soto, A. and Gross-Kanner, H. (2004) Prevalence and clinical characteristics of postictal psychiatric symptoms in partial epilepsy, *Neurology*, **62**, 708–13.

Karis, D., Fabini, M. and Donchin, E. (1984) P300 and memory, *Cognitive Psychology*, **16**, 177–216.

Karlsgodt, K.H., Sanz, J., van Erp, T.G. *et al.* (2009) Re-evaluating dorsolateral prefrontal cortex activation during working memory in schizophrenia, *Schizophrenia Research*, **108**, 143–50.

Karlsson, P., Farde, L., Halldin, C. *et al.* (2002) PET study of D(1) dopamine receptor binding in neuroleptic-naive patients with schizophrenia, *American Journal of Psychiatry*, **159**, 761–7.

Karlsson, P., Smith, L., Farde, L. *et al.* (1995) Lack of apparent antipsychotic effect of the D1-dopamine receptor antagonist Sch39166 in acutely ill schizophrenic patients, *Psychopharmacology (Berl)*, **121**, 309–16.

Kathol, R.G., Noyes, R., Slyman, D.J. *et al.* (1980) Propranolol in chronic anxiety disorders, *Archives of General Psychiatry*, **37**, 1361–5.

Kathol, R.G., Noyes, R., Slyman, D.J. *et al.* (1981) Propranolol in chronic anxiety disorders. In D.F. Klein and J. Rabkin (eds.), *Anxiety, New Research and Changing Concepts*, Raven Press, New York, NY, pp. 81–93.

Kato, T., Takahashi, S., Shioiri, T. *et al.* (1993) Alterations in brain phosphorous metabolism in bipolar disorder detected by *in vivo* ^{31}P and ^{7}LI MRS, *Journal of Affective Disorders*, **27**, 53–60.

Katona, C.L.E., Hale, A.S., Theodorus, S.L. *et al.* (1985) Which depressives have blunted growth hormone responses to clonadine? *Abstracts, Autumn Quarterly Meeting of the Royal College of Psychiatrists*, 6–7.

Kaufman, R.E., Ostacher, M.J., Marks, E.H. *et al.* (2009) Brain GABA levels in patients with bipolar disorder, *Progress in Neuro-psychopharmacology and Biological Psychiatry*, **33**, 427–34.

Kay, D.W.K., Foster, E.M., McKenchnie, A.A. *et al.* (1970) Mental illness and hospital use in the elderly: a random sample followed up, *Comprehensive Psychiatry*, **11**, 26–35.

Keele, N.B. (2005) The role of serotonin in impulsive and aggressive behaviors associated with epilepsy-like neuronal hyperexcitability in the amygdala, *Epilepsy and Behavior*, **7**, 325–35.

Keitner, G.I., Brown, W.A., Qualls, C.B. *et al.* (1985) Results of DST in psychiatric patients with and without weight loss, *American Journal of Psychiatry*, **142**, 246–8.

Keller, J., Shen, L., Gomez, R.G. *et al.* (2008) Hippocampal and amygdalar volumes in psychotic and nonpsychotic unipolar depression, *American Journal of Psychiatry*, **165**, 872–80.

Kellner, C.H., Jolley, R.R., Holgate, R.C. *et al.* (1991) Brain MRI in obsessive–compulsive disorder, *Psychiatric Research*, **36**, 45–9.

Kendler, K.S. (1983) Overview: a current perspective on twin studies of schizophrenia, *American Journal of Psychiatry*, **140**, 1413–25.

Kendler, K.S. and Robinette, C.D. (1983) Schizophrenia in the National Academy of Sciences, *American Journal of Psychiatry*, **140**, 1557–63.

Kendler, K.S., Gruenberg, A.M. and Strauss, T.S. (1981) An independent analysis of the Danish adoption study of schizophrenia, *Archives of General Psychiatry*, **38**, 973–87.

Kendrick, J.F. and Gibbs, F.A. (1957) Origin, spread and neurosurgical treatment of the psychomotor type of seizure discharge, *Journal of Neurosurgery*, **14**, 270–84.

Kepe V., Huang, S.C., Small, G.W. *et al.* (2006) Visualizing pathology deposits in the living brain of patients with Alzheimer's disease, *Methods Enzymology*, **412**, 144–60.

Keshavan, M.S., Prasad, K.M. and Pearlson, G. (2007) Are brain structural abnormalities useful as endophenotypes in schizophrenia?, *International Review of Psychiatry*, **19**, 397–406.

Kessler, R.C. and Walters, E.E. (1998) Epidemiology of DSM III-R major depression and minor depression among adolescents and young adults in the national comorbidity survey, *Depression and Anxiety*, **7**, 3–14.

Kessler, S.R., Garrett, A., Bender, B. *et al.* (2004) Amygdala and hippocampal volumes in Turner's syndrome: a high resolution MRI study of X-monosomy, *Neuropsychologia*, **42**, 1971–8.

Kessler, R.M., Woodward, N.D., Riccardi, P. *et al.* (2009) Dopamine D2 receptor levels in striatum, thalamus, substantia nigra, limbic regions, and cortex in schizophrenic subjects, *Biological Psychiatry*, **65**(12), 1024–31.

Ketter, T.A., George, M.S., Ring, H.A. *et al.* (1994) Primary mood disorders: structural and resting functional studies, *Psychiatric Annals*, **24**, 637–42.

Kety, S.S. (1983) Mental illness in the biological and adoptive relations of schizophrenic adoptees, *American Journal of Psychiatry*, **140**, 720–7.

Kety, S.S. and Schmidt, C.F. (1948) The nitrous oxide method for the quantitative determination of cerebral blood flow in man: theory procedure and normal values, *Journal of Clinical Investigation*, **27**, 476–83.

Kety, S.S., Wender, P.H., Jacobsen, B. *et al.* (1994) Mental illness in the biological and adoptive relatives of schizophrenic adoptees, *Archives of General Psychiatry*, **51**, 442–55.

Kiehl, K.A., Hare, R.D., Liddle, P.F. *et al.* (1999) Reduced P330 responses in criminal psychopaths during a visual oddball task, *Biological Psychiatry*, **45**, 1498–1507.

Kiehl, K.A., Smith, A.M., Hare, R.D. *et al.* (2000) An event-related potential investigation of response inhibition in schizophrenia and psychopathy, *Biological Psychiatry*, **48**, 210–21.

Kilpatrick, C., Burns, R. and Blumbergs, P.C. (1983) Identical twins with Alzheimer's disease, *Journal of Neurology, Neurosurgery and Psychiatry*, **46**, 421–5.

Kilts, C.D. (1994) Recent pharmacologic advances in antidepressant therapy, *American Journal of Medicine*, **97** (Suppl. 6A), S3–S12.

Kim, B., Choi, E.Y., Kim, C.Y. *et al.* (2008) Could HTR2a T102c and DRD3 SER9gly predict clinical improvement in patients with acutely exacerbated schizophrenia? Results from treatment responses to risperidone in a naturalistic setting, *Hum Psychopharmacol*, **23**, 61–7.

King, J.R. and Hullin, R.P. (1983) Withdrawal symptoms from lithium, *British Journal of Psychiatry*, **143**, 30–5.

Kirov, G., Rujescu, D., Ingason, A. *et al.* (2009) Neurexin 1 (NRXN1) deletions in schizophrenia, *Schizophrenia Bulletin* , **35**, 851–4.

Kishi, T., Kitajima, T., Ikeda, M. *et al.* (2009) Association study of clock gene (clock) and schizophrenia and mood disorders in the Japanese population, *European Archives of Psychiatry and Clinical Neuroscience*, **259**(5), 293–7.

Kline, N.S., Li, C.H., Lehmann, H.E. *et al.* (1977) Beta endorphin induced changes in schizophrenic and depressed patients, *Archives of General Psychiatry*, **34**, 1111–14.

Kling, A., Orbach, J., Schwartz, N.B. *et al.* (1960) Injury to limbic system and associated structures in cats, *Archives of General Psychiatry*, **3**, 391–420.

Klüver, H. and Bucy, P.C. (1939) Preliminary analysis of functions of the temporal lobes in monkeys, *Archives of Neurology*, **42**, 979–1000.

Ko, G.N., Elsworth, J.D., Roth, R.H. *et al.* (1983) Panic induced elevation of plasma MHPG levels in phobic anxious patients, *Archives of General Psychiatry*, **40**, 425–30.

Koenigs, M. and Grafman, J. (2009) Posttraumatic stress disorder: the role of medial prefrontal cortex and amygdala, *Neuroscientist*, **15**(5), 540–8.

Koenigs, M., Huey, E.D., Raymont, V. *et al.* (2008) Focal brain damage protects against posttraumatic stress disorder in combat veterans. *Nature Neuroscience*, **11**, 232–7.

Kolakowska, T., Orr, M., Gelder, M. *et al.* (1979) Clinical significance of plasma drug and prolactin levels during acute chlorpromazine treatment: a replication study, *Psychological Medicine*, **135**, 352–9.

Kolakowska, T., Williams, A.O., Jambor, K. *et al.* (1985) Schizophrenia with good and poor outcome, *British Journal of Psychiatry*, **146**, 348–57.

Kolbinger, H.M., Hoflich, G., Hufnagel, A. *et al.* (1995) Transcranial magnetic stimulation (TMS) in the treatment of major depression: a pilot study, *Human Psychopharmacology*, **10**, 305–10.

Kopecek, M., Sos, P., Brunovsky, M. *et al.* (2007) Can prefrontal theta cordance differentiate between depression recovery and dissimulation?, *Neuroendocrinology Letters*, **28**, 524–6.

Kopelman, M.D. (1985) Multiple memory deficits in Alzheimer-type dementia, *Psychological Medicine*, **15**, 527–41.

Korb, A.S., Cook, I.A., Hunter, A.M. *et al.* (2008) Brain electrical source differences between depressed subjects and healthy controls, *Brain Topogr*, 138–46.

Korf, E.S., Wahlund, L.O., Visser, P.J. *et al.* (2004) Medial temporal lobe atrophy on MRI predicts dementia in patients with mild cognitive impairment, *Neurology*, **63**, 94–100.

Kotler, M., Cohen, H., Segman, R. (1997) Excessive dopamine D4 receptor (DRD4) exon 111 seven repeat allele in opiod dependent subjects, *Molecular Psychiatry*, **2**, 251–4.

Kovelman, J.A. and Scheibel, A.B. (1984) A neurohistological correlate of schizophrenia, *Biological Psychiatry*, **19**, 1601–22.

Kozel, F.A. and George, M.S. (2002) Meta-analysis of left prefrontal repetitive transcranial magnetic stimulation (rTMS) to treat depression, *Journal of Psychiatric Practice*, **8**, 270–5.

Kozel, F.A., Johnson, K.A., Mu, Q. *et al.* (2005) Detecting deception using functional magnetic resonance imaging, *Biological Psychiatry*, **58**, 605–13.

Kozel, F.A., Nahas, Z., Debrux, C. *et al.* (2000) How the distance from coil to cortex relates to age, motor threshold and possibly the antidepressant response to repetitive transcranial magnetic stimulation, *Journal of Neuropsychiatry And Clinical Neurosciences*, **12**, 376–84.

Kraepelin, E. (1904) *Lectures on Clinical Psychiatry*, William Wood, New York, NY.

Kraepelin E (1923) *Psychiatrie: Band 3*, Johann Ambrosius Barth, Leipzig.

Krauthammer, C. and Klerman, G.L. (1978) Secondary mania, *Archives of General Psychiatry*, **35**, 1333–9.

Kringlen, E. (1965) Obsessional neurotics, *British Journal of Psychiatry*, **111**, 709–22.

Krishnamoorthy, E.S., Trimble, M.R. and Blumer, D. (2007) The classification of neuropsychiatric disorders in epilepsy: a proposal by the ILAE Commission on Psychobiology of Epilepsy, *Epilepsy Behavior*, **10**, 349–53.

Krishnan, K.R.R., McDonald, W.M., Escalona, P.R. *et al.* (1992) MRI of the caudate nuclei in depression, *Archives of General Psychiatry*, **49**, 553–7.

Kristensen, O. and Sindrup, E.H. (1978) Psychomotor epilepsy and psychosis, *Acta Neurologica Scandinavica*, **57**, 361–70.

Krystal, J.H., Seibyl, J.P., Price, L.H. *et al.* (1993) M-CPP effects in neuroleptic free schizophrenics, *Archives of General Psychiatry*, **50**, 624–35.

Kugaya, A. and Sanacora, G. (2005) Beyond monoamines: glutamatergic function in mood disorders, *CNS Spectrums*, **10**, 808–19.

Lader, M.H. (1969) Psychophysiological aspects of anxiety. In M.H. Lader (ed.), *Studies of Anxiety*, Headley Bros., Kent, pp. 53–61.

Lake, C.R., Pickar, D., Ziegler, M.G. *et al.* (1982) High plasma norepinephrine levels in patients with major affective disorders, *American Journal of Psychiatry*, **139**, 1315–16.

Lammertsma, A.A., Jones, T., Frackowiak, R.S.J. *et al.* (1981) A theoretical study of the steady-state model for measuring rCBF and oxygen utilisation using oxygen-15, *Journal of Computer Assisted Tomography*, **5**, 544–50.

Landis, S. and Insel, T.R. (2008) The 'neuro' in neurogenetics, *Science*, **322**, 821.

Landolt, H. (1958) Serial electroencephalographic investigations during psychotic episodes in epileptic patients and during schizophrenic attacks. In Lorenz de Haas (ed.), *Lectures on Epilepsy*, Elsevier, London, pp. 91–133.

Lange, J. (1929) *Verbrechen als Schicksal*, Thomas, Leipzig.

Lapierre, D., Braun, C.M. and Hodgkins, S. (1995) Ventral frontal deficits on psychopathy: neuropsychological test findings, *Neuropsychologia*, **33**, 139–51.

Laplane, D., Levasseur, M., Pillon, B., Dubois, B. *et al.* (1989) Obsessive–compulsive and other behavioural changes with bilateral basal ganglia lesions, *Brain*, **112**, 699–725.

Lauterbur, P.C. (1973) Image formation by induced local interactions: examples employing NMR, *Nature*, **242**, 190–1.

Lawrence, K.M., De Paermentier, F., Cheetham, S.C. *et al.* (1990) Brain 5-HT uptake sites labelled with ³H-paroxetine in antidepressant-free depressed suicides, *Brain Research*, **526**, 17–22.

Lawrie, S.M., Hall, J., McIntosh, A.M. *et al.* (2008a) Neuroimaging and molecular genetics of schizophrenia: pathophysiological advances and therapeutic potential, *British Journal of Pharmacology*, **153**, Suppl. 1, S120–4.

Lawrie, S.M., McIntosh, A.M., Hall, J. *et al.* (2008b) Brain structure and function changes during the development of schizophrenia: the evidence from studies of subjects at increased genetic risk, *Schizophrenia Bulletin*, **34**, 330–40.

Lazare, A., Klerman, G.L. and Armor, D.J. (1970) Oral, obsessive and hysterical personality patterns, *Journal of Psychiatric Research*, **7**, 275–90.

Leckman, J.F., Gershon. E.S., Nichols, A.S. *et al.* (1977) Reduced MAO activity in first degree relatives of individuals with bipolar affective disorders, *Archives of General Psychiatry*, **34**, 601–8.

Leckman, J.F., Goodman, W.K., North, W.G. *et al.* (1994) Elevated CSF oxytocin in obsessive–compulsive disorder, *Archives of General Psychiatry*, **51**, 782–92.

LeDoux, J.E. (1992) Emotion and the amygdala. In Aggleton, J.P. (ed.) *The Amygdala*, Wiley Liss, New York, NY, pp. 339–51.

LeDoux, J.E., Iwata, J., Cicchetti, P. *et al.* (1988) Differential projections of the central amygdaloid nucleus mediate autonomic and behavioural correlates of conditioned fear, *Journal of Neuroscience*, **8**, 2517–29.

Lee, H.Y., Kim, D.J., Lee, H.J. *et al.* (2009) No association of serotonin transporter polymorphism (5-HTTVNTR and 5-HTTLPR) with characteristics and treatment response to atypical antipsychotic agents in schizophrenic patients, *Progress in Neuro-psychopharmacol Biological Psychiatry*, **33**, 276–80.

Lefaucheur, J.P. (2004) Transcranial magnetic stimulation in the management of pain, *Supplements to Clinical Neurophysiology*, **57**, 737–48.

Lefaucheur, J.P., Drouot, X. and Nguyen, J.P. (2001) Interventional neurophysiology for pain control: duration of pain relief following repetitive transcranial magnetic stimulation of the motor cortex, *Neurophysiologie Clinique*, **31**, 247–52.

Leonard, B.E. (1992) *Fundamentals of Psychopharmacology*, John Wiley and Sons, Chichester.

Leonard, H.L., Swedo, S.E., Lenane, M.C. *et al.* (1993) A 2–7 year follow up study of 54 obsessive–compulsive children and adolescents, *Archives of General Psychiatry*, **50**, 429–39.

Leonhard, K. (1957) *Aufteilung der Endogenen Psychosen*, Akademie Verlag, Berlin.

Leonhard, K. (1980) Contradictory issues in the origin of schizophrenia, *British Journal of Psychiatry*, **136**, 437–44.

Lenze, E., Cross, D., McKeel, D. *et al.* (1999) White matter hyperintensities and gray matter lesions in physically healthy depressed subjects, *American Journal of Psychiatry*, **156**(10), 1602–7.

Lesch, E.P., Hoh, A., Disselkamp-Tietze, J. *et al.* (1991) 5-HT$_{1a}$ receptor responsivity in obsessive–compulsive disorder, *Archives of General Psychiatry*, **48**, 540–7.

Leweke, F.M., Giuffrida, A., Koethe, D. *et al.* (2007) Anandamide levels in cerebrospinal fluid of first-episode schizophrenic patients: impact of cannabis use, *Schizophrenia Research*, **94**, 29–36.

Lewis, A. (1934) Melancholia: a clinical survey of depressive states, *Journal of Mental Science*, **80**, 277–378.

Lewis, A. (1970) Paranoia and paranoid: a historical perspective, *Psychological Medicine*, **1**, 2–12.

Lewis, A. (1971) 'Endogenous' and 'exogenous': a useful dichotomy, *Psychological Medicine*, **1**, 191–6.

Lewis, D.A. and McChesney, C. (1985) Tritiated imipramine binding distinguishes among subtypes of depression, *Archives of General Psychiatry*, **42**, 485–8.

Lewis, D.A., Campbell, M.J., Foote, S.L. *et al.* (1986) The dopaminergic innervation of primate neocortex is widespread, yet regionally specific, *Society of Biological Psychiatry Abstracts*, Washington, DC, May, p. 1.

Leysen, J. and Niemegeers, C.J.E. (1985) Neuroleptics. In A. Lagtha (ed.), *Handbook of Neurochemistry*, Vol. **9**, Plenum, New York, NY, pp. 331–61.

Li, D. and He, L. (2007) Meta-analysis supports association between serotonin transporter (5-HTT) and suicidal behavior, *Molecular Psychiatry*, **12**, 47–54.

Li, X., Teneback, C.C., Nahas, Z. *et al.* (2002) Lamotrigine inhibits the functional magnetic resonance imaging response to transcranial magnetic stimulation in healthy adults, *Biological Psychiatry*, **51**.

Lichtenstein, P., Yip, B.H., Bjork, C. *et al.* (2009) Common genetic determinants of schizophrenia and bipolar disorder in Swedish families: a population-based study, *Lancet*, **373**, 234–9.

Lidberg, L., Tuck, J.R., Åsberg, M. *et al.* (1985) Homicide, suicide and CSF 5-HIAA, *Acta Psychiatrica Scandinavica*, **71**, 230–6.

Lieberman, J.A., Kane, J.M., Sarantakos, S. *et al.* (1985) Dexamethasone suppression tests in patients with obsessive–compulsive disorder, *American Journal of Psychiatry*, **142**, 747–51.

Lim, M.M., Wang, Z., Olazabel, D.E. *et al.* (2004) Enhanced partner preference in a promiscuous species by manipulating the expression of a single gene, *Nature*, **429**, 754–7.

Lin, P.I. and Mitchell, B.D. (2008) Approaches for unraveling the joint genetic determinants of schizophrenia and bipolar disorder, *Schizophrenia Bulletin*, **34**, 791–7.

Linnoila, M. and Martin, P.R. (1983) Benzodiazepines and alcoholism. In M.R. Trimble (ed.), *Benzodiazepines Divided*, John Wiley and Sons, Chichester, pp. 291–306.

Linnoila, M., Karoum, F., Rosenthal, N. *et al.* (1983a) ECT and lithium carbonate, *Archives of General Psychiatry*, **40**, 677–80.

Linnoila, M., Virkkunen, M., Scheinin, M. *et al.* (1983b) Low CSF 5-HIAA concentration differentiates impulsive from non-impulsive violent behaviour, *Life Science*, **33**, 2609–14.

Lipsey, J.K., Robinson, R.G., Pearlson, G.D. *et al.* (1985) The DST and mood following stroke, *American Journal of Psychiatry*, **142**, 318–22.

Lishman, A. (1987) *Organic Psychiatry*, 2nd edition, Blackwell, Oxford.

Livesley, W.J. and Jang, K.L. (2008) The behavioral genetics of personality disorder, *Annual Review of Clinical Psychology*, **4**, 247–74.

Lloyd, K.G., Parley, I.J., Deck, J.H.N. *et al.* (1974) Serotonin and 5-HIAA in discrete areas of the brainstem of suicide victims and control patients, *Advances in Biochemical Psychopharmacology*, **11**, 387–97.

Lodge, D.J., Behrens, M.M. and Grace, A.A. (2009) A loss of parvalbumin-containing interneurons is associated with diminished oscillatory activity in an animal model of schizophrenia, *The Journal of Neuroscience*, **29**, 2344–54.

Logsdail, S.J. and Toone, B.K. (1988) Post-ictal psychoses: a clinical and phenomenological description, *British Journal of Psychiatry*, **152**, 246–52.

Lomarev, M., Denslow, S., Nahas, Z. *et al.* (2002) Vagus nerve stimulation (VNS) synchronized bold fMRI suggests that VNS in depressed adults has frequency/dose dependent effects, *Journal of Psychiatric Research*, **36**, 219–27.

Lucey, J.V., Butcher, G., Clare, A.W. *et al.* (1993) Elevated growth hormone responses to pyridostigmine in obsessive–compulsive disorder, *American Journal of Psychiatry*, **150**, 961–2.

Luxenberg, J.S., Swedo, S.E., Flament, M.F. *et al.* (1988) Neuroanatomical abnormalities in OCD with quantitative X-ray CT, *American Journal of Psychiatry*, **145**, 1089–93.

Maas, J.W., Fawcett, J.A. and Dekirmenjian, H. (1972) Catecholamine metabolism, depressive illness and drug response, *Archives of General Psychiatry*, **26**, 252–62.

Macciardi, F., Petronis, A., van Tol, H. *et al.* (1994) Analysis of the D$_4$ dopamine receptor gene variant in an Italian schizophrenic kindred, *Archives of General Psychiatry*, **51**, 288–93.

MacDonald, R.T. (1982) Drug treatment of senile dementia. In D. Wheatley (ed.), *Psychopathology of Old Age*, Oxford University Press, Oxford, pp. 113–37.

Mackay, A. (1979) Self poisoning: a complication of epilepsy, *British Journal of Psychiatry*, **134**, 277–82.

MacLean, P.D. (1990) *The Triune Brain in Evolution: Role in Paleocerebral Functions*, Plenum Press, New York, NY.

MacLean, P.D. and Ploog, D.W. (1962) Cerebral representation of penile erection, *Journal of Neurophysiology*, **25**, 29–55.

Mahendra, B. (1984) *Dementia*, MTP Press, Lancaster.

Maher, B.S., Riley, B.P. and Kendler, K.S. (2008) Psychiatric genetics gets a boost, *Nature Genetics*, **40**, 1042–4.

Maheu, F.S., Mazzone, L., Merke, D.P. *et al.* (2008) Altered amygdala and hippocampus function in adolescents with hypercortisolemia: a functional magnetic resonance imaging study of cushing syndrome, *Development And Psychopathology*, **20**, 1177–89.

Maier, M., Mellers, J. and Toone, B. (2000) Schizophrenia, temporal lobe epilepsy and psychosis, *Psychological Medicine*, **30**, 571–80.

Maletsky, B.M. (1978) Seizure duration and clinical effect in ECT, *Comprehensive Psychiatry*, **19**, 541–50.

Malitz, S. and Sackeim, H.A. (eds.), (1986) *ECT*, Annals of the New York Academy of Sciences, p. 462.

Malonek, D. and Grinvald, A. (1996) Interactions between electrical activity and cortical microcirculation revealed by imaging spectroscopy: implications for functional brain mapping, *Science*, **272**, 551–4.

Mamounas, L.A., Blue, M.E., Siuciak, J.A. *et al.* (1995) Brain derived neurotrophic factor promotes the survival and sprouting of serotonergic axons in rat brain, *Journal of Neuroscience*, **15**(2), 7929–39.

Mann, J. (1979) Altered platelet MAO activity in affective disorders, *Psychological Medicine*, **9**, 729–36.

Mann, J.J. and Malone, K.M. (1997) Cerebrospinal fluid amines and higher-lethality suicide attempts in depressed in-patients, *Biological Psychiatry*, **41**, 162–71.

Mann, D.M.A., Lincoln, J., Yates, P.O. *et al.* (1980) Changes in monoamine containing neurones of the human CNS in senile dementia, *British Journal of Psychiatry*, **136**, 533–41.

Mann, J.J., Stanley, M., McBride, A. *et al.* (1986) Increased serotonin-2 and beta adrenergic receptor binding in the frontal cortices of suicidal victims, *Archives of General Psychiatry*, **43**, 954–9.

Mann, J.J., McBride, A., Anderson, G.M. *et al.* (1992) Platelet and whole blood serotonin content in depressed inpatients, *Biological Psychiatry*, **23**, 243–57.

Mann, K., Agartz, I., Harper, C. *et al.* (2001) Neuroimaging in alcoholism: ethanol and brain damage, *Alcoholism: Clinical and Experimental Research*, **25**, S104–9.

Manschreck, T.C. and Ames, D. (1984) Neurological features and psychopathology in schizophrenic disorders, *Biological Psychiatry*, **19**, 703–19.

Mantovani, A., Lisanby, S.H., Pieraccini, F. *et al.* (2006) Repetitive transcranial magnetic stimulation (rTMS) in the treatment of obsessive–compulsive disorder (OCD) and Tourette's syndrome (TS), *International Journal of Neuropsychopharmacology*, **9**, 95–100.

Marangell, L.B., George, M.S., Callahan, A.M. *et al.* (1997) Effects of intrathecal thyrotropin-releasing hormone (protirelin) in refractory depressed patients, *Archives of General Psychiatry*, **54**, 214–22.

Marsden, C.D. and Harrison, M.J.G. (1972) Outcome of investigation of patients with presenile dementia, *British Medical Journal*, **ii**, 249–52.

Martin, J.L.R., Barbanoj, M.J., Schlaepfer, T.E. *et al.* (2002) Transcranial magnetic stimulation for treating depression (Cochrane Review), *The Cochrane Library*, Oxford, Update Software.

Masters, C.L., Harris, J.O., Gajdusek, D.C. *et al.* (1979) Creutzfeldt–Jakob disease: patterns of worldwide occurrence and significance of familial and sporadic clustering, *Annals of Neurology*, **5**, 177–88.

Mathers, C.D. and Loncar, D. (2006) Projections of global mortality and burden of disease from 2002 to 2030, *Plos Medicine*, **3**, E442.

Mathew, R.J., Ho, B.T., Kralik, P. *et al.* (1980a) COMT and catecholamines in anxiety and relaxation, *Psychiatry Research*, **3**, 85–91.

Mathew, R.J., Meyer, J.S., Semchuk, K.M. *et al.* (1980b) CBF in depression, *Lancet*, **i**, 1308.

Mathew, R.J., Ho, B.T., Khan, M.M. *et al.* (1982) True and pseudocholinesterases in depression, *American Journal of Psychiatry*, **139**, 125–7.

Mathew, S.J., Manji, H.K. and Charney, D.S. (2008) Novel drugs and therapeutic targets for severe mood disorders, *Neuropsychopharmacology: Official Publication of the American College of Neuropsychopharmacology*, **33**, 2080–92.

Matsuzaki, S. and Tohyama, M. (2007) Molecular mechanism of schizophrenia with reference to disrupted-in-schizophrenia 1 (Disc1), *Neurochemistry International*, **51**, 165–72.

Mayberg, H.S. (1994) Functional imaging studies in secondary depression, *Psychiatric Annals*, **24**, 643–7.

Mayberg, H.S., Robinson, R.G., Wong, D.F. *et al.* (1988) PET imaging of cortical S2 serotonin receptors after stroke: lateralized changes and relationship to depression, *American Journal of Psychiatry*, **145**(8), 937–43.

Mayberg, H.S., Brannan, S.K., Mahurin, R.K. *et al.* (1997) Cingulate function in depression: a potential predictor of treatment response, *Neuroreport*, **8**, 1057–61.

Mayberg, H.S., Liotti, M., Brannan, S.K. *et al.* (1999) Reciprocal limbic–cortical function and negative mood: converging PET findings in depression and normal sadness, *American Journal of Psychiatry*, **156**(5), 675–82.

Mayberg, H.S., Lozano, A.M., Voon, V. *et al.* (2005) Deep brain stimulation for treatment-resistant depression, *Neuron*, **45**, 651–60.

Mayeux, R., Stern, Y., Cote, L. *et al.* (1984) Altered serotonin metabolism in depressed patients with Parkinson's disease, *Neurology*, **34**, 642–6.

Mazzola-Pomietto, P., Azorin, J.-M., Tranoni, V. *et al.* (1994) Relation between lymphocyte β-adrenergic responsivity and the severity of depressive disorders, *Biological Psychiatry*, **35**, 920–6.

McBride, P.A., Brown, R.P., de Meo, M., Keilp, J. *et al.* (1994) Relationship of platelet 5-HT$_2$ receptor indices to major depressive disorder, personality traits and suicidal behaviour, *Biological Psychiatry*, **35**, 295–308.

McClung, C.A. (2007a) Clock genes and bipolar disorder: implications for therapy, *Pharmacogenomics*, **8**, 1097–100.

McClung, C.A. (2007b) Role for the clock gene in bipolar disorder, *Cold Spring Harbor Symposia on Quantitative Biology*, **72**, 637–44.

McClung, C.A. and Nestler, E.J. (2003) Regulation of gene expression and cocaine reward by creb and deltafosb, *Nature Neuroscience*, **6**, 1208–15.

McConnell, K.A., Nahas, Z., Shastri, A. *et al.* (2001) The transcranial magnetic stimulation motor threshold depends on the distance from coil to underlying cortex: a replication in healthy adults comparing two methods of assessing the distance to cortex, *Biological Psychiatry*, **49**(5), 454–9.

McCreadie, R.G., Dingwall, J.M., Wiles, D.H. *et al.* (1980) Intermittent pimozide versus fluphenazine as maintenance therapy in chronic schizophrenia, *British Journal of Psychiatry*, **137**, 510–17.

McDonald, C. (1969) Clinical heterogeneity in senile dementia, *British Journal of Psychiatry*, **115**, 267–71.

McGowan, P.O., Meaney, M.J. and Szyf, M. (2008) Diet and the epigenetic (re)programming of phenotypic differences in behavior, *Brain Research*, **1237**, 12–24.

McGrath, J., El-Saadi, O., Grim, V. *et al.* (2002) Minor physical anomalies and quantitative measures of the head and face in patients with psychosis, *Archives of General Psychiatry*, **59**, 458–64.

McGuffin, P. (1984) Genetic influences on personality, neurosis and psychosis. In P. McGuffin, M.F. Shanks and R.J. Hodgson (eds.), *The Scientific Principles of Psychopathology*, Grune and Stratton, London, pp. 191–228.

McGuffin, P., Farmer, A.E. and Yonance, A.H. (1981) HLA antigens and subtypes of schizophrenia, *Psychiatry Research*, **5**, 115–22.

McGuffin, P., Farmer, A.E., Gottesman, I.I. *et al.* (1984) Twin concordance for operationally defined schizophrenia, *Archives of General Psychiatry*, **41**, 541–5.

McGuire, P.K., Bench, C.J., Frith, C.D. *et al.* (1994) Functional anatomy of obsessive–compulsive phenomena, *British Journal of Psychiatry*, **164**, 459–68.

McKeon, J., McGuffin, P. and Robinson, P. (1984) Obsessive–compulsive neurosis following head injury: a report of four cases, *British Journal of Psychiatry*, **144**, 190–2.

McNamara, B., Ray, J.L., Arthurs, O.J. *et al.* (2001) Transcranial magnetic stimulation for depression and other psychiatric disorders, *Psychological Medicine*, **31**, 1141–6.

Meador-Woodruff, J.H., Grunhaus, L., Haskett, R.F. *et al.* (1986) Post-dexamethasone cortisol levels in major depressive disorder, *Society of Biological Psychiatry Abstracts*, **177**, Washington, DC, 7–11 May.

Meana, J.J., Barturen, F. and Garcia-Sevilla, J.A. (1992) α2-adrenoceptors in the brain of suicide victims, *Biological Psychiatry*, **31**, 471–90.

Mehlman, P.T., Higley, J.D., Faucher, I. *et al.* (1994) Low CSF 5-HIAA concentrations and severe aggression and impaired impulse control in non-human primates, *American Journal of Psychiatry*, **151**, 1485–91.

Meldrum, B.S. (1976) Neuropathology and pathophysiology. In J. Laidlaw and A. Richens (eds.), *A Textbook of Epilepsy*, Churchill Livingstone, Edinburgh, pp. 314–54.

Meltzer, H.Y. and Fang, V.S. (1983) Cortisol determination and the DST, *Archives of General Psychiatry*, **40**, 501–5.

Meltzer, H.Y. and Maes, M. (1994) Effects of buspirone on plasma prolactin and cortisol levels in major depressed and normal subjects, *Biological Psychiatry*, **35**, 316–23.

Meltzer, H.Y., Ross-Stanton, J. and Schlessinger, S. (1980) Mean serum creatine kinase activity in patients with functional psychoses, *Archives of General Psychiatry*, **37**, 650–5.

Meltzer, H.Y., Arora, R.C., Baber, R. *et al.* (1981) Serotonin uptake in blood platelets of psychiatric patients, *Archives of General Psychiatry*, **38**, 1322–6.

Meltzer, H.Y., Kolakowska, T., Fang, V.S. *et al.* (1984) Growth hormone and prolactin response to apomorphine in schizophrenia and the major affective disorder, *Archives of General Psychiatry*, **41**, 512–19.

Mendez, M.F. and Shapira, J.S. (2008) The spectrum of recurrent thoughts and behaviors in frontotemporal dementia, *CNS Spectrums*, **13**, 202–8.

Mendez, M.F. and Shapira, J.S. (2009) Altered emotional morality in frontotemporal dementia, *Cognitive Neuropsychiatry*, **14**, 165–79.

Mendez, M.F., Cummings, J.L. and Benson, D.F. (1986) Depression in epilepsy: significance and phenomenology, *Archives of Neurology*, **43**, 766–70.

Mendez, M.F., Doss, R.C., Taylor, J.L. *et al.* (1993) Relationship of seizure variables to personality disorders in epilepsy, *Journal of Neuropsychiatry Clinical Neuroscience*, **5**, 283–6.

Mendlewicz, J. and Rainer, J.D. (1977) Adoption-studies supporting genetic transmission in manic depressive illness, *Nature*, **268**, 327–9.

Mendlewicz, J. and Youdim, M.B.H. (1983) L-deprenil: a selective MAOB inhibitor, in the treatment of depression: a double-blind evaluation, *British Journal of Psychiatry*, **142**, 508–11.

Mendlewicz, J., Linkowski, P. and Wilmotte, J. (1980) Linkage between glucose-6-phosphate dehydrogenase deficiency and manic depressive psychosis, *British Journal of Psychiatry*, **137**, 337–42.

Mendlewicz, J., Charles, G. and Franckson, J.M. (1982) The dexamethasone suppression test in affective disorders: relationship to clinical and genetic subgroups, *British Journal of Psychiatry*, **141**, 464–70.

Mendlewicz, J., Kerkhofs, M., Hoffman, G. *et al.* (1984) DST and REM sleep in patients with major depressive disorder, *British Journal of Psychiatry*, **145**, 383–8.

Merikangas, K.R. and Low, N.C. (2005) Genetic epidemiology of anxiety disorders, *Handbook of Experimental Pharmocology*, 163–79.

Merskey, H. and Trimble, M.R. (1979) Personality, sexual adjustment and brain lesions in patients with conversion symptoms, *American Journal of Psychiatry*, **136**, 179–82.

Meyer, M.K., Shea, A., Hendrie, H. C *et al.* (1981) Plasma tryptophan and five other amino acids in depressed and normal subjects, *Archives of General Psychiatry*, **38**, 642–6.

Meyer-Lindenberg, A., Buckholtz, J.W., Kolachana, B. *et al.* (2006) Neural mechanisms of genetic risk for impulsivity and violence in humans, *Proceedings of the National Academic of Science U S A*, **103**, 6269–74.

Miczek, K.A., Altman, J.L., Appel, J.B. *et al.* (1975) Para-chlorophenylalanine, serotonin, and killing behavior, *Pharmacology, Biochemistry and Behavior*, **3**, 355–61.

Middeldorp, C.M., Cath, D.C., van Dyck, R. *et al.* (2005) The co-morbidity of anxiety and depression in the perspective of genetic epidemiology: a review of twin and family studies, *Psychological Medicine*, **35**, 611–24.

Middeldorp, C.M., Cath, D.C. and Boomsma, D.I. (2006) A twin-family study of the association between employment, burnout and anxious depression, *Journal of Affective Disoder*, **90**, 163–9.

Middeldorp, C.M., Hottenga, J.J., Slagboom, P.E. *et al.* (2008) Linkage on chromosome 14 in a genome-wide linkage study of a broad anxiety phenotype, *Molecular Psychiatry*, **13**, 84–9.

Mikkelsen, J.D., Woldbye, D., Kragh, J. *et al.* (1994) ECS increases the expression of neuropeptide Y mRNA in the piriform cortex and the dentate gyrus, *Molecular Brain Research*, **23**, 317–22.

Miller, H.L., Delgado, P.L., Salomon, R.M. *et al.* (1992) Acute tryptophan depletion: a method of studying antidepressant action, *The Journal of Clinical Psychiatry*, **53**, Suppl, 28–35.

Mindham, R.H.S., Steele, C., Folstein, M.F. *et al.* (1985) A comparison of the frequency of major affective disorder in Huntington's disease and Alzheimer's disease, *Journal of Neurology, Neurosurgery and Psychiatry*, **48**, 1172–4.

Mindus, P. and Nyman, H. (1991) Normalisation of personality characteristics in patients with incapacitating anxiety disorders after capsulotomy, *Acta Psychiatrica Scandinavica*, **83**, 283–91.

Minzenberg, M.J., Fan, J., New, A.S. *et al.* (2007) Fronto-limbic dysfunction in response to facial emotion in borderline personality disorder: an event-related fMRI study, *Psychiatry Research*, **155**, 231–43.

Mirow, A.L., Krisatbjanarson, H., Egeland, J.A. *et al.* (1994) A linkage study of distal chromosome 5q and bipolar disorder, *Biological Psychiatry*, **36**, 223–9.

Mitchel, P. (2002) 15 Hz and 1 Hz TMS have different acute effects on cerebral blood flow in depressed patients, *International Journal of Neuropsychopharmacology*, **5**, S7–S.08.

Mitchell-Heggs, N., Kelly, D. and Richardson, A. (1976) Stereotactic limbic leucotomy: a follow up at 16 months, *British Journal of Psychiatry*, **128**, 226–40.

Modai, I., Apter, A., Golomb, A.M. *et al.* (1979) Response to amitriptyline and urinary MHPG in bipolar depressed patients, *Neuropsychobiology*, **5**, 181–4.

Moffitt, T.E., Caspi, A. and Rutter, M. (2005) Strategy for investigating interactions between measured genes and measured environments, *Archives of General Psychiatry*, **62**, 473–81.

Mogenson, G.J., Jones, D.L. and Yim, C.Y. (1980) From motivation to action: functional interface between the limbic system and the motor system, *Progress in Neurobiology*, **14**, 69–97.

Møller, S.E., Kirk, L. and Honoré, P. (1979) Free and total plasma tryptophan in endogenous depression, *Journal of Affective Disorders*, **1**, 69–76.

Money, J. (1975) Human behavioural cytogenetics: review of psychopathology in three syndromes: 47XXY, 47XYY and 45X, *The Journal of Sex Research*, **11**, 181–200.

Moniz, E. (1936) *Tentatives Operatroires dans le Traitment de Certaines Psychoses*, Masson, Paris.

Monroe, R. (1970) *Episodic Behaviour Disorders*, Harvard Press, Harvard.

Montigny, C. de and Blier, P. (1985) Electrophysiological aspects of serotonin neuropharmacology. In A.R. Green (ed.), *Neuropharmacology of Serotonin*, Oxford University Press, Oxford, pp. 181–92.

Moore, C.M., Breeze, J.L., Gruber, S.A. *et al.* (2000) Choline, myo-inositol and mood in bipolar disorder: a proton magnetic resonance spectroscopic imaging study of the anterior cingulate cortex, *Bipolar Disorders*, **2**, 207–16.

Morselli, P.L., Bossi, L., Henry, J.F. *et al.* (1980) On the therapeutic action of SL76002, a new GABA-mimetic agent, *Brain Research Bulletin*, **5**, Suppl. 2, 411–15.

Mosimann, U.P., Marre, S.C., Werlen, S. *et al.* (2002) Antidepressant effects of repetitive transcranial magnetic stimulation in the elderly: correlation between effect size and coil–cortex distance, *Archives of General Psychiatry*, **59**, 560–1.

Mu, Q., Bohning, D.E., Nahas, Z. *et al.* (2004) Acute vagus nerve stimulation using different pulse widths produces varying brain effects, *Biological Psychiatry*, **55**, 816–25.

Mueller, F.S., Heninger, G.R. and MacDonald, R. (1969) Insulin tolerance test in depression, *Archives of General Psychiatry*, **21**, 587.

Muggleton, N.G., Postma, P., Moutsopoulou, K. *et al.* (2006) TMS over right posterior parietal cortex induces neglect in a scene-based frame of reference, *Neuropsychologia*, **44**, 1222–9.

Mula, M., Jauch, R., Cavanna, A. *et al.* (2010) Interictal dysphoric disorder and periictal dysphoric symptoms in patients with epilepsy, *Epilepsia*, [Epub ahead of print].

Mula, M., Trimble, M.R., Thompson, P. *et al.* (2003) Topiramate and word-finding difficulties in patients with epilepsy, *Neurology*, **60**, 1104–7.

Munafo, M.R., Brown, S.M. and Hariri, A.R. (2008) Serotonin transporter (5-HTTLPR) genotype and amygdala activation: a meta-analysis, *Biological Psychiatry*, **63**, 852–7.

Murphy, D.L., Brodie, H.K.H., Goodwin, F.R. *et al.* (1971) Regular induction of hypomania by L-dopa in bipolar manic depressive patients, *Nature*, **229**, 135–6.

Murphy, D.L., Belmaker, R. and Wyatt, R.J. (1974) Monoamine oxidase in schizophrenia and other behavioural disorders, *Journal of Psychiatric Research*, **11**, 221–47.

Murphy, D.L., Belmaker, R.H., Buchsbaum, M. *et al.* (1977) Biogenic amine related enzymes and personality variables in normals, *Psychological Medicine*, **7**, 149–57.

Myslobodsky, M., Mintz, M. and Tomer, R. (1979) Asymmetric reactivities of the brain and components of hemispheric imbalance. In J. Gruzelier and P. Flor-Henry (eds.), *Hemisphere Asymmetries of Function in Psychopathology*, Elsevier, North Holland, pp. 125–48.

Naguib, M. and Levy, R. (1982) Prediction of outcome in senile dementia: a CT study, *British Journal of Psychiatry*, **140**, 263–7.

Nahas, Z., Lomarev, M., Roberts, D.R. *et al.* (2001) Unilateral left prefrontal transcranial magnetic stimulation (TMS) produces intensity-dependent bilateral effects as measured by interleaved bold fMRI, *Biological Psychiatry*, **50**(9), 712–20.

Nahas, Z., Marangell, L.B., Husain, M.M. *et al.* (2005) Two-year outcome of vagus nerve stimulation (VNS) therapy for major depressive episodes, *Journal of Clinical Psychiatry*, **66**, 1097–104.

Nasrallah, H.A. (2008) Atypical antipsychotic-induced metabolic side effects: insights from receptor-binding profiles, *Molecular Psychiatry*, **13**, 27–35.

Nasrallah, H.A., McCalley-Whitters, M. and Jacoby, C.G. (1982a) Cortical atrophy in schizophrenia and mania: a comparative CT study, *Journal of Clinical Psychiatry*, **43**, 439–41.

Nasrallah, H.A., McCalley-Whitters, M. and Jacoby, C.G. (1982b) Cerebral ventricular enlargement in young manic males, *Journal of Affective Disorders*, **4**, 15–19.

Nauta, W.J.H. (1964) Some efferent connections of the prefrontal cortex in the monkey. In J.M. Warren and K. Akert (eds.), *The Frontal Granular Cortex and Behaviour*, McGraw Hill, New York, NY, pp. 397–407.

Nauta, W.J.H. (1986) Circuitous connections linking cerebral cortex limbic system and corpus striatum. In B.K. Doane and K.E. Livingstone (eds.), *The Limbic System*, Raven Press, New York, NY, pp. 43–54.

Nauta, W.J.H. and Domesick, V.B. (1982) Neural associations of the limbic system. In A. Beckman (ed.), *The Neural Basis of Behaviour*, Spectrum Inc., New York, NY, pp. 175–206.

Naylor, G.J., McNamee, H.B. and Moody, J.P. (1970) Erythrocyte sodium and potassium in depressive illness, *Journal of Psychosomatic Research*, **14**, 173–7.

Naylor, G.J., Dick, D.A.T. and Dick, E.G. (1976) Erythrocyte membrane cation carrier, relapse rate of manic depressive illness and response to lithium, *Psychological Medicine*, **6**, 257–63.

Naylor, G.J., Smith, A.H.W., Bryce-Smith, D. *et al.* (1984) Tissue vanadium levels in manic depressive illness, *Psychological Medicine*, **14**, 767–72.

Neal, J.B. (1942) *Encephalitis*, H.K. Lewis, London.

Neary, D., Snowden, J.S., North, B. *et al.* (1988) Dementia of the frontal lobe type, *Journal of Neurology, Neurosurgery and Psychiatry*, **51**, 353–61.

Nemeroff, C.B., Krishnan, K.C.R., Reed, D. *et al.* (1992) Adrenal gland enlargement in major depression: a CT study, *Archives of General Psychiatry*, **49**, 384–7.

Nemeroff, C.B., Mayberg, H.S., Krahl, S.E. *et al.* (2006) VNS therapy in treatment-resistant depression: clinical evidence and putative neurobiological mechanisms, *Neuropsychopharmacology*, **31**, 1345–55.

Nesse, R.M., Cameron, O.G., Curtis, G.C. *et al.* (1984) Noradrenergic function in patients with anxiety, *Archives of General Psychiatry*, **41**, 771–6.

Neumann, C.S., Hare, R.D. and Newman, J.P. (2007) The super-ordinate nature of the psychopathy checklist-revised, *Journal of Personality Disorder*, **21**, 102–17.

Neumeister, A., Hu, X.Z., Luckenbaugh, D.A. *et al.* (2006) Differential effects of 5-HTTLPR genotypes on the behavioral and neural responses to tryptophan depletion in patients with major depression and controls, *Archives of General Psychiatry*, **63**, 978–86.

Newmark, M.E. and Penry, J.K. (1980) *Genetics of Epilepsy: A Review*, Raven Press, New York, NY.

Ni, X., Chan, K., Bulgin, N. *et al.* (2006) Association between serotonin transporter gene and borderline personality disorder, *Journal of Psychiatric Research*, **40**, 448–53.

Ni, X., Sicard, T., Bulgin, N. *et al.* (2007) Monoamine oxidase a gene is associated with borderline personality disorder, *Psychiatric Genetics*, **17**, 153–7.

Ni, X., Chan, D., Chan, K. *et al.* (2009) Serotonin genes and gene–gene interactions in borderline personality disorder in a matched case-control study, *Progress in Neuro-Psychopharmacology and Biological Psychiatry* , **33**, 128–33.

Nielsen, H. and Kristensen, O. (1981) Personality correlates of sphenoidal EEG foci in temporal lobe epilepsy, *Acta Neurologica Scandinavica*, **64**, 289–300.

Nielsen, D.A., Goldman, D., Virkkunen, M. *et al.* (1994) Suicidality and 5-HIAA concentration associated with tryptophan hydrolase polymorphism, *Archives of General Psychiatry*, **51**, 34–8.

Nieuwenhuys, R. (1996) The greater limbic system, the emotional motor system and the brain. In H.J. Groenewegen, R. Bandler, C.B. Saper (eds.), *The Emotional Motor System*, Elsevier, Amsterdam.

Ninan, P.T., van Kammen, D.P., Scheinin, M. *et al.* (1984) CSF 5-HIAA levels in suicidal schizophrenic patients, *American Journal of Psychiatry*, **141**, 566–9.

Nobler, M.S. and Sackeim, H.A. (1993) ECT stimulus dosing. In C.E. Coffey (ed.), *The Clinical Science of ECT*, APA Press, Washington, DC, pp. 229–52.

Nobler, M.S., Sackeim, H.A., Prohovnik, I. *et al.* (1994) Regional cerebral blood flow in mood disorders: III. Treatment and clinical response. *Archives of General Psychiatry*, **51**, 884–97.

Nobler, M.S., Roose, S.P., Prohovnik, I. *et al.* (2000) Regional cerebral blood flow in mood disorders. V: Effects of antidepressant medication in late-life depression, *American Journal of Geriatric Psychiatry*, **8**, 289–96.

Nobler, M.S., Oquendo, M.A., Kegeles, L.S. *et al.* (2001) Decreased regional brain metabolism after ECT, *American Journal of Psychiatry*, **158**, 305–8.

Nordstrom, A.-L., Farde, L., Wiesel, F.A. *et al.* (1993) Central D_2-dopamine receptor occupancy in relation to antipsychotic drug effects, *Biological Psychiatry*, **33**, 227–36.

Norton, N., Williams, H.J. and Owen, M.J. (2006) An update on the genetics of schizophrenia, *Current Opinion in Psychiatry*, **19**, 158–64.

Nothen, M.M., Erdmann, J., Korner, J. *et al.* (1992) Lack of association between dopamine D_1 and D_2 receptor genes and bipolar affective disorder, *American Journal of Psychiatry*, **149**, 199–201.

Nudmamud-Thanoi, S., Piyabhan, P., Harte, M.K. *et al.* (2007) Deficits of neuronal glutamatergic markers in the caudate nucleus in schizophrenia, *Journal of Neural Transmission*, Suppl., 281–5.

Nuechterlein, K.H., Luck, S.J., Lustig, C. *et al.* (2009) CNTRICS final task selection: control of attention, *Schizophrenia Bulletin*, **35**, 182–96.

Nutt, D.J. and Glue, P. (1993) The neurobiology of ECT animal studies. In C.E. Coffey (ed.), *The Clinical Science of ECT*, APA Press, Washington, DC, pp. 213–35.

Nutt, D. and Lawson, C. (1992) Panic attacks, *British Journal of Psychiatry*, **160**, 154–64.

Nyback, H., Walters, J.R., Aghajanian, G.K. *et al.* (1975) Tricyclic antidepressants: effect on the firing rate of noradrenergic neurones, *European Journal of Pharmacology*, **32**, 302–12.

O'Donoghue, M.F., Goodridge, D.M., Redhead, K. *et al.* (1999) Assessing the psychosocial consequences of epilepsy: a community-based study, *Br J Gen Pract*, **49**, 211–14.

O'Donovan, M.C., Craddock, N., Norton, N. *et al.* (2008) Identification of loci associated with schizophrenia by genome-wide association and follow-up, *Nature Genetics*, **40**, 1053–5.

O'Keefe, J. and Nadel, L. (1978) *The Hippocampus as a Cognitive Map*, Oxford University Press, Oxford.

Olajide, D. and Lader, M. (1984) Depression following withdrawal from long-term benzodiazepine use: a report of four cases, *Psychological Medicine*, **14**, 937–40.

Olds, J. and Milner, P. (1954) Positive reinforcement produced by electrical stimulation of septal area and other regions of rat brain, *Journal of Comparative and Physiological Psychology*, **47**, 419–27.

Onyike, C.U., Sheppard, J.M., Tschanz, J.T. *et al.* (2007) Epidemiology of apathy in older adults: the Cache County study, *American Journal of Geriatric Psychiatry*, **15**, 365–75.

O'Reardon, J.P., Solvason, H.B., Janicak, P.G. *et al.* (2007) Efficacy and safety of transcranial magnetic stimulation in the acute treatment of major depression: a multi-site randomized controlled trial, *Biological Psychiatry*, **62**, 1208–16.

Oreland, L., von Knorring, L., von Knorring, A.L. *et al.* (1984) Studies on the connection between alcoholism and low platelet MAO. In S. Parvez *et al.* (eds.), *Alcohol, Nutrition and the Nervous System*, International Science Press, Utrecht.

Otterson, O.P. (1981) Afferent connection to the amygdaloid complex of the rat with some observations in the cat: III. Afferents from lower brainstem, *Journal of Comparative Neurology*, **202**, 335.

Ottosson, J.O. (1960) Experimental studies in the mode of action of ECT, *Acta Psychiatrica Scandinavica*, **35**, Suppl. 135, 1–141.

Owen, F., Bourne, R.C., Crow, T.J. *et al.* (1981) Platelet MAO in acute schizophrenia: relationship to symptomatology and neuroleptic medication, *British Journal of Psychiatry*, **139**, 16–22.

Owens, D.G. and Johnstone, E.C. (2006) Precursors and prodromata of schizophrenia: findings from the Edinburgh high risk study and their literature context, *Psychological Medicine*, **36**, 1501–14.

Owens, D.G.C., Johnstone, E.C., Crow, T.J. *et al.* (1985) Lateral ventricular size in schizophrenia: relationship to the disease process and its clinical manifestations, *Psychological Medicine*, **15**, 27–41.

Ozaki, N., Rosenthal, N.E., Mazzola, P. *et al.* (1994) Platelet paroxetine binding, 5-HT-stimulated Ca^{++} response, and 5-HT content in winter seasonal affective disorder, *Biological Psychiatry*, **36**, 458–66.

Padberg, F., Zwanzger, P., Keck, M.E., *et al.* (2002) Repetitive transcranial magnetic stimulation (rTMS) in major depression: relation between efficacy and stimulation intensity, *Neuropsychopharmacology*, **27**, 638–45.

Palmini, A. and Gloor, P. (1992) The localising value of auras in partial seizures, *Neurology*, **42**, 801–8.

Palomino, A., Gonzalez-Pinto, A., Aldama, A. *et al.* (2007) Decreased levels of plasma glutamate in patients with first-episode schizophrenia and bipolar disorder, *Schizophrenia Research*, **95**, 174–8.

Pandey, G.N., Dysken, M.W., Garter, D.L. *et al.* (1979) Beta adrenergic receptor function in affective illness, *American Journal of Psychiatry*, **136**, 675–8.

Pandey, S.C., Kim, S.W., Davis, J. *et al.* (1993) Platelet S_2 receptors in obsessive–compulsive disorder, *Biological Psychiatry*, **37**, 367–72.

Papp, L.A., Klein, D.F. and Gorman, J.M. (1993) Carbon dioxide hypersensitivity, hyperventilation, and panic disorder, *American Journal of Psychiatry*, **150**(8), 1149–57.

Pare, C.M.B. (1985) The present state of MAOI, *British Journal of Psychiatry*, **146**, 576–84.

Parent, C.I. and Meaney, M.J. (2008) The influence of natural variations in maternal care on play fighting in the rat, *Developmental Psychobiology*, **50**, 767–76.

Paterson, A.D., Sunohara, G.A. and Kennedy, J.L. (1999) Dopamine D4 receptor gene: novelty or nonsense?, *Neuropsychopharmacology*, **21**, 3–16.

Paul, M.I., Cramer, H. and Bunney, W.E. (1971a) Urinary adenosine 3,5 monophosphate in the switch process from depression to mania, *Science*, **171**, 300–5.

Paul, M.I., Cramer, H. and Goodwin, F.K. (1971b) Urinary cyclic AMP excretion in depression and mania, *Archives of General Psychiatry*, **24**, 327–33.

Paus, T., Castro-Alamancos, M.A. and Petrides, M. (2001) Cortico–cortical connectivity of the human mid-dorsolateral frontal cortex and its modulation by repetitive transcranial magnetic stimulation, *European Journal of Neuroscience*, **14**, 1405–11.

Paykel, E.S. and Hollyman, J.A. (1984) Life events and depression: a psychiatric view, *Trends in Neurosciences*, **7**, 475–80.

Pearlson, G.D. and Verloff, A.E. (1981) CT scan changes in manic-depressive illness, *Lancet*, **ii**, 470.

Pearlson, G.D., Wong, D.F., Tune, L.E. *et al.* (1995) *In vivo* D_2 dopamine receptor density in psychotic and non-psychotic patients with bipolar disorder, *Archives of General Psychiatry*, **52**, 471–7.

Penry, J.K. and Dean, J.C. (1990) Prevention of intractable partial seizures by intermittent vagal nerve stimulation in humans: preliminary results, *Epilepsy*, **31**, S40–3.

Peralta, V. and Cuesta, M.J. (1999) Dimensional structure of psychotic symptoms: an item level analysis of SAPS and SANS symptoms in psychotic disorders, *Schizophrenia Pesearch*, **38**, 13–26.

Perez, M.M. and Trimble, M.R. (1980) Epileptic psychosis: diagnostic comparison with process schizophrenia, *British Journal of Psychiatry*, **137**, 245–9.

Perris, C. (1974) A study of cycloid psychosis, *Acta Psychiatrica Scandinavica*, Suppl., 253.

Perris, H., von Knorring, L., Oreland, L. *et al.* (1984) Life events and biological vulnerability, *Psychiatry Research*, **12**, 111–20.

Perry, E.K. and Perry, R.H. (1980) The cholinergic system in Alzheimer's disease. In P.J. Roberts (ed.), *Biochemistry of Dementia*, John Wiley and Sons, Chichester, pp. 135–83.

Perry, B.D., Southwick, S.M., Yehuda, R. *et al.* (1990) Adrenergic receptor regulation in post-traumatic stress disorder. In E.L. Giller (ed.), *Biological Assessment and Treatment of PTSD*, APA Press, Washington, DC, pp. 84–114.

Petrides, G., Fink, M., Husain, M.M. *et al.* (2001) ECT remission rates in psychotic versus nonpsychotic depressed patients: a report from core, *Journal of ECT*, **17**, 244–53.

Pezawas, L., Meyer-Lindenberg, A., Drabant, E.M. *et al.* (2005) 5-HTTLRP polymorphism impacts human cingulate-amygdala interactions: a genetic susceptibility mechanism for depression, *Nature Neuroscience*, **8**, 828–34.

Picard, F. and Brodtkorb, E. (2007) Familial frontal lobe epilpesies. In J. Engel and T. Pedley (eds.), *Epilepsy: A Comprehensive Textbook*, 2nd edition, Lippincott Williams & Wilkins, New York, NY, pp. 2495–502.

Pickar, D., Labarca, T., Linnoila, M. *et al.* (1984) Neuroleptic induced decrease in plasma HVA and antipsychotic activity in schizophrenic patients, *Science*, **225**, 954–6.

Pickar, D., Woen, R.R., Litman, R.E. *et al.* (1992) Clinical and biologic response to clozapine in patients with schizophrenia, *Archives of General Psychiatry*, **49**, 345–53.

Pillmann, E., Rohde, A., Ullrich, S. *et al.* (1999) Violence, criminal behaviour, and the EEG: significance of left hemisphere focal abnormalities, *Journal of Neuropsychiatry and Clinical Neuroscience*, **11**, 454–7.

Pilowsky, L.S., Costa, D.C., Ell, P.J. *et al.* (1992) Clozapine, SPET and D_2 dopamine receptor blockade hypothesis of schizophrenia, *Lancet*, **340**, 199–202.

Pisani, F., Narbone, M.C., Fazio, A. *et al.* (1984) Increased serum carbamazepine levels with viloxazine in epileptic patients, *Epilepsia*, **25**, 482–3.

Pitts, F. and McClure, J.N. (1967) Lactate metabolism in anxiety neurosis, *New England Journal of Medicine*, **277**, 1329–36.

Pope, A. and Keck, M.E. (2001) TMS as a therapeutic tool in psychiatry: what do we know about neurobiological mechanisms?, *Journal of Psychiatric Research*, **35**, 193–215.

Porges, S.W. (1995) Orienting in a defensive world: mammalian modifications of our evolutionary heritage: a polyvagal theory, *Psychophysiology*, **32**, 301–18.

Porges, S.W. (2007) The polyvagal perspective, *Biological Psychology*, **74**, 116–43.

Porteous, D. (2008) Genetic causality in schizophrenia and bipolar disorder: out with the old and in with the new, *Current Opinion in Genetics and Development*, **18**, 229–34.

Post, R.M. and Goodwin, F.K. (1975) Time dependent effects of phenothiazines on dopamine turnover in psychiatric patients, *Science*, **190**, 488–9.

Post, R.M. and Goodwin, F.K. (1978) Approaches to brain amines in psychiatric patients, *Handbook of Psychopharmacology*, **13**, 147–85.

Post, R.M. and Uhde, T.W. (1986) Anticonvulsants in nonepileptic psychosis. In M.R. Trimble and T.G. Bolwig (eds.), *Aspects of Epilepsy and Psychiatry*, John Wiley and Sons, Chichester, pp. 177–212.

Post, R.M., Gordon, E.K., Goodwin, F.K. *et al.* (1973) Central norepinephrine metabolism in affective illness: MHPG in the CSF, *Science*, **179**, 1002–3.

Post, R.M., Jimerson, D.C., Ballenger, J.C. *et al.* (1985) CSF norepinephrine and its metabolites in manic depressive illness. In R.M. Post and J.C. Ballenger (eds.), *Neurobiology of Mood Disorders*, Williams and Wilkins, Baltimore, pp. 539–51.

Post, R.M., Rubinow, D.R., Uhde, T.W. *et al.* (1986) Dopaminergic effects of carbamazepine, *Archives of General Psychiatry*, **43**, 392–6.

Prange, A., Wilson, I., Lynn, C.W. *et al.* (1974) L-tryptophan in mania: contribution to a permissive hypothesis of affective disorder, *Archives of General Psychiatry*, **30**, 52–62.

Prata, D.P., Mechelli, A., Fu, C.H. *et al.* (2008a) Effect of disrupted-in-schizophrenia-1 on pre-frontal cortical function, *Molecular Psychiatry*, **13**, 915–7.

Prata, D.P., Mechelli, A., Fu, C.H. *et al.* (2008b) The Disc1 Ser704Cys polymorphism is associated with prefrontal function in healthy individuals, *Molecular Psychiatry*, **13**, 909.

Preece, N.A., Jackson, G.D., Houseman, J.A. *et al.* (1994) NMR detection of elevated cortical GABA in the vigabatrin-treated rat *in vivo*, *Epilepsia*, **35**, 431–6.

Preter, M. and Klein, D.F. (2008) Panic, suffocation false alarms, separation anxiety and endogenous opioids, *Progress in Neuropscholopharmacol and Biological Psychiatry*, **32**, 603–12.

Price, J. (1968) The genetics of depressive disorder. In A. Coppen and A. Walk (eds.), *British Journal of Psychiatry Special Publication*, No. 2, pp. 37–54.

Price, J.L. (1981) The efferent projections of the amygdaloid complex in the rat, cat and monkey. In Y. Ben-Ari (ed.), *The Amygdaloid Complex*, Elsevier, North Holland, pp. 121–32.

Pridmore, S. (2000) Substitution of rapid transcranial magnetic stimulation treatments for electro-convulsive therapy treatments in a course of electroconvulsive therapy, *Depress Anxiety*, **12**(3), 118–23.

Pridmore, S. and Oberoi, G. (2000) Transcranial magnetic stimulation applications and potential use in chronic pain: studies in waiting, *Journal of the Neurological Sciences*, **182**, 1–4.

Procci, W.R. (1976) Schizoaffective psychosis: fact or fiction, *Archives of General Psychiatry*, **33**, 1167–78.

Prusiner, S.B. (1987) Prions and neurodegenerative disease, *New England Journal of Medicine*, **317**, 1571–81.

Qin, P., Xu, H., Laursen, T.M. *et al.* (2005) Risk for schizophrenia and schizophrenia-like psychosis among patients with epilepsy: population based cohort study, *British Medical Journal*, **331**, 23.

Quednow, B.B., Jessen, F., Kuhn, K.U. *et al.* (2006) Memory deficits in abstinent MDMA (ecstasy) users: neuropsychological evidence of frontal dysfunction, *Journal of Psychopharmacol*, **20**, 373–84.

Quednow, B.B., Kuhn, K.U., Hoppe, C. *et al.* (2007) Elevated impulsivity and impaired decision-making cognition in heavy users of MDMA ('ecstasy'), *Psychopharmacology (Berl)*, **189**, 517–30.

Quiske, A., Helmstaedter, C., Lux, S. *et al.* (2000) Depression in patients with temporal lobe epilepsy is related to mesial temporal sclerosis, *Epilepsy Research*, **39**, 121–5.

Rabkin, J.G., Steward, J. and Klein, D.F. (1985) Overview on the relevance of the DST to differential diagnosis. In R.M.A. Hirschfeld (ed.), *Clinical Utility of the Dexamethasone Suppression Test*, NIH, MD, pp. 12–33.

Raine, A. and Yang, Y. (2006) Neural foundations to moral reasoning and antisocial behavior, *Social and Affective Neuroscience*, **1**, 203–13.

Raine, A., Venables, P.H. and Williams, M. (1990) Relationships between central and autonomic measures of arousal at age 15 years and criminality at age 24 years, *Archives of General Psychiatry*, **47**, 1003–7.

Raine, A., Buchsbaum, M.S., Stanley, J. *et al.* (1994) Selective reductions in prefrontal glucose metabolism in murderers, *Biological Psychiatry*, **36**, 365–73.

Raine, A., Phil, D., Stoddard, J. *et al.* (1998) Prefrontal glucose deficits in murderers lacking psychosocial deprivation, *Neuropsychiatry Neuropsychology and Behavioural Neurology*, **11**, 1–7.

Raine, A., Lencz, T., Bihrle, S. *et al.* (2000) Reduced prefrontal gray matter volume and reduced autonomic activity in antisocial personality disorder, *Archives of General Psychiatry*, **57**, 119–27.

Raine, A., Lencz, T., Yaralian, P. *et al.* (2002) Prefrontal structural and functional deficits in schizotypal personality disorder, *Schizophrenia Bulletin*, **28**, 501–13.

Raine, A., Lencz, T., Taylor, K. *et al.* (2003) Corpus callosum abnormalities in psychopathic antisocial individuals, *Archives of General Psychiatry*, **60**, 1134–42.

Randrup, A., Munkvad, I., Fog, R. *et al.* (1975) Mania, depression and brain dopamine. In L. Valzelli (ed.), *Current Development in Psychopharmacology*, Vol. **2**, Spectrum Publications, New York, NY, pp. 207–48.

Rangel-Guerra, R.A., Perez-Payan, H., Minkoff, L. *et al.* (1983) NMR in bipolar affective disorders, *American Journal of Neuroradiology*, **4**, 229–32.

Rao, S.M., Devinsky, O., Grafman, J. *et al.* (1992) Viscosity and social cohesion in temporal lobe epilepsy, *Journal of Neurology, Neurosurgery and Psychiatry*, **55**, 149–52.

Rapoport, J.L. (1992) Animal models of obsessive compulsive disorder, *Clinical Neuropharmacol*, **15**, Suppl. 1, Pt A, A261–2.

Rapoport, J.L., Ryland, D.H. and Kriete, M. (1992) Drug treatment of canine acral lick: an animal model of obsessive–compulsive disorder, *Archives of General Psychiatry*, **49**, 517–21.

Rapoport, J., Chavez, A., Greenstein, D. *et al.* (2009) Autism spectrum disorders and childhood-onset schizophrenia: clinical and biological contributions to a relation revisited, *Journal of the American Academy of Child and Adolescent Psychiatry*, **48**, 10–18.

Rauch, S.L., Jenike, M.A., Alpert, N.M. *et al.* (1994) Regional CBF measured during symptom preoccupation in OCD using O^{15}-labelled CO_2 and PET, *Archives of General Psychiatry*, **51**, 62–70.

Rauch, S.L., Savage, C.R., Alpert, N.M. *et al.* (1995) A positron emission tomographic study of simple phobic symptom provocation, *Archives of General Psychiatry*, **52**, 20–8.

Reiman, E.M., Raichle, M.E., Robins, E. *et al.* (1989) Neuroanatomical correlates of a lactate induced anxiety attack, *Archives of General Psychiatry*, **46**, 493–500.

Reisine, T.D. and Bell, G.I. (1993) Molecular biology of opiate receptors, *TINS*, **16**, 506–10.

Reveley, M.A., Glover, V., Sandler, M. *et al.* (1981) Increased platelet MAO activity in affective disorders, *Psychopharmacology*, **73**, 257–60.

Reveley, M.A., Reveley, A.M., Clifford, C.A. *et al.* (1983) Genetics of platelet MAO activity in discordant schizophrenia and normal twins, *British Journal of Psychiatry*, **142**, 560–5.

Reynolds, E.H. (1976) Neurological aspects of folate and vitamin B12 metabolism, *Clinics in Haematology*, **5**, 661–96.

Reynolds, E.H. (1981) Biological factors in psychological disorders associated with epilepsy. In E.H. Reynolds and M.R. Trimble (eds.), *Epilepsy and Psychiatry*, Churchill Livingstone, Edinburgh, pp. 264–90.

Reynolds, G.P. and Harte, M.K. (2007) The neuronal pathology of schizophrenia: molecules and mechanisms, *Biochemical Society Transactions*, **35**, 433–6.

Reynolds, E.H., Carney, M.W.P. and Toone, B.K. (1984) Methylation and mood, *Lancet*, **ii**, 196–7.

Rhodes, R.A., Murthy, N.V., Dresner, M.A. *et al.* (2007) Human 5-HT transporter availability predicts amygdala reactivity *in vivo*, *Journal of Neuroscience*, **27**, 9233–7.

Ribeiro, S., Tandon, R., Greenhaus, L. *et al.* (1993) The DST as a predictor of outcome in depression: a meta analysis, *American Journal of Psychiatry*, **150**, 1618–29.

Riding, B.E.J. and Munroe, A. (1975) Pimozide in monosymptomatic psychosis, *Lancet*, **ii**, 400–1.

Rihmer, Z., Gonda, X., Akiskal, K.K. *et al.* (2007) Affective temperament: a mediating variable between environment and clinical depression?, *Archives of General Psychiatry*, **64**, 1096–7.

Riley, B. and Kendler, K.S. (2006) Molecular genetic studies of schizophrenia, *European Journal of Human Genetics*, **14**, 669–80.

Riley, G.J. and Shaw, D.M. (1976) Total and non-bound tryptophan in unipolar illness, *Lancet*, **ii**, 1249.

Ring, H.A., Trimble, M.R., Costa, D.C. *et al.* (1992) Effect of vigabatrin on striatal dopamine receptors: evidence in humans for interactions of GABA and dopamine systems, *Journal of Neurololgy, Neurosurgery and Psychiatry*, **55**, 758–61.

Ring, H.A., Trimble, M.R., Costa, C.D. *et al.* (1993) Striatal dopamine receptor binding in epileptic psychoses, *Biological Psychiatry*, **35**, 375–80.

Ring, H.A., Bench C., Trimble, M.R. *et al.* (1994) Depression in Parkinson's disease, *British Journal of Psychiatry*, **165**, 333–9.

Robbins, T.W. and Arnsten, A.F. (2009) The neuropsychopharmacology of fronto-executive function: monoaminergic modulation, *Annual Review of Neuroscience*, **32**, 267–87.

Roberts, G.W., Polak, J.M. and Crow, T.J. (1984) Peptide circuitry of the limbic system. In M.R. Trimble and E. Zarifian (eds.), *Psychopharmacology of the Limbic System*, Oxford University Press, Oxford, pp. 226–43.

Roberts, G.W., Done, D.J., Bruton, C. *et al.* (1990) A 'mock up' of schizophrenia, *Biological Psychiatry*, **28**, 127–43.

Roberts, J.K.A. (1984) *Differential Diagnosis in Neuropsychiatry*, John Wiley and Sons, Chichester.

Robertson, M.M. (1986) Ictal and interictal depression in patients with epilepsy. In M.R. Trimble and T. Bolwig (eds.), *Aspects of Epilepsy and Psychiatry*, John Wiley and Sons, Chichester, pp. 211–32.

Robertson, M.M. (1998) Forced normalisation and the aetiology of depression in epilepsy. In M.R. Trimble and B. Schmitz (eds.), *Forced Normalisation and Alternative Psychoses of Epilepsy*, Wrightson Biomedical Publishing, Petersfield, pp. 143–67.

Robertson, M.M. and Trimble, M.R. (1983) Depressive illness in patients with epilepsy: a review, *Epilepsia*, **24**, Suppl. 2, S109–16.

Robertson, M.M., Trimble, M.R. and Townsend, H.R.A. (1987) The phenomenology of depression in epilepsy, *Epilepsia*, **28**, 364–72.

Robinson, R.G. and Szetala, B. (1981) Mood change following left hemisphere brain injury, *Annals of Neurology*, **9**, 447–53.

Robinson, R.G., Starr, L.B. and Price, T.R. (1984) A two year longitudinal study of mood disorders following stroke, *British Journal of Psychiatry*, **144**, 256–62.

Robinson, D., Wu, H., Munne, R.A. *et al.* (1995) Reduced caudate nucleus volume in OCD, *Archives of General Psychiatry*, **52**, 393–8.

Rodin, E. and Schmaltz, S. (1983) Folate levels in epileptic patients. In M. Parsonage *et al.* (eds.), *Advances in Epileptology: The 14th Epilepsy International Symposium*, Raven Press, New York, NY, pp. 143–53.

Rodrigues, S.M., Ledoux, J.E. and Sapolsky, R.M. (2009) The influence of stress hormones on fear circuitry, *Annual Review of Neuroscience*, **32**, 289–313.

Roffman, J.L., Weiss, A.P., Goff, D.C. *et al.* (2006) Neuroimaging-genetic paradigms: a new approach to investigate the pathophysiology and treatment of cognitive deficits in schizophrenia, *Harvard Review Of Psychiatry*, **14**, 78–91.

Rollnik, J.D., Huber, T.J., Mogk, H. *et al.* (2000) High frequency repetitive transcranial magnetic stimulation (rTMS) of the dorsolateral prefrontal cortex in schizophrenic patients, *Neuroreport*, **11**(18), 4013–15.

Rollnik, J.D., Wustefeld, S., Dauper, J. *et al.* (2002) Repetitive transcranial magnetic stimulation for the treatment of chronic pain: a pilot study, *European Neurology*, **48**, 6–10.

Rolls, E.T. (2001) The rules of formation of the olfactory representations found in the orbitofrontal cortex olfactory areas in primates, *Chem Senses*, **26**, 595–604.

Ron, M.A., Acker, W. and Lishman, W.A. (1979) Dementia in chronic alcoholism. In J. Obiols *et al.* (eds.), *Biological Psychiatry Today*, Elsevier, North Holland, pp. 1146–50.

Ross, C.A., Margolis, R.L., Reading, S.A. *et al.* (2006) Neurobiology of schizophrenia, *Neuron*, **52**, 139–53.

Rossor, M.N. (1981) Parkinson's disease and Alzheimer's disease as disorders of the isodendritic core, *British Medical Journal*, **283**(ii), 1588–90.

Rossor, M.N., Iversen, L.L., Mountjoy, C.Q. *et al.* (1980) AVP and ChAT in brains of patients with Alzheimer-type senile dementia, *Lancet*, **ii**, 1367–8.

Rossor, M.N., Iversen, L.L., Reynolds, G.P. *et al.* (1984) Neurochemical characteristics of early and late onset types of Alzheimer's disease, *British Medical Journal*, **288**(i), 961–4.

Rosvold, H.E., Mirsky, A.F. and Pribram, K.H. (1954) Influence of amygdalectomy on social behaviour in monkeys, *Journal of Comparative and Physiological Psychology*, **47**, 173–80.

Rotarska-Jagiela, A., Oertel-Knoechel, V., Demartino, F. *et al.* (2009) Anatomical brain connectivity and positive symptoms of schizophrenia: a diffusion tensor imaging study, *Psychiatry Research*, **174**(1), 9–16.

Roy, A., Pickar, D., Linnoila, M. *et al.* (1985) Plasma norepinephrine levels in affective disorders, *Archives of General Psychiatry*, **42**, 1181–5.

Roy, A., Pickar, D., Douillet, P. *et al.* (1986a) Urinary monoamines and monoamine metabolites in sub-types of unipolar depressive disorder and normal controls, *Psychological Medicine*, **16**, 541–6.

Roy, A., Pickar, D., Linnoila, M. *et al.* (1986b) CSF monoamine and metabolite levels and the DST in depression, *Archives of General Psychiatry*, **43**, 356–60.

Roy, A., Karoum, F. and Pollack, S. (1992) Marked reduction in indices of dopamine metabolism among patients with depression who attempt suicide, *Archives of General Psychiatry*, **49**, 447–50.

Roy-Byrne, P., Uhde, T.W., Gold, P.W. *et al.* (1985a) Neuroendocrine abnormalities in panic disorder, *Psychopharmacology Bulletin*, **21**, 546–50.

Roy-Byrne, P., Bierer, L.M. and Uhde, T.W. (1985b) The DST in panic disorder, *Biological Psychiatry*, **20**, 1237–40.

Rubin, E., Sackhein, H.A., Nobler, M.S. *et al.* (1994) Brain imaging studies of antidepressant treatments, *Psychiatric Annals*, **24**, 653–8.

Rubinow, D.R., Gold, P.W., Post, R.M. *et al.* (1985) Somatostatin in patients with affective illness and normal volunteers. In R.M. Post and J.C. Ballenger (eds.), *Neurobiology of Mood Disorders*, Williams and Wilkins, Baltimore, MD, pp. 369–87.

Ruby, N.F., Hwang, C.E., Wessells, C. *et al.* (2008) Hippocampal-dependent learning requires a functional circadian system, *Proceeding of the national Academic of Sciences' U S A*, **105**(15), 593–8.

Rudorfer, M.V., Hwu, H. and Clayton, P.J. (1982) DST in primary depression: significance of family history and psychosis, *Biological Psychiatry*, **17**, 41–8.

Rudorfer, M.V., Risby, E.D., Hsiao, J.K. *et al.* (1988) ECT alters human monoamines in a different manner from antidepressant drugs, *Psychopharmacology Bulletin*, **24**, 396–9.

Ruocco, A.C. (2005) The neuropsychology of borderline personality disorder: a meta-analysis and review, *Psychiatry Research*, **137**, 191–202.

Ruocco, A.C. *et al.* (2006) Clinical presentation of juvenile Huntington disease, *Arquivos de Neuro-Psiquiatr*, **64**(1), doi: 10.1590/S0004-282X2006000100002.

Rüsch, N., Tebartz van Elst, L., Baeumer, D. *et al.* (2004) Absence of cortical gray matter abnormalities in psychosis of epilepsy: a voxel-based MRI study in patients with temporal lobe epilepsy, *Journal of Neuropsychiatry Clinical neuroscience*, **16**(2), 148–55.

Rush, A.J., Giles, D.E., Roffwarg, H.P. *et al.* (1982) Sleep EEG and DST findings in out patients with unipolar major depressive disorders, *Biological Psychiatry*, **17**, 327–41.

Rush, A.J., George, M.S., Sackeim, H.A. *et al.* (2000) Vagus nerve stimulation (VNS) for treatment-resistant depressions: a multicenter study, *Boilogical Psychiatry*, **47**, 276–86.

Rush, A.J., Marangell, L.B., Sackeim, H.A. *et al.* (2005) Vagus nerve stimulation for treatment-resistant depression: a randomized, controlled acute phase trial, *Biological Psychiatry*, **58**, 347–54.

Rush, A.J., Trivedi, M.H., Wisniewski, S.R. *et al.* (2006) Bupropion-SR, sertraline, or venlafaxine-XR after failure of SSRIs for depression, *New England Journal of Medicine*, **354**, 1231–42.

Rutecki, P. (1990) Anatomical, physiological and theoretical basis for the antiepileptic effect of vagus nerve stimulation, *Epilepsia*, **31**, S1–36.

Rutter, M. (1994) Psychiatric genetics: research challenges and pathways forward, *American Journal of Medical Genetics*, **54**, 185–98.

Rutter, M. and McGuffin, P. (2004) The social, genetic and developmental psychiatry centre: its origins, conception and initial accomplishments, *Psychological Medicine*, **34**, 933–47.

Sabelli, H.C., Fawcett, J., Gusovsky, F. *et al.* (1983) Urinary phenyl acetate: a diagnostic test for depression, *Science*, **220**, 1187–8.

Sabol, S.Z., Nelson, M.L., Fisher, C. *et al.* (1999) A genetic association for cigarette smoking behavior, *Health Psychology*, **18**, 7–13.

Sachar, E.J., Hellman, L., Roffwarg, H. *et al.* (1973) Disrupted 24 hour patterns of cortisol secretion in psychotic depression, *Archives of General Psychiatry*, **28**, 19–24.

Sachdev, P.S., McBride, R., Loo, C.K. *et al.* (2001) Right versus left prefrontal transcranial magnetic stimulation for obsessive–compulsive disorder: a preliminary investigation, *Journal of Clinical Psychiatry*, **62**, 981–4.

Sackeim, H.A., Keilp, J.G., Rush, A.J. *et al.* (2001a) The effects of vagus nerve stimulation on cognitive performance in patients with treatment-resistant depression, *Neuropsychiatry Neuropsychol Behavioral Neurology*, **14**, 53–62.

Sackeim, H.A., Rush, A.J., George, M.S. *et al.* (2001b) Vagus nerve stimulation (VNS) for treatment-resistant depression: efficacy, side effects, and predictors of outcome, *Neuropsychopharmacology*, **25**, 713–28.

Sackeim, H.A., Prudic, J., Nobler, M.S. *et al.* (2008) Effects of pulse width and electrode placement on the efficacy and cognitive effects of electroconvulsive therapy, *Brain Stimulation*, **1**, 71–83.

Sacks, O. (1973) *Awakenings*, Duckworth, London.

Saleem, P.T. (1984) Dexamethasone Suppression Test in depressive illness: its relation to anxiety symptoms, *British Journal of Psychiatry*, **144**, 181–4.

Saletu, B., Grunberger, J. and Rajna, P. (1983) Pharmaco-EEG profiles with antidepressants, *British Journal of Clinical Pharmacology*, **15**, S 369–84.

Salinsky, M.C., Uthman, B.M., Ristanovic, R.K. *et al.* for the Vagus Nerve Stimulation Study Group (1996) Vagus nerve stimulation for the treatment of medically intractable seizures: results of a 1-year open-extension trial, *Archives of Neurology*, **53**, 1176–80.

Sanacora, G., Fenton, L.R., Fasula, M.K. *et al.* (2006) Cortical gamma-aminobutyric acid concentrations in depressed patients receiving cognitive behavioral therapy, *Biological Psychiatry*, **59**, 284–6.

Sanacora, G., Mason, G.F., Rothman, D.L. *et al.* (2002) Increased occipital cortex GABA concentrations in depressed patients after therapy with selective serotonin reuptake inhibitors, *American Journal of Psychiatry*, **159**, 663–5.

Sanacora, G., Zarate, C.A., Krystal, J.H. *et al.* (2008) Targeting the glutamatergic system to develop novel, improved therapeutics for mood disorders, *Nature Reviews: Drug Discovery*, **7**, 426–37.

Sandler, M. (1983) Benzodiazepines: studies on a possible endogenous ligand. In M.R. Trimble (ed.), *Benzodiazepines Divided*, John Wiley and Sons, Chichester, pp. 139–47.

Sandler, M., Bonham Carter, S., Cuthbert, M.F. *et al.* (1975) Is there an increase in monoamine oxidase activity in depressive illness?, *Lancet*, **i**, 1045–8.

Santarelli, L., Saxe, M., Gross, C. *et al.* (2003) Requirement of hippocampal neurogenesis for the behavioral effects of antidepressants, *Science*, **301**, 805–9.

Saper, C. (1996) The role of the cerebral cortex in cerebral expression. In G. Holstege, R. Bandler and C.B. Saper (eds.), *The Emotional Motor System*, Elsevier, Amsterdam.

Sapolsky, R.M. (1996) Why stress is bad for your brain, *Science*, **273**, 749–50.

Sapolsky, R.M., Krey, L.C. and McEwen, B.S. (1985) Prolonged glucocorticoid exposure reduces hippocampal neurone number, *Journal of Neuroscience*, **5**, 1222–7.

Saver, J.L. and Rabin, J. (1997) The neural substrates of religious experience, *Journal of Neuropsychiatry and Clinical Neuroscience*, **9**, 498–510.

Savitz, J., Lucki, I. and Drevets, W.C. (2009) 5-HT(1A) receptor function in major depressive disorder, *Progress Neurobiology*, **88**, 17–31.

Sawyer, C.H. (1957) Triggering of the pituitary by the CNS. In P. Bullock (ed.), *Physiological Triggers*, Waverly Press, Baltimore, MD, pp. 164–74.

Scatton, B. and Zivkovic, B. (1984) Neuroleptics and the limbic system. In M.R. Trimble and E. Zarifian (eds.), *Psychopharmacology of the Limbic System*, Oxford University Press, Oxford, pp. 174–97.

Schaer, M. and Eliez, S. (2007) From genes to brain: understanding brain development in neurogenetic disorders using neuroimaging techniques, *Child Adolescent Psychiatric Clinic of North America*, **16**, 557–79.

Schatzberg, A.F. and Lindley, S. (2008) Glucocorticoid antagonists in neuropsychiatric [corrected] disorders, *European Journal Of Pharmacology*, **583**, 358–64.

Schatzberg, A.F., Rothschild, A.J., Gershon, B. *et al.* (1985) Toward a biochemical classification of depressive disorders, *British Journal of Psychiatry*, **146**, 633–7.

Schmahmann, J.D. (1991) An emerging concept: the cerebellar contribution to higher functions, *Archives of Neurology*, **48**, 1178–87.

Scarpa, A. and Raine, A. (1997) Psychophysiology of anger and violent behavior, *Psychiatric Clinics of North America*, **20**, 375–94.

Scher, M., Krieg, J.N. and Juergens, S. (1983) Trazadone and priapism, *American Journal of Psychiatry*, **140**, 1362–3.

Scher, A.I., Xu, Y., Korf, E.S. *et al.* (2007) Hippocampal shape analysis in Alzheimer's disease: a population-based study, *Neuroimage*, **36**, 8–18.

Schildkraut, J.J. and Kety, S.S. (1967) Biogenic amines and emotion, *Science*, **156**, 21–30.

Schildkraut, J.J., Orsulak, P.J., Schatzberg, A.F. *et al.* (1984) Urinary MHPG in affective disorders. In R.M. Post and J.C. Ballenger (eds.), *Neurobiology of Mood Disorders*, Williams and Wilkins, Baltimore, MD, pp. 519–628.

Schipper, H.M. (2007) The role of biologic markers in the diagnosis of Alzheimer's disease, *Alzheimers Dement*, **3**, 325–332.

Schipper, H.M. (2009) Apolipoprotein E: implications for Alzheimer's Disease neurobiology, epidemiology and risk assessment, Neurobiol Aging (epub ahead of print, PMID: 19482376).

Schmitz, B. and Trimble, M.R. (2007) Psychoses. In P. Engel *et al.*, *Epilepsy: A Comprehnesive Textbook*, 2nd edition, Lippincott Williams & Wilkins, New York, NY.

Schmitz, B. and Wolf, P. (1991) Psychoses in epilepsy. In O. Devinsky and W.H. Theodore (eds.), *Epilepsy and Behaviour*, Wiley-Liss, New York, NY, pp. 97–128.

Schmitz, B. and Wolf, P. (1995) Psychosis with epilepsy: frequency and risk factors, *Journal of Epilepsy*, **8**, 295–305.

Schmitz, B., Moriarty, J., Costa, D.C. *et al.* (1997) Psychiatric profiles and patterns of cerebral blood flow in focal epilepsy: interactions between depression, obsessionality, and perfusion related to the laterality of the epilepsy, *Journal of Neurological Neurosurgery Psychiatry*, **62**, 458–63.

Schmitz, B., Robertson, M. and Trimble, M.R. (1999) Depression and schizophrenia in epilepsy: social and biological risk factors, *Epilepsy Research*, **35**, 59–68.

Schneider, K. (1957) Primary and secondary symptoms in schizophrenia. In S.R. Hirsch and M. Shepherd (eds.), *Themes and Variations in European Psychiatry*, John Wright, Bristol, pp. 40–6.

Schneider, K. (1959) *Clinical Psychopathology* (Translated by M.W. Hamilton and E.W. Anderson), Grune and Stratton, New York, NY.

Schooler, C., Zahn, T.P., Murphy, D.I. *et al.* (1978) Psychological correlates of monoamine oxidase activity in normals, *Journal of Nervous and Mental Disease*, **166**, 177–86.

Schreiner, L. and Kling, A. (1956) Rhinencephalon and behaviour, *American Journal of Psychiatry*, **184**, 486–90.

Schwartz, J.H. (1981) Chemical basis of synaptic transmission. In E.R. Kandel and J.H. Schwartz (eds.), *Principles of Neural Science*, Elsevier, North Holland, pp. 106–20.

Schwartz, M.F., Bauman, J.E. and Masters, W.H. (1982) Hyperprolactinaemia and sexual disorders in men, *Biological Psychiatry*, **17**, 861–76.

Seeman, P. (1992) Dopamine receptor sequences: therapeutic levels of neuroleptics occupy D_2 receptors, clozapine occupies D_4, *Neuropsychopharmacology*, **7**, 261–84.

Severino, G., Manchia, M., Contu, P. *et al.* (2009) Association study in a Sardinian sample between bipolar disorder and the nuclear receptor REV-ERBalpha gene, a critical component of the circadian clock system, *Bipolar Disorders*, **11**, 215–20.

Shagass, C. (1972) *Evoked Brain Potentials in Psychiatry*, Plenum Press, New York, NY.

Shagass, C., Roemer, R.A., Straumanis, J.J. *et al.* (1979) Evoked potential evidence of lateralised hemispheric dysfunction in the psychoses. In J. Gruzelier and P. Flor-Henry (eds.), *Hemisphere Asymmetries of Function in Psychopathology*, Elsevier, North Holland, pp. 293–316.

Shagass, C., Roemer, R.A., Straumanis, J.J. *et al.* (1981) Differentiation of depressive and schizophrenic psychoses by evoked potentials, *Advances in Biological Psychiatry*, **6**, 173–9.

Shah, S.A., Doraiswany, P.M., Hussain, M.M. *et al.* (1992) Posterior fossa abnormalities in major depression, *Acta Psychiatrica Scandinavica*, **85**, 474–9.

Shajahan, P.M., Glabus, M.F., Steele, J.D. *et al.* (2002) Left dorso-lateral repetitive transcranial magnetic stimulation affects cortical excitability and functional connectivity, but does not impair cognition in major depression, *Progress in Neuropsychopharmacology and Biological Psychiatry*, **26**, 945–54.

Shalev, A.Y., Videlock, E.J., Peleg, T. *et al.* (2008) Stress hormones and post-traumatic stress disorder in civilian trauma victims: a longitudinal study: part I. HPA axis responses, *International Journal Neuropsychopharmacol*, **11**, 365–72.

Shane, M.S., Stevens, M., Harenski, C.L. *et al.* (2008) Neural correlates of the processing of another's mistakes: a possible underpinning for social and observational learning, *Neuroimage*, **42**, 450–9.

Shapira, B., Lerer, B., Kindler, S. *et al.* (1992) Enhanced serotonergic responsivity following ECT in patients with major depression, *British Journal of Psychiatry*, **16**, 233–9.

Shapiro, D. (1999) *Neurotic Styles*, New York, NY, Basic Books.

Shaw, D.M., Camps, F.E. and Eccleston, E.G. (1967) 5-hydroxytryptamine in the hind-brains of depressive suicides, *British Journal of Psychiatry*, **113**, 1407–11.

Sheline, Y.I., Sanghavi, M., Mintun, M.A. *et al.* (1999) Depression duration but not age predicts hippocampal volume loss in medically healthy women with recurrent major depression, *Journal of Neuroscience*, **19**, 5034–43.

Shelley, B.P. and Trimble, M.R. (2004) The insular lobe of Reil – its anatamico-functional, behavioural and neuropsychiatric attributes in humans – a review, *World Journal of Biological Psychiatry*, **5**, 176–200.

Shelley, B.P., Trimble, M.R. and Boutros, N.N. (2008) Electroencephalographic cerebral dysrhythmic abnormalities in the trinity of nonepileptic general population, neuropsychiatric, and neurobehavioral disorders, *Journal of Neuropsychiatry of Clinical Neuroscience*, **20**, 7–22.

Shen, D., Liu, D., Liu, H. *et al.* (2004) Automated morphometric study of brain variation in XXY males, *Neuroimage*, **23**, 648–53.

Sher, L., Mann, J.J., Traskman-Bendz, L. *et al.* (2006) Lower cerebrospinal fluid homovanillic acid levels in depressed suicide attempters, *Journal of Affective Disorder*, **90**, 83–9.

Shi, J., Wittke-Thompson, J.K., Badner, J.A. *et al.* (2008) Clock genes may influence bipolar disorder susceptibility and dysfunctional circadian rhythm, *American Journal of Medical Genetics. Part B: Neuropsychiatric Genetics*, **147b**, 1047–55.

Shibasaki, J., Barrett, G., Halliday, E. *et al.* (1980) Components of the movement-related cortical potential and their scalp topography, *Electroencephalography and Clinical Neurophysiology*, **49**, 213–26.

Shields, J. (1954) Personality differences and neurotic traits in normal twin schoolchildren, *Eugenics Review*, **45**, 213–46.

Shields, J. (1962) *Monozygotic Twins Brought Up Apart and Brought Up Together*, Oxford University Press, London.

Shihabuddin, L., Buchsbaum, M.S., Brickman, A.M. *et al.* (2001) Diffusion tensor imaging in Kraepelinian and non-Kraepelinian Schizophrenia, *Biological Psychiatry*, **49**, 19–67.

Shoghi-Jadid, K., Barrio, J.R., Kepe, V. *et al.* (2005) Imaging beta-amyloid fibrils in Alzheimer's disease: a critical analysis through simulation of amyloid fibril polymerization, *Nuclear Medical Biology*, **32**, 337–51.

Shopsin, B., Friedman, E. and Gershon, S. (1976) Parachlorophenylalanine reversal of tranylcypramine effects in depressed patients, *Archives of General Psychiatry*, **33**, 811–19.

Shorvon, S.D. and Reynolds, E.H. (1982) Early prognosis of epilepsy, *British Medical Journal*, **ii**, 1699–701.

Sibley, D.R. and Monsma, F.J. (1992) Molecular biology of dopamine receptors, *TIPS*, **13**, 61–9.

Siegel, A., Edinger, H. and Dotto, M. (1975) Effects of electrical stimulation of the lateral aspects of the pre-frontal cortex upon attack behaviour in cats, *Brain*, **93**, 473–84.

Siegel, B.V.J., Buchsbaum, M.S., Bunney, W.E.J. *et al.* (1993) Cortical-striatal-thalamic circuits and brain glucose metabolic activity in 70 unmedicated male schizophrenic patients, *American Journal of Psychiatry*, **150**, 1325–36.

Siesjo, B.K. (1978) *Brain Energy Metabolism*, John Wiley and Sons, Chichester.

Siever, L.J. and Coursey, R.D. (1985) Biological markers for schizophrenia and the biological high-risk approach, *Journal of Nervous and Mental Disease*, **173**, 4–16.

Siever, L.J. and Uhde, T.W. (1984) New studies and perspectives on the noradrenergic receptor system in depression: effects of the alpha-2 adrenergic agonist clonidine, *Biological Psychiatry*, **19**, 131–56.

Siever, L.J., Insel, T.R., Jimerson, D.C. *et al.* (1983) Growth hormone response to clonidine in obsessive–compulsive patients, *British Journal of Psychiatry*, **142**, 184–7.

Silbersweig, D., Clarkin, J.F., Goldstein, M. *et al.* (2007) Failure of frontolimbic inhibitory function in the context of negative emotion in borderline personality disorder, *American Journal of Psychiatry*, **164**, 1832–41.

Sim, M. (1979) Early diagnosis of Alzheimer's disease. In A. Glen and L.J. Whalley (eds.), *Alzheimer's Disease*, Churchill Livingstone, Edinburgh, pp. 78–85.

Skare, S.S., Dysken, M.W. and Billington, C.J. (1994) A review of the GHRH stimulation test in psychiatry, *Biological Psychiatry*, **36**, 249–65.

Skuse, D. (2006) Genetic influences on the neural basis of social cognition, *Philosophical Transactions of the Royal Society London B Biological Science*, **361**, 2129–41.

Skuse, D.H. (2007) Rethinking the nature of genetic vulnerability to autistic spectrum disorders, *Trends Genet*, **23**, 387–95.

Slade, A.P. and Checkley, S.A. (1980) A neuroendocrine study of the mechanism of action of ECT, *British Journal of Psychiatry*, **137**, 217–21.

Slater, E. and Beard, A.W. (1963) The schizophrenia-like psychoses of epilepsy, *British Journal of Psychiatry*, **109**, 95–150.

Slater, E. and Roth, M. (1960) *Clinical Psychiatry*, 1st edition, Baillière Tindall and Cassell, London.

Slater, E. and Roth, M. (1969) *Clinical Psychiatry*, 3rd edition, Baillière Tindall and Cassell, London.

Small, J.G. (1970) Small sharp spikes in a psychiatric population, *Archives of General Psychiatry*, **22**, 277–84.

Small, J.G., Small, I.F., Milstein, V. *et al.* (1975) Familial associations with EEG variants in manic depressive disease, *Archives of General Psychiatry*, **32**, 43–8.

Small, J.G., Milstein, V., Klapper, M.H. *et al.* (1986) ECT for manic episodes. In S. Malitz and H.A. Sackeim (eds.), *ECT*, Annals of the New York Academy of Science, Vol. **462**, pp. 37–49.

Small, G.W., Ercoli, L.M., Silverman, D.H. *et al.* (2000) Cerebral metabolic and cognitive decline in persons at genetic risk for Alzheimer's disease, *Proceedings of National Academy of Sciences, U S A*, **97**(11), 6037–42.

Smith, D.A. and Lantos, P.L. (1983) A case of combined Pick's disease and Alzheimer's disease, *Journal of Neurology, Neurosurgery and Psychiatry*, **46**, 675–7.

Smolka, M.N., Buhler, M., Schumann, G. *et al.* (2007) Gene–gene effects on central processing of aversive stimuli, *Molecular Psychiatry*, **12**, 307–17.

Smythies, J.R. (1976) Recent progress in schizophrenia research, *Lancet*, **ii**, 136–9.

Smythies, J. (2002) *The Dynamic Neuron*, MIT Press, Cambridge, MA.

Snyder, S.H., Banerjee, S.P., Yamamura, H. I *et al.* (1974) Drugs, neurotransmitters and schizophrenia, *Science*, **184**, 1243–53.

Sobin, C., Blundell, M.L., Weiller, F., Gavigan, C. *et al.* (2000) Evidence of a schizotypy subtype in OCD, *Journal of Psychiatry Research*, **34**, 15–24.

Soeteman, D.I., Hakkaart-Van Roijen, L., Verheul, R. *et al.* (2008) The economic burden of personality disorders in mental health care, *Journal of clinical Psychiatry*, **69**, 259–65.

Sohal, V.S., Zhang, F., Yizhar, O. *et al.* (2009) Parvalbumin neurons and gamma rhythms enhance cortical circuit performance, *Nature*, **459**(7247), 698–702.

Sokoloff, L.M., Reivich, C., Kennedy, M.H. *et al.* (1977) The 14C deoxyglucose method for the measurement of local cerebral glucose utilisation, *Journal of Neurochemistry*, **28**, 897–916.

Soloff, P.H., Meltzer, C.C., Greer, P.J. *et al.* (2000) A fenfluramine-activated FDG-PET study of borderline personality disorder, *Biological Psychiatry*, **47**, 540–7.

Soloff, P.H., Price, J.C., Meltzer, C.C. *et al.* (2007) 5HT2A receptor binding is increased in borderline personality disorder, *Biological Psychiatry*, **62**, 580–7.

Sørensen, B., Kragh-Sørensen, P., Larsen, N.E. *et al.* (1978) The practical significance of nortriptyline plasma control: a prospective evaluation under routine conditions in endogenous depression, *Psychopharmacology (Berl)*, **59**(1), 35–9.

Southwick, S.M., Krystal, J.H., Morgan, A. *et al.* (1993) Abnormal noradrenergic function in post-traumatic stress disorder, *Archives of General Psychiatry*, **50**, 266–74.

Soyka, M., Preuss, U.W., Koller, G. *et al.* (2002) Dopamine D 4 receptor gene polymorphism and extraversion revisited: results from the Munich gene bank project for alcoholism, *Journal of Psychiatric Research*, **36**, 429–35.

Spar, J.E. and Gerner, R. (1982) Does the DST distinguish dementia from depression?, *American Journal of Psychiatry*, **139**, 238–40.

Speer, A.M., Kimbrell, T.A., Wasserman, E.M. *et al.* (2000) Opposite effects of high and low frequency rTMS on regional brain activity in depressed patients, *Biological Psychiatry*, **48**(23), 1133–41.

Spiegelhalder, K., Hornyak, M., Kyle, S.D. *et al.* (2009) Cerebral correlates of heart rate variations during a spontaneous panic attack in the fMRI scanner, *Neurocase*, 1–8.

Squire, L.R., Shimamura, A.P. and Amaral, D.G. (1989) Memory and the hippocampus. In J. Byrne and W. Berry (eds.), *Neural Models of Plasticity*, Academic Press, New York, NY, pp. 208–40.

Stafford-Clarke, D. and Taylor, F.H. (1949) Clinical and EEG studies of prisoners charged with murder, *Journal of Neurology, Neurosurgery and Psychiatry*, **12**, 325–30.

Stanley, M. and Mann, J.J. (1983) Increased serotonin-2 binding sites in frontal cortex of suicide victims, *Lancet*, **i**, 214–16.

Stanley, B., Molcho, A., Stanley, M. *et al.* (2000) Association of aggressive behavior with altered serotonergic function in patients who are not suicidal, *American Journal of Psychiatry*, **157**, 609–14.

Stanton, P.K. and Sejnowsky, T.J. (1989) Associative long-term depression in the hippocampus induced by Hebbian covariance, *Nature*, **339**, 215–18.

Stark, A.K., Uylings, H.B., Sanz-Arigita, E. *et al.* (2004) Glial cell loss in the anterior cingulate cortex, a subregion of the prefrontal cortex, in subjects with schizophrenia, *American Journal of Psychiatry*, **161**, 882–8.

Starkman, M.N., Giordani, B., Gebarski, S.S. *et al.* (1999) Decrease in cortisol reverses human hippocampal atrophy following treatment of Cushing's disease, *Biological Psychiatry*, **46**, 1595–602.

Starkstein, S.E. and Robinson, R.G. (1993) Depression in cerebrovascular disease. In S.E. Starkstein and R.G. Robinson (eds.), *Depression in Neurologic Disease*, Johns Hopkins Press, Baltimore, MD, pp. 28–49.

Starkstein, S.E., Preziosi, T.J., Bolduc, P.L. *et al.* (1990) Depression in Parkinson's disease, *Journal of Nervous and Mental Disease*, **178**, 27–31.

St Clair, D.M., Blackwood, D.H.R. and Christie, J.E. (1985) P3 and other long latency auditory evoked potentials in presenile dementia, Alzheimer-type and the alcoholic Korsakoff syndrome, *British Journal of Psychiatry*, **147**, 702–6.

Stefansson, S.B., Olafsson, E. and Hauser, W.A. (1998) Psychiatric morbidity in epilepsy: a case controlled study of adults receiving disability benefits, *Journal of Neurology, Neurosurgery and Psychiatry*, **64**, 238–41.

Stefansson, H., Ophoff, R.A., Steinberg, S. *et al.* (2009) Common variants conferring risk of schizophrenia, *Nature*, **460**, 744–7.

Stein, D.J. and Ythilingum, B. (2009) Love and attachment: the psychobiology of social bonding, *CNS Spectrums*, **14**(5), 239–42.

Stern, R.S. and Cobb, J.P. (1978) Phenomenology of obsessive compulsive neurosis, *British Journal of Psychiatry*, **132**, 233–9.

Stern, E., Silbersweig, D.A., Chee, K.Y. *et al.* (2000) A functional neuroanatomy of tics in tourette syndrome, *Archives in General Psychiatry*, **57**, 741–8.

Stevens, J.R. (1979) All that spikes is not fits. In C. Shagass, S. Gershon and A.J. Friedhoff (eds.), *Psychopathology and Brain Dysfunction*, Raven Press, New York, NY, pp. 183–98.

Stevens, J.R. (1986) Epilepsy and psychosis: neuropathological studies of six cases. In M.R. Trimble and T. Bolwig (eds.), *Aspects of Epilepsy and Psychiatry*, John Wiley and Sons, Chichester, pp. 117–45.

Stevens, J.R. and Hermann, B.P. (1981) Temporal lobe epilepsy, psychopathology and violence; the state of the evidence, *Neurology*, **31**, 1127–32.

Stevens, J.R. and Livermore, A. (1978) Kindling in the mesolimbic dopamine system: animal model of psychosis, *Neurology*, **28**, 36–46.

Stewart, L., Walsh, V., Frith, U. *et al.* (2001) TMS produces two dissociable types of speech disruption, *Neuroimage*, **13**, 472–8.

Strafella, A.P., Paus, T., Barrett, J. *et al.* (2001) Repetitive transcranial magnetic stimulation of the human prefrontal cortex induces dopamine release in the caudate nucleus, *Journal of Neuroscience*, **21**, RC157.

Strakowski, S.M., Woods, B.T., Tohen, S.M. *et al.* (1993) MRI subcortical hyperintensities in mania at first hospitalisation, *Biological Psychiatry*, **33**, 204–6.

Struve, F.A. and Willner, A.E. (1983) Cognitive dysfunction and tardive dyskinesia, *British Journal of Psychiatry*, **143**, 597–600.

Struve, F.A., Saraf, K.R., Arko, R.S. *et al.* (1979) Relationships between paroxysmal electroencephalographic dysrythmia and suicide ideation and attempts in psychiatric patients. In C. Shagass, S. Gershon and A.J. Friedhoff (eds.), *Psychopathology and Brain Dysfunction*, Raven Press, New York, NY, pp. 199–221.

Stuss, D.T. and Benson, D.F. (1984) Neuropsychological studies of the frontal lobes, *Psychological Bulletin*, **95**, 3–28.

Su, Y., Burke, J., O'Neill, A. *et al.* (1993) Exclusion of linkage between schizophrenia and the D_2 dopamine receptor gene region, *Archives of General Psychiatry*, **50**, 205–11.

Sulser, F. (1984) Regulation and function of noradrenaline receptor in systems in brain, *Neuropharmacology*, **23**(2B), 255–61.

Svrakic, D.M., Whitehead, C., Przybeck, T.R. *et al.* (1993) Differential diagnosis of personality disorders by the seven-factor model of temperament and character, *Archives of General Psychiatry*, **50**, 991–9.

Swedo, S.E., Rapoport, J.L., Cheslow, D.L. *et al.* (1989a) High prevalence of obsessive–compulsive symptoms in patients with Sydenham's chorea, *American Journal of Psychiatry*, **146**, 246–9.

Swedo, S.E., Schapiro, M.B., Grady, C.L. *et al.* (1989b) Cerebral glucose metabolism in childhood onset OCD, *Archives of General Psychiatry*, **46**, 518–23.

Swedo, S.E., Leonard, H.L., Kraesi, M.J.P. *et al.* (1992) CSF neurochemistry in children and adolescents with obsessive–compulsive disorder, *Archives of General Psychiatry*, **49**, 29–36.

Sydenham, T. (1740) *The Whole Works*, 11th edition, J. Pechey, Ware, London.

Symonds, C. (1962), The schizophrenia-like psychoses of epilepsy: discussion, *Proceedings of the Royal Society of Medicine*, **55**, 311.

Szasz, T.S. (1976) Schizophrenia: the sacred symbol of psychiatry, *British Journal of Psychiatry*, **129**, 308–16.

Szigethy, E., Conwell, Y., Forbes, N.T. *et al.* (1994) Adrenal weight and morphology in victims of completed suicide, *Biological Psychiatry*, **36**, 374–80.

Szyf, M., McGowan, P. and Meaney, M.J. (2008) The social environment and the epigenome, *Environmental and Molecular Mutagenesis*, **49**, 46–60.

Tajima, K., Diaz-Marsa, M., Montes, A. *et al.* (2009) Neuroimaging studies in borderline personality disorder, *Actas Espanolas de Psiquiatria*, **37**, 123–7.

Takahashi, S., Kondo, H. and Kato, N. (1975) Effect of L-5HTP on brain monoamine metabolism and evaluation of its clinical effect in depressed patients, *Journal of Psychiatric Research*, **12**, 177–87.

Talairach, J., Bancaud, J., Geier, S. *et al.* (1973) The cingulate gyrus and human behaviour, *Electroencephalography and Clinical Neurophysiology*, **34**, 45–52.

Tamminga, R.C., Smith, R.C. *et al.* (1976) Depression associated with oral choline, *Lancet*, **ii**, 905.

Tan, H.Y., Callicott, J.H. and Weinberger, D.R. (2008) Intermediate phenotypes in schizophrenia genetics redux: is it a no brainer?, *Molecular Psychiatry*, **13**, 233–8.

Tandon, R., Keshavan, M.S. and Nasrallah, H.A. (2008) Schizophrenia, 'just the facts': what we know in 2008: 2. Epidemiology and etiology, *Schizophrenia Research*, **102**, 1–18.

Targum, S.D., Rosen, L. and Capodanno, A.E. (1983a) The dexamethasone suppression test in suicidal patients with unipolar depression, *American Journal of Psychiatry*, **140**, 877–9.

Targum, S.D., Rosen, L.N., Delisi L.E. *et al.* (1983b) Cerebral ventricular size in major depressive disorder: association with delusional symptoms, *Biological Psychiatry*, **18**, 329–36.

Taylor, D.C. (1975) Factors influencing the occurrence of schizophrenia-like psychosis in patients with TLE, *Psychological Medicine*, **5**, 249–54.

Taylor, J. (1958) *Selected Writings of John Hughlings Jackson*, Basic Books, New York, NY.

Taylor, M.A. and Abrams, R. (1984) Cognitive impairment in schizophrenia, *American Journal of Psychiatry*, **141**, 196–201.

Taylor, P. and Fleminger, J.J. (1980) ECT for schizophrenia, *Lancet*, **i**, 1380–3.

Tebartz van Elst, L., Woermann, F., Lemieux, L. *et al.* (2000) Affective aggression in patients with temporal lobe epilepsy: a quantitative magnetic resonance study of the amygdala, *Brain*, **123**, 234–43.

Tebartz van Elst, L. and Thiel, T. (2001) Subtle prefrontal neuropathology in a pilot MRS study in patients with borderline personality disorder, *Journal of Neuropsychiatry and Clinical Neuroscience*, **13**, 511–14.

Tebartz van Elst, L., Hesslinger, B., Thiel, T. *et al.* (2003) Frontolimbic brain abnormalities in patients with borderline personality disorder: a volumetric magnetic resonance imaging study, *Biological Psychiatry*, **54**, 163–71.

Tellez-Zenteno, J.F., Patten, S.B. and Wiebe, S. (2005) Pychiatric comorbidity in epilepsy: a population-based analysis, *Epilepsia*, **46**, Suppl. 8, 264.

Temkin, O. (1971) *The Falling Sickness*, Johns Hopkins Press, Baltimore, MD.

Teneback, C.C., Nahas, Z., Speer, A.M. *et al.* (1999) Two weeks of daily left prefrontal rTMS changes prefrontal cortex and paralimbic activity in depression, *Journal of Neuropsychiatry Clinical Neuroscience*, **11**, 426–35.

Thaker, G.K. (2008) Neurophysiological endophenotypes across bipolar and schizophrenia psychosis, *Schizophrenia Bulletin*, **34**, 760–73.

Thaker, G.K., Tamminga, C.A., Alphs, L.D. *et al.* (1987) Brain GABA abnormality in tardive dyskinesia, *Archives of General Psychiatry*, **44**, 522–31.

Theodore, W.H., Hasler, G., Giovacchini, G. *et al.* (2007) Reduced hippocampal 5HT1A PET receptor binding and depression in temporal lobe epilepsy, *Epilepsia*, **48**, 1526–30.

Thome, J., Weijers, H.G., Wiesbeck, G.A. *et al.* (1999) Dopamine D3 receptor gene polymorphism and alcohol dependence: relation to personality rating, *Psychiatr Genet*, **9**, 17–21.

Thompson, P.J. and Trimble, M.R. (1982a) Anticonvulsant drugs and cognitive functions, *Epilepsia*, **23**, 531–44.

Thompson, P.J. and Trimble, M.R. (1982b) Non-MAOI antidepressant drugs and cognitive function: a review, *Psychological Medicine*, **12**, 539–48.

Thoren, P., Åsberg, M., Cronholm, B. *et al.* (1980a) Clomipramine treatment of obsessive–compulsive disorder: I. Controlled clinical trial, *Archives of General Psychiatry*, **37**, 1281–5.

Thoren, P., ÅAsberg, M., Bertilsson, L. *et al.* (1980b) Clomipramine treatment of obsessive–compulsive disorder: II. Biochemical aspects, *Archives of General Psychiatry*, **37**, 1289–94.

Thorgeirsson, T.E., Geller, F., Sulem, P. *et al.* (2008) A variant associated with nicotine dependence, lung cancer and peripheral arterial disease, *Nature*, **452**, 638–42.

Tienari, P. (1963) Psychiatric illness in identical twins, *Acta Psychiatrica Scandinavica*, **391**, Suppl. 171.

Todes, C.J. and Lees, A.J. (1985) The premorbid personality of patients with Parkinson's disease, *Journal of Neurology, Neurosurgery and Psychiatry*, **48**, 97–100.

Todrick, A. and Tait, A.C. (1969) The inhibition of human platelet 5HT uptake by tricyclic antidepressive drugs, *Journal of Pharmacy and Pharmacology*, **21**, 751–62.

Tomlinson, B.E. (1982) Plaques, tangles and Alzheimer's disease, *Psychological Medicine*, **12**, 449–59.

Toone, B. (1981) Psychoses of epilepsy. In E.H. Reynolds and M.R. Trimble (eds.), *Epilepsy and Psychiatry*, Churchill Livingstone, Edinburgh, pp. 113–37.

Toone, B.K., Dawson, J. and Driver, M. (1982a) Psychoses of epilepsy: a radiological evaluation, *British Journal of Psychiatry*, **140**, 244–8.

Toone, B.K., Garralda, M.E. and Ron, M.A. (1982b) The psychosis of epilepsy and the functional psychoses: a clinical and phenomenological comparison, *British Journal of Psychiatry*, **141**, 256–61.

Torgersen, S. (2000) Genetics of patients with borderline personality disorder, *Psychiatrical Clinics of north America*, **23**, 1–9.

Torgersen, S., Lygren, S., Oien, P.A. *et al.* (2000) A twin study of personality disorders, *Comprehensive Psychiatry*, **44**, 416–25.

Toulopoulou, T., Quraishi, S., McDonald, C. *et al.* (2006) The Maudsley family study: premorbid and current general intellectual function levels in familial bipolar I disorder and schizophrenia, *Journal of Clinical and Experimental Neuropsychology*, **28**, 243–59.

Träskman, L., Tybring, G., ÅAberg, M. *et al.* (1980) Cortisol in the CSF of depressed and suicidal patients, *Archives of General Psychiatry*, **37**, 761–7.

Treffert, D.A. (1964) The psychiatric patient with an EEG temporal lobe focus, *American Journal of Psychiatry*, **120**, 765–71.

Trimble, M. (1978) Serum prolactin in epilepsy and hysteria, *British Medical Journal*, **2**, 1682.

Trimble, M.R. (1980) New antidepressant drugs and the seizure threshold, *Neuropharmacology*, **19**, 1227–8.

Trimble, M.R. (1981a) *Neuropsychiatry*, John Wiley and Sons, Chichester.

Trimble, M.R. (1981b) *Post-traumatic Neurosis*, John Wiley and Sons, Chichester.

Trimble, M.R. (1986a) PET in epilepsy. In M.R. Trimble and T. Bolwig (eds.), *Aspects of Epilepsy and Psychiatry*, John Wiley and Sons, Chichester, pp. 147–60.

Trimble, M.R. (1986b) Recent contributions of benzodiazepines to the management of epilepsy, *Epilepsia*, **27**, Suppl. 1.

Trimble, M.R. (1986c) Hypergraphia. In M.R. Trimble and T. Bolwig (eds.), *Aspects of Epilepsy and Psychiatry*, John Wiley and Sons, Chichester, pp. 75–87.

Trimble, M.R. (1988) *Biological Psychiatry*, 1st edition, John Wiley and Sons, Chichester.

Trimble, M.R. (1991) *The Psychoses of Epilepsy*, Raven Press, New York, NY.

Trimble, M.R. (1996) *Biological Psychiatry*, 2nd edition, John Wiley and Sons, Chichester.

Trimble, M.R. (1997) Clinical consequences of pharmacology. In J. Engel and T. Pedley (eds.), *Epilepsy: A Comprehensive Textbook*, 2nd edition, Lippincott Williams & Wilkins, New York, NY, pp. 2161–70.

Trimble, M.R. (1998) Forced normalisation and the role of anticonvulsants. In M.R. Trimble and B. Schmitz (eds.), *Forced Normalisation and Alternative Psychoses of Epilepsy*, Wrightson Biomedical Publishing, Petersfield, pp. 169–78.

Trimble, M.R. (2000) Cognitive and personality profiles in patients with juvenile myoclonic epilepsy. In M.R. Trimble and B. Schmitz (eds.), *Juvenile Myoclonic Epilepsy: The Janz Syndrome*, Wrightson Biomedical Publishing, Petersfield, pp. 101–9.

Trimble, M.R. (2007a) Personality disorders in epilepsy. In S.C. Schachter, G.L. Holmes *et al.*, *Behavioral Aspects of Epilepsy*, Demos, New York, NY, pp. 253–60.

Trimble, M.R. (2007b) *The Soul in the Brain: The Cerebral Basis of Language, Art and Belief*, Johns Hopkins Press, Baltimore, MD.

Trimble, M.R. and Freeman, A. (2006) An investigation of religiosity and the Gastaut–Geschwind syndrome in patients with temporal lobe epilepsy, *Epilepsy and Behavior*, **9**, 407–14.

Trimble, M.R. and Meldrum, B.S. (1979) Monoamines, epilepsy, and schizophrenia. In J. Obiols *et al.* (eds.), *Biological Psychiatry Today*, Elsevier, Amsterdam, pp. 470–5.

Trimble, M.R. and Reynolds, E.H. (1976) Anticonvulsant drugs and mental symptoms: a review, *Psychological Medicine*, **6**, 169–78.

Trimble, M.R. and Reynolds, E.H. (1984) Neuropsychiatric toxicity of anticonvulsant drugs. In W.B. Matthews (ed.), *Recent Advances in Clinical Neurology*, Churchill Livingstone, Edinburgh, pp. 261–80.

Trimble, M.R. and Robertson, M.M. (1986) The psychopathology of tics. In C.D. Marsden (ed.), *Movement Disorders*, Vol. **2**, Butterworths, Kent, pp. 406–20.

Trimble, M.R. and Thompson, P. (1985) Neuropsychiatric aspects of epilepsy. In I. Grant and K. Adams (eds.), *Neuropsychological Assessment of Neuropsychiatric Disorders*, Oxford University Press, Oxford, pp. 321–48.

Trimble, M.R., Corbett, J.A. and Donaldson, J. (1980) Folic acid and mental symptoms in children with epilepsy, *Journal of Neurology, Neurosurgery and Psychiatry*, **43**, 1030–4.

Tsaung, M.T. (1993) Genotypes, phenotypes, and the brain, *British Journal of Psychiatry*, **163**, 299–307.

Tschanz, J.T., Welsh-Bohmer, K.A., Lyketsos, C.G. *et al.* (2006) Conversion to dementia from mild cognitive disorder: the Cache County study, *Neurology*, **67**, 229–34.

Tsunoda, T., Yoshino, A., Furusawa, T. *et al.* (2008) Social anxiety predicts unconsciously provoked emotional responses to facial expression, *Psychological Behavior*, **93**, 172–6.

Tucker, G., Detre, T., Harrow, M. *et al.* (1965) Behaviour and symptoms of psychiatric patients and the EEG, *Archives of General Psychiatry*, **12**, 278–86.

Tuke, D.H. (1894) Imperative ideas, *Brain*, **17**, 179–97.

Tuominen, H.J., Tiihonen, J., Wahlbeck, K. (2006) Glutamatergic drugs for schizophrenia, *Cochrane Database Syst Rev*, doi: CD003730.

Tyrer, P. (1976) Towards rational therapy with MAOI, *British Journal of Psychiatry*, **128**, 354–60.

Tyrer, P.J. and Lader, M.H. (1974) Response to propranolol and diazepam in somatic and psychic anxiety, *British Journal of Psychiatry*, **2**, 14–16.

Tyrer, P.J., Owen, R. and Dawling, S. (1983) Gradual withdrawal of diazepam after long-term therapy, *Lancet*, **i**, 1402–6.

Uhde, T.W., Boulenger, J.-P., Vittone, B. *et al.* (1985) Human anxiety and noradrenergic function. In P. Pichot (eds.), *Psychiatry: The State of the Art*, Vol. **2**, Plenum, New York, NY, pp. 693–8.

Ungerstedt, U. (1971) Stereotaxic mapping of the monoamine pathways in the rat brain, *Acta Physiologica Scandinavica*, **197**, Suppl. 367, 1–48.

Uthman, B.M., Wilder, B.J., Penry, J.K. *et al.* (1993) Treatment of epilepsy by stimulation of the vagus nerve, *Neurology*, **43**, 1338–45.

Vagus Nerve Stimulation Study Group (1995) A randomized controlled trial of chronic vagus nerve stimulation for treatment of medically intractable seizures, *Neurology*, **224**, 230.

Valli, I., Howes, O., Tyrer, P. *et al.* (2008) Longitudinal PET imaging in a patient with schizophrenia did not show marked changes in dopaminergic function with relapse of psychosis, *American Journal of Psychiatry*, **165**, 1613–14.

Vallortigara, G. (2006a) Cerebral lateralization: a common theme in the organization of the vertebrate brain, *Cortex*, **42**, 5–7.

Vallortigara, G. (2006b) The evolutionary psychology of left and right: costs and benefits of lateralization, *Developmental Psychobiological*, **48**, 418–27.

van Asselt, A.D., Dirksen, C.D., Arntz, A. *et al.* (2007) The cost of borderline personality disorder: societal cost of illness in BPD-patients, *European Psychiatry*, **22**, 354–61.

van der Kolk, B.A. (1994) The body keeps the score: memory and the evolving psychobiology of post-traumatic stress, *Harvard Review of Psychiatry*, **1**, 253–65.

van Haren, N.E., Bakker, S.C. and Kahn, R.S. (2008) Genes and structural brain imaging in schizophrenia, *Current Opinion in Psychiatry*, **21**, 161–7.

van Os, J., Rutten, B.P. and Poulton, R. (2008) Gene–environment interactions in schizophrenia: review of epidemiological findings and future directions, *Schizophrenia Bulletin*, **34**, 1066–82.

van Praag, H.M. (1977a) Significance of biochemical parameters in the diagnosis, treatment and presentation of depressive disorders, *Biological Psychiatry*, **12**, 101–31.

van Praag, H. M (1977b) The significance of dopamine for the mode of action of neuroleptics and the pathogenesis of schizophrenia, *British Journal of Psychiatry*, **130**, 463–74.

van Praag, H.M. (1980a) Central monoamine metabolism in depressions: 1. Serotonin and related compounds, *Comprehensive Psychiatry*, **21**, 30–43.

van Praag, H.M. (1980b) Central monoamine metabolism in depressions: 11. Catecholamines and related compounds, *Comprehensive Psychiatry*, **21**, 44–54.

van Praag, H.M., van den Burg, W., Bos, E. *et al.* (1974) 5HTP in combination with clomipramine in 'therapy resistant' depression, *Psychopharmacologia*, **38**, 267–9.

van Rijn, S., Aleman, A., Swaab, H. *et al.* (2006) Klinefelter's syndrome and schizophrenia-spectrum pathology, *British Journal of Psychiatry*, **189**, 459–61.

van Rijn, S., Aleman, A., Swaab, H. *et al.* (2008) Effects of an extra X chromosome on language lateralization: an fMRI study with Klinefelter men (47,XXY), *Schizophrenia Research*, **101**, 17–25.

van 't Ent, D., Lehn, H., Derks, E.M. *et al.* (2007) A structural MRI study in monozygotic twins concordant or discordant for attention/hyperactivity problems: evidence for genetic and environmental heterogeneity in the developing brain, *Neuroimage*, **35**, 1004–20.

van Winkel, R., Stefanis, N.C. and Myin-Germeys, I. (2008) Psychosocial stress and psychosis: a review of the neurobiological mechanisms and the evidence for gene–stress interaction, *Schizophrenia Bulletin*, **34**, 1095–105.

Vertes, R.P. (1990) Fundamentals of brainstem anatomy. In W.R. Klemm and R.P. Vertes (eds.), *Brainstem Mechanisms of Behaviour*, John Wiley and Sons, Chichester, pp. 33–104.

Victoroff, J.I., Benson, F., Grafton, S.T. *et al.* (1994) Depression in complex partial seizures: electroencephalography and cerebral metabolic correlates, *Archives of Neurology*, **51**, 155–63.

Volkow, N.D., Hitzemann, R., Wang, G.J. *et al.* (1992) Decreased brain metabolism in neurologically intact healthy alcoholics, *American Journal of Psychiatry*, **149**(8), 1016–22.

Volkow, N.D., Wang, G.J., Hitzemann, R. *et al.* (1994) Recovery of brain glucose metabolism in detoxified alcoholics, *American Journal of Psychiatry*, **151**, 178–83.

Völlm, B.A., Taylor, A.N., Richardson, P. *et al.* (2006) Neuronal correlates of theory of mind and empathy: a functional magnetic resonance imaging study in a nonverbal task, *Neuroimage*, **29**, 90–8.

Völlm, B., Richardson, P., McKie, S. *et al.* (2007) Neuronal correlates of reward and loss in cluster B personality disorders: a functional magnetic resonance imaging study, *Psychiatry Research*, **156**, 151–67.

von Economo, C. (1931) *Encephalitis Lethargica* (Translated by K.O. Newman), Oxford University Press, Oxford.

von Schantz, M. (2008) Phenotypic effects of genetic variability in human clock genes on circadian and sleep parameters, *Journal of Genetics*, **87**, 513–19.

Waddington, J.L., Youssef, H.A., Molloy, A.G. *et al.* (1985) Association of intellectual impairment, negative symptoms, and aging with tardive dyskinesia: clinical and animal studies, *Journal of Clinical Psychiatry*, **46**, 29–33.

Waddington, J.L., Weller, M.P., Crow, T.J. *et al.* (1992) Schizophrenia, genetic retrenchment and epidemiologic renaissance, *Archives of General Psychiatry*, **49**, 990–4.

Walinder, J., Skott, A., Carlsson, A. *et al.* (1976) Potentiation of the antidepressant action of clomipramine by tryptophan, *Archives of General Psychiatry*, **33**, 1384–9.

Walsh, V. and Cowey, A. (2000) Transcranial magnetic stimulation and cognitive neuroscience, *Nature Reviews Neuroscience*, **1**, 73–9.

Walzer, S., Wolff, P.H. and Bowen, D. *et al.* (1978) A method for the longitudinal study of behavioural development in infants and children: the early development of XXY children, *Journal of Child Psychology and Psychiatry*, **19**, 213–29.

Wassermann, E.M. (1997) Report on risk and safety of repetitive transcranial magnetic stimulation (RTMS): suggested guidelines from the international workshop on risk and safety of rTMS (June 1996), *Electroencephalo Clinical Neurology*, **108**, 1–16.

Wassermann, E.M., Cohen, L.G., Flitman, S.S. *et al.* (1996) Seizures in healthy people with repeated safe trains of transcranial magnetic stimuli, *Lancet*, **347**, 825–6.

Watis, L., Chen, S.H., Chua, H.C. *et al.* (2008) Glutamatergic abnormalities of the thalamus in schizophrenia: a systematic review, *Journal of Neural Transmission*, **115**, 493–511.

Waxman, S.G. and Geschwind, N. (1975) The interictal behaviour syndrome of temporal lobe epilepsy, *Archives of General Psychiatry*, **32**, 1580–6.

Webster, N.J., Green, K.N., Peers, C. *et al.*, Institute for Cardiovascular Research, University of Leeds, Leeds, UK (2002) Altered processing of amyloid precursor protein in the human neuroblastoma SH-SY5Y by chronic hypoxia, *Journal of Neurochemistry*, **83**(6), 1262–71.

Wegner, J.T., Catalano, F., Gibralter, J. *et al.* (1985) Schizophrenics with tardive dyskinesia, *Archives of General Psychiatry*, **42**, 860–5.

Weickert, C.S., Webster, M.J., Gondipalli, P. *et al.* (2007) Postnatal alterations in dopaminergic markers in the human prefrontal cortex, *Neuroscience*, **144**, 1109–19.

Weinberg, S.M., Jenkins, E.A., Marazita, M.L. *et al.* (2007) Minor physical anomalies in schizophrenia: a meta-analysis, *Schizophrenia Research*, **89**, 72–85.

Weinberger, D.R. (2009) Janssen Lecture, Institute of Psychiatry, London, 4 November; and personal communication.

Weiner, R.D. (1986) Electrical dosage, stimulus parameter and electrode placement, *Psychopharmacology Bulletin*, **22**, 499–502.

Weingartner, H. and Silberman, S. (1985) Cognitive changes in depression. In R.M. Post and J. Ballenger (eds.), *Psychobiology of Mood Disorders*, Williams and Wilkins, Baltimore, MD, pp. 121–35.

Weinstein, D.D., Diforio, D., Schiffman, J. *et al.* (1999) Minor physical anomalies, dermatoglyphic asymmetries, and cortisol levels in adolescents with schizotypal personality disorder, *American Journal of Psychiatry*, **156**, 617–23.

Weissman, J.D., Epstein, C.M. and Davey, K.R. (1992) Magnetic brain stimulation and brain size: relevance to animal studies, *Electroencephalo Clinical Neurology*, **85**, 215–19.

Wells, C.E. (1979) Pseudodementia, *American Journal of Psychiatry*, **136**, 895–900.

Whalen, P.J., Rauch, S.L., Etcoff, N.L. *et al.* (1998) Masked presentations of emotional facial expressions modulate amygdala activity without explicit knowledge, *Journal of Neuroscience*, **18**, 411–18.

Whalley, L.J., Borthwick, N., Copolov, D. *et al.* (1986) Glucocorticoid receptors and depression, *British Medical Journal*, **292**, 859–61.

White, L.E. (1981) Development and morphology of human nucleus accumbens. In R.B. Chronister and J.F. de France (eds.), *The Neurobiology of the Nucleus Accumbens*, Haer Institute, Brunswick, NJ, pp. 198–209.

Whitlock, F.A. and Evans, L.E.J. (1978) Drugs and depression, *Drugs*, **15**, 53–71.

Whittle, S., Chanen, A.M., Fornito, A. *et al.* (2009) Anterior cingulate volume in adolescents with first-presentation borderline personality disorder, *Psychiatry Research*, **172**, 155–60.

Whitwell, J.L., Jack, C.R., Jr, Parisi, J.E. *et al.* (2007) Rates of cerebral atrophy differ in different degenerative pathologies, *Brain*, **130**, 1148–58.

Wieck, A., Kumar, R., Hirst, A.D. *et al.* (1991) Increased sensitivity of dopamine receptors and recurrence of affective psychosis after childbirth, *British Medical Journal*, **303**, 613–16.

Wiesel, F., Fyro, B., Nyback, H. *et al.* (1982) Relationship in healthy volunteers between secretion of monoamine metabolites in urine and family history of psychiatric morbidity, *Biological Psychiatry*, **17**, 1403–13.

Wieser, H.G. (1983) *Electroclinical Features of the Psychomotor Seizure*, Gustav Fischer, Stuttgart.

Williams, D. (1956) The structure of emotions reflected in epileptic experiences, *Brain*, **79**, 29–67.

Williams, D. (1969) Neural factors related to habitual aggression, *Brain*, **92**, 503–20.

Willner, P. (1983) Dopamine and depression: a review of recent evidence, *Brain Research Reviews*, **6**, 225–36.

Wilson-Barnett, J. and Trimble, M.R. (1985) An investigation of hysteria using the IBQ, *British Journal of Psychiatry*, **146**, 601–8.

Wing, J.K., Cooper, J.E. and Sartorius, N. (1974) *Description and Classification of Psychiatric Symptoms*, Cambridge University Press, Cambridge.

Wingenfeld, K., Rullkoetter, N., Mensebach, C. *et al.* (2008) Neural correlates of the individual emotional stroop in borderline personality disorder, *Psychoneuroendocrinology*, **34**(4), 571–86.

Winokur, G. (1977) Delusional disorder, *Comprehensive Psychiatry*, **18**, 511–21.

Winokur, G. (1982) The development and validity of familial subtypes in primary unipolar depression, *Pharmacopsychiatrica*, **15**, 142–6.

Winokur, G. and Tanna, V.L. (1969) Possible role of X-linked dominant factor in manic depressive disease, *Diseases of the Nervous System*, **30**, 87–94.

Winokur, A., Amsterdam, J., Caroff, S. *et al.* (1982) Variability of hormonal responses to a series of neuro-endocrine challenges in depressed patients, *American Journal of Psychiatry*, **139**, 39–44.

Winslow, R.S., Stillner, V., Coons, D.J. *et al.* (1986) Prevention of acute dystonic reactions in patients beginning high-potency neuroleptics, *American Journal of Psychiatry*, **143**, 706–10.

Wirz-Justice, A. (1977) Theoretical and therapeutic potential of indolamine precursors in affective disorders, *Neuropsychobiology*, **3**, 199–233.

Woermann, F., Tebartz van Elst, L., Koepp, M.J. *et al.* (2000) Reduction of frontal neocortical grey matter associated with affective aggression in patients with temporal lobe epilepsy: an objective voxel-by-voxel analysis of automatically segmented MRI, *Journal of Neurology, Neurosurgery and Psychiatry*, **68**, 162–9.

Wolf, P. (1982) Manic episodes in epilepsy. In H. Akimoto, H. Kazamatsuri, M. Seino and A.A. Ward, Jr (eds.), *Advances in Epileptology: XIIIth Epilepsy International Symposium*, Raven Press, New York, NY, pp. 237–40.

Wolf, P. and Trimble, M.R. (1985) Biological antagonism and epileptic psychosis, *British Journal of Psychiatry*, **146**, 272–6.

Wolpert, L. (1984) DNA and its message, *Lancet*, **ii**, 853–6.

Wong, D.F., Wagner, H.N., Pearlson, G. *et al.* (1985) Dopamine receptor binding of C-11-3-N-methylspiperone in the caudate in schizophrenia and bipolar disorder, *Psychopharmacology Bulletin*, **21**, 595–8.

Wood, P.L., Suranyi-Cadotte, B., Schwartz, G. *et al.* (1983) Platelet 3H-imipramine binding and red blood cell choline in affective disorders, *British Medical Journal*, **18**, 715–20.

Wood, J., Birmaher, B., Axelson, D. *et al.* (2009) Replicable differences in preferred circadian phase between bipolar disorder patients and control individuals, *Psychiatry Research*, **166**, 201–9.

World Health Organization (1973) *Report of the International Pilot Study of Schizophrenia*, WHO, Geneva.

World Health Organization (1993) *The ICD-10 Classification of Mental and Behavioural Disorders: Diagnostic Criteria for Research*, WHO, Geneva.

Wu, J.C., Buchsbaum, M.S., Hershey, T.S. *et al.* (1991) PET in generalised anxiety disorder, *Biological Psychiatry*, **29**, 1181–99.

Wu, J.C., Gillin, J.C. *et al.* (1992) Effect of sleep deprivation on brain metabolism of depressed patients, *American Journal of Psychiatry*, **149**, 538–43.

Wuerfel, J., Krishnamoorthy, E.S., Brown, R.J. *et al.* (2004) Religiosity is associated with hippocampal but not amygdala volumes in patients with refractory epilepsy, *Journal of Neurology, Neurosurgery and Psychiatry*, **75**, 640–2.

Wyatt, R.J., Termini, B.A. and Davis, J. (1971) Biochemical and sleep studies of schizophrenia: a review of the literature 1960–1970, *Schizophrenia Bulletin*, **4**, 10–66.

Yadalam, K.G., Jain, A.K. and Simpson, G. (1985) Mania in two sisters with similar cerebral disturbance, *American Journal of Psychiatry*, **142**, 1067–9.

Yamamoto, K. and Hornykiewicz, O. (2004) Proposal for a noradrenaline hypothesis of schizophrenia, *Prog Neuropsychopharmacol Biol Psychiatry*, **28**, 913–22.

Yang, Y., Raine, A., Lencz, T. *et al.* (2005a) Prefrontal white matter in pathological liars, *British Journal of Psychiatry*, **187**, 320–5.

Yang, Y., Raine, A., Lencz, T. *et al.* (2005b) Volume reduction in prefrontal gray matter in unsuccessful criminal psychopaths, *Biological Psychiatry*, **57**, 1103–8.

Yang, Y., Raine, A., Narr, K.L. *et al.* (2007) Localisation of increased prefrontal white matter in pathological liars, *British Journal of Psychiatry*, **190**, 174–5.

Yang, Y., Glenn, A.L. and Raine, A. (2008) Brain abnormalities in antisocial individuals: implications for the law, *Behavioral Scientific Law*, **26**, 65–83.

Yang, Y., Raine, A., Colletti, P. *et al.* (2009) Abnormal temporal and prefrontal cortical gray matter thinning in psychopaths, *Molecular Psychiatry*, **14**, 561–2, 555.

Yatham, L.N. (1994) Buspirone induced prolactin release in mania, *Biological Psychiatry*, **35**, 553–6.

Yehuda, R. (1997) Stress and glucocorticoids, *Science*, **275**, 1662–3.

Yehuda, R. and Golier, J. (2009) Is there a rationale for cortisol-based treatments for PTSD?, *Expert Review of Neurotherapeautics*, **9**, 1113–15.

Yehuda, R., Morris, A., Labinsky, E. *et al.* (2007) Ten-year follow-up study of cortisol levels in aging holocaust survivors with and without PTSD, *J Trauma Stress*, **20**, 757–61.

Young, A.B., Greenamayr, J.T., Hollingsworth, Z. *et al.* (1988) NMDA receptor losses in putamen from patients with Huntington's disease, *Science*, **241**, 981–3.

Young, K.A., Liu, Y. and Wang, Z. (2008) The neurobiology of social attachment: a comparative approach to behavioral, neuroanatomical, and neurochemical studies, *Comp Biochem Physiol C Toxicological Pharmacology*, **148**(4), 401–10.

Young, L.T., Warsh, J.J., Kish, S.J. *et al.* (1994) Reduced brain 5-HT and elevated NA turnover and metabolites in bipolar affective disorder, *Biological Psychiatry*, **35**, 121–7.

Young, A. and Breslau, N. (2007) Troublesome memories: reflections on the future, *Journal of Anxiety Disorder*, **21**, 230–2.

Young, E.A. and Breslau, N. (2004) Saliva cortisol in posttraumatic stress disorder: a community epidemiologic study, *Biological Psychiatry*, **56**, 205–9.

Zabara, J. (1985a) Peripheral control of hypersynchronous discharge in epilepsy, *Electroencephalography and Clinical Neurophysiology*, **61**, S162.

Zabara, J. (1985b) Time course of seizure control to brief, repetitieve stimuli, *Epilepsia*, **26**, 518.

Zabara, J. (1992) Inhibition of experimental seizures in canines by repetitive vagal stimulation, *Epilepsia*, **33**, 1005–12.

Zametkin, A.J. and Liotta, W. (1998) The neurobiology of attention-deficit/hyperactivity disorder, *Journal of Clinical Psychiatry*, **59**, Suppl. 7, 17–23.

Zammit, S., Allebeck, P., Andreasson, S. *et al.* (2002) Self-reported cannabis use as a risk factor for schizophrenia in swedish conscripts of 1969: historical cohort study, *British Medical Journal*, **325**, 1199.

Zanetti, M.V., Soloff, P.H., Nicoletti, M.A. *et al.* (2007) MRI study of corpus callosum in patients with borderline personality disorder: a pilot study, *Progress in Neuropsychopharmacol Biological Psychiatry*, **31**, 1519–25.

Zardetto-Smith, A.M. and Gray, T.S. (1990) Organization of peptidergic and catecholaminergic efferents from the nucleus of the solitary tract to the rat amygdala, *Brain Research Bulletin*, **25**, 875.

Zifkin, B.G., Guerrini, R. and Plouin P. (2007) Reflex seizures. In J. Engel and T. Pedley (eds.), *Epilepsy: A Comprehensive Textbook*, 2nd edition, Lippincott Williams & Wilkins, New York, NY, pp. 2559–72.

Zilboorg, G. (1941) *A History of Medical Psychology*, W.W. Norton, New York, NY.

Index

References to tables are given in bold type.

5-HIAA *see* hydroxyindoleacetic acid
5-HT *see* serotonin

abecarnil 306
abulia 227
accumbens 38, 58–59, 217
acetylcholine 25, 188
    receptors 20–21
    see also cholinergic systems
action potential 11
acute schizophrenia-like psychotic disorder
        149
addictive disorders 215
    benzodiazepines 307
    brain damage 224–226
    conditioning 217–219
    cravings 226–227
    electroencephalographic data 223
    genetic factors 219–220
    imaging studies 223–226
    medication for 317–318
    neurological disease and 227
    see also alcoholism
adenosine 3,5-monophosphate
        (AMP) 8
adenosine diphosphate (ADP) 8
adenosine triphosphate (ATP) 8
adrenaline 135
adrenoceptors 18, 289
adrenocorticotropic hormone (ACTH) 193,
        194–195, 195–196
affective disorders
    aetiology 190–193, 210–212
        noradrenaline hypothesis 188–189

permissive amine hypothesis 211
        serotonin 187–188
    cerebrospinal fluid investigations 198–203
    cerebrovascular accidents and 208
    classification 183–184, 209–210
    computerized axial tomography (CAT)
            203–204
    electroconvulsive therapy (ECT) 319
    electroencephalagraphic (ECG) studies
            200–203
    epilepsy and 245
    genetics 184–186
    hormonal data 193–196, 196–198
    magnetic resonance imaging (MRI)
            203–204
    metabolic factors 186–187
    neurochemistry 200
    neurological data 206–207
    neuropsychological disturbances 208–209
    neurotransmitters and 212
    pharmacological treatment
            antidepressants *see* antidepressants
            lithium 309–310
    sleep deprivation therapy 329
    sleep studies 203
    see also bipolar disorder; depression
aggression 122–123
    epilepsy and 244–245
    neurophysiological factors 74
agoraphobia 132
agranular cortex 34
agranulocytosis 303
AIDS-dementia complex 272–273
akathisia 301